W0043602

Textbook of Developmental Pediatrics

Textbook of Developmental Pediatrics

Edited by

Marvin I. Gottlieb, M.D., Ph.D.

Director, Institute for Child Development.
Hackensack Medical Center
Professor, Department of Pediatrics
University of Medicine and Dentistry of New Jersey–New Jersey Medical School
Hackensack, New Jersey

and

John E. Williams, M.D.

Chief, Section of Developmental Pediatrics
Associate Director, Institute for Child Development
Hackensack Medical Center
Clinical Assistant Professor, Department of Pediatrics
University of Medicine and Dentistry of New Jersey–New Jersey Medical School
Hackensack, New Jersey

Plenum Medical Book Company
New York and London

Library of Congress Cataloging in Publication Data

Textbook of developmental pediatrics.

Includes bibliographies and index.
1. Developmental disabilities. I. Gottlieb, Marvin I. II. Williams, John E. (John Edward),
1951–   . [DNLM: 1. Child Behavior—in infancy & childhood. 2. Child Development
Disorders—in infancy & childhood. 4. Nervous System Diseases—in infancy & childhood. 5.
Speech Disorders—in infancy & childhood. WS 350.6 T355]
RJ135.T47   1987   618.92   86-30411
ISBN-13: 978-1-4612-9006-3   e-ISBN-13: 978-1-4613-1797-5
DOI: 10.1007/ 978-1-4613-1797-5

© 1987 Plenum Publishing Corporation

Softcover reprint of the hardcover 1st edition 1987

233 Spring Street, New York, N.Y. 10013

Plenum Medical Book Company is an imprint of Plenum Publishing Corporation

All rights reserved

No part of this book may be reproduced, stored in a retrieval system, or transmitted
in any form or by any means, electronic, mechanical, photocopying, microfilming,
recording, or otherwise, without written permission from the Publisher

Contributors

William C. Adamson, M.D. • Professor, Department of Mental Health Sciences, Hahnemann University, Philadelphia, Pennsylvania 19102

Lorian Baker, Ph.D. • Associate Research Psycholinguist, UCLA Neuropsychiatric Institute, Los Angeles, California 90024

George W. Brown, M.D. • Director, Los Lunas Hospital and Training School, Los Lunas, New Mexico 87031

Dennis P. Cantwell, M.D. • Joseph Campbell Professor, UCLA Neuropsychiatric Institute, Los Angeles, California 90024

Arnold J. Capute, M.D., M.P.H. • Vice President for Medical Affairs, The Kennedy Institute for Handicapped Children, Department of Pediatrics, The Johns Hopkins University Medical Institutions, Baltimore, Maryland 21205

Herbert J. Cohen, M.D. • Professor, Departments of Pediatrics and Rehabilitation Medicine, Director, Rose F. Kennedy University Affiliated Facility and Children's Evaluation and Rehabilitation Center, Albert Einstein College of Medicine, Bronx, New York 10805

Sylvia M. Davis, Ph.D. • Professor, Department of Communication Disorders, Louisiana State University Medical Center, New Orleans, Louisiana 70112

Marion P. Downs, M.A., D.H.S. • Professor Emerita, Department of Otolaryngology, University of Colorado Health Sciences Center, Denver, Colorado 80262

Bill R. Gearheart, Ed.D. • Professor, Department of Special Education, University of Northern Colorado, Greeley, Colorado 80639

Gerald S. Golden, M.D. • Shainberg Professor, Department of Pediatrics, Professor and Acting Chairman, Departments of Pediatrics and Neurology, University of Tennessee Center for the Health Sciences, Memphis, Tennessee 38105

Marvin I. Gottlieb, M.D., Ph.D. • Director, Institute for Child Development, Hackensack Medical Center, and Professor, Department of Pediatrics, University of Medicine and Dentistry of New Jersey–New Jersey Medical School, Hackensack, New Jersey 07601

Roger L. Hiatt, M.D. • Professor and Chairman, Department of Ophthalmology, University of Tennessee Center for the Health Sciences, Memphis, Tennessee 38163

Paul King, M.D. • Clinical Assistant Professor, Child and Adolescent Psychiatry, Director, Adolescent Services, Charter Lakeside Hospital, University of Tennessee Center for the Health Sciences, Memphis, Tennessee 38103

Marcel Kinsbourne, M.D. • Adjunct Professor, Department of Psychology, Brandeis University, and Director, Department of Behavioral Neurology, Eunice Kennedy Shriver Center for Mental Retardation, Waltham, Massachusetts 02254

Dorothy Kletzkin, Ed.D. • Chief, Section of Learning Disabilities, Institute for Child Development, Hackensack Medical Center, Hackensack, New Jersey 07601

Theresa E. Laurie, Ph.D. • Education Director, TRANSACT Health Systems, Forbes Regional Health Center, Monroeville, Pennsylvania 15146

Craig B. Liden, M.D. • Medical Director, TRANSACT Health Systems, Forbes Regional Health Center, Monroeville, Pennsylvania 15146

Frederick B. Palmer, M.D. • Developmental Pediatrician, The Kennedy Institute for Handicapped Children, Associate Professor, Department of Pediatrics, The Johns Hopkins University Medical Institutions, Baltimore, Maryland 21205

Donald L. Rampp, Ph.D. • Professor and Head, Department of Communication Disorders, Louisiana State University Medical Center, New Orleans, Louisiana 70112

Bruce K. Shapiro, M.D. • Developmental Pediatrician, The Kennedy Institute for Handicapped Children, Associate Professor, Department of Pediatrics, The Johns Hopkins University Medical Institutions, Baltimore, Maryland 21205

Rachel E. Stark, Ph.D. • Associate Professor, Department of Neurology, John F. Kennedy Institute, Johns Hopkins University School of Medicine, Baltimore, Maryland, 21205

Emily A. Tobey, Ph.D. • Assistant Professor, Department of Communication Disorders, Louisiana State University Medical Center, New Orleans, Louisiana 70112

Abby L. Wasserman, M.D. • Director, Division of Psychiatry and Psychology, St. Jude Children's Research Hospital, Memphis, Tennessee 38101

John E. Williams, M.D. • Chief, Section of Developmental Pediatrics, Associate Director, Institute for Child Development, Hackensack Medical Center, and Clinical Assistant Professor, Department of Pediatrics, University of Medicine and Dentistry of New Jersey–New Jersey Medical School, Hackensack, New Jersey 07601

Peter W. Zinkus, Ph.D. • Director, Child Psychology Division, Le Bonheur Children's Medical Center, Memphis, Tennessee 38103

Preface

Child/adolescent development and behavior have been a traditional "concern" of primary health care providers. However, it was not until the mid-1960s that attempts were made to consolidate developmental–behavioral issues into an identifiably distinct fund of medical knowledge. During the ensuing two decades, *developmental–behavioral pediatrics* was recognized as a clinical and research subspecialty, within the framework of comprehensive health care for children. The influence of public advocacy groups, topic-dedicated journals, national professional specialty societies, subject-related continuing education programs, and federal legislation (PL94-142) has served to crystallize developmental–behavioral pediatrics as a specialized field of study. As a consequence, during the past ten years significant modifications have restructured medical student and pediatric resident education, providing an emphasis on developmental–behavioral issues. The focus on neurodevelopmental, educational, and psychosocial issues reflects changing priorities in traditional health care for children. The postgraduate training of pediatric fellows, in two- and three-year training programs, was initiated to accommodate professional manpower needs in both academic and practice settings.

Many of the problems in childhood development and behavior frequently span the traditional areas of child neurology, child psychiatry, and general pediatrics. As a result there has been some confusion in demarcating professional responsibilities in diagnosis and management, as well as poorly defined terminology and classification schemas. With the birth of *developmental pediatrics* as a pediatric specialty, a more cohesive fund of knowledge has been accumulated and more meaningful strategies have been designed for prevention, diagnosis, and management. Although originally an "offshoot" of professional interest in mental retardation, developmental–behavioral pediatrics has significantly broadened its clinical perspective to include such topics as: learning disabilities, communication handicaps, cognitive disorders, neuromotor problems, behavioral problems (e.g., hyperkinesis), and adjustment reactions—to mention only a few.

Within this framework, these disorders are of critical concern to the developmental pediatrician. Although confusions in terminology and classification persist, a "working" definition of developmental–behavioral disorders might best be conceptualized as *any* disorder which is potentially capable of producing a chronic handicap that adversely affects the *quality* of the child/adolescent's life. Perhaps the key component of this definition of developmental–behavioral disorders relates to the recognition that, in association with most of the problems for which intervention is not provided, there is a negative effect on the child's self-concept, self-esteem, and self-confidence. Poor self-concept can in turn jeopardize the course of childhood, adolescence, and adult life. As these negative psychosocial variables persist, they may significantly impede neurodevelopment and behavior. Often the superimposed personality and behavioral disorder can present a greater management problem than the original pathology. For the child, the family, the educational system, the community, and the professional team, developmental–behavioral problems generally encompass problems associated with emotional and financial strains. These variables further impact on the course of the neurodevelopmental or neurobehavioral disorder. Because of their special skills, pediatricians have been assigned a significant and critical role in developmental–behavioral medicine. However, the complex nature of these disorders generally necessitates a well-coordinated intervention by an interdisciplinary team.

The scope of developmental concerns has been dramatically expanded during the past decade. To cover *all* of the developmental–behavioral disorders in depth would require a work encyclopedic in nature, perhaps consisting of several volumes. Therefore, we have not made an attempt to cover the broad area of *developmental–behavioral pediatrics* entirely in this book. We have, instead, compiled what we feel to be many of the essential and timely topics that confront the pediatric health care provider in the area of child development and behavior. Effort has been made to present this information in a concise text, with a more extensive appendix that includes useful tables and information for quick reference. Although we hope that medical students, pediatric residents, fellows, and practitioners will find this book particularly useful, we have dedicated this work to all professionals who help families and their children who have developmental disabilities.

Marvin I. Gottlieb
John E. Williams

Hackensack, New Jersey

Contents

1

*Neurological Aspects of
Developmental Pediatrics*

Developmental Disabilities: A Pediatrician's Perspective

Herbert J. Cohen

HISTORICAL BACKGROUND

During the past two decades, major changes have occurred in the care and treatment of children with developmental disabilities. These changes have altered the role of the pediatrician considerably in the management of children with disabilities.

The history and evolution of services for the developmentally disabled in Western societies, and in the United States in particular, reflect the changes in attitudes about mental disability, as well as the level of scientific understanding of the causes and possible treatment of the disorder. As the 1976 report of the President's Committee on Mental Retardation pointed out,[1] service delivery, and especially development of institutional care, have undergone substantial changes. Attitudinal changes range from a retarded or disabled individuals being viewed as a *sick person*—a subhuman organism, a potential menace, an object of pity, a burden of charity, or a holy innocent—to the current more progressive view, which has resulted in these persons being treated as individuals capable of learning and change. Perspectives about the changeability of the retarded or mentally handicapped have varied from extreme optimism to marked pessimism, the latter most significantly influenced by theories of genetic inferiority. The current and more hopeful

Herbert J. Cohen • Departments of Pediatrics and Rehabilitation Medicine, Rose F. Kennedy University Affiliated Facility and Children's Evaluation and Rehabilitation Center, Albert Einstein College of Medicine Bronx, New York 10805

ideologies blend a realistic view of the handicapped individual's potential with the commendable idealism about achieving more normal patterns of everyday life.

A significant aspect of the early history of services for the developmentally disabled in the United States can be traced to the development of institutional care. Based on the work of Howe[2] and Sequin,[3] institutions were founded for the mentally retarded during the same era that facilities were developed for other deviant groups. The hopeful objective was to render the resident populations "undeviant." Facilities for the mentally retarded were called "state schools," since they were viewed as training institutions. In 1851, at the founding of what was to become the Fernald State School, Howe stated: "This establishment, being intended as a school, should not be converted into an establishment for incurables."[4] However, as the nineteenth century progressed, attitudes and influences surfaced that resulted in the increased isolation and segregation of the institutions. During this era, the objective varied from protecting deviant individuals from the undeviant to preventing exploitation and sheltering society from mentally defectives. The nature and characteristics of institutional philosophy passed through different stages. An initial goal was to provide benevolent isolation in the rural countryside. Eventually this was replaced by the creation of new, large asylums or the modification of existing facilities, which could provide as cardinal objectives isolation and an economical method of offering subsistence. The focus shifted from what might be the best interests of the child to what was more convenient for the staff or community.

The philosophy of *custodial care* appeared to be spurred on by the concerns of eugenicists and the growth of state or local bureaucracies with vested interests in preserving an institutional system of care. During the early twentieth century, larger and increasingly more crowded institutions were developed that provided dehumanizing care and little or no training or treatment.

The major factors influencing changes in the system, from institutional modalities of care to a greater emphasis on education, habilitation, and/or community living, occurred after World War II. The concepts of the civil rights movement and the rise of consumerism melded together and generated the creation of consumer associations. These groups were composed primarily of parents, but concerned professionals were important collaborators. Parents and relatives demanded changes and the development of new service options, insisting upon improved and expanded special education programs, outpatient clinical services, day treatment programs, and better-quality institutional care.

The largest and most active advocacy group involved those concerned about the mentally retarded. Local community, state, and national associations were organized to promote the interests of retarded children. Groups interested in other types of disabilities were also founded, eventually resulting in the creation of lobbying groups for individuals with cerebral palsy, learning disabilities, autism, and a variety of other chronic handicapping disorders. Services for the disabled population gradually began to expand at local levels, while simultaneous efforts continued to upgrade institutional care. Three major objectives emerged from consumer advocacy groups: (1) better care for institutionalized relatives, (2) more services for the disabled living at home with their families; and (3) the development of smaller homelike residential alternatives within communities in which the handicapped persons resided.

During the early 1960s, the movement to improve and expand special services received considerable impetus; it gained momentum with help of important allies. At that time, President Kennedy publicly acknowledged having a mentally retarded sister in his family. The publicity surrounding this disclosure provided an important psychological boost to parents and relatives who harbored feelings of shame or guilt about a retarded family member. Perhaps of greater significance and long-range impact was the Kennedy administration's legislative efforts. The passage of landmark legislation, P.L. 88-164, initiated new research, training, and services in the field of mental retardation. This was the initial component of what became series of legislative actions that continued through the 1970s. These measures led to improved public services and authorization of new entitlements guaranteeing legal rights, provided access to public facilities, and made free public education available for all handicapped children. Appropriate services and rights of handicapped adults were, in part, also assured through many of the legislative actions.

Over the past 20 years, numerous influential individuals contributed to improving the lives of the disabled. The list includes federal and state legislators, legal advocates, public interest attorneys, and individuals from varied professional backgrounds. In addition, professional and public associations have lobbied in behalf of disabled citizens.

THE ROLE OF THE PHYSICIAN

During the nineteenth century, physicians were instrumental in founding institutions as a result of their interest in treating mentally retarded and disabled individuals. Institutional directors during this era were physicians, a general pattern that persisted during the early 1970s. During the twentieth century, psychiatrists assumed these roles in facilities serving the mentally ill and the mentally retarded. In many states, the two populations were intermingled in state hospitals.

During the post-World War II era, very few facility directors were pediatricians. In general, physicians working in institutions had few ties with the medical community, particularly with academic institutions and/or teaching hospitals. A notable exception was Dr. Herman Yannet who, while located at Southbury Training School in Connecticut, had a formal affiliation with the Yale Medical School. The major focus of medical concern and intervention was for the basic medical needs of the institutionalized population. Educational activities were similarly based, to a significant extent, on the determination or categorization of the child's medical diagnosis. Physicians formulated the decisions. Then, other professionals (or nonprofessionals) followed the directives. This approach, the "medical model," provided accountability. Participation of other professionals was secondary, however, and their potential constructive role in program development was muted. The model has recently been widely criticized.

However, modifications of this traditional "medical model" occurred as new leadership roles emerged during the 1960s. Pediatricians and other specialists were designated leaders and members of a key planning group, the President's Panel of Mental Retardation. This Committee was given an advisory role on issues relating to mental retardation, in order to develop legislation to effect change. The original group's successor, the President's Committee on Mental Retardation, became an important advisory committee to presidents for the past two decades. Leadership of this Committee has included physicians from the academic community, as well as from institutional backgrounds. Some leaders were parents of retarded children. Recognizing the needs, many of these pediatricians lobbied for changes in the field, stressing the necessity for increased involvement of academic centers and teaching hospitals in research and training. These objectives were supported by consumers and other concerned professionals. Eventually, after P.L. 88-164 became law, this led to the establishment of a national network of 46 University Affiliated Facilities for training in mental retardation (see Appendix). In addition, funds were made available to create 12 mental retardation research centers. Both types of facilities were established to foster improvements in the care and treatment of the mentally retarded and developmentally disabled.

Concomitant with changes in service delivery for the mentally disabled were alterations in the patterns of physician involvement. The dominance of psychiatrists in the field diminished, in part resulting from the resentment that stemmed from their political control over the archaic institutional system. Relatively few new psychiatrists entered the field of mental retardation. Pediatric specialists assumed increasing responsibilities for serving the needs of children with disabilities. In various academic settings, they became known as developmental pediatricians. Many of the initial group of specialists were self-trained. Some developmental pediatricians received formal training in the diagnosis, care, and treatment of developmental disabilities, whereas others focused primarily on diagnostic issues or research in normal or aberrant child development.

The new breed of pediatricians specializing in developmental disabilities founded or worked in special diagnostic and evaluation clinics, developing teaching and research roles in medical school departments of pediatrics and in teaching hospitals. Developmental pediatricians worked in institutions and as consultants to voluntary agencies and school systems. While many assumed full-time positions in the field, others remained in private practice, offering their specialized skills on a part-time basis. Many of the early leaders in developmental pediatrics became advocates for change or were themselves "change agents." They worked with representative local and national organizations to adopt more progressive positions about care for children with mental retardation and developmental disorders. The developmental pediatricians gained national recognition serving in leadership roles as presidents of national associations, such as the American Association of Mental Deficiency and the American Academy for Cerebral Palsy. They participated as chairpersons of key committees of the American Academy of Pediatrics, as well as on the boards of directors of various state, local, and national organizations or advisory groups. Within a relatively short time, the field of developmental pediatrics was established as a major component of comprehensive health care for children.

THE CURRENT ROLE OF THE PEDIATRICIAN

Two major categories of pediatric practitioners provide care for children with disabilities. One group includes a relatively small number of pediatricians, identified as "specialists" in developmental disabilities, practicing either on a full- or part-time basis. The other, and much larger, group consists of general pediatric practitioners who serve disabled children as a component of their primary health care practice.

The number of specialists in developmental disabilities has increased substantially from a few practitioners in the 1960s to several hundred in the 1980s. The growth of the specialty reflects the success of federally supported training programs, primarily sponsored by the Division of Maternal and Child Health (U.S. Public Health Service), Department of Health and Human Services. These specialists have become significant contributors to the service, teaching, and research activities in medical schools, hospitals, institutions, outpatient clinics, and school settings. Developmental pediatricians often provide leadership within the context of a multidisciplinary/interdisciplinary team of medical and nonmedical specialists. During the past two decades, the medical model has been modified to allow for a greater sharing of responsibility and decision-making with all professional disciplines, recognizing the particular skills and roles of each professional discipline in the diagnosis and management of children with disabilities. The pediatrician in an interdisciplinary setting makes an important medical contribution. The leadership role, however, may be limited to administrative responsibilities and/or representation of a particular area of knowledge, rather than as in the past when his or her views were accepted as "the final word" merely because of the leader's status as a physician. The team of professionals share responsibilities, particularly since management recommendations frequently address nonmedical issues including educational, behavioral, and developmental goals. The "medical model" has been replaced by a "developmental model," based on results of the interdisciplinary process and a more dynamic perspective of the programmatic needs and potentials of the affected child.

In some cases, as a member of the team, the pediatrician may assume case-management responsibilities, serving as major advocate for the child and primary communicator with the parents, relatives, and treatment agencies. In other situations, other professionals may assume these roles and/or may share these responsibilities.

Developmental pediatricians are important advocates for individual patients and for groups of patients with particular types of handicaps. Their leadership roles in the community, among concerned professionals, parents, legislators, or political groups, has helped modify the formerly hostile attitude toward the medical profession. It is now appreciated that pediatricians can be very effective in assisting parents and patients obtain improved services for the developmentally disabled.

The role of practicing pediatricians, without specialized training in developmental disabilities, is changing. Various surveys and reports[5,6] have indicated that pediatricians do not feel adequately prepared to assist children with chronic handicaps. It is obvious that modified and improved graduate training programs in pediatrics are necessary in order to accommodate the increasing involvement of pediatric practitioners with developmentally disabled children. There is an expanding population of handicapped children remaining in the community, cared for by their families and requiring general health care. The practicing pediatrician is increasingly called upon to provide this comprehensive care. Early identification efforts stimulated by "child find," Early Periodic Screening and Diagnostic Testing (EPSDT), and heightened public awareness mandate that pediatricians more closely monitor early development and increase their diagnostic acumen in assessing developmental problems.

The implementation of P.L. 94-142, the Education for All Handicapped Children Act, has brought demands on practitioners to work more closely with schools and to assure provision of noneducational "related services" for children attending special educational programs. In some areas, the educational system has assumed total responsibility for the management of children with special needs, including *all* their needs while in school. Practitioners and organizations in these areas have become more outspoken about the importance of physicians in the management of children with disabilities. The major national medical organization representing pediatricians, the American Academy of Pediatrics, has asserted itself in the area by (1) developing an extensive national continuing education network of training programs and courses in developmental disabilities for practicing pediatricians, (2) providing a leadership role in amalgamating a consortium of organizations to define respective professional roles in implementing "related services" components of P.L. 94-142, (3) ensuring that pediatricians will be prominent participants in various advocacy roles representing children with developmental disabilities, and (4) making specific recommendation about the Pediatrician's important role in the provision of "related services" under P.L. 94-142.[7] During the past decade, practicing pediatricians and their representative organizations have become increasingly involved with all aspects of care of children with chronic disabilities. Pediatricians in particular have become leading participants in various primary and secondary prevention efforts in local communities and on a national level. As a result, most practitioners are generally more knowledgeable about the diagnostic/management problems and the psychosocial and educational needs of the developmentally disabled.

Despite the overall progress, the record of training for physicians in the care of children with disabilities has not always been exemplary. A key Task Force, including representatives from most national organizations with which practitioners and academically oriented pediatricians are affiliated, analyzed the curricula of graduate training programs in pediatrics. The Task Force found it necessary to recommend expanded training in developmental and behavioral pediatrics with a greater emphasis on care of the chronically handicapped child.[8] In several pediatric training centers, this expanded curriculum has been implemented, along with similar programs for medical students.[9,10] Unfortunately, not all training programs for pediatricians include a systematic training experience in the care of the chronically ill and/or developmentally disabled child.

FUTURE ROLES

Several trends in the delivery of services for the developmentally disabled appear to be significant factors in determining the future role of pediatricians. Although accurate predictions cannot be guaranteed, it appears that the trend toward increased community care and a de-emphasis on institutionalization should continue. An increasing number of families wish to keep their disabled children at home. These families are demanding an array of services to assist them in providing their children with as normal a life as possible both at home and in the community. These families, as a combined voice in local and national organizations, are becoming a stronger lobbying force. Their cause has been increasingly recognized as an economically justifiable option in view of the escalating costs of institutional care. As the disabled children living at home grow older, the demand increases for more community residential living opportunities, such as group homes. More physicians are being called upon to provide medical supervision for these children and adolescents while these patients live in the community and attend preschool and public school programs.

It is anticipated that pediatricians will be increasingly involved with expanded efforts in primary and secondary prevention. This involvement will be stimulated by technological advances and the cost effectiveness of prevention efforts. Primary prevention activities will include a greater focus on prevention of prematurity, improvement of perinatal care, and prevention of accidental poisonings or exposure to environmental toxins or contaminations. Secondary prevention will emphasize early identification of developmental disabilities and the provision of intervention programs. The rapid growth and sophistication of neonatal intenstive care and the concomitant survival of very low-birth-weight infants should lead to better mechanisms to identify brain dysfunction in infants and to earlier, more sophisticated means of conducting developmental assessments for high-risk infants. Pediatricians will be required to offer comprehensive care with attention to both the medical and nonmedical needs of all infants and children at risk.

In order to fulfill their responsibilities in the prevention and provision of comprehensive care for children, pediatricians will again require more and improved training in developmental diagnosis and greater familiarity with the problems involved in the care of chronically ill and disabled children. It is very likely that there will be a continued growth of developmental pediatrics as a subspecialty. There may also be a continued expansion of training programs for general pediatricians designed to emphasize the developmental and behavioral areas. A decade ago, it was a relative rarity to find a developmental pediatrician (or a division of developmental pediatrics or child development) as part of the organizational framework of an academic pediatric department. During the past decade, this has changed significantly. It is likely that the growth of this field will continue. Developmental/behavioral pediatricians are essential instructors for both the future general practitioners who provide generic care, as well as the experts who will provide diagnostic assessments, who will deal with the specialized medical needs of the handicapped children, or who will provide consultation to others on prevention and anticipatory guidance for families.

Pediatricians and pediatric associations have an obvious key role as advocates, lobbying for the needs of the developmentally disabled. The American Academy of Pediatrics (AAP) is already playing an active role in this regard during recent years. The AAP has offered strong testimony in Congress on behalf of handicapped children. The AAP has (1) demanded improved quality of pediatric services for the developmentally disabled, (2) stressed the need to improve the quality of *all* types of services, and (3) offered educational opportunities for pediatric practitioners to become more expert in developmental disabilities.

An optimistic view of the future would envision pediatricians as leaders in local, state, and national efforts to assure that developmentally disabled children receive the necessary care, training, or rehabilitation that will enable them to fulfill their maximum potential and permit as many as possible to become useful and productive adults.

REFERENCES

1. Wolfensberger, W.: The origin and nature of our institutional models, in Kugel, R. (ed.): *Changing Patterns in Residential Services for the Mentally Retarded.* President's Committee on Mental Retardation, DHEW Publication No. (OHD) 76-21015, 1976, pp. 35–82.
2. Howe, S. G.: *Report Made to Legislature of Massachusetts Upon Idiocy.* Collidge and Wiley, Boston, 1848.
3. Seguin, E.: *New Facts and Remarks Concerning Idiocy.* William Wood, New York, 1870.

4. Howe, S. G.: Address at institution dedication. *J. Insanity* 270, 1852.
5. Burg, F., and Wright, F. H.: Evaluation of pediatric residents and their training programs. *J. Pediatr.* **80:**183–189, 1972.
6. Christy, R. A., *et al.: Lengthening Shadows.* A Report of the Council on Pediatric Practice of the American Academy of Pediatrics on the Delivery of Health Care to Children. AAP, Evanston, Illinois, 1970.
7. AAP Committee on Children with Disabilities: Provision of related services for children with chronic disabilities. *Pediatrics* **75:**796–797, 1985.
8. Kempe, C. H., *et al.: The Future of Pediatric Education.* A Report by the Task Force on Pediatric Education, Evanston, Illinois, 1979.
9. Guralnick, M. J., and Richardson, H. B.: *Pediatric Education and the Needs of Exceptional Children.* University Park Press, Baltimore, 1980.
10. Cohen, H. J., and Diamond, D.: Training and preparing physicians to care for mentally retarded and handicapped children. *Appl. Res. Ment. Retard.* **5:**279–291, 1984.

Cerebral Palsy
History and State of the Art

Bruce K. Shapiro, Frederick B. Palmer, and Arnold J. Capute

HISTORICAL BACKGROUND

Motor disability in childhood has been recognized since the earliest of recorded history. However, the recognition of individual disease entities that cause motor disability is more recent. Cerebral palsy, poliomyelitis, muscular dystrophy, and spinal muscular atrophy were all described during the nineteenth century.

Cerebral palsy was first described by William John Little, an orthopedic surgeon. Little had talipes equinovarus, and this is credited with determining his career choice and becoming the foremost authority on clubfoot and its treatment.[1] As a result of his clinical experience, Little described the type of cerebral palsy known as spastic diplegia, which bears his name. Little's interest in cerebral palsy extended beyond surgical management. The results of his attempts to define the etiology of cerebral palsy are found in, "On the Influence of Abnormal Parturition, Difficult Labor, Premature Birth, and Asphyxia Neonatorum, on the Mental and Physical Condition of the Child, Especially in Relations to Deformities," initially presented to the Obstetrical Society of London in 1861.[2]

Bruce K. Shapiro, Frederick B. Palmer, and Arnold J. Capute • The Kennedy Institute for Handicapped Children, Department of Pediatrics, The John Hopkins University Medical Institutions, Baltimore, Maryland 21205.

Since Little's pioneering work, the concept of cerebral palsy has developed along several lines. Further classification of various cerebral palsy syndromes predominated late in the nineteenth century. In a series of lectures entitled "The Cerebral Palsies of Children," Sir William Osler, described the clinical findings in 150 cases of cerebral palsy, grouped them according to presumed etiology, and speculated upon pathophysiological mechanisms.[3] Osler is credited with the first use of the term "cerebral palsy," derived from the German *Cerebrale Kinderlahung* (cerebral child paralysis). Sigmund Freud, known initially as a neurologist and neuropathologist, further classified clinical manifestations of the bilateral cerebral palsies and attempted to relate these to anatomical lesions.[4]

Although taxonomy was progressing, there were very few advances in the habilitation of the cerebral palsied child, from the time of Little until the early twentieth century—when Bronson Crothers established a clinic for the muscle training of children with paralysis.[5] Winthrop Phelps, professor of orthopedics at Yale University, established the Children's Rehabilitation Institute (Baltimore) in 1936. Phelps was exposed to muscle education techniques while serving as a fellow in orthopedic surgery. He expanded on these techniques and developed a school of treatment stressing (1) a specific diagnostic classification, (2) specific modalities of therapy for each class prescribed for the individual child, and (3) bracing and adaptive equipment, in addition to muscle education.[6] Cognizant of and sensitive to the influence of associated neurological deficits on habilitation, Phelps fostered multidisciplinary teams. (In 1961, the Board of the Johns Hopkins University approved an affiliation with the Children's Rehabilitation Institute and this agreement evolved into the John F. Kennedy Institute for Handicapped Children.)

Cerebral palsy became a recognized field of study following World War II. Advances in genetic and metabolic studies permitted delineation of disorders previously categorized under the broad heading of "cerebral palsy." A specific etiology—hyperbilirubinemia—was established for a cerebral palsy syndrome consisting of choreoathetoid cerebral palsy, hearing loss, limitation of upward gaze, and staining of primary teeth. New therapies were proposed (e.g., those suggested by Bobath and Bobath[7]; Rood[8]; Kabat and Knott[9]; Vojta[10]; and Petö[11]) de-emphasizing individual muscles and focusing on movement and maintenance of posture. The rapid expansion of knowledge resulted in confusion as to what constituted cerebral palsy and how to classify it. In 1957, a conference was assembled to address issues of terminology and classification of cerebral palsy. From these discussions, several factors regarding cerebral palsy were proposed: (1) it was a disorder of movement and posture; (2) "early years of life" or "early brain development" was preferable to mentioning an exact age; (3) knowledge of the brain's control of movement and posture was incomplete, preventing further localization; and (4) cerebral palsy was progressive, with peripheral manifestations changing despite the static nature of the pathological lesion. The following definition was proposed:

> Cerebral palsy is a persistent but not unchanging disorder of movement and posture, appearing in the early years of life and due to a nonprogressive disorder of the brain, the result of interference during its development. . . . Persistence of the infantile type of motor control, such as may be seen in intellectually handicapped children, is not considered to be "cerebral palsy."[12]

In 1964 a group of professionals met to review the terminology and classification of cerebral palsy. They recognized the need to develop a common terminology of investigators from different countries. The group reached agreement on a definition of cerebral palsy as "a disorder of movement and posture due to a defect or lesion of the immature brain.''[13] However, agreement could not be reached on the various types of cerebral palsy.

CLASSIFICATION

As a diagnostic entity, "cerebral palsy" makes no inference as to etiology, pathophysiology, degree of handicap, therapy, or prognosis. This limitation has led to the suggestion that the term "cerebral palsy" be abandoned. Nevertheless, the term does have value as a generic descriptor referring to a group of heterogeneous disorders in which static motor encephalopathy is a common feature. The further classification of cerebral palsy (CP) syndromes is useful for treatment, research, and prognosis.

Despite multiple classifications systems for CP, no one system has proved entirely successful. In the nineteenth century, attempts were made to define the pathological anatomy of CP. Although unable to correlate neuropathological with clinical findings, Freud[4] proposed a clinical classification that recognized the major syndromes: hemiplegia, generalized cerebral spasticity, paraplegic spasticity, generalized chorea and double athetosis, and double spastic hemiplegia.

Etiological classifications originated with Little, whose paper alluded to "the suspected cause of spastic diplegia."[2] A system assigning disorders to prenatal, natal, or postnatal factors was proposed by Sachs[14] and by Sachs and Hausman.[15] Etiological classifications were as unsatisfactory as were neuropathological classifications because similar clinical syndromes appeared to result from different etiologies and were associated with different neuropathological findings.

Additional neurological deficits frequently accompanied cerebral palsy.[16] Little, Osler, and Freud all noted that mental deficiency was commonly observed in association with cerebral palsy. Speech and language disorders, auditory and visual problems, seizures, sensory disturbances, and behavioral disorders are also noted with greater frequency in the CP population. Similarly, disorders of growth and secondary disorders of the musculoskeletal system are found. Denhoff recognized the associated deficits and defined cerebral palsy as

> One component of a broader brain damage syndrome comprised of neuromotor dysfunction, psychological dysfunction, convulsions and behavior disorders of organic origin . . . .. Cerebral palsy is the neuromotor component of the "brain damage" syndrome. It must always be kept in mind that the CP child may suffer from any other component of the syndrome along with the neuromotor handicap.[17]

The classification currently in use is modified from a system designed by the Americal Academy for Cerebral Palsy, as recommended by W. L. Minear.[18] It represents an amalgamation of the cited classification systems, coupled with measures of functional ability and therapeutic interventions. It is composed of several factors: physiological (motor), topographical, etiological, supplemental (associated deficits), neuroanatomical, functional capacity, and therapeutic. Such a systemic classification system facilitates identification of more homogeneous subgroups and permits the collection of information relating to the epidemiology, mechanisms, and treatment of the various CP syndromes.

Classification according to the type of motor deficit (physiological and topographical) is of assistance to the clinician and researcher. The physiological classification

Table I. Physiological Classification of Cerebral Palsy

Spastic	Tremor
Extrapyramidal	Atonic
Rigidity	Mixed
Ataxia	Unclassified

From Minear[13]

(Tables I and II) is of value as a marker for associated deficits. Patients with extra-pyramidal cerebral palsy are more likely to have feeding and speech problems than are those with spastic CP. Mental retardation, seizures, and orthopedic deformities are more common in spastics. Little change has been noted in the pattern of associated deficits among spastics, whereas extrapyramidal CP has been modified significantly as the incidence of kernicterus has changed.[19]

By contrasting subgroups of motor disability within a physiological class different patterns of associated dysfunctions emerge. Two subgroups of extrapyramidal CP have been identified, dystonic and hyperkinetic, differing as to motor prognosis, mental retardation, and frequency of multiple handicaps. The dystonic subgroup is the more common and is associated with inability to walk (90%), IQ < 50 (41%), and high rates of multiple handicapping conditions. The hyperkinetic (choreatic and athetotic) subgroup is associated with milder motor impairment, greater intelligence (86% >50), but higher rates of hearing loss.[20]

Differences among spastics are usually based on the number of limbs involved (topography) rather than the quality of the movement disorder (Table III). There are clear relationships between the subtypes of spasticity, based on topographical distribution and

Table II. Clinical Signs That Distinguish Spastic from Nonspastic (Extrapyramidal) Cerebral Palsy

Clinical sign	Spastic CP	Extrapyramidal CP
General	Persistent and consistent signs	Variability of signs common
Reflexes	Brisk stretch reflexes, sustained clonus, and/or increase in reflexogenic tone	Normal to moderately hyperreflexic reflexes (unsustained clonus)
Pathological reflexes	Pathological reflexes (i.e., Babinski, Chaddock, Oppenheim, Gordon, or Hoffmann)	Absent pathological reflexes (extensor plantar response may be part of athetoid movements)
Primitive reflexes	May be exaggerated or persistent	Exaggerated and persistent to a greater degree (common)
Tone	Clasp-knife hypertonus, which cannot be shaken out and persists in sleep	Lead pipe or candle wax quality to tone; may be readily "shaken out" and usually disappears with sleep
Contractures	Nonpositional contractures common	Nonpositional contractures uncommon, although contractures may result from prolonged sitting position (wheelchair)

Table III. Topographical Classification of Spastic Cerebral Palsy

Condition	Characteristics
Monoplegia	Involves one limb; usually a forme fruste of hemiplegia or diplegia
Hemiplegia	Lateralized one-half of the body affected; arm usually more affected than the leg
Diplegia	Both legs affected; slight upper extremity involvement noted.
Triplegia	Involves three extremities; may represent either a hemiplegia plus diplegia or incomplete quadriplegia
Quadriplegia	All limbs affected; generally defined as follows: spastic (greatest involvement of the legs), extrapyramidal (greatest involvement of the arms)
Double hemiplegia	Evidence of more spastic involvement of the arms that of the legs (rare)
Paraplegia	Involves the legs only, with normal upper extremity function (term currently reserved for spinal cord injuries)

Adapted from Minear.[13]

associated deficits. The degree of mental retardation is usually increased proportionately to the number of limbs involved. Homonymous hemianopsia, growth arrest, and disorders of cortical sensory function on the affected side are associated with hemiplegia. The evidence suggests that the prognosis for ambulation of hemiplegics is not altered by physical therapy.[21] As many as 40% of children with spastic diplegia are born prematurely. The general diagnosis of CP offers relatively little information. By contrast, subclassification enables the clinician to discern relatively homogeneous groups and to discuss etiology, degree of handicap, therapy, and prognosis.

A major factor for the lack of a satisfactory classification of CP is the inability to predict how an immature nervous system will develop. Although brain dysfunction is said to be static, the peripheral manifestations do change. Consequently the diagnosis of CP is often deferred until the age of 2 years. In a review of data from the Collaborative Perinatal Project of the National Institute of Neurological and Communicative Disorders and Stroke, 51% of children diagnosed as having CP at age 1 year were found to be free of motor handicap by 7 years of age. Among the factors identified with resolution of early motor abnormalities were the following: (1) type of CP (i.e., all monoplegias resolved, whereas spastic hemiplegia and quadriplegia persisted), (2) severity of motor handicap, (3) race (resolved more frequently in blacks than in whites), and (4) sex (more apt to resolve in females than in males). Among an older population, Paine found a high correlation (78–95%, depending on type of CP) between initial diagnosis and follow-up evaluation, with monoplegia (12%) the exception.[23]

Should children who "outgrow" their motor dysfunction be considered cerebral palsied? Clearly, these children demonstrate a disorder of posture and locomotion, with signs of CNS dysfunction. The definition of CP does not qualify the degree of dysfunction. However, motor dysfunction resolves in children, is the use of the term justified? This group of children is at least equal in number to those children with traditional CP. They usually do not come to the attention of the orthopedist, neurologist, developmental pediatrician, or motor therapist. Their motor prognosis is excellent and they "catch up." Nevertheless, children in whom a motor dysfunction resolves may be at risk of additional neurological deficits. The rate of mental retardation, seizures, and speech and behavioral problems is lower than that in the traditional CP palsy population—and somewhat differ-

Table IV. Expanded Classification of Cerebral Palsy

Classification	Rate of motor development	Motor signs	Associated dysfunction
Minimal	Normal; motor quotient (MQ 75–100); qualitative abnormalities only	Transient abnormalities of tone; persistence of some primitive reflexes to a mild degree; deviant postural development; mild neurodevelopmental deficits in fine and gross motor abilities (i.e., clumsy)	Communicative disorder; specific learning disability; Strauss syndrome[a]
Mild	2/3 normal (MQ 50–70); walks by age 24 months	Several abnormalities of traditional neurological examination; unusual primitive reflex development; mildly delayed postural responses; moderate neurodevelopmental deficits in fine and gross motor abilities (i.e., tremor, synkinesias, poor coordination)	Communicative disorder; specific learning disability; mental retardation; Strauss syndrome[a]
Moderate	1/2 normal (MQ 40–50); walks by age 3; may need bracing; usually does not require assistive devices or surgery	Many neurological findings; strong, persistent primitive reflexes with some obligates; delayed postural responses	Mental retardation specific learning disorder; communicative disorder; seizures; expanded Strauss syndrome[b]
Severe/profound	Less than 1/2 normal (MQ < 40); may not walk freely in the community; may need bracing, assistive devices, and orthopedic surgery	Traditional neurological signs predominate; obligatory primitive reflexes; postural reactions absent or markedly delayed in appearance	Mental retardation; seizures; expanded Strauss syndrome[b] + others

[a]Strauss syndrome: hyperkinesis, attentional peculiarities (short attention span to perseveration), distractibility, easily frustrated, temper tantrums.
[b]Expanded Strauss syndrome: components of Strauss syndrome to a greater degree and includes repetitive stereotypical activities (e.g., rocking, head banging, flapping, or spinning and mild self-injurious behavior).

ent in quality However, language and visual perception problems, attentional peculiarities, and hyperkinetic syndromes are more frequent than in the general population.[22,24] The characteristic pattern of development for these children indicates resolution of the motor delay by 2 years of age, but a persistence of clumsiness remains. Language and speech problems are more evident in the preschool age group, commonly persisting into the early school years. Academic underachievement is evident in the primary grades and frequently requires special education placement. The current classification scheme does not recognize these children, inasmuch as they do not fit the traditional concept of CP. Nevertheless, the frequent need for developmental intervention suggests that classification should be expanded. A recommended classification would group children on the basis of (1) degree of motor delay, (2) neuromotor signs, (3) associated dysfunctions, and (4) functional ability.[25] The group designated "minimal to mild" would include children in whom neuromotor signs resolve. Children with persisting motor handicaps would be classified as having "moderate," "severe," or "profound" CP (Table IV).

Children with motor delay and mental retardation can similarly be accommodated in this schema. The traditional definition of CP excludes mentally retarded children who manifest "the infantile type of motor control." However, an attempt to differentiate delayed from abnormal cannot be justified because (1) not all mentally retarded children are motor delayed, (2) the motor delay in mental retardation has been attributed to central hypotonia (e.g., Down syndrome) or delayed onset of postural reactions,[26] and (3) the minimal cognitive level needed for gross motor activities has not been determined.[27,28,29] If these children are regarded as "mildly" or "minimally" cerebral palsied, they can be placed on a spectrum of motor dysfunction.

DIAGNOSIS

Theoretically, it can be argued that there is no need for an early diagnosis of CP because (1) treatment has not been demonstrated to prevent CP before it is clinically manifest, and (2) it is unlikely that significant problems will develop in a child without becoming clinically manifest. Nevertheless, early detection of CP does offer four potential advantages (justifying the effort despite the lack of an efficacious treatment): (1) improved parent–child interaction, through anticipatory guidance; (2) earlier adaptation of the family to the child's handicap with improved functioning; (3) the possible (although unlikely) development of an effective treatment that would prevent the clinical manifestations; and (4) improved assessment of obstetrical and neonatal interventions.

Although early detection may be desirable, it is difficult to achieve because motor abnormality is subtle in infants. The paucity of motor milestones during the first 6 months of life generally eliminates the presenting complaint of "motor delay," precluding a valuable component of the diagnostic process. Prematurity and asphyxia confound the early clinical examination in inconsistent ways. Similarly, signs change with maturation, and their significance is altered. The lack of clinically applicable techniques, with prospective validity, is a major handicap in the early detection of CP.

The pediatric assessment of the motor-delayed child begins with confirmation and quantification of "delay" by comparison of the infant's performance with known motor milestones (Table V).[30] This is best achieved through the use of historical information and observation. The motor examination of infants with delayed attainment of gross motor skills focuses on three components: (1) traditional neurological examination, (2) assessment of primitive reflexes, and (3) elicitation of postural response. Each component does not reliably detect CP except in extreme cases, but combining the parts of the motor examination aids the detection of CP.

The purpose of the traditional neurological examination of infants is to detect signs that are not normally present. Disordered movements, tonal abnormalities (hyper- and hypotonus), sustained clonus of stretch reflexes, and asymmetrical findings are examples of neurological signs associated with CP.

Table V. Mean Age of Gross Motor Attainment in Normal Children

Milestone	Age (month)	SD	% Recall (N = 183)
Rolls prone to supine	3.3	1.3	97
Rolls supine to prone	4.6	1.3	95
Sits supported	5.4	1.0	67
Sits alone	6.2	1.2	95
Creeps	6.5	1.4	92
Pulls to sit	7.4	1.7	78
Crawls	7.6	1.7	96
Pulls to stand	8.0	1.4	99
Cruise	8.8	1.5	98
Walks	11.6	1.6	98
Walks backward	14.5	2.3	83
Runs	14.8	2.5	92

In contrast to the adult and older child, the neurological examination of the infant changes with maturation: (1) moderate left–right asymmetries may disappear; (2) three outcomes may result for the hypotonic child (i.e., continued hypotonia, normalization of tone, and progression to spastic hypertonus and/or choreathetosis); (3) prominent adventitious movements may be present at nine months but not at 15 months; and (4) spastic diplegics may be initially hypotonic in the legs, whereas children with choreathetoid CP may show generalized hypotonia before exhibiting their movement disorder.

Similar findings have different significance when they occur at different ages: (1) flexor hypertonus is normal in term babies but abnormal at about 6 months, (2) Babinski signs may be present at several months of age but should not persist beyond the first year, and (3) increased reflexogenic zone is normal in young infants but is rare after 9 months of age. The traditional neurological examination is of limited use for the early detection of CP because of instability of signs, changing interpretations of similar signs with age, and poor localizing value.

Primitive reflexes are brainstem-mediated reflexes that are present at birth and that diminish in activity during the first year of life.[31] These responses have been associated with the development of normal motor activity[32] and are considered the earliest indicators of significant motor disability.[33,34] Abnormalities of primitive reflex activity can be grouped into four major categories: (1) absence of reflexes that should be present (e.g.,

Table VI. Postural Reactions

Reaction	Age of appearance (months)	Function
Head righting	1	Lifts chin from table top in prone
Landau	2–3	Head up from prone (series of midline righting reactions)
Derotative righting	4–5	Segmental rolling (series of axial righting reactions)
Anterior propping	5	Tripod sits
Lateral propping	7	Sits alone
Posterior propping	10–12	Pivots in sitting

Table VII. The Motor Examination in Infants with Cerebral Palsy

Type of CP	Neurological findings	Primitive reflexes	Postural reactions

Hemiplegia	Early handedness (<1 year)
	Eversion of involved Leg
	Asymmetries predominate
	  Movement
	  Tone
	  Fall away
	  Stretch reflexes
	  Pathological reflexes
	  Growth arrest
		Asymmetries
		  Placing
		  Grasps
		  Asymmetric tonic neck
		    reflex (ATNR)
		  Galant
		  Tonic labyrinthine (TL)
			Asymmetry of propping
			Unilateral derotative
			  righting

Diplegia	Frog position in supine
	  (hypotonic phase)
	Decreased movement in
	  legs
	Discrepancy between tone
	  in arms and legs
	Sits on air (hypotonic
	  phase)
	Hip adductor tone in-
	  creased (hypertonic
	  phase)
	Scissoring/diapering
	  difficulties
	Hyperreflexia of legs
	Pathological reflexes in
	  legs
		Persistence of ATNR, TL
		  in legs
		Absent placing of legs
		Positive absent (hypotonic
		  phase)
		Positive support obligate
		  (hypertonic phase)
		Strong plantar grasps ±
		  withdrawal
			Absent downward
			  parachute
			Upper extremity propping
			  may be delayed

Quadriplegia	Decreased active
	  movement
	Clasp knife spasticity in all
	  limbs
	Generalized hyperreflexia
	  with sustained clonus
	Pathological reflexes
		Absence or incomplete
		  placing
		Increased primitive reflex
		  activity with obligatory
		  responses
			Markedly delayed if pre-
			  sent at all

Extrapyramidal	Generalized hypotonia
	  (early)
	Involuntary movements at
	  rest or difficulty modu-
	  lating active movements
	Variable tone in
	  extremities
	Axial tone often decreased
	Brisk to diminished stretch
	  reflexes
		Exaggerated and/or per-
		  sistent in all limbs
		Prominent signs of oral
		  motor dysfunction-root,
		  snout, jaw jerk, palmo-
		  mental, drooling, hyper-
		  active gag, tongue thrust
			Usually delayed if present
			  at all

Moro at birth), (2) excessive reflex activity for a given age, (3) persistence beyond the usual time of disappearance, and (4) obligatory reflex activity (always imposable or inability to change posture). Except for the most extreme cases, isolated primitive reflexes do not portend motor handicap. Additional research is needed to determine the clinical applicability of combinations of reflexes.[35]

Postural responses include righting and equilibrium responses. As primitive reflexes diminish in activity, postural responses become more evident. Volitional motor activity is closely associated with the appearance of postural responses. Righting responses such as head righting and the Landau response are present from several months of age, whereas the propping responses appear during the second half of the first year (Table VI). The neurological findings and primitive and postural responses for the various types of CP are summarized in Table VII.

It is not sufficient to perform only a motor examination on the child who presents with "motor delay." Gross motor development during early life is reflective of neurological function and developmental syndromes that may not cause motor handicaps; for example, mental retardation, communication disorders, and learning disabilities may present as motor delay. Consequently, a comprehensive neurodevelopmental examination, including assessment of language, cognition, and adaptive skills, in addition to motor skills, is indicated for the child who manifests gross motor delay.

TREATMENT

During the past decade, numerous advances have been made in the prevention of CP. Immunizations, both active (e.g., rubella and rubeola) and passive (e.g., anti-RH immunoglobulin to prevent Rh sensitization and subsequent hemolytic disease of the newborn with kernicterus) have clearly altered the incidence and types of CP. It is in the areas of obstetrics and neonatology, however, that the most dramatic changes have occurred. The concept of organizing "high-risk" obstetrical centers, which have the ability to manage both mothers and infants, reflects the ability to monitor pregnancies and provide meaningful intervention. The fetus and uterus are no longer regarded as *terra incognita*. Ultrasound permits visualization of the fetus and placenta, measurement of certain physiological factors, and the establishment of the duration of pregnancy. Amniocentesis permits detection of chromosomal abnormalities, culture of fetal cells (to detect certain metabolic derangements), and detection of spina bifida through α-fetoprotein (AFP) analysis. Stress tests and biochemical measures, such as human placental lactogen (hPL), permit indirect measurement of the fetoplacental unit.

Monitoring of the fetal heart rate (FHR) in relationship to uterine contractions has altered the conduct of labor. Previously undetectable disorders are now more easily identified. Measurement of fetal scalp pH can be used to measure acid–base metabolism and, indirectly, asphyxia. Although the effects of these interventions on the incidence of CP remains to be demonstrated, their use in selected risk populations is warranted.

During the past decade, the intensive care of sick newborns has advanced significantly. New techniques are continually being introduced for the detection and management of problems of prematurity and deficient intrauterine growth. Although the beneficial effect of intensive care on neonatal mortality is clear, the effect on the incidence of CP remains controversial.[36-39]

Cerebral palsy is not curable. There is no scientific evidence that any intervention effectively alters the natural history of CP, although there is a plethora of anecdotal clinical impressions. The key question is not whether a child makes progress but whether the rate of progress is greater than would be expected by maturation. Although therapy has been given to CP patients for about a century, only a few scientifically designed studies have been attempted.[37-39] The reasons for this paucity are multiple, in view of two major roadblocks. First, the developmental outcome of a disordered nervous system cannot be predicted accurately; therefore, randomized control studies are required to determine whether the rate of skill acquisition is enhanced. Second, it is difficult to ensure comparable study groups for randomized control studies because of the many patterns of motor deficiency and associated deficits that may result in discarding a beneficial therapy or in falsely endorsing an ineffective treatment.

A complete developmental diagnosis, which includes investigation of associated dysfunctions in addition to the motor disability is more than of academic interest, however. Treatment of CP without the benefit of awareness of the associated deficits usually results in incomplete habilitation. For example, to focus on enabling a child to ambulate while ignoring the child's mental retardation is obviously a disservice. On the other hand, to treat only the signs and symptoms of a disordered nervous system without understanding the underlying cause could result in inappropriate expectations and parental frustration.

Before instituting treatment of the cerebral palsied child, quantifiable short-term and long-term objectives should be defined. Once this is established, the therapist and parent can honestly appraise whether the objectives are being reached; they can also ensure that provision of therapy per se is not the end objective. Many factors must be considered in setting goals for the CP patient:

Cerebral palsy factors: These factors relate to the motor deficit and the associated deficits. Most children with minimal and mild CP do not require specific motor therapy, although language and educational therapies are frequently necessary. For example, a blind child with severe spastic diplegia would be treated differently than would a child with normal vision. Language therapy would probably not be recommended if a hemiplegic's expressive and receptive language abilities are in keeping with the remainder of the child's cognitive abilities.

Child factors: These relate to the child and include age, individual goals, and self-image. An example is an adolescent with diplegia who decides that it requires too much effort to walk with canes (or that it looks ungainly) and who elects to use a wheelchair instead (to the consternation of parents and therapists). Another example is the limited ability of the young child to participate in programs designed to stimulate cognition, upper extremity development, language, gross motor development, independence, and "appropriate" behaviors.

Family factors: A number of variables are included: (1) parents' perception of the handicap, (2) influence of other family members (both nuclear and extended), (3) parents priorities and their expectations for success, and (4) stressors of finance, work, marriage, and transitions.

Environmental factors: Availability of service, ability of the family to secure services, and distance are frequently major issues for the infant and the toddler (although PL 94-142, the Education for All Handicapped Children Act, mandates an appropriate education for handicapped children).

The goals of therapists can generally be divided into two major categories: (1) to maintain function (secondary prevention), and (2) to maximize or develop new functions. Activities directed toward maintenance of function may include (1) motor therapy to prevent contractures, (2) positioning to ensure symmetry and prevent scoliosis, and (3) soft tissue surgery to prevent hip dislocation. Nonmotor activities frequently are directed toward maintenance of self-esteem and prevention of secondary behavioral disturbances, including (1) parental counseling to make for appropriate expectations, (2) school placement consonant with the child's abilities, and (3) opportunities for social interaction. Activities directed toward maximization of function and for the development of new skills focus on communication, activities of daily living, and mobility.

The ability to communicate effectively permits the patient with CP to overcome many of the limitations imposed by the motor deficits. Difficulty in communicating was initially believed to be synonymous with cognitive limitation. Subsequently, disordered oral motor control was seen as the etiology for the communicative disorder. As experience with cerebral palsied children increased, central language disorders joined hearing loss, cognitive limitation, and poor oral motor control as an etiology for communicative failure. Many children with CP benefit from speech therapy; but there are many who will not be able to communicate through traditional means. Augmentive methods for communication for these children have been developed over the past decade.[40,41] These methods range from simple eye blinks and signs to computers that speak. Initially there was concern that augmentative methods might hinder speech development in children; the contrary seems to be true. Currently children are matched to an augmentative system, on a trial-and-error basis. Although some of the factors that determine the success of a system are known (e.g., cognition, motor dysfunction, and the fashion in which the system is to be used), additional research is needed to identify the determinants of successful utilization.

Performing activities of daily living enables the cerebral palsied individual to be independent.[42] These skills (feeding, dressing, toileting, and bathing) depend on upper extremity abilities, vision, and cognition. For successful completion of activities of daily living, the individual must be positioned so as to diminish the effects of primitive reflexes and permit maximal functioning of the extremities. This commonly requires adaptations to chairs or car seats for infants. Additional assistance may be obtained through the use of techniques that decrease tone or alter movement (e.g., physical therapy, pharmacotherapy, neurosurgery, or biofeedback) or that prevent or correct the deformity (e.g., physical therapy or orthopedic surgery). However, not all cerebral palsied individuals are able to perform activities of daily living successfully; some will require adaptive equipment. Special equipment is often designed by parents because of the lack of systematic approaches in this area.

Mobility is usually the primary concern of parents when they learn that their child has CP. Nevertheless, mobility is only of limited importance to ultimate adaptation. There is a continuum of ambulatory abilities, ranging from walking freely in the community (e.g., at shopping centers) to walking about the house, and to ambulation for exercise purposes;

there is also the nonwalker who has arm function. Neurodevelopmental, modified neurodevelopmental therapy, bracing, and orthopedic surgery are therapeutic modalities commonly employed to assist mobility. Ambulation depends on the successful integration of motor components, but the ability to use a walker and canes is, in large measure, dependent on arm function. If the development of effective ambulatory skills fails, alternative methods of transportation must be utilized, such as the use of a wheelchair, which may be adapted to diminish the effects of the gross motor disability.

Transportation is an outgrowth of mobility. Infants and small children pose no problems in transportation, as they travel in car seats or strollers (which may be adapted). Many hemiplegics can drive without difficulty. Diplegics may require hand controls to operate a motor vehicle. More severely involved cerebral palsied individuals are restricted because of the lack of accommodations for wheelchairs. Although attempts are being made to improve this situation, it remains a major impediment to habilitation.

OUTCOME

The determinants of a successful social adjustment are unknown. Minimal, mild, and even moderate disorders may not be considered CP. Consequently, their success, or lack thereof, cannot be ascertained. The prognosis for CP remains "guarded"—even the most optimistic report found only 60% to be gainfully employed or expected to be so after training.[43,44] Factors that influence outcome include motor capabilities, associated dysfunctions, personality factors, and family function.[45] Whether the approaches used during the late 1960s and 1970s have altered this prognosis remains to be demonstrated.

SUMMARY

During the nineteenth century, CP was distinguished from other causes of motor handicap. Initially defined by orthopedic deformities, less handicapping forms of CP were recognized as experience increased. It was not until well into the twentieth century that the role of additional associated neurological dysfunctions was appreciated. More recently it has been recognized that children who demonstrate early motor abnormalities can normalize with maturation. These children would not be referred to the orthopedist, neurologist, or developmental pediatrician as "motor delayed," but they frequently have additional neurological dysfunctions requiring habilitation. Consequently thay can be considered at the mild/minimal end of the spectrum of CP.

Cerebral palsy is the most common motor disorder of infants and children. Despite almost a century of experience, the treatment of CP is empirical. This is because of our inability to predict outcomes for the developing nervous system and because the variety of subtypes of motor handicap and associated dysfunctions precludes a "garden variety" of CP. Technology has facilitated the development of circumvention strategies that permit the severely cerebral palsied to transcend their motor limitations. The long-term social functioning of persons treated during the 1960s and 1970s and the effect of the therapy on function remain questions that require additional study.

REFERENCES

1. Bishop, W. J.: William John Little, 1810–94 A Brief Biography. *Cerebral Palsy Bull.* **1**:3–4, 1958.
2. Little, W. J.: On the influence of abnormal parturition, difficult labors, premature birth, and asphyxia neonatorum, on the mental and physical condition of the child, especially in relation to deformities. *Trans. Obstet. Soc. Lond.* **3**:293–344, 1861–1862.
3. Osler, W.: The cerebral palsies of children. *Med. News* **53**:29–35, 57–66, 85–90, 113–116, 141–145, 1888.
4. Freud, S.: *Infantile Cerebral Paralysis*, Russin, L. (Trans.), University of Miami Press, Coral Gables, Florida, 1968.
5. Keats, S.: *Cerebral Palsy*. Charles C. Thomas, Springfield, Illinois, 1965.
6. Levitt, S.: Stimulation of movement: A review of therapeutic techniques, in Holt, K. (ed.): *Movement and Child Development. Clinics in Developmental Medicine 55.* Lippincott, Philadelphia, 1975.
7. Bobath, K., and Bobath, B.: The neurodevelopmental treatment, in Scrutton, D. (ed): *Management of the Motor Disorders of Children with Cerebral Palsy. Clinics in Developmental Medicine No. 90.* Lippincott, Philadelphia, 1984, pp. 6–18.
8. Cited in Stockmyer, S. A.: The Rood Approach. *Am. J. Phys. Med.* **46**:900, 1967.
9. Cited in Levitt, S.: *Treatment of Cerebral Palsy and Motor Delay*, 2nd ed. Blackwell Scientific, Boston, 1982.
10. Vojta, V.: The basic elements of treatment according to Vojta, in Scrutton, D. (ed.): *Management of the Motor Disorders of Children with Cerebral Palsy. Clinics in Developmental Medicine No. 90.* Lippincott, Philadelphia, 1984, pp. 75–85.
11. Cited in Hari, M., and Tillemans, T.: Conductive education, in Scrutton, D. (ed.): *Management of the Motor Disorders of Children with Cerebral Palsy. Clinics in Developmental Medicine No. 90.* Lippincott, Philadelphia, 1984, pp. 19–35.
12. MacKeith, R. C., Mackenzie, I. C., and Polani, P. E.: The Little Club memorandum on terminology and classification of "cerebral palsy." *Cerebral Palsy Bull.* **5**:27–35, 1959.
13. Bax, M. C. O.: Terminology and classification of cerebral palsy. *Dev. Med. Child Neurol.* **6**:295–297, 1964.
14. Sachs, B.: Contributions to the pathology of infantile cerebral palsies. *N.Y. Med. J.* **53**:503–510, 1891.
15. Sachs, B., and Hausman, L.: *Nervous and Mental Disorders from Birth through Adolescence.* Hoeber, New York, 1926.
16. Shapiro, B. K., Palmer, F. B., Wachtel, R. C., *et al.:* Cerebral palsy: Associated dysfunctions. in Thomson, G., Rubin, I. L., Bilenker, R. M. (eds.). *Comprehensive Management of Cerebral Palsy.* Grune & Stratton, New York, 1982.
17. Denhoff, E.: Cerebral palsy: Medical aspects, in: Cruickshank, W., and Raus, G. (eds.): *Cerebral Palsy. Its Individual and Community Problems.* Syracuse University Press, Syracuse, New York, 1955.
18. Minear, W. L.: A classification of cerebral palsy. *Pediatrics* **8**:841–852, 1956.
19. Marquis, P., Palmer, F. B., Mahoney, W. S., and Capute, A. J.: Extrapyramidal cerebral palsy: A changing view. *J. Dev. Behav. Pediatr.* **3**:65–68, 1982.
20. Kyllerman, M., Bager, B., Bensch, J., et al.: Dyskinetic cerebral palsy. I. Clinical categories, associated neurological abnormalities and incidences. *Acta Pediatr. Scand.* **71**:543–550, 1982.
21. Paine, R. S.: On the treatment of cerebral palsy: The outcome of 177 patients, 74 totally untreated. *Pediatrics* **29**:605–616, 1962.
22. Nelson, K. B., and Ellenberg, J. H.: Children who "outgrew" cerebral palsy. *Pediatrics* **69**:529–536, 1982.
23. Crothers, B. S., and Paine, R. S.: *The Natural History of Cerebral Palsy.* Harvard University Press, Cambridge, Massachusetts, 1958.
24. Drillien, C. M.: Abnormal neurologic signs in the first year of life in low birthweight infants: Possible prognostic significance. *Dev. Med. Child Neurol.* **14**:575–584, 1972.
25. Capute, A. J., Shapiro, B. K., and Palmer, F. B.: Spectrum of developmental disabilities: Continuum of motor dysfunction. *Orthop. Clin. North A.* **12**:3–22, 1981.
26. Molnar, G.: Motor deficits of retarded infants and young children. *Arch. Phys. Med. Rehabil.* **55**:393–398, 1974.

27. Shapiro, B. K., Capute, A. J., and Accardo, P. J.: Factors affecting walking in a profoundly retarded population. *Dev. Med. Child Neurol.* **21:**369–373, 1979.
28. Hreidarsson, S. J., Shapiro, B. K., and Capute, A. J.: Age of walking in the cognitively impaired, *Clin. Pediatr.* **22:**248–250, 1983.
29. Capute, A. J., Shapiro, B. K., Palmer, F. B., *et al.:* Cognitive motor interactions: The relationship of infant gross motor attainment to IQ at three years. *Clin. Pediatr.* **24:**671–675, 1985.
30. Capute, A. J., and Shapiro, B. K.: The motor quotient: A method for the early detection of motor delay, *Am. J. Dis. Child.* **139:**940–942, 1985.
31. Capute, A. J., Palmer, F. B., Shapiro, B. K., *et al.:* Primitive reflex profile: A quantitation of primitive reflexes in infancy, *Develop. Med. Child Neurol.* **26:**375–383, 1984.
32. Capute, A. J., Shapiro, B. K., Accardo, P. J., et al.: Motor functions: Associated primitive reflexes profiles. *Dev. Med. Child. Neurol.* **24:**662–669, 1982.
33. Paine, R. S., Brazelton, T. B., Donovan, D. E., et al.: Evolution of postural reflexes in normal infants and in the presence of chronic brain syndromes. *Neurology (N.Y.)* **14:**1036–1048, 1964.
34. Capute, A. J.: Identifying cerebral palsy in infancy through study of primitive-reflex profiles. *Pediatr. Ann.* **8:**10–15, 1979.
35. Palmer, F. B., Shapiro, B. K., Wachter, R. C., *et al.:* Primitive reflex profile: Clinical applications in: Thompson, G., Rubin, I. L., Bilenker, R. M. (eds.), *Comprehensive Management of Cerebral Palsy.* Grune & Stratton, New York, 1982.
36. Kiely, J. L., Paneth, N., Stein, Z., and Susser, M.: Cerebral palsy and newborn care: III. Estimated prevalence rules of cerebral palsy under differing rates of mortality and impairment of low birthweight infants. *Dev. Med. Child Neurol.* **23:**801–806, 1981.
37. Capute, A. J., Palmer, F. B., Shapiro, B. K., *et al.:* Motor effects of physical therapy (PT) in infants with spastic diplegia (abs.), *Pediatr. Res.* **20:**460A, 1986.
38. Goldkamp, O.: Treatment effectiveness in cerebral palsy, *Arch. Phys. Med. Rehabil.* **65:**232–234, 1984.
39. Scherzer, A. L., Mike, V., and Ilson, J.: Physical therapy as a determinant of change in the cerebral palsied infant, *Pediatrics* **58:**47–51, 1976.
40. Vanderheiden, G. C.: Augmentative modes of communication for the severely speech- and motor-impaired. *Clin. Orthop. and Rel. Res.* **148:**70–86, 1980.
41. Desch, L. W.: High technology for handicapped children, *Pediatrics* **77:**71–87, 1986.
42. Finnie, N. R.: *Handling the Young Cerebral Palsied Child at Home,* 2nd ed. Dutton, New York, 1975.
43. Pollock, G. A., and Stark, G.: Long term results in the management of 67 children with cerebral palsy. *Dev. Med. Child Neurol.* **11:**17–34, 1969.
44. O'Grady, R. S., Nishimura, D. M., Kohn, J. G., *et al.:* Vocational predictions compared with present vocational status of 60 young adults with cerebral palsy, *Develop. Med. Child Neurol.* **27:**775–784, 1985.
45. Jones, M. H.: Differential diagnosis and natural history of the cerebral palsied child, in: Samilson, R. L. (ed.): *Orthopedic Aspects of Cerebral Palsy. Clinics in Developmental Medicine,* Vols. 52/53. Lippincott, Philadelphia, 1975.

Common Neuromotor Disorders

Gerald S. Golden

COMMON NEUROMOTOR DISORDERS

Parents generally lack detailed knowledge of adaptive, linguistic, and cognitive development. Motor milestones are more widely appreciated, however, and parents often recognize when their child appears to have delays. It is therefore not uncommon for motor delays to be recognized relatively early and for delays in other areas to be overlooked for some time. A baby who appears weak and "floppy" or who is not sitting and pulling to stand within the first year of life is readily identified by parents and professionals as abnormal. These abnormalities are categorized as neuromotor disorders.

    The neuromotor disorders are generally divided into two major categories: (1) pri-

Gerald S. Golden • Departments of Pediatrics and Neurology, University of Tennessee Center for the Health Sciences, Memphis, Tennessee 38105.

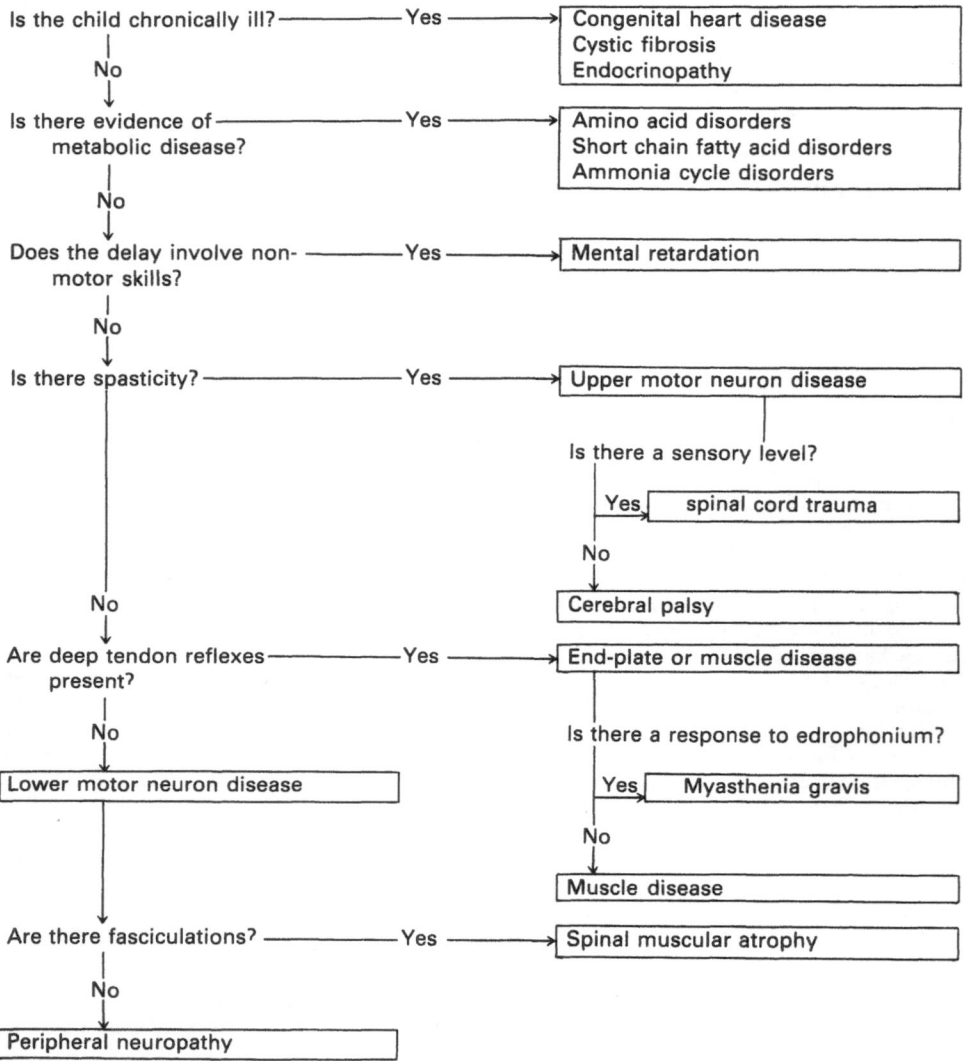

Figure 1 Initial diagnostic approach to neuromotor disorders

mary, due to pathological anatomical, biochemical or physiological processes involving the central or peripheral nervous systems or the muscles and (2) secondary, a manifestation of chronic illness or generalized metabolic disease. A diagnostic schema of the major processes to be considered when a child manifests a neuromotor delay is outlined in Figure 1. A child may fit into more than one of the diagnostic categories outlined. The questions and examination results schematized in Figure 1 serve as general guidelines. They are not intended to be used as absolute diagnostic criteria. This chapter focuses on a brief review

Table I. Muscle Diseases

Muscular dystrophy
  Progressive (Duchenne) muscular dystrophy
  Late onset (Becker) X-linked dystrophy
  Fascioscapulohumeral dystrophy
  Limb-girdle dystrophy
  Myotonic dystrophy
Inflammatory myopathies
  Polymyositis
  Dermatomyositis
  Trichinosis
  Infections
Congenital myopathies
  Central core disease
  Myotubular myopathy
  Mitochondrial myopathies
  Nemaline myopathy
  Lipid myopathies
  Congenital fiber-type disproportion

---

of several of the common neuromotor disorders and their developmental–behavioral implications,

MUSCULAR DYSTROPHY

Muscular dystrophy refers to a group of disorders that share several common features: (1) primarily involving muscle, (2) progressive disability, and (3) hereditary pattern. Although progressive (Duchenne) and myotonic muscular dystrophies have been well known for more than a century, specialized histological techniques have defined a number of conditions referred to as the congenital myopathies. The congenital myopathies are also primary hereditary disorders of muscle. Some are progressive, others are not. Table I outlines the major muscle diseases affecting children.

Progressive Muscular Dystrophy: Duchenne

Progressive muscular dystrophy (PMD) is the prototype of a clearly hereditary, obviously progressive, disease of muscle. The incidence is approximately 30 in 100,000 male births. The disorder is transmitted in an X-linked recessive pattern (virtually restricted to males). Girls are rarely affected clinically. The few documented female cases have been associated with Turner's syndrome or with cases that raise complex discussions concerning the biology of the X chromosome.

The clinical manifestations of PMD are uniquely uniform, and the course of the illness is highly stereotyped. The constancy of rate and pattern of progression of the disorder allow for assignment into clinical stages[1] (Table II). The child generally appears normal during the first year of life, although there may be slight delays in independent walking. Between 18 and 24 months of age, it becomes evident that the child stumbles

Table II. Functional Classification of Muscular Dystrophy[a]

Class	Ambulation	Rising from chair	Stair climbing
1	Independent	Yes	Yes
2	Independent	Yes	With railing
3	Independent	Yes	Slowly, with railing
4	Independent	Yes	No
5	Independent	No	No
6	Independent with braces	No	No
7	Assistance of one person; braces	No	No
8	Stands in braces; cannot walk, even with assistance	No	No
9	Wheelchair bound	No	No

[a]From Harris and Cherry.[1]

and falls more frequently than do other children of the same age. Weakness in the legs becomes obvious between 2 and 4 years of age. This weakness is particularly striking in tasks requiring the use of hip girdle muscles, such as climbing stairs. Toe walking is a common feature of the disorder and is frequently the presenting complaint. Involvement of the shoulder girdle muscles is less apparent, but the patient may be unable to keep his hands held over his head or hang from a jungle gym. Examination at this stage of the disorder does not demonstrate prominent muscle atrophy. Some muscles, especially the gastrocnemius and deltoids, may appear enlarged (pseudohypertrophy). However, on palpation of the affected muscles, an abnormal firm woody consistency is noted. Weakness is most pronounced at the hips.[2] The gait is characterized by a gluteal lurch, in which the hip drops on the side on which the leg is lifted to step forward. The weakness is demonstrated as the Trendelenburg sign: with the child standing on one foot, the hip on that side drops. Gower's sign is also noted with PMD: when rising from a supine position, the child rolls to the prone position, gets onto hands and knees, and then places his hands on his thighs, pushing the trunk upright with the arms. Shoulder weakness can be demonstrated by having the child attempt to support his weight on his hands while the examiner holds the legs. A normal child can execute this maneuver quite well. Lumbar lordosis is a prominent sign. Deep tendon reflexes are maintained in this stage of the disorder.

Weakness is inexorably progressive, and most affected children are confined to a wheelchair by the age of 12 years. The shoulder and arm weakness becomes progressively severe. The patient has difficulty with combing hair, brushing teeth, and self-feeding. However, movements of the hands and fingers are not impaired.

In most cases the child is virtually helpless by the age of 15 years. Muscle atrophy is marked, and voluntary motion is severely limited; sitting is no longer possible, and progressive scoliosis impairs respiratory function. Death due to pulmonary compromise, infection, and cardiomyopathy occurs between 15 and 30 years of age.[3] Cardiomyopathy is clinically significant in approximately 50% of patients. Sepsis from infected decubitus ulcers also contributes significantly to mortality. Progressive impairment of cognitive function does not occur, even during the terminal stages of the disorder.

During the later stages of the disease, examination demonstrates progressive muscle atrophy, although the appearance of pseudohypertrophy may persist, especially in the

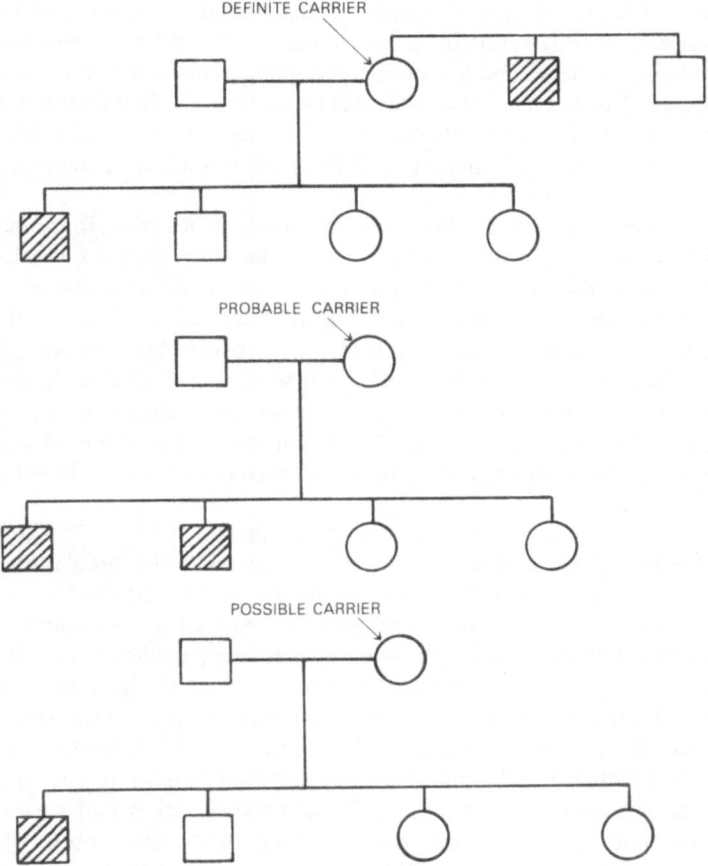

Figure 2. Carrier status in progressive muscular dystrophy. Definite carrier: The patient's mother who has an affected brother (or sister has an affected son). Probable carrier: The woman who has two affected sons. Possible carrier: The mother of any affected boy.

gastrocnemius. Joint contractures become increasingly prominent and are progressive. Deep tendon reflexes can be elicited, however, until the joints become fixed.

An association of PMD and mental retardation is present in some children.[4] The average intelligence quotient (IQ) of patients is slightly less than that of affected siblings. Some patients are obviously retarded; this appears to be specific to certain families. If the child with PMD is retarded, siblings who have PMD will also be retarded. The converse is true as well: if the affected individual has normal intelligence, siblings will be cognitively normal. It is not known whether this is due to a closely linked gene or to a different allele of the gene producing PMD.

The genetic pattern of inheritance is clearly that of an X-linked recessive trait. If the mother is a carrier, 50% of male children will be affected, and 50% of female children will be carriers. The rate of new mutations is fairly high, however, and discussion of genetic risk depends on differentiating a new mutation from the same condition transmitted from a maternal carrier.[5] The most important genetic tool is a detailed analysis of the patient's pedigree. Three levels of certainty can be set (Fig. 2). In the case of a possible or probable carrier, serum enzyme levels provide some diagnostic assistance. If the mother is a carrier, her creatinine phosphokinase (CPK) level will be elevated in approximately 80% of cases.

Although the clinical course is highly characteristic, other conditions must be considered at the time of initial presentation. Spinal muscular atrophies are typically associated with fasciculations of the tongue, early prominent muscle atrophy, and absent reflexes. Serum enzyme activity is generally normal. Electrodiagnostic studies reveal fibrillations and fasciculations. Inflammatory myopathies[6] (polymyositis, dermatomyositis) should be considered if skin rash, muscle pain, or muscle tenderness are present. In the absence of these findings, muscle biopsy is necessary to rule out an inflammatory myopathy. Congenital myopathies are not generally associated with marked elevation of serum enzyme levels. Diagnosis of the congenital myopathies ultimately depends on histological examination of the muscle.

Laboratory studies can virtually confirm the diagnosis of PMD. The abnormal muscle releases relatively large amounts of various enzymes into the circulation. CPK is the most commonly measured, and levels are 10–100 times normal. Most of the activity is due to the muscle isozyme.[7] Aldolase and serum glutamic-oxaloacetic transaminase (SGOT) are also markedly elevated and similarly provide confirmatory evidence. Levels are highest early in the disease process and are elevated before clinical signs and symptoms are present. A definitive diagnosis of PMD depends on muscle biopsy. The major histological features include destruction and fragmentation of muscle fibers, increase in connective tissue around and within muscle bundles, replacement of muscle by fat, and large basophilic fibers that represent attempts at muscle regeneration. Biopsy of severely involved muscles demonstrates mainly fibrous tissue and fat, with few muscle fibers and no evidence of attempted regeneration. CPK levels begin to fall in the later stages of the disease and actually may return to normal levels as the muscle mass decreases.

There is no specific treatment to alter the progression of the disease. Digitalis, anabolic steroids, glucocorticoids, and other pharmacological agents have been used but have never been proved efficacious in controlled studies. Several profound developmental–behavioral issues are associated with PMD. The disabling nature of the disorder often necessitates a multidisciplinary management approach. Physical therapy is an important therapeutic interaction in order to maintain general conditioning and to minimize joint contractures. Occupational therapy can assist in the design of adaptive devices, allowing the child to maintain independence in self-help skills and activities of daily living. Strict attention must be paid to skin care and to the use of padding and cushions to prevent the development of decubitus ulcers. A manually propelled wheelchair will become necessary and eventually must be replaced by a motorized wheelchair when weakness becomes profound. Hand and finger motion are maintained until very late in the course of PMD, permitting mobility for as long as the child can be maintained in a sitting position.

Respiratory therapy is essential, especially late in the course of the illness, as atelectasis and pneumonia are the major causes of death. The role of orthopedic surgery is limited, however, and surgery is reserved for those situations that will provide functional improvement or facilitation of nursing care. Early in the course of PMD, surgery is effective in lengthening the Achilles tendon to permit plantigrade gait. A procedure has been developed that minimizes the amount of postoperative time spent in bed. Children with PMD do very poorly with bed rest, rapidly losing muscle strength and the ability to walk. Ambulation is encouraged even during serious intercurrent illnesses. It is readily apparent that counseling of the child and family members (including genetic counseling) is a critical support service. Counseling is an essential adjunct in the management of these chronic handicapping disorders.

Treatment requirements are obviously very expensive. In most states children with neuromotor disorders are eligible for services through the Crippled Children's Program. In addition, the Muscular Dystrophy Association sponsors specialized care clinics that can provide some assistance in obtaining equipment such as wheelchairs and suction machines.

Myotonic Muscular Dystrophy

Myotonic muscular dystrophy, less common than PMD, has an incidence of 2.4–4.9 in 100,000 persons. Early diagnosis of this disorder is important for appropriate genetic counseling. Characteristically, myotonic dystrophy presents in early adulthood with progressive muscle weakness, myotonia, striking atrophy of the temporalis muscles ("hatchet face" appearance), frontal balding, endocrine dysfunctions (including gonadal atrophy), and behavioral and psychiatric problems. The diagnostic clinical feature is myotonia, manifested by an inability to rapidly relax muscles following a sustained voluntary contraction (e.g., closing the eyelids tightly or shaking hands). Similar findings can be elicited by direct percussion of the muscle, which produces a slow, sustained, involuntary contraction. Children are occasionally affected at birth, presenting as a hypotonic infant with little or no facial movement. This weakness causes major problems in sucking and swallowing.[8] Orthopedic deformities (e.g., clubfoot) are frequently associated with the disorder. The condition is transmitted as an autosomal dominant disorder with high penetrance.

Although myotonic muscular dystrophy is transmitted by a dominant gene, it only presents at birth if the affected parent is the mother.[9] There is currently no satisfactory explanation for this phenomenon. The child's mother must be examined carefully, as the condition is often difficult to diagnosis in its early stages and is not clinically obvious. Electromyography is a useful diagnostic tool, with characteristic findings of myotonia. CPK levels are moderately elevated in the mother. Muscle biopsy is diagnostic, demonstrating centrally placed nuclei in the muscle fibers, subsarcolemmal pads, and peculiar ring-shaped muscle fibers.

As is the case in the majority of the neuromotor disorders, no specific treatment is available. Weakness increases as the child becomes older. Atrophy of the muscles occurs particularly in the distal portions of the limbs and the temporalis muscles. Additional features of the condition, such as cataracts, baldness, and gonadal atrophy, may be delayed until the third decade of life. There is an increased incidence of mental retardation associated with childhood-onset myotonic dystrophy.[8]

Congenital Myopathies

The congenital myopathies constitute a heterogeneous group of disorders that vary in their course and associated clinical features.[10] All the congenital myopathies are hereditary primary diseases of muscle. Diagnosis can be suspected clinically but ultimately depends on muscle biopsy. Muscle biopsy should be restricted to diagnostic centers that can provide special techniques and expertise. The minimal criteria for an acceptable muscle biopsy include the following: (1) the muscle biopsied should be moderately involved, (2) an adequate specimen should be removed isometrically, (3) a frozen sample should be used for histochemical staining, and (4) a pathologist with special experience should examine the specimen. Electron microscopic evaluation may be required for the more difficult diagnostic problems.

SPINAL MUSCULAR ATROPHIES

The spinal muscular atrophies are a group of conditions that share the following features: (1) loss of anterior horn cells, (2) progressive course, and (3) hereditary pattern. The spinal muscular atrophies are genetically related conditions. The severe early-onset forms are transmitted in an autosomal recessive mode. Autosomal recessive, X-linked recessive, and autosomal dominant patterns have been reported for the form with later onset. The anterior horn cells, located in the ventral column of the spinal cord, provide the final common pathway for the neural control of muscle. Acute destruction of these cells, as in poliomyelitis, or the progressive loss associated with spinal muscular atrophies, is manifested clinically by reduction of muscle strength and eventual paralysis. This is accompanied by decreased muscle tone, muscle atrophy, and loss of deep tendon reflexes.

Progressive Infantile Spinal Muscular Atrophy: Werdnig-Hoffman Disease

The best known condition in this group is progressive infantile spinal muscular atrophy, or Werdnig-Hoffman disease. In the classic presentation, the mother may note decreased or weak fetal movements during the last trimester of pregnancy. At birth the infant experiences difficulty in initiating respirations, is hypotonic, and lies in a "pithed frog" position. Proximal limb movements are diminished or absent, but strength and movement in the fingers and toes are preserved. There is a poor or absent traction response and virtually no head control when the infant is pulled to a sitting position.

On examination, the tongue shows a shimmering surface caused by fasciculations of the underlying muscle bundles. Swallowing is impaired. Paradoxical respirations, collapse of the chest and expansion of the abdomen during inspiratory effort, are present due to weakness of intercostal muscles and diaphragmatic breathing. Deep tendon reflexes cannot be elicited. Eye movements are intact despite the severe neuromotor involvement. The child appears bright, alert, and fully aware of the environment. The course is relentless. Nasogastric feedings or a permanent gastrostomy become necessary. Death due to respiratory infections generally occurs during the first year of life.

Juvenile Spinal Muscular Atrophy: Kugelberg-Welander Disease

A juvenile form of spinal muscular atropy, Kugelberg-Welander disease, begins in late preschool or school-age children. Slowly progressive weakness of the limb girdles provides the rationale for the initial use of the term pseudodystrophy. Muscle tone is decreased, and deep tendon reflexes become difficult to elicit. Small-amplitude jerking movement of the fingers is observed when the hands are held outstretched (polyminimyo-clonus). The course is generally progressive, although there may be long periods of stability. Many patients survive well into the adult years, requiring many specialized services during childhood and adolescence.

Numerous cases of spinal muscular atrophy do not fit either of these classic pictures but are intermediate as to age of presentation, severity of symptoms, rapidity of progression, and duration of life.[11,12] A general rule is useful: the later the onset, the slower the course. The maximum level of gross motor performance attained (sitting, standing, walking, running) appears to correlate well with severity of the disability and the life-span. The concept of a continuum of severity is important for effective patient management and counseling.

The differential diagnosis is in part resolved by electrodiagnostic studies; electromyography reveals fasciculations and fibrillations in all muscle groups. Serum enzyme values are not significantly elevated. A definitive diagnosis requires a muscle biopsy, which characteristically shows group atrophy. As each anterior horn cell innervates a group of muscle fibers in close anatomical proximity, groups of small, atrophic, angulated fibers are interspersed with groups of normal muscle fibers. Signs of inflammation, fibrosis, or fatty infiltration are absent. Postmortem examination of the central nervous system (CNS) reveals changes limited to the large motor neurons in the ventral horns of the spinal cord and cranial nerve motor nuclei. Cellular loss is seen without necrosis, inflammation, or gliosis. The associated ventral roots and motor nerves are atrophic; myelin disappears.

As with the muscular dystrophies, specific therapy is not available; the limited goals of physical and occupational therapy and orthopedic surgery are the same. Involvement of the bulbar musculature necessitates tube or gastostomy feeding, generally earlier in the course than muscular dystrophy. Respiratory therapy and prompt treatment of pulmonary infections are the keys to survival.

JUVENILE MYASTHENIA GRAVIS

Myasthenia gravis is encountered less frequently than the disorders previously described. Myasthenia gravis is a debilitating disorder and may be fatal unless a diagnosis is made early in its course. Specific therapy is available for this disorder. Three variants of myasthenia gravis in childhood have been described.[13]

Juvenile myasthenia gravis does not differ from forms of the disorder occurring later in life.[14] The child, previously in good health, presents with weakness involving extraocular, bulbar, and peripheral musculature, in any combination of locations and with variations in severity. Symptoms are less marked at the beginning of the day, becoming increasingly apparent as the day progresses or following exercise. Muscle fatigue can be demonstrated during the neurological examination and is an important diagnostic clue. Repetitive exercise of any muscle leads to rapid weakening. Improvement of muscle strength following a test dose of edrophonium confirms the diagnosis. Electrodiagnostic studies reveal a decremental muscle response following rapid stimulation of a motor nerve. This response can also be reversed by edrophonium. Serum enzyme levels and routine muscle biopsy are nonrevealing. Management of juvenile myasthenia gravis presents a difficult problem. Administration of long-acting acetylcholine esterase (AChE) inhibitors is the basis for therapy. Inadequate drug levels provide insufficient recovery of strength, and excessive doses produce weakness due to cholinergic blockade. A dosage sufficient for one muscle group may provide inadequate treatment for a second group and may be excessive for a third. Drug dosages, therefore, must be titrated to determine the "compromise dosage," which provides the best functional outcome. Side effects of these drugs present additional problems: blurred vision, sialorrhea, bronchospasm, and abdominal cramps.

Patients refractory to standard therapy are treated with corticosteroids or immunosuppressive drugs. Experimental approaches such as plasmapheresis have been used to reduce the level of circulating antibodies. Controversy surrounds the role of thymectomy in management.[14] If a thymoma is present, this is clearly required, but other indications for surgery have not been well defined.

THE "FLOPPY" INFANT

The term "floppy infant" refers to infants who are hypotonic and who have a reduction in the amount and range of spontaneous movements, but who have no evidence of a definable neuromotor disorder. The diagnostic schema in Figure 1 outlines the major etiological possibilities for this disorder. Systemic disease, metabolic disorders, and CNS abnormalities must be considered in the differential diagnosis. If none of these is found, attention is then focused on the neuromotor system.

The evaluation, following physical and neurological examination, consists of serum enzyme levels, electrodiagnostic studies, and an edrophonium test. If the results of these studies are normal, a muscle biopsy should be considered. If deep tendon reflexes are absent, an early biopsy is indicated, since the genetic and prognostic implications of spinal muscular atrophy are crucial. The child should be carefully monitored and muscle biopsy postponed if reflexes are intact and gains in motor strength and motor performance can be documented. Biopsy is indicated when substantial gains cannot be documented by the age of 9–12 months.

BRACHIAL PLEXUS PALSY

The brachial plexus is susceptible to trauma during the process of birth. Traction on the arm or any maneuver that forcibly moves the shoulder and head in opposite directions can stretch the plexus or tear nerve roots where they emerge from the spinal cord.

Erb Palsy

Erb palsy predominantly involves the upper brachial plexus, supplied by nerve roots C4–C6. The affected arm is held abducted and internally rotated at the shoulder, extended and pronated at the elbow, and flexed at the wrist and fingers. The abnormal position of the arm can be accentuated, and the paralysis demonstrated, by attempts to elicit a Moro response. It is asymmetrical, with little movement of the affected arm. Involvement of C4 can cause paralysis of the hemidiaphragm on that side, although there is generally no significant respiratory embarrassment.

Klumpke Paralysis

Klumpke paralysis occurs following injury to the lower brachial plexus, with predominant involvement of the roots of C7–C8 and T1. Flexors and extensors of the fingers are involved, and the child has a flail hand. Disruption of innervation to the superior cervical ganglion can occur; if so, the child will have a Horner syndrome. The eye on the involved side manifests ptosis and a small pupil, and sweating on that side of the face may be decreased.

Recovery depends on whether the lesion was due to stretch, typical in Erb's palsy, or to avulsion of roots, more common in Klumpke's palsy. Stretch injuries generally make a full recovery over a period of weeks to months. On the other hand, if there is an avulsion, recovery is not possible. Therapy is directed toward preventing joint contractures and, with Erb palsy, preventing dislocation of the shoulder. There is no evidence that either physical therapy or electrical stimulation of nerve or muscle hastens, recovers, or improves the final outcome. In later childhood, various types of joint fusions may improve function when incomplete recovery occurs. In rare instances, the entire plexus is damaged and the arm and hand are flail and anesthetic. The paralyzed limb can become an impediment to the extent that amputation must be considered.

MOVEMENT DISORDERS

A group of disorders whose major manifestations are involuntary movements result from pathological or functional abnormalities of the basal ganglia. Some of these conditions are restricted to the motor system (e.g., tic disorders), while others are associated with more global brain dysfunction (e.g., Wilson disease, Huntington chorea). Tic disorders are the only common movement disorders occurring in childhood.[15]

Tic Disorders

Tics are rapid, irregular, repetitive, involuntary, highly stereotyped movements. Simple tics are common, involving as many as 15–30% of all children at some time. They are manifested most frequently as eye blinking, facial grimacing, head turning, or shoulder shrugging. Only a single tic is present during any time period, and most resolve within 3 months. Although traditional teaching is that this symptom is a response to psychological tension, that is not easily proved. There is no evidence that the rate of resolution or final outcome is changed by psychotherapy.

Complex tic disorder encompasses a broad group of conditions ranging from chronic motor tic disorder (the presence of one or more tics persisting for longer than one year) to Tourette syndrome.

The basic defining criteria of Tourette syndrome are the presence of multiple motor and vocal tics that become apparent during childhood, a changing repertory, waxing and waning severity, and persistence for longer than 1 year. The individual motor tics are indistinguishable from transient simple tics. The most frequent vocalizations are coughing, sniffing, and throat clearing. Some patients progress to producing loud inarticulate noises, and in 25–30% of children echolalia or coprolalia will develop. Coprolalia, the involuntary utterance of obscenities, is a dramatic symptom but is not required for diagnosis. In many affected individuals bizarre stereotyped mannerisms develop, such as jumping, compulsive touching, and smelling objects. Early diagnosis is difficult because of the unimpressive nature of the initial symptoms. It is the development and progression of the disorder that raises the possibility of Tourette syndrome.

Neurochemical investigations point toward hypersensitivity of dopamine receptors as the major pathogenetic factor. This hypothesis is supported by the therapeutic response to haloperidol, a potent postsynaptic dopamine antagonist. The drug provides good control of symptoms in 80–85% of patients but is associated with side effects, such as sedation and cognitive blunting, in 50% of patients. The central role of dopamine is also supported by the adverse effects of psychostimulants (methylphenidate, dextroamphetamine, pemoline) on 50% of the patients who take them. These drugs can produce dramatic exaggeration of the symptoms; discontinuing the medication reverses this effect. A number of cases of Tourette syndrome appear to have been precipitated by these drugs, suggesting that children for whom psychostimulants are prescribed must be carefully monitored during treatment. If tics occur, the drug should be discontinued.

The relationship between chronic motor tic disorder and Tourette syndrome is supported by the occurrence of both syndromes in the same families. The response to medication is also identical in both groups. Whether transient simple tics are part of the same spectrum is a matter of speculation. It is interesting to note, however, that the frequency of various individual tics, age of onset, male preponderance, and response to haloperidol are the same for transient simple tics, chronic motor tic disorder, and Tourette syndrome.

Sydenham Chorea

Chorea is manifested by rapid, random, irregular involuntary movements. They are most prominent in the distal portion of the extremities, and the face is often involved. The decline in incidence of acute rheumatic fever has brought with it a parallel decrease in the occurrence of Sydenham chorea. This condition, characterized by the subacute onset of chorea, is often associated with emotional lability. The child tries to mask the dyskinesia by converting the movements into what appear to be voluntary actions. In severe cases, however, the movements are constant and uncontrollable and can make walking and activities of daily living impossible. Full recovery usually takes many months, and some children continue to have behavioral problems or difficulties with fine motor coordination..

The sudden onset of chorea in adolescents can be precipitated by the use of oral contraceptives. Some of these girls have a past history of Sydenham chorea. Symptoms resolve when the medication is discontinued.

Tremor

Tremor refers to rhythmical, regular, rapid oscillating movements at a joint. Essential tremor can begin at any age. It is most obvious when the hand is held extended against gravity and a superimposed element of intention tremor is noted. A family history, suggesting autosomal dominant inheritance, is often found. If the symptoms are severe, they can often be controlled by the administration of propranalol.

Spasmus nutans presents in early childhood with a head-nodding tremor, head tilt, and nystagmus. Any combination of these findings may be seen; the nystagmus is often monocular. The condition is self-limited and is rarely associated with other neurological disorders. There have been occasional reports of spasmus nutans in children with brain tumors, however.

Wilson disease is rare, but is important, as early diagnosis and treatment can prevent serious progressive neurological disease. Fifty percent of cases present with neurological signs and symptoms, 50% with hepatic disease. The most typical presentation is with acute pseudobulbar signs and rigidity. Cirrhosis and portal hypertension produce hepatic dysfunction.

Diagnosis depends on the demonstration of low serum ceruloplasmin and copper levels, increased urinary copper excretion, and increased tissue copper. Mobilization and excretion of copper occur with the administration of penicillamine. Despite many problems with the use of this drug, treatment can reverse pre-existing neurological deficits and the long-term prognosis is good.

SUMMARY

Neuromotor disorders and movement disorders can have profound effects on a child's development and behavior. The age of onset, severity, and rate of progression will variably influence motor, language, cognitive, and personal-social skills. The child and family will require multidisciplinary support services to meet the immediate and long-range needs produced by the disorder. A neuromotor disorder is a catastrophic illness and will have a significant impact on the child, the family, the educational system, and the community.

As a group, the neuromotor disorders necessitate interdisciplinary services for child and family. In most cases a physician will be required to coordinate these services in order to recommend changes based on the clinical course of the disorder. Support systems must include resources in medical, educational, and social areas. The chronic nature of the neuromotor disorders demands strong family supports, including consideration of the devastating financial implications. Perhaps no other group of disorders has so great a need for coordinated comprehensive services involving multiple professional disciplines. The nonfatal neuromotor disorders (e.g., Erb palsy, Klumpke paralysis) and movement disorders cannot be managed with lesser concerns. These disorders may necessitate additional interventions in vocational guidance and possible counseling for the parents and the patient (when indicated) to aid in emotional adjustment to their chronic disabilities.

REFERENCES

1. Harris, S. E., and Cherry, D. B.: Childhood progressive muscular dystrophy and the role of physical therapy. *Phys. Ther.* **54**:4–12, 1974.
2. Ziter, F. A., Allsop, K. G., and Tyler, F. H.: Assessment of muscular dystrophy. *Neurology (N.Y.)* **27**:981–984, 1977.
3. Burke, S. S., Grove, N. M., Houser, C. R., *et al.:* Respiratory aspects of pseudohypertrophic muscular dystrophy. *Am. J. Dis. Child.* **121**:230–234, 1974.
4. Karagan, N. J.: Intellectual functioning in Duchenne muscular dystrophy: A review. *Psychol. Bull.* **86**:250–259, 1979.
5. Roses, A. D., Roses, M. J., Metcalf, B. S., *et al.:* Pedigree testing in Duchenne muscular dystrophy. *Ann. Neurol.* **2**:271–278, 1977.
6. Carpenter, S., Karpati, G., Rothman, S., *et al.:* The childhood type of dermatomyositis. *Neurology (N.Y.)* **26**:952–962, 1976.
7. Silverman, L. M., Mendell, J. R., Sahenk, Z., *et al.:* Significance of creatine phosphokinase isoenzymes in Duchenne dystrophy. *Neurology (N.Y.)* **26**:561–564, 1976.
8. Harper, P. S.: Congenital myotonic dystrophy in Britain. I. Clinical aspects. *Arch. Dis. Child.* **50**:505–513, 1975.
9. Harper, P. S.: Congenital myotonic dystrophy in Britain. II. Genetic basis. *Arch. Dis. Child.* **50**:514–521, 1975.
10. Gardner-Medwin, D., and Tizard, J. P. M.: Neuromuscular disorders in infancy and early childhood, in Walton, J. (ed.): *Disorders of Voluntary Muscle,* 4th ed. Churchill Livingstone, New York, 1981, pp. 625–663.
11. Benady, S. G.: Spinal muscular atrophy in childhood: Review of 50 cases. *Dev. Med. Child. Neurol.* **20**:746–757, 1978.
12. Pearn, J.: Classification of spinal muscular atrophies. *Lancet* **1**:919–922, 1980.
13. Fenichel, G. M.: Clinical syndromes of myasthenia in infancy and childhood. *Arch. Neurol.* **35**:97–103, 1978.
14. Snead, O. C., Benton, J. W., Dwyer, D., *et al.:* Juvenile myasthenia gravis. *Neurology (N.Y.)* **30**:732–739, 1980.
15. Golden, G. S.: Movement disorders in children: Tourette syndrome. *Dev. Behav. Pediatr.* **3**:209–216, 1982.

4

Common Seizure Disorders

Gerald S. Golden

The International Classification of the Epilepsies, revised in 1981, has been successful in replacing the numerous terms commonly utilized in clinical practice.[1] An advantage of this classification is that it provides a synthesis of the electrophysiological and clinical aspects of seizures. This is an extremely important feature, inasmuch as various types of seizures may appear clinically identical. However, there are wide variations in underlying pathology and choice of drugs for treatment. Table I provides an outline of the major types of seizures, and a compendium of some of the older clinical terms. Table II outlines the important associated features.

GENERALIZED CONVULSIONS: GRAND MAL SEIZURES

A generalized convulsion begins without an obvious aura. Some patients, however, may experience a vague and peculiar "rising" feeling in the abdomen or chest. The onset of seizure activity is bilateral; therefore, loss of consciousness is the first clinical mani-

Gerald S. Golden • Departments of Pediatrics and Neurology, University of Tennessee Center for the Health Sciences, Memphis, Tennessee 38105.

Table I. Classification of Seizure Disorders

International League against Epilepsy[a]	Traditional clinical classification
Partial seizures (initially focal EEG discharge)	Focal cortical seizures
Simple partial seizures (consciousness not impaired)	
With motor signs	Focal motor seizures
With sensory signs	Sensory seizures
With autonomic signs	Autonomic seizures
Complex partial seizures (consciousness impaired)	Psychomotor seizures
Partial seizures with secondary generalization	
Generalized seizures (initially bilateral EEG discharges; consciousness generally impaired)	Centrencephalic seizures
Absence seizures	
Typical	Petit mal
Atypical	Atypical petit mal
Myoclonic seizures	Myoclonic seizures
Clonic seizures	Grand mal seizures
Tonic seizures	Grand mal seizures
Tonic–clonic seizures	Grand mal seizures
Atonic seizures	Akinetic seizures

[a]From the Commission on Classification and Terminology of the International League Against Epilepsy.[1]

festation. Characteristically, the patient will cry out, stiffen, and fall to the floor. The rigid *tonic phase* is replaced by rhythmical contractions of the extremities, the *clonic phase,* which become progressively slower and then cease. Respirations may be briefly impaired and there is associated perioral cyanosis, stertorous breathing, and frothing at the mouth. Occasionally, the tongue is bitten. Bladder, or less frequently bowel, incontinence may occur. When the seizure stops the individual is generally somnolent and confused and if undisturbed will sleep for a short period of time. Common postictal complaints include backache, muscle soreness, and headache. The patient has amnesia for the event.

    Specific precipitating factors are rarely found, although psychological stress or sleep deprivation appears to lower the seizure threshold in some patients. Some children are most susceptible to seizures either after awakening in the morning or when they are drowsy. Alcoholic beverages, antihistamines, and tranquilizers also appear to lower the seizure threshold. Seizures that occur during sleep present a diagnostic problem because they may escape observation.

    Primary generalized seizures rarely have a definable cause, in contrast to seizures

Table II. Features Associated with Seizure Disorders

Type of seizure	Familial occurrence	Associated disabilities	Relapse rate (%)
Tonic–clonic	Approximately 3% risk in first-degree relatives	Uncommon	14
Absence	12% risk	Rare	>10
Partial complex	Slight increase	Behavioral disorders	31
Infantile spasms	Depends on underlying etiology	Mental retardation, 80–85%	High
Febrile seizures	7.3% in first-degree relatives	Rare	1.1

Table III. Anticonvulsant Drugs.

Drug	Daily dosage (mg/kg per day)	Therapeutic blood concn. (μg/ml)	Seizure types (primary indication)	Toxicity
ACTH	40u (IM) (Total dose)	—	Myoclonic in infancy	Weight gain, peptic ulcer, adrenal suppression
Carbamazepine	8–30	5–12	Complex partial	Lethargy, ataxia, rash leukopenia
Clonazepam	0.03–0.1	—	Myoclonic, atonic, absence	Lethargy, ataxia, hyper-salivation
Clorazepate	0.3–1.0	—	Complex partial	Lethargy
Diazepam	0.3 (IV)	—	Status epilepticus	Lethargy, respiratory arrest
Ethosuximide	20–40	50–100	Absence	Leukopenia
Phenobarbital	3–10	15–40	Partial, tonic, clonic, tonic–clonic, febrile	Lethargy, ataxia, personality change
Phenytoin	3–8	10–20	Partial, tonic, clonic tonic–clonic	Ataxia, hypersensitivity, gum hypertrophy, rickets, macroytic anemia, nystagmus
Primidone	12–20	8–15	Complex partial, tonic, clonic, tonic–clonic	Lethargy, ataxia personality change
Trimethadione	20–40	500–1200	Absence	Rash, agranulocytosis, nephrosis
Valproic acid	15–60	50–100	Generalized, especially absence	Gastrointestinal distress, hepatic·damage, thrombocytopenia, tremor, weight gain

with a focal onset and secondary generalization. There is an increased incidence of seizure disorders in families, suggesting a genetic basis for a lowered seizure threshold.[2] Generalized seizures may result from a variety of metabolic disorders and often cease when homeostasis is restored.

Few studies are required to establish the diagnosis of generalized seizures. The electroencephalogram (EEG) documents that the seizure has a generalized, rather than a focal, onset.[3] Metabolic studies are required only if there are clinical reasons to suspect the presence of these specific disorders. There is little or no rationale for obtaining skull radiographs, brain scans, or a computed tomography (CT) scan in most cases. Additional studies are indicated when there is a change in the seizure pattern, abnormal signs on neurological examination, or inability to obtain control with the usual drugs.

The medications used to treat major types of seizures are outlined in Table III. The general principles for drug use are basically the same, regardless of the specific agent selected: (1) use only one drug if possible; (2) use this drug at the lowest dose that is effective; (3) use the drug at its maximum dose, as documented by blood levels, before discontinuing it if it is not effective; and (4) carefully assess the child for subtle behavioral changes as well as more obvious side effects. A more rational basis for the treatment of seizures has been formulated with the development of accurate and easily available blood anticonvulsant level determinations. Blood levels are not obtained "routinely" but are indicated in certain circumstances: (1) 2–3 weeks after starting a drug, to document the blood level; (2) after a second drug is added, to evaluate drug interaction; (3) if seizure control is inadequate; (4) if any side effects are suspected, and (5) if there is concern about compliance.

Thurston et al.[4] documented the prognosis for the major types of seizure disorders. These investigators found certain factors to correlate with a good prognosis. Others predicted a return of seizures when medication was discontinued after 4 years of treatment with no seizures. A good prognosis was associated with a short duration of seizures before control was obtained and a normal neurological status. A high risk of recurrence was associated with Jacksonian or mixed seizures. The relapse rate for generalized seizures was 14%.[4]

PARTIAL COMPLEX SEIZURES: PSYCHOMOTOR

This category includes seizures that present with a variety of clinical manifestations. Common features include a decreased level of alertness, changed interaction with the environment, motor manifestations, and behavioral phenomena. Behavioral phenomena may either be internal experiences (e.g., visual or auditory sensations, unusual thoughts) subsequently reported by the patient or observable inappropriate behaviors. The range of behaviors can vary and include motor actions such as rising out of a chair and running.

There is a controversy regarding whether planned, directed, aggressive behavior can occur as part of a partial complex seizure.[5] At this time the evidence suggests that this happens extremely rarely, if at all. Attempts to restrain a confused patient during a seizure could provoke nonspecific lashing out, but this is a different situation.

A much more complex problem is the extent to which behavioral and psychiatric abnormalities are found in patients who have partial complex seizures. This specifically refers to problems in the interictal state and is discussed under Seizures and Development—Interictal EEG abnormalities.

Partial complex seizures, by definition, are associated with a focal electrophysiological abnormality. The functional abnormality implies that there may be an underlying structural lesion. Examination of temporal lobe tissue, removed from patients for the surgical treatment of drug-resistant intractable seizures, frequently reveals definable pathological abnormalities. Small vascular malformations, benign tumors, and a form of scarring known as incisural sclerosis are the most common findings. The origin of incisural sclerosis is controversial: some believe it is due to birth trauma or perinatal asphyxia; others postulate that it is a sequela of febrile seizures.

Although the chance of finding a lesion that is progressive or amenable to direct surgical treatment is small, computed tomography (CT) is frequently performed because of the focal nature of the underlying pathology.[6] Additional indications for CT include seizures of recent onset, changes in the seizure pattern, abnormalities detected on neurological examination, and progressive behavioral changes. More invasive studies are rarely indicated, although angiography is necessary to define the vascular anatomy of arteriovenous malformations.

Electroencephalography confirms the focal nature of the seizure discharge. A normal EEG during the interictal period does not rule out the diagnosis of a seizure disorder. The focus, in some patients with partial complex seizures, may be in deep areas of the brain that are not well represented on the clinical EEG. Repeated recordings, both asleep and awake, special provocative techniques, or long duration monitoring to record a seizure are required if the diagnosis is not clinically clear.

Treatment, as with all seizure disorders, is primarily pharmacological. The prognosis for complete remission after discontinuing medication is 69%.[4]

INFANTILE SPASMS (MYOCLONIC SEIZURES)

This seizure type almost always has its onset during the first year of life. The child presents with seizures consisting of sudden rapid movements, which can be any combination of flexion or extension of the head, trunk, arms, and legs. The most common pattern is flexion in all areas, often accompanied by an expiratory grunt. The seizures occur singly or in flurries of several spasms over a period of a few minutes. There is greater susceptibility soon after the child has awakened from sleep or when he is drowsy. After the seizure, the patient is often irritable and lethargic. Studies using combined EEG and videotape monitoring have clearly demonstrated that these children often have hundreds of seizures each day, well beyond the estimates of most observers.

A large number of structural and metabolic conditions have been associated with infantile spasms.[7] The most frequent are perinatal trauma and asphyxia, tuberous sclerosis, and phenylketonuria (PKU). Despite the multiplicity of etiological factors, the outcome is generally quite uniform. Approximately 80–85% of these children are mentally retarded on long-term follow-up, and in many cases other types of seizure disorders develop.[8]

The restricted age of onset, varied etiological factors, and predictable prognosis suggest that infantile spasms result from a severe insult to an immature brain. Diagnostic studies are targeted toward defining a structural defect or metabolic problem. This is of major importance, as many of the underlying conditions have a genetic basis, and appropriate counseling must be offered to the family. The basic evaluation includes EEG, CT scan, metabolic screening studies, and amino acid chromatography. In approximately 85% of cases, the EEG shows a characteristic pattern referred to as hypsarrhythmia. The electrical activity is severely disorganized, with a changing pattern of high-voltage spikes and slow waves.

The initial treatment of infantile spasms is parenteral administration of adrenocorticotropic hormone (ACTH). This approach was developed empirically, without a sound theoretical base. Recent work suggests that ACTH acts directly on the brain, and not only by stimulating adrenal secretion of corticosteroids. Studies suggest that ACTH is more effective than the administration of steroid compounds. The seizures usually respond well and the EEG may normalize, but in most cases the prognosis for intellectual outcome remains poor.

Other seizure disorders often develop as the child grows older, a common one being the Lennox–Gastaut syndrome. This is the combination of mental retardation, an EEG that shows 2–2.5-Hz spike and wave, and a mixed pattern of seizures (akinetic, myoclonic, partial complex, generalized). These children rarely respond adequately to anticonvulsants.

FEBRILE SEIZURES

Seizures in young children during the course of a febrile illness are a common occurrence in pediatric practice. The child is well except for a minor illness with fever. The sudden appearance of a generalized convulsion is dramatic and frightening.

Typically, the child with a febrile seizure is between 1 and 5 years of age. There is usually a respiratory infection early in the illness, associated with a sharp rise in body temperature to 102°F or higher; a generalized convulsion then occurs. The seizure typically lasts less than 5 min. After a period of postictal somnolence, the child appears well. There are no neurological abnormalities either before or after the episode. The convulsion has no focal features, and focal signs cannot be identified on the neurological examination performed after the seizure. The child's recovery is rapid and complete.

The underlying pathophysiology of febrile seizures is not clear, but there does appear to be a genetic component producing a lowered seizure threshold with the stress of fever. A family history of other children or a parent with febrile seizures is found in approximately 7.3% of cases. There is an age-related factor, as febrile seizures are rare before 1 year of age and after age 5 years.

An EEG is generally obtained, which is expected to be normal during the interictal period. In the face of a seizure with fever and no atypical features, there is a question of the necessity for obtaining an EEG. Additional diagnostic procedures are not indicated if the neurological examination is normal.

There is also controversy concerning the need for a lumbar puncture at the time of the first febrile seizure. If the child is seen some time after the seizure, is awake and alert, and manifests no signs of meningeal irritation, lumbar puncture would not appear necessary. Clinical judgment should prevail.

Treatment and prognosis are intricately interwoven issues. A review of available data, including long-term follow-up studies from the Collaborative Study for Cerebral Palsy, was carried out at a National Institutes of Health (NIH) Consensus Development Conference.[9] The general consensus at this time may be summarized as follows:

1. Febrile seizures, strictly defined, have a high recurrence rate but are not associated with any detectable residua.
2. The recurrence risk can be decreased with continuous anticonvulsant prophylaxis. The most effective drug is phenobarbital, given in sufficient doses to ensure a therapeutic blood level of at least 15 μg/ml.
3. Phenobarbital is associated with adverse behavioral effects (hyperactivity, irritability, sleep disturbance) in 40% of cases.
4. Under most circumstances, anticonvulsant prophylaxis is not required. During illness, attention should be paid to control of body temperature.
5. Anticonvulsant prophylaxis is recommended when the following clinical features are present:
   a. Abnormal neurological development
   b. Seizure longer than 15 min in duration, focal, or followed by a transient or persistent neurological abnormality
   c. History of a nonfebrile seizure
   d. Seizures of genetic origin in a parent or sibling

Using these guidelines, children manifesting none of these factors have a risk of 1.1% for developing subsequent nonfebrile seizures. In the presence of any of these factors, the risk is 9.2%. This compares with a risk of 0.5% for a child who has never had a febrile seizure.[10]

SEIZURES AND DEVELOPMENT

The relationship of seizure disorders to developmental problems is exceedingly complex. The major factors to be considered in the analysis include the following effects:

Seizures

The effect of the seizures per se, independent of the underlying brain pathology, is difficult to define. At one extreme, seizures can be repeated so frequently that the child spends a large portion of the day somnolent or in a state of postictal confusion. Seizures that are poorly controlled can cause repeated episodes of anoxia and minor head injuries, as well as excessive school absence and the necessity for additional anticonvulsant medications in higher doses. A study of identical twins with different seizure frequencies revealed greater disability in intelligence, academic achievement, neuropsychological function, and emotional and social adjustment in the more severely involved of the pair.[11]

Underlying Neurological Abnormality

If a neurological abnormality is apparent, such as mental retardation or cerebral palsy, the behavioral aspects can probably be attributed to the organic component. It is now recognized that there is an increased incidence in *all* types of behavioral and psychological problems in children with any type of neurological abnormality involving the brain.[12] The psychological/behavioral difficulties appear to be independent of the degree of functional disability and seem to relate most closely to the severity of brain damage. It is assumed that an abnormal brain would have difficulty processing and responding appropriately to social and interpersonal stimuli, as it would to cognitive and sensory stimuli.

Interictal EEG Abnormalities

Most studies have focused on the interictal behavioral problems in patients with partial complex (psychomotor) seizures. Catastrophic rages and attention deficit are the most common associated problems of partial complex seizures in children. Adult patients with this disorder exhibit rage attacks and have a higher incidence of psychoses, including schizophrenia. It is important to note, however, that these patients make up only a relatively small percentage of individuals with major psychiatric disorders. A long-term follow-up study of children with partial complex seizures demonstrated that although 85% had psychiatric problems during childhood, only 20% of the group (who were not severely retarded) continued to have these problems as adults.[13] The most serious outcome was the development of schizophrenia in 10% of the children. Males with continuing seizures and an epileptic focus in the left temporal lobe were at highest risk. Of the total group of children with partial complex seizures, 14% had problems with antisocial behavior.

Learning disabilities associated with seizures have been documented and described. Neuropsychological studies are currently being used to investigate the more subtle degrees of impairment. Partial complex seizures, especially when associated with a left temporal EEG focus, appear to be associated with deficits in verbal learning and memory.

Anticonvulsant Medication

Clinically evident sedation will obviously produce behavioral and cognitive problems and should be avoided if at all possible. A behavioral counterpart to sedation can occur in response to barbiturate therapy, especially in young children. Manifestations include attention deficit disorder with hyperactivity, aggressiveness, irritability, and sleep disturbances. These problems have been estimated to occur in 40% of preschool children. Drugs such as phenytoin, which are not usually associated with clinically evident changes in most children, can produce subtle cognitive deficits.

Family and Social Responses

In addition to the psychosocial, educational, and financial problems associated with chronic illness, the families of children with seizure disorders face two additional problems. The first is the unpredictable and dramatic nature of the seizures per se. There is constant apprehension and anxiety concerning their occurrence during sleep, in the bathtub, while crossing streets, and in any situation in which the child's safety might be compromised. The parents are concerned about the child having a seizure in a public place and the reaction of passers-by and their ability to provide proper emergency management. The social embarrassment of seizures in school (or in any public place) is a constant source of tension. The second factor is related to the psychosocial development of the child with seizures. Seizures still carry a heavy burden of social stigma. There are often difficulties in obtaining employment, even if the seizures are controlled or occur infrequently. Employers are concerned about "appearances" if an employee has a seizure in view of customers and about the liability for job-related injuries. Numerous occupational restrictions are necessary and narrow opportunities for employment. These include restrictions on driving and flying, working in high exposed places, and working around heavy machinery.

Psychosocial management of the child with seizures and the family must be initiated as soon as the diagnosis is made.[14] Comprehensive services are required, and anticipatory guidance is most important. Acceptance of the disability and need for treatment will ease the child's way in life as well as the family's adjustment.

LIMITATIONS ON THE CHILD WITH SEIZURES

The child with a seizure disorder has a number of limitations imposed by the threat of seizures per se in addition to others resulting from the attitudes of the family and society.

Until control of seizures has been achieved, defined as 3–6 months without any seizures, the child should not be permitted to participate in any activity that could result in serious harm to himself or others if a seizure should occur. These activities include riding a bicycle in traffic, climbing ropes or ladders, and swimming. These restrictions can be lifted when it is clear that seizures are well controlled, although swimming should always be carefully supervised.

If it is clear that seizures are refractory to control, compromises will have to be made so that the range of permissible activities is increased while the danger of significant harm is minimized. Factors to take into consideration include the frequency of seizures; their nature, severity, and length; the duration of the postictal period; and superimposed drug toxicity. If seizures only occur during sleep, no limitations are necessary.

There is no absolute restriction on contact sports when seizures are controlled. They should be prohibited, however, for any child who has seizures as a result of a head injury and for any child in whom seizures are precipitated by contact during the game. Restriction would also be warranted for the child who is lethargic from anticonvulsant medication.

Restrictions on driving vary with the state in which the child resides. Most states allow an operator's permit to be issued if seizures have been under complete control for at least 1 year and the patient is under a physician's care. The application for an operator's permit asks whether seizures have occurred; if so, the child's physician will be requested to provide a medical report. Whether the physician must report a patient known to have seizures is determined by state statute. If reporting is not required, the physician could be liable for legal action based on breach of confidentiality and invasion of privacy. The question of the physician's liability if the patient should be involved in an accident resulting from a seizure is complex and unresolved.

Alcohol use should be avoided, as there is a risk of precipitating seizures in some patients. Alcohol and barbiturates have a synergistic effect, enhancing the depressant action of alcohol. There is little information concerning illicit drug use and seizures. In general, their use should be discouraged.

REFERENCES

1. Commission on Classification and Terminology of the International League Against Epilepsy: Proposal for revised classification of epileptic seizures. *Epilepsia* 2:489–501, 1981.
2. Jennings, M. T., and Bird, T. D.: Genetic influences in the epilepsies. *Am. J. Dis. Child.* 135:450–457, 1981.
3. Lewis, D. V., and Freeman, J. M.: The electroencephalogram in pediatric practice: Its use and abuse. *Pediatrics* 60:324–330, 1977.
4. Thurston, J. H., Thurston, D. L., Hixon, B. B., *et al.:* Prognosis in childhood epilepsy. *N. Engl. J. Med.* 306:831–836, 1982.
5. Delgado-Escueta, A. V., Mattson, R. H., King, L., *et al.:* The nature of aggression during epileptic seizures. *N. Engl. J. Med.* 305:711–716, 1981.
6. Bachman, D. S., Hodges, F. J., and Freeman, J. M.: Computerized axial tomography in chronic seizure disorders of childhood. *Pediatrics* 58:828–832, 1976.
7. Riikonen, R., and Donner, M.: Incidence and aetiology of infantile spasms from 1960 to 1976: A population study in Finland. *Dev. Med. Child. Neurol.* 21:333–343, 1979.
8. Matsumoto, A., Watanabe, K., Negoro, T., *et al.:* Long-term prognosis after infantile spasms: A statistical study of prognostic factors in 200 cases. *Dev. Med. Child. Neurol.* 23:51–65, 1981.

9. Consensus Development Conference: Febrile seizures: Long-term management of children with fever-associated seizures. *Pediatrics* **66:**1009–1012, 1980.
10. Nelson, K. B., and Ellenberg, J. H.: Prognosis in children with febrile seizures. *Pediatrics* **61:**720–727, 1978.
11. Dodrill, C. B., and Troupin, A. S.: Seizures and adaptive abilities. *Arch. Neurol.* **33:**604–607, 1976.
12. Rutter, M., Graham, P., and Yule, W.: A neuropsychiatric study in childhood. *Clin. Dev. Med.* **35/36:**1–272, 1970.
13. Lindsay, J., Ounsted, C., and Richards, P.: Long-term outcome in children with temporal lobe seizures. III. Psychiatric aspects in childhood and adult life. *Dev. Med. Child. Neurol.* **21:**630–636, 1979.
14. Voeller, K. K. S., and Rothenberg, M. B.: Psychosocial aspects of the management of seizures in children. *Pediatrics* **51:**1072–1082, 1973.

II

*Psychoeducational Aspects of
Developmental Pediatrics*

Specific Learning Disabilities and Attention-Deficit Disorder with Hyperactivity

Marcel Kinsbourne

Marcel Kinsbourne • Department of Psychology, Brandeis University, and Department of Behavioral Neurology, Eunice Kennedy Shriver Center for Mental Retardation, Waltham, Massachusetts 02254.

INTRODUCTION

The learning disabilities are developmentally determined delays in children's acquisition of certain mental skills. They are selective—only a subset of mental skills is insufficiently developed; by definition, mental skills are relevant to the educational process. Children vary in the degree to which they are affected along a continuum originating within the normal range. The mental operations affected differ, and the pathogenesis of the disorder is diverse (genetic flaw, genetic diversity, early brain damage). Learning-disabled children are not consistently characterized by evidence of structural brain disorder, metabolic abnormality, or associated neurological signs. Although certain clinical appearances accompany learning disabilities with more than chance frequency, none appears to be of diagnostic use. Diagnosis is made on the basis of the characteristics of the behavioral disorder alone.[2]

The lack of scope for the usual medical diagnostic process sets learning disorders apart. According to the medical model, the surface phenomenology of a disease should suggest an underlying cause. This is verifiable by clinical tests. Treatment is directed at the underlying pathology. If this is corrected successfully, the surface appearances clear. In learning disability, the sequence is not reproducible. The underlying cause can only be inferred and is not subject to verification. No treatment is known to influence the underlying cause. The diagnostic process serves to delineate the surface phenomenology as precisely as possible and to exclude nondevelopmental causes that are capable of converging into similar behavioral manifestations. Treatment is exclusively symptomatic and, instead of altering the situation, is aimed at fostering adaptive functioning.

One approach to the brain basis of learning disabilities is to regard the problem as a special case of brain-based variability of intellect. This is the *individual difference model,* which treats learning disability as representing extremes of normal variation (although acknowledging the possibility that specific focal damage could occasionally result in indistinguishable manifestations). This model has recently replaced in popularity the more time-honored view of learning disabilities as representing a neurological deficit.

The physical basis of variability in intellectual function can hardly be doubted. Physical factors can influence intellectual development. The point of this issue is the continuity–discontinuity distinction. The *deficit model* suggests that properly understood, learning disabilities will break down into a few definable disorders, such as dyslexia and hyperactivity. The continuity approach suggests that these are "spectrum disorders" with gradations across patients, along several behavioral dimensions.

THE SPECIFIC LEARNING DISABILITY–HYPERACTIVITY DISTINCTION

The terms learning disability and hyperactivity are customarily used in a broad fashion and overlap the bulk of mild to moderate childhood psychopathology. *Learning disabilities* refer to cognitive developmental psychopathology: imperfections in mental development falling short of global mental retardation or of the very severe selective deficits such as developmental aphasia. *Hyperactivity* is used in a far broader context than the word suggests, designating the spectrum of developmentally based (as opposed to learned) behavioral disorders that fall short of borderline or actual psychosis, such as infantile autism or childhood schizophrenia. Being less than severe, the manifestations in question are most obtrusive in the most demanding and structured situations, typically at school. Although in general they are often considered school problems, behavior at home and in other nonacademic settings is by no means normal. However, antecedent pathology is apparent well before school age. Similarly, when children outgrow school age, they generally do not cease to show signs of these problems. Instead, the learning disability and the hyperactivity remain present in an age-appropriate form subsequent to leaving school and possibly indefinitely.

Learning disability and hyperactivity are not identical or even overlapping. They represent, however, complementary domains of mental life. Behavior is a composite of two ingredients: selection and processing. The organism has to select, from a rich external and internal stimulus source, what to attend to, and from a rich repertoire of possible actions, what to do. Information processing occurs after having made the selection (adopted perceptual readiness, adopted categorical mental set, prepared for action). The selected input must be analyzed to the extent necessary for adaptive purposes, and planned actions must be performed effectively. Deficient selection and deficient processing converge to the same end point: failed performance. Failure to adopt the appropriate mental set leaves potentially effective processing equipment unused. Adopting that mental set, however, serves little if the processing equipment is ineffective. Hyperactive children fail to deploy their attention in a fashion adaptive to what is expected of them—a problem of selection. Even if they attend efficiently, learning-disabled children find specific forms of processing disproportionately difficult, and they fail in corresponding arenas of achievement. Learning disability is an impairment in the area of the intellect, whereas hyperactivity is an impairment in the area of temperament. Both conditions lead to specific failure in adaptive behavior.

Topics of learning disability and hyperactivity are usually organized around the school experiences. With respect to school performance, the effect of hyperactivity is on attention. From this perspective, hyperactivity has recently been named *attention-deficit disorder*.[1] It cannot be assumed, however, that this difficulty is specific. Behavioral pathology can leave its victim with a different agenda than the usual, and attention in conventional settings such as the classroom necessarily suffers. The failure to pay attention in class is indicative, but does not explain the disorder. In more severe cases, the inattention becomes more flagrant and the child's behavior more at variance with that which is expected. In this way, the diagnosis merges into what has recently been called a *conduct disorder*. The frequent occurrence of depression is not a surprising effect of the pressures on the child, resulting from the misfit between ideal and actual behavior. Some hyperactive children become alienated and exhibit psychopathic behavior.

Cognitive psychopathology (against a background of normal general intelligence) can manifest itself in the classroom as an unexpected difficulty in certain academic subjects or types of learning. In highly selective cases, the difficulty may narrowly invest in one specific area, such as reading and writing. In more severe cases, however, the problem can be broad to the extent of merging into general mental abnormality.

The breadth of definition outlined is far from that intended by the originators of the concepts. Dyslexia was initially conceived as a selected problem in learning to read and write, without an abnormality outside of these domains. Hyperactivity was thought to be a particular medical condition characterized by restlessness. However, as experience accumulated, the supposed selectivity or isolated nature of these two "medical conditions" appeared less impressive. Rather, they appear to arise from a continuum both in terms of depth (severity) within an area of mental function, and in terms of breadth (extent) across areas of mental function. The less specific term *learning disability* was therefore substituted for dyslexia. It included a variety of patterns of disabilities, involving at the very least arithmetic as well as reading and writing and often language-based fields as well, such as social studies and visuospatially based fields, such as art. *Attention-deficit disorder* is also more broadly construed than hyperactivity. It can be diagnosed in the absence of restlessness.

One consequence of this change is that the terms can be used as socially respectable euphemisms for children who would be more properly described as mentally retarded or emotionally disturbed, respectively. More importantly, current practice acknowledges, by implication, that both entities are better described as spectrum disorders rather than as specific diseases.

In an effort to consolidate the two entities, attempts have been made to subtype them. Consequently, subtypes of dyslexia have been repeatedly defined. Similarly, a variety of dichotomies have been proposed for attention-deficit disorder (e.g., pure hyperactivity versus conduct disorder, situational versus pervasive hyperactivity, hyperactivity versus aggressiveness, attention deficit with or without hyperactivity). Subtyping has the obvious advantage of adding clarity and specificity to diagnostic labels. Behavior can be clustered in various ways. However, not until objective correlates of these subtypes become available (and better still, specific treatments) will the definition of syndromes within a broad spectrum of cognitive and behavioral psychopathology become more than descriptively useful. Current methods of treatment—educational, behavioral, or psychopharmacological—are all symptomatic in that they do not change the disordered neural substrate; i.e., they do not cure. The treatment modalities are nonspecific in that they do not address any particular "condition" selectively.

In view of these concepts, the most reasonable approach to the understanding of learning disabilities and hyperactivity is to deal with them in terms of a model of delayed maturation and individual difference, rather than as discrete and delimited deficits. Learning disabilities are characterized by a delay in development in certain facets of mental skill. Within these areas a child behaves like a normal younger child. Behavioral psychopathology is characterized by the overuse of certain types of selective processes and the underuse of others. In the case of neither type of disorder do children actually behave in ways that are qualitatively deviant. Any behavior exhibited by a child will also be exhibited by an unaffected child, to some extent some of the time. The problem resides in the failure of maturation of intellectual skills and the failure of adaptive selection between behavioral options.

We now consider separately first the cognitive, then the behavioral type of psychopathology, with emphasis on its relationship to school achievement and classroom conduct.

LEARNING DISABILITIES: DIAGNOSIS

The learning-disabled child is considered to have a selective difficulty in certain kinds of learning against a background of intact general intelligence. This is usually operationalized in terms of backwardness on certain educational achievement tests exceeding an arbitrary criterion, given normal or better score on certain intelligence tests. Different approaches include (1) requiring the child to be behind by an absolute number of "achievement years" (typically two), given that intelligence is within the normal range; (2) relating the amount of requisite backwardness to the child's grade level (i.e., diagnosing the condition on a lesser amount of absolute delay in the earlier grades); and (3) relating the diagnosis to the child's mental age rather than chronological age. This implies that a child with superior intelligence and a learning disability can be diagnosed, even with achievement approximating the norm. Similarly, a learning disability can be diagnosed in a child of subnormal intelligence if achievement in a certain area is low, even relative to the generally subnormal level of functioning.

An obvious weakness of these formulations is that they do not allow for the fact that relative failure in school can be the final common pathway of a variety of causes, including environmental deprivation, emotional disorder, inadequate schooling, inadequate school attendance, and incomplete command of English as a second language. A variety of exclusionary clauses are usually added to make the definition of the learning disability one that attempts to dispose of these other potential causes. They have not been operationalized, however. Therefore, it often remains a matter of opinion whether non-ideological factors suffice to explain a child's academic handicap. A more fundamental difficulty resides in the implicit assumption that there is something properly termed *general intelligence* against a background of which specific difficulties may occur. This concept is by no means established. A more conservative formulation is to acknowledge that any individual may be more intelligent in some spheres of mental function than in other spheres. Thus intelligence level may be separately evaluated and characterized. From that perspective, the learning-disabled child is one who is more intelligent in areas in which function is not impaired and who is less intelligent in areas in which performance is inadequate. His is a selective mental retardation.

Diagnosis of selective reading disability (dyslexia) is clearly a demanding exercise, requiring a substantial data base about the child that is not always available. Many specialists depart radically from the requisite standards that they themselves assert when making statements about populations rather than individuals. In inferring a familial incidence of dyslexia or postulating dyslexia as a cause of maladaptive behavior, claims made are on the basis of no more than reported illiteracy in people who are not obviously mentally retarded. This practice leads to foolishly proposing grandiose claims for the incidence of dyslexia and its dire consequences. These in turn generate understandable skepticism in the reader. The same skepticism should apply to claims that figures of historical note, such as daVinci, Edison, Rodin, Andersen, Einstein, and Churchill, were dyslexic.

DEFICIT AND DIFFERENCE MODELS

The deficit and the difference model have no differential implication for practical management. Specifically, a child with a deficit who does not respond to regular classroom instruction may well respond to an individualized program. An impaired brain substrate may impair learning to a relative extent only or preclude it only if taught in a particular way. Conversely, the child considered different as a consequence of the vagaries of genetic diversity may be different to an extent prohibitive of successful instruction. Both structural insult and unfavorable genetic programming limit how efficiently the brain works, and a specific lack of behavioral control results. This does not by its nature betray its pathogenesis. Nevertheless, there is a tendency for proponents of "difference" viewpoints to advocate intensive remedial instruction and for advocates of "deficit" models to favor alternative education ("bypass") instead. These viewpoints are more an expression of feeling than an interpretation of fact.

Much has been made of allegations that some poor readers read as well (or as poorly) when the print is upside down as when it is normally oriented. An improvement in reading immediately after turning print upside down has even been claimed. Whether the claims are valid is an empirical issue that remains unresolved. Their theoretical basis is not novel, however. It is analogous to the "ill lateralization" and "right hemisphere dominance" notions. The former, traceable to Orton, regards both hemispheres as in potential control of the reading act.[3] The latter regards the right hemisphere as in control, therefore favoring the right to left scanning direction. Indeed, both are sometimes held at the same time, although they are incompatible with each other. It should be noted in passing that mirror writing appears to be more common among nonrighthanders, although whether this is due to superior skill or simply greater practice in this minority group is not firmly established.

Orton distinguished between *static reversals* (mirror-image reversal of single letters) and *dynamic reversals* (reading words from right to left).[3] Both could represent momentarily reversed directionality of scan. Quite distinct from them is the letter-order error that characterizes the Gerstmann subtype of reading disability. Insofar as this can be referred to any locus in the brain (based on analogy with adult acquired disease), these errors are referrable to dominant parietal lobe dysfunction and are quite distinct from static or dynamic reversals.

LEARNING DISABILITY: BRAIN BASIS OF INTELLECT

Learning disabilities can be viewed as arising from particular patterns of the intellectual profile and related to problems of brain maturation. Consequently, explorations are possible as to the role of various brain structures enabling the normal child to learn under conventional circumstances. Maldevelopment of the brain precludes the learning-disabled child from doing so. Assuming that, with rare exceptions, there is no evidence of structural abnormality in the brain of learning-disabled individuals, it can be hypothesized that there is malfunction or malcoordination of brain areas at an organizational level.[4] In general, the same applies to individual differences in intellect; i.e., the brains of dull, normal, and intellectually superior individuals cannot be shown to differ, by currently avaliable methods. Only when mental retardation is severe or profound is there a high probability that neuropathological study will reveal a gross abnormality. Within the limits of a wide normal range, neither size nor shape of the brain discriminates with respect to level of intellectual function. For these reasons, investigators have attempted to infer the organizational principles of malfunction on the basis of certain frequently associated findings. A miscellany of minor neurological signs and signs of neurological immaturity have been documented in some but by no means all these children. These signs supposedly indicate the influence of nonspecific adverse factors in retarding development, not only of particular parts of the nervous system yielding the signs in question, but also in those areas that subserve higher mental function, the integrity of which cannot be examined in this way. A wide range of miscellaneous variations of waveforms on the electroencephalogram (EEG) have been similarly interpreted. However, the frequent dissociation between these "minimal cerebral dysfunction" signs and learning disability at the cognitive level makes it difficult to infer a pathogenesis. These minor neurological signs are useless for purposes of diagnosis in any individual case.

A perennially intriguing observation is the higher incidence of non-right-handers (ambidexters and sinistrals) among learning-disabled populations. Like all other associates of learning disability, its association with non-right-handedness is purely statistical. This association is in no sense specific, as non-right-handers are also overrepresented in other suboptimally functioning populations, notably the mentally retarded (in proportion to the severity of the retardation) and epileptics (of early onset).

There are several hypotheses about the relationship between non-right-handedness and learning disabilities: (1) the left-hander's brain is organized in a fashion not conducive to optimal learning; (2) left-handers are more vulnerable than others to a variety of forms of early brain damage, potentially leading to learning disability; and (3) early brain damage is antecedent to left-handedness, which in many cases represents a deviation of phenotypic hand use (left) from that in the genotype (right), i.e., "pathological left-handedness."[5]

Whereas the cerebral hemispheres in right-handers are well known to be differentiated (in all but a few cases), such that the left hemisphere is in charge of verbal-sequential and the right hemisphere of spatial-relational function, non-right-handers are known to be very heterogeneous in this respect. A further unusual feature is that in a substantial minority of left handers it would appear that one hemisphere is responsible both for verbal-sequential and spatial-relational function (leaving one wondering what the other hemisphere does). Concepts of brain organization that regard cerebral space as limited postulate a crowding artifact of one function by another, when both are concentrated within the same structure.[6] A more functional approach would regard this as causing a problem only when the individual is attempting to use both skills in question in coordination simultaneously.[7] In any case, the various forms of brain organizations that occur in non-right-handers are frequently represented in the normally reading and writing population. Thus they cannot be regarded as in themselves sufficient to explain the learning problem.

The concept that families of left-handers are subject to a variety of ailments has been proposed repeatedly. The issue remains controversial. However, recent evidence suggests that the probability of having a relatively profoundly retarded child is greater in relatively nonright-handed parental matings. Similarly, it appears that a number of diseases of the immune system (causing autoimmune reaction) are more prevalent in families in whom sinistrality is a feature.[8] What impact such disorders might have on the developing brain is unknown.

The principle of pathological left-handedness has been validated by the observation of patients with focal epileptic seizures, caused by very early left hemisphere damage. Among these patients, lefthandedness is particularly common. The applicability of the concept outside this limited population is more controversial, but evidence has been adduced that a proportion of both mentally retarded and normally functioning left-handers are pathological in origin. This does suggest that adverse influences on the left hemisphere can manifest themselves in this way and further supports the concept that in learning disability the left hemisphere may be impaired in maturation. It does not explain how that comes about.

If the nature of the damage that causes learning disabilities is uncertain, so is the mechanism by which it exerts its effects. The simplest hypothesis is that certain central processing areas are incapacitated. However, the plasticity of the immature nervous system is such that it seems improbable that a limited amount of damage would not be efficiently compensated. An alternative point of view is that the cerebral processors are intact but are not properly activated to fulfill their function when called upon. There is increasing evidence of a brainstem "selector" system responsible for enabling the person to adopt the appropriate mental set when given tasks that require or call for reflective thought. It is possible that children with learning disabilities fail to activate the appropriate left hemispheric areas to the necessary extent (and perhaps activate the right hemisphere instead).[9]

The concepts cited are leads that will fuel further investigation. Some may be useful points to review in discussing the nature of the problem with parents. However, knowledge at this level of analysis is nowhere near the point of being applicable in practice.

LEARNING DISABILITY: NEURODEVELOPMENTAL LAG

Children with gross brain damage, such as cerebral palsy, exhibit abnormalities on classic neurological examination ("hard signs"). By contrast, the diagnosis of minimal brain dysfunction (MBD) is based on findings that are abnormal only with reference to the child's age ("soft signs"). At a younger age, the same findings would be normal. They indicate a relative delay in corresponding aspects of neurological maturation.

Many adverse influences can cause neurodevelopmental lag, and there is no relationship between a pattern of affected functions and any particular pathogenesis. Similarly, the antecedents of MBD do not differ from those of major brain dysfunction, such as cerebral palsy, mental retardation, or infantile autism. Any influence that is deleterious to neurons can retard the pace of some aspect of brain development if it affects territory that has not yet undergone functional differentiation. In that case, differentiation may be delayed in onset, slow in evolution, and limited in ultimate expression. The precise trajectory of development cannot be predicted, however. Whether the insult leads to developmental lag or frank neurological deficit depends on the distribution and severity of its impact. If it impairs mechanisms that would normally be functioning at birth, the resulting clinical picture is abnormal irrespective of the stage of extrauterine life, and MBD is not diagnosed. When a later evolving mechanism is affected, in that its maturation is delayed, MBD may be said to obtain.

It follows that all soft sign indicators of MBD represent the normal state of affairs in younger children. The factors that selectively limit the performance of children with MBD are some that normally limit the performance of younger children. With respect to these factors, young normal children constitute a model for MBD. The context of the inadequate performance, however, is different in the child with MBD, since in other respects he is functioning at a substantially higher level, appropriate to his chronological age; he also has the additional experiences of his greater age at his disposal.

The lag in neural development may affect any component of the nervous system. Sometimes it is inconsequential for the child's daily life and social adjustment, as when it involves some minor reflex abnormality. At other times, it may be of major importance, as when a motor immaturity causes the child to be seen as clumsy for his age, inflexible deployment of attention limits his adaptive potential or immature cognitive processes make him unready to learn to read by the usual methods.

THE LEARNING-DISABLED CHILD: PRINCIPLES OF COGNITIVE DEVELOPMENT

Learning-disabled children differ greatly in terms of the sphere of intellect in which they are most delayed maturationally. However, the form of the immaturity remains fairly constant across cognitive spheres. It conforms to the sequence of development that occurs normally and reveals the learning disabled child as corresponding in his relevant intellectual skills to a younger, normal child.

The overriding principle in cognitive development across perceptual, executive, linguistic, memorial, and reasoning areas is one of progressive differentiation and flexibility of attention. From a base state in which the child is tied to salient and immediately present percepts and concepts, and confined to preprogrammed synergisms of response, he gradually becomes able to attend and respond differentially. The child learns to detach attention from the most salient percept or obvious concept to one more finely tuned to the adaptive issue and is able to use response patterns that increasingly deviate from those that are biologically hard wired.

Perception

Changes during maturation and perception do not relate to elementary visual sensation (e.g., acuity, color discrimination) but to the individual's ability to control the focus and capacity of visual attention, The immature perceptual system is closely tied to whichever visual dimension is most salient in the field. Given bright colors and striking shapes, the infant notices little else, even though the perceptual machinery for discriminating size, location, orientation, and sequence is in place. The more mature individual will still first observe those perceptual dimensions that are highest on the "perceptual hierarchy" but is able to detach ("decenter") attention to less salient dimensions. These less salient dimensions are not only occasionally of adaptive significance in the natural world but are used in conventional signaling systems, such as writing and print. The child's increasing ability to shift attention to less salient perceptual dimensions is one reason why he finds it easier to learn to read as he grows older. The ability of children to search systematically and comprehensively through a multi-item visual array also develops steadily during early childhood.

Language

Language precursors consist in attaching verbal labels to salient objects currently in view. The nature of verbal development is such that until about age 5 years words are used to label and communicate but not for purposes of coding and transforming (reasoning) or reconstituting (remembering) reality. Between ages 5 and 7, the child experiences a rapid increase in the ability to use words instrumentally as a facet of the intellect.

In reading (by means of phonics instruction), the ability of individuals to segment word sounds imaginatively into constituent speech sounds is crucial. This ability does not develop spontaneously but must be taught. It cannot readily be taught to preschool children since they lack the analytical capability to perform this effort of abstraction.

Memory

The ability to remember an episode calls for the detaching of attention from the present, in favor of re-experiencing some aspect of the past. The ability to escape constraints of the here and now takes years to develop. The young child is stimulus bound by his immediate surroundings, and therefore episodic memory is weak until school age.

The ability to learn, i.e., to become more fluent and automatized with respect to performing particular physical and mental operations, is not constrained in this way. This is evident from a very early age, as exemplified by the acquisition of motor skills and language. Differences in language abilities in younger and older children appear to be quantitative rather than qualitative. The younger child requires more practice but nevertheless can ultimately reach the same point.

Motor Skills

The newborn is equipped with a small number of rigidly preformed synergisms involving a multitude of muscle groups in a predetermined pattern: sucking, rooting, crying, startle, and lateral orienting, and so forth. The newborn is unable to depart from these patterns. Although all the muscles are operational, they can be used initially only in a constrained fashion. As motor control becomes more differentiated, synergisms can be broken up and elements of different synergisms recombined in ways not hard wired in the organism. The ability to move differentially involves restraining the rest of the synergism to which that movement "belongs." Thus, the immature nervous system manifests not weakness but overuse of muscles: Unwanted movements join the desired movement in execution. These associated and mirror movements gradually decrease as inhibitory control improves.

These principles are directly applicable to learning disabled children who have trouble, for example, in learning to read, spell, and write. Learning-disabled children manifest (1) rigid adherence of attention to salient percepts, (2) inability to re-experience episodes, (3) failure of a developing ability to use words for purposes of flexible coding, and (4) a problem with finely differentiated movement as called for in writing. All these difficulties are referrable to various stages of the maturation of the relevant development sequences. The nature of the difficulty suggests how it should be handled. The child is provided external structure where he cannot spontaneously provide this for himself.

Similarly, the child is provided more than the usual amount of practice in view of the immature state of the nervous system. Where possible, ''bypass'' techniques are used, enlisting those skills that in fact have already matured in the selectively disabled individual.

DIAGNOSIS OF DYSLEXIA

Inadequate acquisition of reading and writing skills by children of normal general intelligence is the end point of many causes—experiential, motivational, and attentional—as well as specific to the mental operations on which reading readiness is predicated. Dyslexia implies impaired development of some of the latter mental operations. However, their status cannot be measured directly because no acceptable model of reading acquisition exists. The constituent processes are unknown and therefore not measurable. Consequently, dyslexia has to be inferred from (1) the characteristics of the learning failure, and (2) the status of the other possible causes of learning failure in each individual case. Dyslexia implies that reading and writing failures should be selective and that progress in other academic areas should not be deficient. One difficulty in this requirement is that it applies with decreasing force as the child grows older. In higher grades, instruction depends increasingly on the written word. In particular, arithmetic problems are frequently posed in a verbal context, which may not be understood by the dyslexic child. An additional difficulty is that at least one subtype of selective reading impairment includes an impairment in calculation (Gerstmann syndrome). The demoralizing effect of reading failure may lead to a broadening of academic failure. As a consequence of these factors, some cases of dyslexia will not exhibit the selectivity inherent in the diagnosis, at the level of school achievement.

Obvious experimental factors contributing to reading failure are poor teaching, interrupted schooling, lack of sympathy for literacy in the home, and the problems of bilingualism. Motivational factors include sociocultural, personality, and psychiatric aspects. The culturally alienated child, the psychopath, and the thought-disordered child lack motivation to work (and to perform tests used for diagnosis), although for different reasons. Attention deficit, as in the hyperactive child, is a potent cause of school failure. Correspondingly, deficient concentration and disruptive behavior are common among backward readers. Remedial reading specialists often regard this as reactive to the reading failure. To confirm this diagnosis, it must be demonstrated that the inattention is limited to the situation of inadequate performance and that there was no inattention before the academic difficulty declared itself. Dyslexia in the presence of attention deficit is difficult to diagnose, and it can only be convincingly demonstrated if the attention deficit is successfully controlled and the difficulty in learning to read persists.

In view of these confounds, dyslexia is difficult if not impossible to diagnose in the following populations: (1) the culturally deprived, (2) children who are attention deficient, and (3) delinquent children. This is not to say that dyslexia does not occur among these groups. However, it is inadmissible to infer a cognitive processing deficit if motivational or attentional causations cannot be ruled out. A striking example of a mistake in this respect is the frequent claim that delinquency is caused by dyslexia. The coexistence of delinquency and illiteracy is no proof of such a causal relationship. It is necessary to first demonstrate that reading failure preceded any evidence of antisocial or psychopathic personality. This calls for longitudinal investigation, which has not been done.

The limits on our ability to diagnose dyslexia are significant for research purposes, reflecting a difficulty in the acquisition of valid subject samples for study. It makes little difference for practical purposes, as no systematic differences exist between teaching methods for dyslexics and children retarded in reading for other reasons. The main advantage of the dyslexia or kindred brain diagnosis is the effect it may have on the morale of the child and those around him. In a favorable case, it will single out the child for sympathetic individual attention and thus improve his learning experience.

DIFFICULTIES EXPERIENCED BY DYSLEXICS

The mental processes involved in learning to read and write can be classified into those that are specifically linguistic and those that could be at work in any visual–vocal pattern-labeling activity.

The earliest accomplishments in learning to read are probably not specifically linguistic.[10] Discrimination of letter forms and adoption of consistent (left to right) directionality in scanning letter sequences are visual–motor skills. Presumably these skills are operative when the visual targets do not have conventional symbolic significance. Learning letter–letter name and letter group–word associations would be considered a rote exercise in cross-model associations. Outspoken failure at these early levels cannot be explained soley as a linguistic problem. However, success in these activities does not go far toward guaranteeing reading acquisition. Either as a result of explicit teaching or unconsciously in the course of growing familiarization, children extract invariants from letter displays and learn phonological rules. Later, when acquiring fluency, they will similarly learn syntactic rules that they are not explicitly taught. A child whose dyslexia deficit is restricted to a difficulty in learning these rules would be expected to show little deficit during the earlier stages of reading acquisition. However, this child will exhibit increasing difficulty in acquiring the fluency that should naturally follow. Although systematic information is not available, most clinicians would agree that dyslexic children have trouble from the very beginning of learning to read. This could occur because a different subtype of dyslexia is operative (even a "right hemispheric" type, as suggested by Bakker[10]). Another possibility, as in the developmental model offered by Satz and Morris,[16] is that early ("prelinguistic") reading difficulty is succeeded by linguistic problems in the same child.

At least in theory, difficulty in acquiring phonological and syntactical rules, with respect to the written word, could reflect a more general linguistic problem, detectable on examination of speech comprehension. Alternatively, the deficit could be restricted to the decoding of the written word. The concept of reading acquisition as involving the acquisition of phonological skill over and above the items explicitly taught is important in considering the possible impact on children with reading difficulties and of current remedial methods emphasizing phonics instruction. Even if word attack is successfully inculcated, it does not follow automatically that the child will broaden out from this narrow skill to fluency by the acquisition of familiarity with phonological rules. This too may explicitly have to be taught.

TAXONOMY OF LEARNING DISABILITIES

Learning disabilities have been classified as a set of disorders that are isomorphic with their impact on the educational process.[2] Thus if the problem is limited to reading, the term *dyslexia* has been used; if limited to writing, *dysgraphia;* and if limited to arithmetic, *dyscalculia,* with such attached adjectives as developmental or congenital, specific or selective. This rigid application of a medical model encounters two obvious difficulties. First, within any of these academic areas, failure can occur for more than one reason, and there is no evidence that different children find different aspects of the curriculum disproportionately difficult. Second, often the educational problem is not so limited but straddles several academic subjects, at times occurring secondarily, particularly in language skills, which are involved not only in reading and writing but in the higher grades, in history, in social studies, and even in arithmetic, where story problems are increasingly used. But even discounting those problems outside reading and writing, which are secondary to difficulties therein, it is clear that many children have combined syndromes not narrowly delimited as above.

The extreme opposing position is that each learning-disabled child is unique in the particular constellation of his difficulties. This approach emphasizes the complex of interacting processes drawn upon within each educational area and the fact that the deployment of mental processes within any educational area differs radically, depending on the level of instruction (i.e., the child's age and grade level). This approach emphasizes the continuity between the disabled and the able learner, with the disability being a matter of degree, qualified by such factors as the size of the classroom, quality of instruction, motivation to learn transmitted by the family, and so forth.

The two approaches cited have different implications for designing remedial methodologies. The traditional preconception is that a disease should have a particular treatment. The disease model encourages methodologies that purport to be effective for "all such children." An outstanding example is the Orton–Gillingham method for developmental dyslexia, which purports to address virtually all the problems encountered by virtually all the children of this type. The individual difference approach emphasizes the need for individualized prescriptive education. In that sense, it comes closer to the prevailing spirit in the remedial educational field. It encourages eclectic methodologies, with the inclusion of components of a variety of reading instructional methods. These methods are used opportunistically as one follows the course of the child's progress in learning. The first approach has the drawback of rigidity. The second approach has the drawback that little is learned from one case to the next, with each teacher beginning, as it were, anew in attempting to conquer the learning difficulty.

Presumably some middle way between these two extremes is the most appropriate and helpful. It is necessary to delineate what learning disabled children have in common and how they cluster into subtypes. It can be hypothesized that they are divisible into subtypes depending on which part of the brain is underdeveloped. Regardless of the part of the brain that is underdeveloped, the brain state closely approximates that of a normal younger child. The younger child is regarded as a model to understand the difficulties encountered by the older child with a specific learning problem.

SUBTYPES OF DYSLEXIA

Dyslexia has been subtyped according to three organizing principles, or patterns: (1) associated test performance, (2) academic disability across subjects, and (3) errors made in reading and writing. The most frequent attempts to subtype have been based on the implicit assumption that any dyslexic child has a problem of cognitive processing. In addition to impairing the child's ability of learning to read and write, this deficit also has an impact on performance extraneous to reading and writing. By its very nature, this type of classification rejects the concept that pure dyslexia is a defect limited entirely to the acquisition of reading and writing. The subtyping is based on tests for processes that do not involve the child in reading and writing but that do tap abilities thought to be involved in aspects of learning to read and write. The taxonomies have been derived (1) by analogy with known syndromes of adult cerebral brain damage involving reading and/or writing, and (2) empirically by cluster analysis of extensive test battery results.

In the domain of adult neuropsychology, the following syndromes notably affect reading and writing:

1. *Aphasia:* In this dominant hemisphere disorder of language, reading is impaired and writing usually still more impaired. Mistakes made by the patient suggest difficulty in relating the written word to its phonemic equivalents and in analyzing a word sound into its constituent speech sounds.
2. *Gerstmann syndrome:* This dominant hemisphere (posterior parietal) syndrome specifically involves difficulty in spelling (with respect to the sequence of letters rather than the letter choice) and, to a much lesser extent, sequence of sounds in reading. An arithmetic problem in relationship to the place value of digits in multiple digit numbers co-occurs.
3. *Alexia without agraphia:* This syndrome is characterized by an impairment of rapid recognition of visual shapes.[11] As rapid serial recognition is usually only called for in reading, it is reading difficulty that is the presenting complaint.
4. *Right hemisphere dyslexia:* In this variant, a visuospatial problem causes subjects to wander off the printed line across the page and to misread word beginnings. They also have difficulty at the comprehension level with respect to relational propositions.
5. *Apraxic agraphia:* This rare syndrome involves a problem with the skilled forming of written letters and words.
6. *Dysarthria and motor apraxia:* These anterior dominant hemisphere syndromes implicate the motor output of speech and writing, although not the inner speech that is being expressed.

In the past attempts were made to identify "developmental dyslexia" with one or more of these syndromes. In 1962, Kinsbourne and Warrington[11] published illustrative cases to show that at least two of these syndromes have analogues among the population of children with selective reading problems: aphasia and the Gerstmann syndrome. The language-disordered children (1) showed an impairment in learning to read and write with little or no difficulty in arithmetic other than secondary to their language problem, (2) made reading and writing mistakes suggesting inaccurate handling of speech sounds, (3) outside the reading and writing domain, gave history of a slow language development, and (4) on testing demonstrated mild but significant problems in spoken speech comprehension. In the Gerstmann disorder, the child manifested a writing delay greater than that in reading but an arithmetic problem as well. The problem is particularly marked in such procedures as subtracting or multiplying, where one has to carry from column to column. Other problems are finger agnosia (difficulty in recognizing the fingers based on their relative position on the hand) and right–left disorientation. The mistakes in spelling were largely of relative position rather than of letter choice. Mattis *et al.*[12] presented three subtypes of dyslexia. The first two subtypes (probably analogous to those of Kinsbourne and Warrington, although described differently) involve selective language and visuospatial sequential processes. The third type was analogous to the output problems of dysarthria and motor apraxia. Pirozzolo and Rayner[13] replicated the Kinsbourne–Warrington classification, extending knowledge of the Gerstmann type by demonstrating associated difficulties in scanning eye movements intended to follow an orderly series of fixations. Meantime, a number of empirical endeavors to subtype were launched.[14–16] These studies employed extensive test batteries reflecting the investigators' theoretical predilections. Typically one or more language subtypes as well as one or more subtypes of a visuospatial nonverbal kind would emerge.

Both the syndrome analogy approach and the empirical approach are beset by problems that have not yet been fully resolved. The difficulty with syndrome analogies resides in the fact that developmental syndromes must differ from acquired ones because of their different antecedent life history. However, it is not clear exactly how they should differ. Although it has been easy to demonstrate typical cases, it has not proved a simple task to account for the bulk of reading disability in syndrome terms. Finally, because most investigators have used tests of their own choosing rather than ones chosen by their predecessors, the question of overlap between findings remains largely open.

The syndrome approach lacks any objective yardstick for validation, When clusters of test findings emerge within a reading-disabled population, the question of validity remains open. There is no objective test of the proposition that the particular clusters in fact have something to do with the difficulty in reading. Certainly it is quite possible that if normal readers were similarly analyzed, similar clusters might emerge. Thus what the empirical methodology gains in terms of comprehensive coverage of the total population, it loses in terms of interpretability of the findings. It remains possible, for instance, to make the claim that language difficulty is central and the rest irrelevant.[17]

A systematic attempt was made to subtype developmental dyslexia by error pattern, by presenting methodology for error analysis in reading and writing.[18] This approach resulted in subtyping into *dysphonetic* (language type), *dyseidetic* (visuospatial type), and a *combined* syndrome. The Boder test has recently been published in a standard and systematically administerable form and may further advance in the field.[18] Recent endeavors have attempted to demonstrate that dyslexic children are "right hemispheric" in the pattern of their abilities.[9] Gordon proposed that there is a certain reciprocity in the distribution of aspects of intellect; i.e., the two hemispheres are separate packages and, to some extent, when one is in the ascendant the other is on the decline. Children who, for as yet unknown reasons, are adept at right hemisphere performance experience the most selective difficulty in learning to read. This approach does not subtype but can accommodate subtypes within its framework. Variants could be regarded as distinctive left hemisphere syndromes.[11,12]

Beyond persisting difficulties in cross-validating different typologies and resolving the question of transitional cases, the subtyping has been disappointing in that it has not yet resulted in any educational benefit. No one has yet validated differential methodologies for educating children who fall within different subclasses. Indeed it is not clear whether determining a child's dyslexia subtype tells anything more than what the teacher already knows about the child's strengths and weaknesses. Subtyping remains an important area for investigation, possibly relating the cognitive difficulty to its brain basis. However, at the practical level it is not yet useful.

The brain basis of reading disabilities has been attacked from another perspective.[4] A dyslexic individual who died of unrelated reasons revealed abnormalities of neuronal distribution and migration in the classic language area of the left hemisphere of the brain. From this case and other unpublished material it has been argued that, contrary to general belief, dyslexia arises from a structural abnormality of the left hemisphere. Because of the well-known compensatory ability of the immature brain with respect to focal abnormality, this seemed unlikely. However, if cases such as those published by Galaburda and others were to be found with reasonable frequency, a change in perspective would be warranted. Meantime, judgment must be suspended on this hypothesis.

One other possible form of subtyping is beginning to take shape. Geschwind and Behan[8] reported that lefthanders in the general population were not only more likely to be dyslexic than righthanders (as had frequently been claimed in the past) but were also significantly subject to a variety of disorders described as "autoimmune": asthma, eczema, collagen disease, diabetes, and myasthenia. Kinsbourne[19] studied these factors in a learning-disabled population and found that the attributions made by Geschwind and Behan applied to families. Within sinistral families (which include one or more left-handed members), the incidence of autoimmune disease was significantly higher than in dextral families (regardless of whether the affected individual himself was right- or left-handed). This finding supports Geschwind's contention that left-handedness and left hemisphere maturational lags might derive from a common antecedent cause, hypothesizing the effect of testosterone as an explanatory principle. A pleiotrophic gene effect is an alternative explanation.[19]

REMEDIAL EDUCATION

The only validated management approach for specific learning disability is remedial education. The hallmark of an appropriate approach is individualization. The instruction is individualized with respect to the child's level of accomplishment in target academic fields. It is specifically designed to explain issues that are customarily more difficult to understand and materials that are disproportionately difficult to remember. There are some commonalities as well as considerable diversities with respect to the learning requirements of children with learning disabilities.

In a typical case, a child failing in reading and writing will be equipped with a larger number of partially or totally incorrect responses to the written word. It is usually necessary to educate in a highly analytical mode, giving the child an intensive learning experience in fundamental reading and writing relationships. In other words, overtraining is necessary. The response should be correct and rapid (fluent). A number of analytical teaching programs for reading are commercially available, notably the Orton–Gillingham method and Distar. These very systematic and logically progressive programs are also exceedingly monotonous. They are only successful if the child is motivated to persevere, and this in turn depends crucially on the relationship child and teacher. Much of the work relates to training of an analytical approach to word sounds and their decomposition into sounds. This is part of the phonics approach to teaching reading, followed by the necessary acquaintance with phonological rules of language. However, rule learning does not guarantee fluency. At some point, it is necessary to institute specific methodologies for accelerating the child's reading response to a rate sufficient to acquire information that is useful in practice.

Despite numerous claims, it is not clear whether specific teaching programs for dyslexic children are any different than for children who are slow in learning to read and other possible reasons. Although there appear to be different subtypes of dyslexia, it has not been clearly shown that different instructional programs are appropriate for children from different subtypes. Ideally the clinician secures an educational situation in which individual instructional needs are determined and in which instruction is logically graduated with continual feedback.

This type of instruction can generally be obtained in a regular school setting on a "withdrawal" basis or in a resource room. A special school, on a day or boarding basis, is usually necessary only if the local school system cannot provide required resources. In the case of some adolescents who have become emotionally conflicted about their academic difficulty, however, the change of scene into a novel and supportive environment may have excellent effects.

DISORDERS OF ATTENTION

A variety of checklists and questionnaires list generally accepted descriptors of hyperactive behavior. Unfortunately, there is no validated way of organizing them into clusters or into primary and secondary manifestations. In the past, restlessness was accepted as primary. More recently the DSM III classification makes restlessness a subsidiary feature, present or not, to two other descriptors—impulsivity and inattentiveness—nominated as primary, hence *attention deficit disorder* (ADD). In fact, these features are not invariable. Like restlessness, impulsivity or inattentiveness may or may not be observed. ADD is best understood as a spectrum of developmental psychopathology involving anomalies of personality (but not psychosis, which is classified separately). Children with attention deficient occupy extremes (polar opposites) on dimensions of overactivity–underactivity, aggressiveness–impulsivity, sociability–unsociability, under- versus overfocus of attention, impulsivity–compulsivity, and emotional ability–hyperstability. These children have in common a pattern of deviant temperament, are nonconformist to societal demands, and are not susceptible to the usual naturally available reinforcements. ADD children also have in common impairments of attention because this is a secondary feature of the disorder. Across a wide range of personality disorders, children will tend to follow their bent rather than attend to an internally imposed structure.

In view of the miscellany of personality types labeled hyperactive (ADD), it is not surprising that investigators are attempting to subtype these children. This effort does not appear to have clinical value, however. Children are classified together largely because they share certain characteristic responses to a management modality: (1) high probability of favorable stimulant response, (2) poor response to psychotherapy and to behavior management, and (3) good response to interpersonal attention. The stimulant response in particular has been assumed to imply some uniformity of pathophysiology across this spectrum. However, it is as nonspecific as the taxonomic category of hyperactivity is miscellaneous. Some hyperactive children express their personality differences in infancy, others not until later. Colicky restlessness is common, as are short sleep periods. Once ambulatory, the children may be very mobile, in apparent disregard for common hazards. An insatiable need for personal attention emerges and is conspicuous in group settings (in the preschool). The child may fail to exhibit self-regulated behavior. Some preschool children are aggressive at this age, others later. Difficulty in limit setting comes early and becomes increasingly serious as the child achieves greater independence. By school entry, a child has usually declared his personality disorder, but parents often still blame their apparently inadequate child-rearing skills for this outcome.

Hyperactive children fail to conform in the classroom. At this young age, the deviant direction of attention is signaled by shifts in posture and restless movements. Some children act out, some merely let their attention shift. They disrupt verbally and show insensitivity to social cues, thus earning disapproval of their peers and elders. In a sociogram study, it was observed that hyperactive children are very negatively classified by their peers (even when their diagnosis had not been mentioned).[20] Domineering ways also disrupt relationships, with siblings as well as peers. Failure to complete assignments becomes an increasing problem as the child progresses into higher grade levels. Low frustration tolerance and failure to work for long-term goals cumulatively impair academic progress. These signs and symptoms contrast sharply with the excellent attention these children exhibit if they choose to do so, e.g., to a hobby, a favorite subject area, or a favored teacher. Although they usually attend quite poorly, their attentional mechanisms are patently in place but are simply not used in the usual way.

In adolescence, social ineptitude is prominent, which can lead to depression and in some cases delinquent behavior. As adults, the hyperactive outcome is miscellany imperfect, with many failing to maintain steady employment or long-term close relationships. Social intrusiveness characterizes many, but happy vocational choices can turn some not-too-extreme temperamental deviances to advantage. Superimposed on these deviant behavioral patterns is a degree of variability that renders the behavior unpredictable. However, situational factors can be identified that improve or impair the attention of many of these children.

Attention deficit is at its height in monotonous situations, in which children are called upon to respond relatively unvarying input over long periods of time. The nature of the deficit is probably similar to that induced in normal people in extremes of such conditions—the "vigilance decrement." In these circumstances, otherwise normal people exhibit some characteristics of hyperactivity.[21] Attention-deficient children become bored easily. They respond relatively well to vivid, novel, and even stressful situations, such as emergencies. Their inability includes failure to sustain not only constructive efforts but also recrimination and anger. While others are still reeling under the impact of conflict, the ADD child has moved obviously onto the next train of thought.

LABORATORY STUDIES

Two controlled paradigms have been used to collect objective data on hyperactive behavior: (1) comparison of hyperactive with controls, and (2) comparison of the untreated with the treated hyperactive (double-blind drug/placebo design). Hyperactives have been shown, as a group, to perform less well in attention demanding tasks. This is particularly true over extensive periods of time: paired associate and serial learning, vigilance, and continuous performance tests.[22]

Hyperactive children perform better when taking a stimulant drug as compared with a placebo on cognitive tests as well as on tests of avoidance learning, risk taking, and collaborative performance.[21] Normal populations exhibit effects in the same direction on simple (low level) tasks but opposite effects on complex (high level) tasks. Thus whether the stimulus responses causes "normal" or "paradoxical" depends on the task used.[23]

Although group averages vary, there is striking subject diversity in any hyperactive group. Some will overlap controls and some will not respond to stimulants or respond adversely (i.e., with impaired rather than enhanced performance). The reliability of individual findings in a given paradigm, and the extent to which they generalize across situations are unknown. It appears that stimulants are most effective when the patient is doing least well and that the patient does least well when uninterested in the task. The instruction of hyperactives is hard to control by the usual reinforcements. Indeed, the ineffectiveness of motivators is close to the central behavioral mechanism of hyperactivity, and the inconstant attention (DSM III notwithstanding) is probably secondary.

BEHAVIOR OF HYPERACTIVE CHILDREN

Hyperactive children are not simply "children who move a lot." High activity level in itself is no disease. There are reasons for restlessness other than hyperactivity (e.g., nervousness, boredom, lack of motivation, discomfort). Restlessness is not invariably a part of the symptom complex called hyperactivity. In 1980, this realization led the taxonomists of DSM III (American Psychiatric Association) to relabel the disorder ADD. ADD was further subdivided into ADD (H) and ADD, depending on whether "hyperactivity" is displayed. This misconstrues the problem. There is no objective evidence that the presence or absence of motor symptoms is important diagnostically. Any of the descriptions of hyperactive behavior that are reviewed may or may not apply to an individual patient, or may apply to him at one age, but not at another. The diagnosis does not hinge on any one "cardinal" sign or on any "inner circle" of signs (e.g., hyperactivity, impulsivity, and inattentiveness, nominated by DSM III). Instead, the checklist approach implies that the diagnosis (as by Conners questionnaire) is a matter of degree. A criterial amount of behavioral abnormality as rated justifies the diagnosis. Different systems receive equal weight at the present stage of our knowledge, as no one knows whether one is more "central" than another. Hyperactivity may be regarded as a spectrum disorder and, if so, no single manifestation could be expected to appear across the spectrum.

Paradoxical though it may sound, many hyperactive children and most hyperactive adults do not move more than is customary. The label "hyperactivity" is deceptive. It was applied in history of knowledge about the disorder before it was realized that motor restlessness is an inconstant and transient characteristic of these children's behavior.

Children regarded as hyperactive are restless. They continually and unpredictably shift positions and change what they are doing. Overall, they may be very active at times or inactive at other periods. More importantly, they move when others think it wise to be still. Restlessness differs from the repetitive movement patterns of individuals who are anxious and drum their fingers, smooth their hair, straighten their tie, or twitch. Restlessness or hyperactivity within the context of this analysis implies certain characteristics.

1. *Inattentiveness:* Characteristically, these children flit from one thing to another. They are not just distractable, they welcome distractions. This inattentiveness differs from that of the child who is merely bored or preoccupied with other matters.

2. *Hastiness:* These children lack impulse control and crave immediate gratification. They come to conclusions and expect consequences without having done the necessary physical or mental work. This differs from the behavior of children who are merely uninterested or otherwise preoccupied.

3. *Resistance to limit setting:* The child opposes discipline with whining manipulations or temper tantrums of spiraling intensity. Threats and bribes are ineffective, and punishment does not deter. This behavior differs from that of the ill-bred or spoiled child or of the child who is angry or even psychotic.

4. *Emotional instability:* These children lack self-control and express each change in mood and bewilder with mood changes. This differs from the child who has a major affective disorder, such as primary mania or depression.

5. *Inconsequentiality:* These children seem to have trouble in connecting cause with effect. Disapproval of their antisocial behavior perpetually catches them by surprise. This differs from the actions of children who really do not understand because they are poorly raised or mentally retarded.

6. *Accident proneness:* Carelessness and uninhibited curiosity bring physical injury as well as social mishaps to these children. This differs from the adversities that befall those who are inexperienced, untaught, or so preoccupied that they are oblivious to hazards.

7. *Social ineptitude:* These children are friendly but so insensitive and lacking in empathy that their friends soon drift away. This differs from the behavior of "loners," who prefer their own company.

8. *Emotional superficiality:* Their style is bland, defensive, and denying. Relationships are kept at a shallow level. This differs from anxiety, self-centered obliviousness, or the inappropriate interactions of people who are psychotic and have disordered thoughts.

No one of these attributes in itself is diagnostic of hyperactivity. On the other hand, no child is likely to display all these characteristics. Among the younger, preschool children, restlessness, accident proneness, and recalcitrant behavior would be most noticeable. Among gradeschoolers, however, these children would be conspicuous as inattentive, hasty, and disruptive. In high school social ineptitude takes its toll, and the inconsequentiality may lead to antisocial and delinquent behavior. The motor restlessness has usually disappeared by this age. Among adults, failure to consolidate relationships and to maintain jobs may be the most apparent characteristics.

No one symptom is pathognomonic for the diagnosis of hyperactivity. Since a child cannot be expected to exhibit all the associated symptoms, it is necessary to rely on some criterion based on a number of positive entries in a checklist. However, each behavioral attribute can have more than one cause and must be analyzed with respect to its nature, before entering it in the checklist. In addition, it would not be expected that such behaviors would be confined to any one situation, such as the classroom. Children who appear hyperactive in the classroom but who are generally not so at home are unlikely candidates for a diagnosis of hyperactive (the reverse is equally true). Manifestations of hyperactivity are least apparent in familiar, unthreatening, and monotonous situations, common in everyday life. Nevertheless, the hyperactive child's temperament is apparent as a pervasive trait, not only in the child's learning but in psychosocial living.

TREATMENT MODALITIES

Medications

Learning disabilities are not known to be amenable to drug treatment. The agent piracetam, a cerebral activator, has some published claims as a facilitator of memory, however, and is currently undergoing clinical trial. By contrast, attention deficit (hyperactivity) is amenable to treatment by psychoactive drugs, and for most children this is the preferred treatment modality. The drugs most frequently used in hyperactivity are the psychostimulants; occasionally antidepressants and lithium are used.

The most common psychostimulants used are D-amphetamine (Dexedrine), methylphenidate (Ritalin), and pemoline (Cylert). The stimulants are catecholaminergic. Formulations of the nature of stimulant effects usually invoke their action in raising dopamine and norepinephrine levels in the brain. However, other neurotransmitter levels may also be changed. The inference is often made that because most hyperactive children respond at least to some extent to stimulants, they must be suffering from a deficiency in one or more catecholamine neurotransmitters. This inference is unwarranted because there is no evidence for a specific relationship between the therapeutic effect of any stimulant at the behavioral level and the change it induces in any neurotransmitter substance. Similarly, there is no conclusive reason to suppose that hyperactive children have lower than normal resting levels of any of the neurotransmitters. It is not even clear that when stimulants have beneficial effect, they do so by correcting abnormalities in the neurochemical deficiency in hyperactivity. It is equally possible that stimulants exert their effect by enabling other systems to courteract or to hold in check the causative pathology. There is no evidence that the effect of stimulant drugs is highly selective or specific at the level of the brain. This is also true at the level of behavior.

Stimulants are administered orally and are short acting. The half-life of D-amphetamine and methylphenidate in the bloodstream is approximately 2 hr. The behavioral time—response measurement places the maximum length of effect of a single administration at about 4 hr, Pemoline, and the slow-acting forms of methylphenidate and D-amphetamine are active for 4 to 8 hr. In each case multiple administration would be required for a therapeutic effect throughout the waking day. A cumulative action from day to day is not expected. In essence, each child who is on stimulant therapy is off stimulant therapy when he awakens each morning and again several times that day.

There are no restrictions on the use of these medications in terms of cross-reaction. It is felt that methylphenidate should be given in the fasting state (e.g., half an hour before meals). The behavioral effects of the stimulants are evident within half an hour to an hour after the first administration. In most cases, there is apparently little change in the effect across a course of treatment. A single dose is an approximate test case of how the child would react if administered the same agent in the same dosage for a longer term. Some children do appear to become tolerant between 4 and 8 weeks after initiation of stimulant therapy. Except in rare cases, minor upward adjustments of dosage overcome this difficulty. The stimulants have frequent side effects in the form of anorexia with attendant weight loss, and some sleeplessness until the right schedule is established. Conflicting reports assert and deny that growth retardation is a hazard. Where growth retardation is claimed to exist, it is usually stated that this is transitory and subsequently self-correcting. Drug addiction does not appear to be a hazard of stimulant treatment.

Overdose tends to precipitate the child into a state that is opposite of what characterizes him (and is complained of). The restless child becomes inert, the boisterous child socially withdrawn, the risk taker overcautious, the impulsive individual deeply reflective, and the hasty and careless person compulsive. Overdose effects wear off with the termination of the effect of the single dose, and if no further drug is given at the overdose level no ill effects result.

The behavioral effects of stimulant drugs have been extensively studied. They lack uniformity and instead appear to address only those behaviors that are most deviant in the particular individual. The stimulant drugs can apparently have opposite effects on different individuals. Thus they may slow down impulsive responding but accelerate hesitant responding, diminish motor restlessness but counteract hyperactivity, diminish emotional lability, and induce some emotionality in those who are unduly devoid of this characteristic.

Stimulant effects may be measured in terms of behavioral checklists, objective observation, and controlled performance tests. The effects of drugs can be measured in terms of reduction in prominence of complained-of behaviors (over a wide range of possibilities as exemplified in the Conners' questionnaires and DSM III checklists). Objective observation focuses both on the proportionate amount of time on-task and on various acting-out behaviors. Successful use of stimulants has been shown by objective means to counteract such difficulties. Laboratory controlled performance tests involve procedures demanding substained attention, such as continuous performance tasks or learning tests. Hyperactive children who perform poorly on any such test in the placebo state can generally be demonstrated objectively to perform better when taking the drug. It should be noted that there is no uniform improvement performance across the board. Indeed, there is some indication that the otherwise favorably responsive child may do a little less well on things that he is particularly good at—a matter that calls for close monitoring.

It has been suggested that the effect of stimulants on hyperactive children is by no means paradoxical, as has been believed, but is identical with that on normal children. This is not so in the strict sense, as normal children by definition do not show the behavioral deviations exhibited by the hyperactives so that the comparison is not meaningful. However, within the range of normal variation, children are placed outside that range. The effect, howbver, is correspondingly less.

At different stages in the life-span various "target behaviors" call for therapy and correspondingly the stimulant treatment has different effects. There is no evidence however that there is any systematic change in how stimulants act. As children get older or even that a patient's need for stimulant therapy, to foster adaptive functioning, differs across the life span.

Given the purely symptomatic nature of stimulant therapy it comes as no surprise that when the stimulant is discontinued the child generally manifests the same personality characteristics as before. The enduring effects of whatever social learning might have taken place during the course of therapy are not impressive. Follow-up studies indicate that when treatment is discontinued the prognosis is quite mixed. In many cases treatment has been prematurely discontinued (on account of the mistaken belief that the problem naturally resolves at around puberty). There are no good studies available of the prognosis for hyperactive children in whom long-term stimulant therapy is systematically continued.

The most difficult variable encountered in managing stimulant therapy is deciding on the dose to be administered. Although for conventional reasons most research studies use a milligram-per-kilogram formulation, there is no reason to suppose that this is the correct way to calculate dosage. The agent has considerable affinity for brain tissue and is not uniformly distributed through bodily tissues. The growing child does not require an increase in stimulant dosage in parallel with weight gain. Indeed, an adolescent may sometimes require doses that would seem quite small for younger children. At any given age or weight, however, there is a great range of optimal dosage between individuals. There is no short cut for determining this. It is necessary to perform a therapeutic test at each dosage change. A typical schedule would be to increase the dose of methylphenidate by 2.5 mg/week, in conjunction with observation by parents and teachers reported weekly to the clinician. The effect of stimulant therapy at any dose level declares itself quickly and if nothing is accomplished within a week a shift to a higher dose is justified. If a therapeutic effect does appear in a parental and teacher report on ratings, further minor increments are still justified in an attempt to identify the optimal dose level. A typical schedule would begin with 5 mg of methylphenidate three times a day (if control during classroom period time and at home is desired). With pemoline, a typical starting dose might be 37.5 mg in the morning and in midafternoon. Treatment may be initiated at any age including adulthood and there is no arbitrary cutoff age for treatment. Treatment is determined entirely by current clinical necessity. The only reservation is that stimulant therapy below the age of approximately 4, although in principle admissible, tends to be somewhat difficult to manage.

In hyperactivity, the only management option other than stimulant therapy for which any objective support exists is the use of the additive-free diet.[24] This treatment modality has its passionate advocates, as well as vehement opposition both from legitimate sceptics and industrial pressure groups. At the clinical level and the level of the open therapeutic trial, the evidence for beneficial effect of a diet that excludes, to the extent possible, artificial food dyes, flavors, and preservatives is massive. At the level of controlled (i.e., double-blind) experimentation, the beneficial effect of the additive-free diet (compared with control diets or the same diet with additives surreptitiously reintroduced) has been difficult to demonstrate. Challenge studies, which reintroduce, in a placebo-controlled fashion, the presumptively offending additives into the diet of hyperactive children, have also been differently interpreted by different investigators. The issues are presented in some detail by Kinsbourne.[25] For present purposes, a summary statement will suffice.

It is necessary to disassociate the beneficial effects of any treatment modality from the mechanisms of such effects. It is legitimate to doubt whether the effects of an additive-free diet, as reported by parents of hyperactive children, are specific enough to correct a brain metabolic dysfunction. There is less reason to doubt that many families profess themselves "better off" on this treatment. The clinician is not entitled to ignore the latter fact in pursuit of a more intellectually satisfying specific option (which happens not to be available). Indeed, lack of specificity invests all known treatments of hyperactivity. A significant minority of hyperactive children do appear to run into fewer adaptive problems on the Feingold diet, and for this reason it is advised that this option be presented to the parents at the initial interview. They must be warned that the diet, as currently used, is time consuming and expensive, and many families do not wish to burden themselves with this responsibility. Should the family desire to do so, however, the diet treatment should be attempted first (before drugs are instituted). Should it work then the problem is relieved (although adjunct stimulant therapy should still be considered to press home the advantage). Should it not work, the slate has been cleared for a serious consideration of the remaining options. A few weeks will suffice to make it clear whether a given child or family will benefit from this treatment modality.

Behavioral and Educational Options

A variety of behavior modification and cognitive training modalities have been advocated on behalf of hyperactive children. The goal is to help them control impulsive responding and the tendency to drift off task. There is no objective evidence that these measures, by themselves, alleviate the problem to any sufficient extent with generality across life situations. On the other hand, there is reason to believe that in some children these behavioral methods are useful adjuncts to drug and/or diet therapies. The same principle applies to educational measures. There is no known educational method that sufficiently and consistently constrains the attention to an academic task of a significantly hyperactive child. However if the child is receiving an effective stimulant therapy then a variety of educational strategies should be deployed. Clearly, the therapy does not teach but renders the child more receptive to learning. The educational approach may be of a straightforward nature, i.e., helping the child catch up. On the other hand, if the child is learning disabled, individualized techniques suitable to the particular problem can be deployed.

There has been comment that stimulant therapy in the long term fails to significantly advance childrens' educational achievements. An analysis of these studies reveals that these claims are ill founded. It can be concluded that children who are treated with drugs but do not receive educational support cannot learn. In all probability, a child who by virtue of effective stimulant therapy spends more time on task, doing homework, and practicing academic skills will correspondingly benefit in the long term by measurable advances in educational achievement. However, should treatment be terminated prematurely, regression may occur.

Irrational Therapies

Diseases for which there is a cure usually have one treatment. Diseases without a known cure usually have some treatments to offer. The diversity of arbitrary and irrational treatment modalities is particularly great in chronic disorders of childhood. Time is on the therapist's side with children as long as the therapy is sufficiently time consuming. Deficits caused by static lesions tend to ameliorate in almost any child as he grows older, due to superimposed cognitive development. However, despite how much the child falls short of normality, gains relative to the previous situation can usually be demonstrated. These gains are usually due to the normal maturation of the nervous system, but many therapists often claim the credit.

Therapies are unproven if they lack empirical support and irrational if they lack a credible theoretical basis. The practitioner need not necessarily insist on formal empirical support before deploying a treatment modality for a developmental disability. Should he do so, he would find himself singularly bereft of resources for his patients. However, if the clinician is to adopt a treatment modality that is unproven, it should at least be one that makes sense. Claims should be consistent with what is known about the function of the human body. The following is an incomplete listing of some of the better known irrational therapies for learning disabilities, since all lack acceptable theoretical basis as well as empirical validation:

1. *Patterning:* Methodologies developed by Doman and Delacato are now some decades old. They are based on an assumption that the developmental sequence is obligatory for efficient development; i.e., if the child "misses" any developmental stage, subsequent development would be handicapped. It logically follows that the child should be returned to the "missed stage," once that is identified. It is presumed that if the child is helped through that stage, abilities will flourish. A variety of sensory stimulations are applied in order to elicit function from the brain that it previously could not manifest. There is no scientific evidence that the patterning theory and the intense sensory stimulation required have the effects claimed by Doman and Dalacato. It has not been objectively demonstrated that on an empirical basis they do.

2. *Sensory integration therapy:* This methodology is derived from the hypothesis of Ayers, an occupational therapist who attributes learning disabilities to brainstem disorders of sensory integration. These problems include imperfect control of movement, impaired visual orientation to external space, difficulty in auditory processing, and distractibility. Ayers postulates that certain controlled forms of sensory stimulation can facilitate the formation of efficient connections at the brainstem level; i.e., vestibular stimulation improves auditory processes and assists children with language and learning disorders.

Although some clumsy children have impaired maturation of particular brain stem mechanisms, the evidence suggests that in learning disability the problem is at the cerebrocortical level. There is no evidence for the hypothesis that sensory stimulation, provided for an individual who had not been previously artificially deprived of such stimulation, modifies the growth and interconnection of neurons in the brain.

3. *Optometric training:* The obvious fact is that children with impaired vision may have difficulty in seeing and reading print, requiring corrective lenses. However, some optometrists have theorized that certain imbalances of eye movements may affect learning in a broader sense. It has been proposed that this imbalance can be corrected by a variety of eye exercises. However, attempts to validate the efficacy of this approach have consistently failed.

4. *Vestibular–cerebellar dysfunction:* Levinson has asserted that dyslexia is caused by a dysfunction in the relationships between the vestibular (balance) system and the cerebellar (movement control) system. He proposes to correct this imbalance by the administration of sea sickness remedies. The theoretical approach is idiosyncratic and no attempt at objective appraisal of the results of this treatment is apparent in Levinson's writings.

5. *Megavitamins:* Massive doses of vitamins have been recommended for the treatment of a variety of psychiatric disorders. The claim that this treatment helps learning-disabled children remain as unvalidated as the claim that it helps anyone suffering from any disease at all.

6. *Trace elements:* It has been theorized that deficiencies in elements that occur only to a trace extent in the body (e.g., chromium, copper, magnesium, manganese, and zinc) can cause learning disabilities. However, it has never been demonstrated that deficiency of any one or combination of these elements causes learning problems. Replacement therapies are practiced without a validated base.

7. *Hypoglycemia:* It has been claimed that low levels of blood sugars cause learning disabilities. However, no objective double-blind study has yet demonstrated that a corrective diet for hypoglycemia is in any way superior to a placebo. Furthermore, there has been no demonstration of a consistent abnormality in glucose metabolism in learning-disabled children or even a subset of those children.

8. *Allergies:* There are some reports of the effects of allergic reactions on subjective states, specifically in relationship to the so-called tension–fatigue syndrome. When these subjective changes occur in conjunction with more conventional and recognizable hallmarks of allergy (such as hives), the relationship is credible. Attempts to demonstrate that mental symptoms (unaccompanied by other signs of allergy) are allergic in nature have been inconclusive. The incidence of allergies is high in learning-disabled children, but it is also quite substantial in children without such problems; no specific effects have yet been proved.

9. *Negative ion therapy:* It has been claimed that stale, polluted, urban air changes the ionic balance. The deleterious effects of this ionic imbalance affects the child's ability to pay attention and learn. Devices that generate negative ions to replace those lacking under such circumstances have been proposed as a treatment for impaired classroom functioning. The methodology has not been shown to be efficacious.

10. *The phonic ear:* Tomatis proposed a curious set of assumptions about mental development, concluding that learning disabilities may be treated by presenting filtered

sound to children, with emphasis on their right ear (to foster left hemisphere dominance). This import from Europe is currently growing in Canada and will presumably travel south in the natural course of events. It clearly lacks a theoretical basis and its merits have not been empirically demonstrated.

RISK FACTORS AND PRECURSORS

Repeated attempts have been made to define an "at-risk" preschool population for learning and attention problems. The goal would be to institute early preventive measures. However, these risk factors have been exceptionally difficult to define. If school problems could be referred back to a particular etiology or pathogenesis, the problem would simply be one of detecting this. Instead, they represent the final common pathway of expression of many different adverse effects on the brain. Some of these factors include birth damage, toxic ingestion, and malnutrition. It is impressive from existing research how little of the learning-disabled and hyperactive population can be shown to have such antecedents. If birth damage is severe, it seems to result in the more complete disorders of mental retardation, cerebral palsy, and epilepsy. Milder birth damage is of very uncertain prognostic implication. Sameroff and Chandler[26] suggested that the outcome following mild birth injury is modulated by the socioeconomic setting in which the child is reared. They find that these children, reared in high socioeconomic contexts, do well. On the other hand, children of comparable early history reared in poverty may have bad outcomes. They refer to a "continuum of caretaker casualty," expressing their view that it is the *quality of caretaking* which makes the difference. Learning disabilities and hyperactivity have not been shown to be more prevalent in low socioeconomic circles. Malnutrition seems either to have no long-term effect or otherwise to have a rather diffusely retarding effect on mental development. The most impressive evidence identifies genetic factors. Numerous pedigrees of inheritance of dyslexia within families have been well defined. Recently it has been claimed that dyslexia is associated with a deletion in the short arm of chromosome 15.[27] In the case of hyperactivity, several adoption studies have indicated a familial tendency. It has been claimed that adult temperamental traits arguably analogous to hyperactivity in children are more prevalent with normal parents of these children (alcoholism, psychopathy, and hysteria). Recently, Deutsch *et al.*[28] showed that hyperactivity is far more prevalent among adopted than natural children in families and has further demonstrated that the reason for this has to be sought in biological factors (such as the parent's temperament or circumstances attending the pregnancy, usually that of an unwed teenager). In fact, nonrelative adoption is the most substantial risk factor for hyperactivity yet identified.

In contrast to biological determinants, it has never been satisfactorily demonstrated that the nature of interaction within the family is associated with the genesis of learning disabilities and hyperactivity. Hyperactivity and other behavioral problems might be overidentified based on the testimony of parents with a highly structured life-style and obsessive temperament. On the other hand, it may be underdiagnosed when parents' temperaments are the reverse. Part of the problem is that appraisals of parental temperament and child-rearing practices are made, retrospectively, and in ways lacking objectivity. Cause and effect can easily be confused. Parents who seem cold, negative, and withholding may indeed be so (or that may be the end point of lengthy, unhappy, and frustrating experiences with an intractable child). Parents who seem disorganized and incapable of setting proper limits may indeed be so (or this may be for them a survival tactic given the impossibility of enforcing any structure on a child who is exceptionally difficult to raise). Mental health professionals in general do well in refraining from attributing the causation of a child's problem (and the guilt that comes with it) to a parent, because (1) they can rarely be sure this is justified, and (2) even if they could be, there is nothing to be gained by doing so.

Precursors of learning and attention problems can be classified into those that are nonspecific associates and those that perhaps occupy early points on a developmental sequence that concentrates in cognitive processes relative to the area of difficulty. Thus the observation that minor congenital anomalies are more common in learning disabled children than controls is of research interest. The relationship is purely statistical, however, and too vague to be of clinical help.

Measurements of infant temperament are too controversial, and the opportunity of such temperamental traits across the passive changes of the early years of development is so ill established that little can be concluded of a practical nature.

Learning disability involving substantial general language development delay can usually be diagnosed well before school entry. Where there is substantial visuomotor difficulty, the clumsiness of the preschooler will often be apparent. The child of impulsive, inattentive, or emotionally labile temperament will similarly attract attention. In the absence of such major precursors, there is little of a screening nature that is worthwhile. Readiness for school entry is normally achieved at age 5 or 6, which presumably is why the beginning of grade school is so timed. If readiness skills are found lacking in younger children, this could be quite normal by the time of school entry by no more than a month or two is apt to make a damaging false-positive identifications. The child for whom school failure is predicted might, in a self-fulfilling prophecy, accomplish such failure.

One form of early identification is possible but is rarely attempted. It is the usual practice not to attempt to teach children academic subjects in preschool or kindergarten. The intention is to protect the children from undue pressure. This goal underestimates the natural curiosity and eagerness of young children. It is perfectly possible to teach the rudiments of school subjects before grade school entry in an unthreatening, noncompetitive, and appealing manner for short periods of time each day. Only such trial teaching can reveal the beginnings of problems within any such areas, should they exist.

PROGNOSIS

Valid prognostication is exceptionally difficult in the field of school problems. Management decisions such as the provision of individualized prescriptive education for a learning-disabled child or the clinically effective use of stimulant therapy for a hyperactive child often appear not to be attended by the anticipated improvement in educational task completion and increased achievement level. By contrast, some children for whom no promising management regimen has been implemented seem to improve spontaneously. Many factors presumably interact to determine the long-range prospects of a child with school problems: (1) the severity of the initial difficulty, (2) its relevance to adaptive behavior (which may differ, depending on the stage of the life span), (3) the extent and rate of ongoing maturation of the neural substrate of the disabled performance, (4) the provision of educational facilities appropriate to the child's difficulties, (5) the ability of teachers to motivate, (6) the degree of support obtained from the various relevant adults, (7) the nature and quality of the unaffected cognitive abilities, and (8) ultimately the vocational choice, the expectations of others.

It is well beyond the range of our present methodologies to measure any one, let alone all, of these, in interaction. Even the most common-sense educational provisions that all specialists in the field would agree on have never been objectively shown to be effective in the medium or long range. Instead of prognosticating, the clinician should confine himself to pointing out the wide range of possible outcomes: (1) a learning-disabled child may become a normally accomplished reader and writer or may remain functionally illiterate throughout life (specialized instruction notwithstanding); (2) the hyperactive individual may become a productive member of society, particularly in a vocation suited to an impulsive and sensation-seeking temperament, or may become an impulse offender, social isolate, or ineffectual employee and spouse. By default, our management options must always rely on the facts of the situation that prevails, rather than any that might be anticipated for the future. Neither what has happened in the past nor what is believed will happen in the future is of much use in determining what to do. Within the area of school failure, the closer the test is to the actual performance expected of the child, the greater its validity as a predictor. The best predictor for how a child will learn to read is how he learns to read! The necessary data base is a current description of the child's strength and weaknesses in intellect and temperament.

THE MEDICAL ROLE

In many areas of the country it is customary to refer children who suffer unexpected school failure for medical examination. What is asked of the physician is often not clear. A cure in the strict medical sense can hardly be envisaged. Prognosis is simply impossible. Failing the availability of useful steps in the three major areas of medical functioning, what is the physician to do? A diagnosis that specifies the cause of the irregularity of mental developmental is almost always conjectural and in any case has no practical application.

The physician's role may either be conceived narrowly or broadly. A narrow construction is as follows: (1) to scrutinize the child's general health to determine whether some factor extraneous to intellect is impairing performance (e.g., subclinical epileptic seizures, anemia, or even progressive degeneration of the brain); (2) to document of the child's neurodevelopmental status; (3) to make a diagnosis, for purposes of satisfying formal requirements of third party insurers, and of public agencies charged with providing resources for the learning disabled; and (4) to manage psychoactive medication regimens, when indicated.

In addition to the measures cited, the physician who wishes to intervene in a broader sense (1) coordinates the cross-disciplinary assessment of the child's learning difficulty and its socioemotional context, (2) interprets findings for family and school, (3) puts the child in contact with the appropriate multimodel remedial program, and (4) acts as part of the program counsel family and child.

Medical intervention involves two distinct lines: (1) the gathering of information about relevant aspects of the child's current function, and procuring appropriate help for him now, and (2) documenting the past, predicting the future, and responding to inquiries from parents, schools, and agencies. Only actions under the first category are of practical value to the patient. Actions in the second line address the needs of parties other than the child. Once the child's present status and needs have been sufficiently documented, the gathering of further information is unnecessary and detrimental in that it confuses the situation and distracts attention from the child's actual learning requirements.

THE INDIVIDUALIZED EDUCATIONAL PLAN

Under P.L. 94-142 and comparable laws at the state level, local school systems are mandated to provide an appropriate and adequate individualized educational plan (IEP) for every child with special needs, including children who are learning disabled. It is further required that such a plan be implemented in the least restrictive setting possible. The process by which these plans are formulated and implemented usually involves a physician only if it goes awry. When parents dispute the provisions of the IEP and refuse to accept it, the physician's opinion is often enlisted as to the plan's adequacy and practibility by one or other of the sides in the dispute. For this specialized purpose, the usual medical moves of diagnosing and recommending management options are insufficient. Differences of opinion about the IEP rarely revolve around such matters. Instead, the clinician is expected to show detailed familiarity with the provisions of the IEP, on the basis of which he is required to give an opinion as to whether (1) the IEP provides for individualized instruction at the child's developmental level (in other words at a level to which the child can relate); (2) the school system is able to deliver the program that it has offered, (3) the proposed instructor is capable of adopting a goal-oriented rather than rote approach to instruction, consistent with principles of individualization, and (4) the IEP makes provision for controlling any behavioral or emotional symptoms a child might have and safeguarding both him and other children against any adverse consequences of his conduct.

REFERENCES

1. Diagnostic and Statistical Manual of Mental Disorders, 3rd ed., American Psychiatric Association, 1981.
2. Kinsbourne, M., and Caplan, P. J.: *Children's Learning and Attention Problems*. Little, Brown, Boston, 1979.
3. Orton, S.: *Reading, Writing and Speech Problems in Children*. Norton, New York, 1937.
4. Galaburda, A. M., and Kemper, T. L.: Cytoarchitectonic abnormalities in developmental dyslexia; a case study. *Ann. Neurol.* **6:**94–100, 1979.
5. Satz, P.: Pathological left-handedness: An explanatory model. *Cortex* **8:**121–135, 1972.
6. Witelson, S. F.: Developmental dyslexia: Two right hemispheres and none left. *Science* **195:**309–311, 1977.
7. Kinsbourne, M.: *A model for the ontogeny of cerebral organization in nonrighthanders*, in Herron, J. (ed.): *Neuropsychology of Left-handedness*. Academic, New York, 1980, pp. 177–185.
8. Geschwind, N., and Behan, P.: Left-handedness: Association with immune disease, migraine, and developmental learning disorder. *Proc. Natl. Acad. Sci. U.S.A.* **79:**5097–5100, 1982.

9. Gordon, H. W.: The learning disabled are cognitively right, in Kinsbourne, M. (ed.): *Brain Basis of Learning Disability. Topics in Learning and Learning Disabilities*, Vol. 3. Aspen, Gaithersburg, Maryland, 1983, pp. 29–39.

10. Bakker, D. J.: Hemispheric differences and reading strategies: Two dyslexias? *Bull. Orton Soc.* **29**:84–100, 1979.

11. Kinsbourne, M., and Warrington, E. K.: Developmental factors in reading and writing backwardness. *Br. J. Psychol.* **54**:145–156, 1963.

12. Mattis, S., French, J. H., and Rapin, I.: Dyslexia in children and young adults: Three independent neuropsychological syndromes. *Dev. Med. Child Neurol.* **17**:150–163, 1975.

13. Pirozzolo, F. J., and Rayner, K.: Disorders of oculomotor scanning and graphic orientation in developmental Gerstmann syndrome. *Brain Language* **5**:119–126, 1978.

14. Doehring, D. G., and Hoshko, I. M.: Classification of reading problems by the Q-technique of factor analysis. *Cortex* **13**:281–294, 1977.

15. Petrauskas, R., and Rourke, B.: Identification of subgroups of retarded readers: A neuropsychological, multivariate approach. *J. Clin. Neuropsychol.* **1**:17–37, 1979.

16. Satz, P., and Morris, R.: Learning disability subtypes: A review, in Pirozzolo, F. J., and Wittrock, M. C. (eds.): *Neuropsychological and Cognitive Processes in Reading*. Academic, New York, 1981.

17. Vellutino, F. R.: *Dyslexia: Theory and Research*. MIT Press, Cambridge, Massachusetts, 1979.

18. Boder, E.: Developmental dyslexia. A diagnostic approach based on three atypical reading patterns. *Dev. Med. Child Neurol.* **15**:663–687, 1973.

19. Kinsbourne, M.: Sinistrality and risk for immune diseases and learning disorders: A pleiotropic gene effect? *Ann. Neurol.* **20**:416, 1986.

20. Pelham, W. E., and Bender, M. E.: Peer relationships in hyperactive children: Description and treatment. *Adv. Learning Behav. Disabilities* **1**:365–436, 1982.

21. Kinsbourne, M.: Toward a model for the attention deficit disorder. in Perlmutter, M. (ed.): *The Minnesota Symposium in Child Development*, 1983, pp. 137–166.

22. Douglas, V. I., and Peters, K. G.: Toward a clearer definition of the attentional deficit of hyperactive children, Hale, G. A., and Lewis, M. (eds.): in *Attention and the Development of Cognitive Skills*. Plenum, New York, 1980.

23. Kinsbourne, M., Swanson, J. M., and Herman, D.: Laboratory measurement of hyperactive children's response to stimulant medication, in Denhoff, E., and Stern, L. (eds.): *Minimal Brain Dysfunction: A Developmental Approach*. Masson, New York, 1979, pp. 81–106.

24. Feingold, B. F.: *Why Your Child is Hyperactive*. Random House, New York, 1975.

25. Kinsbourne, M.: Hyperactivity management: The impact of special diets, in Levine, M., and Satz, P. (eds.): *Middle Childhood: Developmental Variation and Dysfunction between Six and Fourteen Years*. Appleton-Century-Crofts, East Norwalk, Connecticut, 1984, pp. 487–499.

26. Sameroff, A. J., and Chandler, M. J.: Reproduction risk and the continuum of caretaking casualty, in Horowitz, F. D., Hetherington, E. M., Scarr-Salapatek, S., and Siegel, G. M. (eds.): *Review of Child Development Research*, Vol. 4. University of Chicago Press, Chicago, 1975, pp. 187–244.

27. Smith, S. D., Kimberling, W. J., Pennington, B. J., *et al.:* Specific reading disability: Identification of an inherited form through linkage analysis. *Science* **219**:1345–1347. 1983.

28. Deutsch, C. K., Swanson, J. M., Bruell, J. H., *et al.:* Overrepresentation of adoptees in children with the attention deficit disorder. *Behav. Genet.* **12**:231–238, 1982.

Dyslexia
An Ophthalmologist's Perspective

Roger L. Hiatt

OVERVIEW

The role of vision in learning is well known. It has been estimated that 85% of a child's learning involves the visual modality. In general, parents and teachers almost automatically first suspect vision difficulties as the cause of impaired reading skills. This chapter focuses on the child who has a reading problem but whose visual acuity is intact.

TERMINOLOGY/INCIDENCE/ETIOLOGY

Reading problems generally do not exist in isolation. Dyslexia (often used synonymously with "reading problem") in fact is only one form of reading disorder. Dyslexia has been defined as a family of CNS defects that share among other manifestations a handicapped ability to process the abstract symbols of language despite normal intelligence and adequate education. The terminology and classifications of the specific reading disabilities of dyslexia are extensive, reflecting the complexity of the problem.

Roger L. Hiatt • Department of Ophthalmology, University of Tennessee Center for the Health Sciences, Memphis, Tennessee 38163.

Among the terms more commonly used are central nervous system dysfunction, minimal brain dysfunction, and neurological dysfunction, pinpointing the cause of the reading disorders as a CNS disorder. Other diagnostic labels that have been used include hyperactive child and hyperkinetic child, implying either a secondary or primary behavioral manifestation of the reading disorder. Perception disability, perceptual handicap, visuomotor perceptual disability, or congenital word blindness suggest that the difficulty lies in the decoding of the visual image and in computerizing the visual data, rather than in the distortion of the visual input per se. Other terms encountered include reading disability, reading retardation, mirror vision, language disability, learning disability, and educational handicap, all of which refer to either the behavioral manifestations or the educational difficulty per se. Finally a term, with an anatomical/physiological connotation, strephosymobolia (''difficulty in handling symbols'') has been used to clarify the pathogenesis of the reading disorder. It has been estimated that in an average urban population approximately 8% of all children in the elementary grades have significant reading problems. Only 1% will have a specific reading disorder or dyslexia. The etiology of dyslexia is unknown, but multiple origins of reading problems have been defined. The range of etiologies associated with impaired reading skills is broad. Reading problems may be a consequence of overcrowding of (or transient) populations, which tax the child with marginal reading potential. Compulsory promotion and inadequate teaching have also been implicated as causes of reading deficiences. Emotional, psychological, and/or psychiatric disorders may be manifested as reading problems as well as organic deficits. Despite the voluminous accumulation of discussion, description, and theory about dyslexia, little progress has been made in understanding the basic causes of the disorder. The extensive literature on dyslexia reflects multidisciplinary interest and views of ophthalmology, psychology, speech/language, neurology, education, behavior science, psychiatry, audiology, pediatrics, physical therapy, and optometry.

A quotation from one of Hinshelwood's early reports (in 1900) in *Lancet* illustrates our progress:

> His difficulty in learning to read is no doubt due to some defect in his visual memory center which makes it much more difficult for him to retain and store the visual memories of words. This is the real explanation of the difficulty. It is not owing to any defect in his general intelligence or in any diminution of visual acuity.[1]

It has been estimated that 60% of schoolchildren will learn to read, regardless of the instructional system or method used. Another 20% will learn with a moderate investment of special assistance time, within the classroom situation. The remaining 20% with reading problems require special educational remediation, but less than one-half will require tutorial instruction or specific resource class participation. The relatively small residue of children will be diagnosed as having primary developmental dyslexia, perhaps 1% at the most. It has been suggested that dyslexia is inherited as a monohybrid autosomal dominant trait. It is most likely, however, that there is more than one mode of inheritance.

CHARACTERISTICS OF DYSLEXIA

There appears to be a higher incidence of reading disorders among children whose parents or grandparents exhibited similar problems. Neither the etiology of dyslexia nor the basis for the male predilection (male to female ratio is approximately 8 : 1) is understood. The children characteristically have at least average intelligence. There is no differential incidence based on socioeconomic factors. The dyslexic child characteristically reads one to two grades below the expected achievement level. The dyslexic child usually performs better in nonreading subjects such as mathematics, and an obvious disparity is noted between math and reading scores. The child rarely reads as a hobby or for enjoyment. Characteristically there is evidence of emotional confusion, dissatisfaction, and anxiety when the child is challenged in reading situations. Frequently mirror writing or reversal of letters, such as a *d* for *b* or *b* for *d,* is observed. Spelling is usually poor and writing is irregular and unattractive. Impaired concentration and a short attention span, are usually associated with dyslexia. A higher incidence of "dominance problems" (e.g., right-eyed and left-handed or left-handed and right-eyed) has been suggested, but the etiology is unknown. Visuomotor coordination deficits are frequently associated with dyslexia; the child may exhibit difficulties in drawing geometric shapes, and poor handwriting (dysgraphia) may be noted.

There is increasing evidence that a deficit or immaturity in the ability to equate or translate perceptions from one sensory system to another is an important factor in this reading disability syndrome. A child with a specific reading disability may fail tasks of visually and auditorally matching a letter with the alphabet; i.e., the child is unable to match items by looking, feeling, and/or listening. Direct confusion is generally a problem in understanding opposites, such as in and out, back and front, before and after, and yesterday and tomorrow. The conceptual problem is much more complex and involves the mechanisms of concept formation and processing. For example, the individual with a reading disability syndrome may be able to perceive a cup, whatever point of the compass it faces, and whether it is missing a handle. However, this same individual does not appreciate that alphabet characters and words change their significance when their direction or sequence is modified. The remedial program for severe cases of reading disabilities usually requires years of special therapeutic intervention. In some cases, little or no progress is made despite intensive therapy. Most affected children make some progress. For most, however, the ultimate reading level may be below that of their peers. Children with significantly above-average intelligence may become college graduates and appear to read normally. Their reading speed, however, is probably below that which is expected on the basis of their intelligence. Interest and skill in reading as a recreation will likely be . quite low.

The dyslexic child frequently exhibits a poor visual memory for language symbols. By repetitive drill, the child may learn that C A T spells cat, failing to recognize the word when it is presented at a later time. The traditional educational strategy of look-and-tell or flash-and-tell systems (teaching reading by flash cards) may be a disaster for the child with dyslexia. By contrast, phonetic augmentation of visual presentation may be of considerable value as an educational approach.

Basically, there are two groups of individuals with reading retardation. One group reflects an underlying neurological dysfunction, despite the absence of a history or signs of brain injury, referred to as a primary reading retardation or developmental dyslexia. The second category includes individuals with a reading retardation as a reaction to other pathology problems.

Gubbay *et al.*[2] noted a high incidence of agnosia, constructional apraxia, and electroencephalographic (EEG) abnormalities in children with severe clumsiness. Developmental dyslexia may arise from multiple anatomical sites. The existence of a congenital Gerstmann syndrome has been postulated. Perception apparently occurs in Brodmann's areas 18 and 19, which surrounds the visual cortex and communicates with the angular gyrus in the area of the parietal lobe. Perceptual development, a function of maturity, is important in (1) enabling the child to detect clues in printed works, and (2) permitting reading with speed, fluency, and understanding. Perception is not synonymous with vision or sight. Ocular acuity (resolving power) is the first step in the complex process of visual perception. The focused image on the retina is converted into an electrochemical stimulus that is transmitted from the optic nerve to the lateral geniculate body, along the optic radiations to the occipital cortex. The impulse is projected from the gray matter of the occipital lobe (with numerous synapses and cross-connections) into the angular gyrus in the parietal lobe. From the parietal lobe, the visually derived stimuli continue to the frontal lobe. These regions of the cerebral cortex are apparently associated with the ability to "intellectualize" or appreciate symbolic meaning of visual images (visual perception). In summary, meaningful utilization of the symbol (visual pictures), i.e., the printed word, depends on vision, perception, and conception.[3]

CLASSIFICATION OF DYSLEXIA

No single classification system of dyslexia has received universal acceptance. The following outline demonstrates the difficulty encountered in devising an all-inclusive categorization schema[4]:

Specific dyslexia or developmental dyslexia (strephosymbolia, dyssymbolia)
Secondary dyslexias (symptomatic, secondary reading retardation)
  Secondary to organic brain pathology
    Brain damage (cerebral dysfunction, encephalopathy, cerebral palsy, mental retardation, low IQ; perceptual disorders, word blindness, visual agnosia, anomia, soft neurological stigma)
    Genetic
    Post-traumatic
      Prenatal
      Natal
      Postnatal
    Postinflammatory (intrauterine, extrauterine)
      Encephalitis
      Meningitis
    Asphyxic (hypoxic) (intrauterine, extrauterine)
      Placenta previa
      Cord strangulation
      Maternal circulatory collapse
      Excessive maternal narcosis; drugs
      Circulatory collapse, cardiac arrest, cerebrovascular accident
    Prematurity
    Other specific brain lesions (e.g., aneurysm, cyst)

Secondary to slow maturation (''late bloomer''; developmental delay); associated with impaired lateralization and dominance
Secondary to emotional disturbances
  Hyperactivity, short concentration span
  Depression
  Anxiety
Secondary to uncontrolled seizure states
Secondary to environmental disturbances
  Cultural deprivation
  Poor motivation (extrinsic or intrinsic)
  Poor instruction
Slow readers (handicapped without symbolic confusion), bradylexia
  Asthenopia, visual handicaps (hyperopia, heterophoria, astigmatism, binocular control abnormalities)
  Auditory impairments
  Hypothyroid states
Acquired dyslexia (lesions of dominant hemisphere, angular gyrus, and splenium)
Mixed

EXAMINATION/SPECIAL TESTING

There is no evidence of an increased incidence of eye problems (visual acuity or motility) in patients with dyslexia. There is no special ophthalmological examination for dyslexia, but the examination should include as assessment of all components of vision and motility. The history deserves special attention, particularly to neurosensory signs and problems in behavior.

Special testing should be performed, by the primary care provider or the ophthalmologist, for any child suspected of having a reading disability. Special tests such as reading tasks using reading cards with appropriate questions can be used to screen for comprehension. It is important to establish an ongoing communication with the teacher to determine the quality of school performance. The Benton Visual Retention Test is a useful inventory that can be performed by office personnel (administration time approximately 15–20 min). This test of visual retention is scored according to grade level and age, providing clues of possible visual perceptual deficits. The eye track machine is avaliable primarily as a research tool, representing an improvement of the ophthalmograph tracking movement of the eye during reading. The apparatus provides an indication of reading speed, eye movements, the number of regressions, and the general ability to undergo pursuit movements necessary for reading.

DIAGNOSIS/TREATMENT

The role frequently assumed by the ophthalmologist is to provide a presumptive diagnosis of a reading disorder. In general the ophthalmologist is discouraged from assuming responsibility as ''captain of the team,'' a role more properly the responsibility of the pediatrician or primary care physician. The child should have complete physical and neurological examinations, with initiation of management strategies for organic psychological disorders. Obviously, if there are general health deficiencies or specific deficits in hearing or sight, these should be corrected. Psychological and/or psychiatric aspects of the child's problem should receive prompt remedial care. No evidence is available to date that motor treatment of the eyes per se has a specific benefit on improving the reading disorder. Decisions regarding group or individual reading therapy are primarily an educational consideration. Group (class) programs may be located in the regular school setting or in special facilities. The child may require individual tutorial support, (general educators or a special educator) in addition to resource assistance in school.

SPECIAL COMMENTS ON MANAGEMENT

In May 1979, Elmer B. Staats, Comptroller General of the United States, in reporting to both House and Senate Appropriation Committees, noted the widely different opinions between ophthalmologists and optometrists about the medical value of perceptual and visual training in treating visual disorders. He noted that officials at the National Institute of Health, National Eye Institute, reported that no existing scientific evidence conclusively proved the medical value of such treatment. The American Association of Ophthalmology, the American Academy of Ophthalmology and Otolarynology, and the American Academy of Pediatrics issued a joint organization statement (1971), *The Eye and Learning Disabilities*. The statement maintained that dyslexia and learning disabilities require a multidisciplinary management, involving at least medicine, education, and psychology. Eye care should never be instituted in isolation. There is no known scientific evidence supporting claims for improving the academic learning of disabled or dyslexic children based solely on (1) visual training, or (2) perceptual training. In 1981 the American Association of Pediatric Ophthalmology and Strabismus and the American Academy of Ophthalmology made the following statements:

1. Dyslexia and related learning disabilities, as well as other forms of learning underachievement, require a multidisciplinary approach from medicine, education, and psychology in evaluation, diagnosis, and treatment. Certain symptoms may be detected during infancy and early childhood through the use of screening techniques by educational specialists. Children with potential problems include those with speech defects, emotional problems, or family history of learning disability. These individuals should be assessed by educational and psychological specialists as early as possible to identify individuals who may exhibit indications of learning disabilities.
2. Eye care should never be instituted in isolation when a person does have dyslexia or a related learning disability. Children identified as having such problems should be evaluated for general medical, neurological, psychological, visual, and hearing defects. Any problems of this nature should be corrected as early as possible.
3. Since clues in word recognition are transmitted through the eyes to brain, it has, unfortunately, become common practice to attribute reading difficulties to subtle ocular abnormalities, presumed to cause faulty perception. Although eyes are

necessary for vision, the brain encodes visual information, resulting in "visual perception." Attention directed to the eyes would not be expected to have any effect on the brain's processing of visual stimuli. Indeed, children with dyslexia or related learning disabilities have the same incidence of ocular abnormalities, e.g., refractive errors and muscle imbalance (including near point of convergence and binocular fusion deficiencies) as children without. There is no peripheral eye defect that produces dyslexia and associated learning disabilities. Indeed, recent studies suggest that dyslexia and associated learning disabilities may be related to genetic, biochemical, and/or structural brain changes. Further controlled research is warranted.

4. No known scientific evidence supports claims for improvement of the academic abilities of dyslexic or learning-disabled children or modification of delinquent or criminal behavior with treatment based on

   a. Visual training, including muscle exercises, ocular pursuit or tracking exercises, or glasses (with or without bifocals or prisms)

   b. Neurological organizational training (laterality training, balance board, perceptual training)

   Furthermore, such training frequently yields deleterious effects. A false sense of security is created that may delay or prevent proper instruction or remedial therapy. The expense of such procedures is unwarranted, and appropriate remedial educational techniques may be omitted. Improvement claimed for visual training or neurological organizational training typically result from those remedial education techniques with which they are combined.

5. Excluding correctable ocular defects, glasses (with or without bifocals or prisms) have no value in the specific treatment of dyslexia or a related learning disability. In fact, unnecessarily prescribed glasses may create a false sense of security, delaying treatment.

6. The teaching of dyslexic and learning-abled children and adults is a problem of educational science. Proper, proven, expert educational psychological testing should be performed to identify the type of learning disability. Since remediation may be more effective during early years, especially before the development of a pattern of failure, early diagnosis is paramount. As mental and psychological factors contribute to a child's success or failure, no single educational approach is applicable to all children. A change in any variable may result in improved performance and reduced frustration (including placebo benefits).[5-13]

The identification and management of patients with dyslexia are difficult indeed, but with persistence on the part of the child, parents, and those working with them, most children can be helped. Patience is key to dealing with such children—and remember always that time is on their side.

REFERENCES

1. Hinshelwood, J.: Congenital word blindness. *Lancet*, **1**:1506–1508, 1900.
2. Gubbay, S. S., Ellis, E., Walton, J. N., *et al.*: Clumsy children—A study of apraxic and agnosic defects in 21 children. *Brain* **88**:295–312, 1965.

3. Goldberg, H. K.: Vision, perception, and related facts in dyslexia, in Keeney, A. H., and Keeney, V. T. (eds.): *Dyslexia.* C. V. Mosby, St. Louis, 1968, pp. 90–109.
4. Keeney, A. H.: Comprehensive classification of the dyslexias, in Keeney, A. H., and Keeney, V. T. (eds.): *Dyslexia.* C. V. Mosby, St. Louis, 1986, pp. 174–175.
5. Flax, N.: Visual function in dyslexia. *Am. J. Optom.* **45:**574–586, 1968.
6. Bettman, J. W., Jr., Stern, E. L., Whitsell, L. J., *et al.:* Cerebral dominance in developmental dyslexia: Role of ophthalmology. *Arch. Ophthalmol.* **78:**722–730, 1967.
7. Norn, M. S., Rindziunsky, E., and Skydsgaard, H.: Ophthalmologic and orthoptic examinations of dyslectics. *Acta Ophthalmol.* **47:**147–160, 1969.
8. Goldberg, H. K., and Drash, P. W.: The disabled reader. *J. Pediatr. Ophthalmol.* **5:**11–24, 1968.
9. University of Miami: Chromosome 15 may cause dyslexia. *Med. World News.* Dec. 22, 1980, p. 24.
10. Shaywitz, S. E., Cohen, D. J., and Shaywitz, B. A.: The biochemical basis of minimal brain dysfunction. *J. Pediatr.* **92:**179–187, 1978.
11. Galaburda, A. M., and Kemper, T. L.: Cytoarchitectonic abnormalities in development dyslexia. *Ann. Neurol.* **6(2):**96–100, 1979.
12. Cohen, H. J., Birch, H. G., and Taft, L. T.: Some considerations for evaluating the Doman–Delacato patterning method. *Pediatrics* **45:**302–314, 1970.
13. Committee on Handicapped Child: Doman–Delacato treatment of neurologically handicapped children. *Am. Acad. Pediatr. Newsl.* 1968.

7

Learning Disabilities
New Perspectives from an Educational Specialist

Dorothy Kletzkin

PROBLEMS RELATING TO DESCRIPTION AND DEFINITION OF LEARNING DISABILITIES

The cognitive development of the child identified as "learning disabled" has been the subject of varying hypotheses, considerable research, and controversy, for many decades. Interest in learning disabilities has been sparked by concerns of parents and professionals that some children may have difficulty acquiring and applying information presented in the traditional academic environment. In 1970, the United States Office of Education defined children with specific learning disabilities as

> Those children who have a disorder in one of the more basic psychological processes involved in understanding, or in using language, spoken or written, which disorder may manifest itself in imperfectability to listen, think, speak, read, write, spell or do mathematical calculations. Such disorders include perceptual handicaps, brain injury, minimal brain dysfunction, dyslexia, and developmental asphasia. Such terms do not include children who have learning problems which

Dorothy Kletzkin • Section of Learning Disabilities, Institute for Child Development, Hackensack Medical Center, Hackensack, New Jersey 07601.

are primarily the result of visual, hearing or motor handicaps, of mental retardation, or of emotional disadvantages.[1]

The term *general learning disabilities* has been similarly defined, but it also includes children who are mentally retarded. These definitions are in agreement with those proposed and accepted by the Council for Exceptional Children.[2] The concept of *exceptional* includes children outside the ''normal range,'' both gifted and retarded, as well as children with all types of handicaps. National recognition of the problem followed the enactment in 1975 of federal legislation (P.L. 94-142), which mandated appropriate identification and education for *all* handicapped children.

The ''spirit'' of P.L. 94-142 deserves recognition because it is an effort meant to improve services for the handicapped, including children with chronic disabling conditions and those with learning disabilities.

The initial concept and definition of learning disabilities was regarded as too restrictive and has been variously enlarged in scope. Cruickshank[3] defined learning disabilities within a developmental framework of acquisition of academic skills and social/emotional growth. He proposed that inasmuch as learning disabilities resulted from perceptual and linguistic processing problem deficits, it should be redefined without regard for etiology, age and level of intellectual functioning. The National Joint Committee for Learning Disabilities (NJCLD), a confederation of many professional organizations, proposed the following definition for learning disabilities:

> Learning disabilities is a generic term that refers to a heterogeneous group of disorders in the acquisition and use of listening, speaking, reading, reasoning or mathematical abilities. These disorders are intrinsic to the individual and perceived to be due to central nervous system dysfunctions.
>
> Even though a learning disability may occur concommitantly with other handicapping conditions (e.g., sensory impairment, mental retardation, social and emotional disturbance) or environmental influences (e.g., cultural differences, insufficient/inappropriate instruction, psychogenic factors) it is not the direct result of those conditions or influences.[4]

The field of study is thus compromised by a multiplicity of criteria and limited ability in identifying the maladaptive behaviors that characterize a learning disability. There is even less agreement about treatment or remediation strategies, although considerable interest and research has been generated in this area. The wide diversities in professional orientations and approaches has been responsible for significant divisions within the field. These disparities are reflected educationally, scientifically, and politically. The myriad of professional and parent organizations, journals, and symposia devoted to the cause of helping these children is a manifestation of diverse concepts and approaches. However, despite the variations in definitions, classifications, and treatment strategies, a basic and consistent hypothesis is that learning disabilities are caused by limitation in the basic psychological processes required to achieve successful academic performance. Paradoxically, although intelligence tests were designed to predict academic performance, IQ tests are regarded as inadequate for the measurement of learning deficits. Another hypothesis concerning the etiology of learning disabilities suggests that the problem is not the fault of the student or the teacher but is rather the result of varying neurological approaches that cause the disability or cognitive limitations. Each child therefore requires special treatment or remediation based on the individual characteristics, etiology, and prognosis. The objective is to identify the basic subtypes or models allowing for some commonality of diagnosis and intervention.

On the basis of these assumptions, fueled by concerns of parents and government, special education programs and research have been devoted to identification of substrates characteristic of the learning-disabled child. Research and results of various remedial practices suggested several specific theories and models about the causes of learning disabilities. However, numerous hypotheses, although fashionable for varying periods, have subsequently fallen into disfavor because of insufficient reliability and/or validity, or from failure to help the child.

REVIEW OF MAJOR LEARNING DISABILITY THEORIES

Analysis of the myriad of descriptions and definitions of learning disabilities generally reveals two fundamental approaches: (1) biological or neurophysiological, and (2) behavioral. Educators and psychologists favor the behavioral approach because analyses of tasks and situational variables are more useful in attempting to remedy the child's learning disabilities. The behavioral approach emphasizes an association between learning disabilities and deficiencies in learning behavior. This approach suggests that etiological factors have little relevance to the intervention process. Some educators view a focus on etiology as an excuse for educational failure. Greater significance is placed on the formulation of behavioral objectives and organizing subtasks and teachable units. The latter can be assessed by examination of the effectiveness of the teaching techniques and materials. Comparisons are made with baseline data obtained before initiating intervention strategies. Behaviorists postulate the effective teaching of a sequential hierarchy of skills (from the simple to the more complex), with constant feedback and encouragement, is the key to successful educational remediation.

By contrast, the neurophysiological model focuses on the child's deficits. It depicts learning disabilities as resulting from perceptual processing deficits (PPD); i.e., since perceptual processes are the result of central neural activity, neurological deficits must be a major factor in dysfunction.

Orton[5] proposed an alternative neurophysiological concept. He postulated that cerebral dominance (inappropriate cerebral dominance) causes problems such as "dyslexia." Orton advocated "training" to strengthen the left cerebral hemisphere—his successors are still promoting this approach, but in modified forms. The Orton Dyslexia Society has grown into a national organization whose specific objective is to assist the numerous children and adults with "learning" difficulties (dyslexia).

Several research studies suggest that there may be a genetic predisposition for specific types of learning disabilities. Reading disabilities, spelling, mathematical disabilities, and/or hyperactivity are frequently found in several family members.[6]

Calanchini and Traut[7] have proposed a concept that amalgamates the neurophysiological and behavioral models, relating learning theory to brain function. The hypothesis proposes that learning disabilities is cortical in origin, resulting from inefficient function in the phylogenetically and autogenetically newest and most complex areas of the brain. It has been postulated that the prefrontal, inferior parietal, and inferior temporal regions are the last regions to mature in the developing brain and would most likely vary in degree of development. Therefore, learning disabilities result from inefficient function in these or adjacent cortical areas. However, a more sophisticated understanding of brain anatomy and physiology and their relationship to function is necessary to appreciate the child's learning disability, regardless of etiology. Calanchini and Traut[7] noted that it is "possible to relate the neurology of learning to diagnostic appraisal and educational remediation of children with neurological learning disabilities. What is known about the brain and learning can be incorporated in the selection of a diagnostic test battery, in outlining guidelines for the interpretation of test data and behavior, and in determining the selection of remediation materials and techniques."

MODELS OF LEARNING DISABILITIES

Before examining various models of learning disabilities, some general observations on identification and evaluation are in order. It is generally agreed that biological and environmental factors contribute to the complex nature of a learning disability. Therefore, it is anticipated that some children will manifest only neurophysiological deficiencies or behavioral deficiencies, while others may exhibit both deficits.

Regardless of the significance attached to specific causative factors, children are identified as learning disabled only if they have a learning problem. Evaluation of the relative contributions of biological and environmental factors aids in classifying the student and, it is hoped, in providing an optimal remediation program. Although the particular preference of a model of learning disabilities may well influence assessment and therapy, the present state of knowledge mandates flexibility and pragmatism in dealing with the learning disabled student.

Neurophysiological Perceptual-Deficit Models

The studies of Strauss and Lehtinen[8] with brain-damaged mentally retarded children are credited with differentiating learning disabilities as distinct and separate from mental retardation. Their observations defined the similarities in behavioral and biological characteristics of certain groups of children and brain-injured soldiers (World War I). These children were classified as exogenously retarded, in contrast to endogenously retarded children due to genetic or familial factors. The children in the former group manifested perceptual disorders, conceptual problems, and behavioral dysfunctions. These neurodevelopmental deficits are suggestive of underlying brain damage when associated with (1) soft neurological signs, (2) a history of neurological impairment, and (3) absence of familial mental retardation.

Although their studies and hypotheses have been critized, Strauss and Lehtinen had a profound influence on strategies for remediation and research in learning disabilities. Kephart,[9] Getman,[10] Cruickshank,[11] Barsch,[12] and Frostig et al.[13] adopted the basic neurological–physiological orientation of learning disabilities. The focus of their research was on the learning-disabled child who was not retarded but who evidenced impairment in one or more underlying perceptual processing abilities. These perceptual processes include (1) auditory abilities (auditory discrimination and memory), (2) visual abilities (visual discrimination and spatial relationships), (3) cross-sensory perceptual abilities (auditory–visual integration), and (4) psycholinguistic abilities (auditory sequential memory and linguistic verbal expression). Kirk and Kirk[14] characterized these problems as follows:

> Children with perceptual disorders are those whose sensory abilities are intact but do not perceive, discriminate or recognize efficiently in one or more of the sense modalities. A child who can hear sounds but is unable to discriminate or recognize them is said to have an auditory perceptual problem. A child who cannot recognize the faces of his classmates until he hears their voices is one who has a visual perceptual disorder. . . . In addition, there are disturbances in speed of perception, figure-ground discrimination, closure ability or other difficulties dealing primarily with auditory and visual nonsymbolic perceptual problems.

"Deficit" proponents suggest remedial interventions based on the hypothesis that (1) impairments in processing skills are related to inability in mastering basic academic skills, such as use of language or reading; (2) remediation is a prerequisite to successful academic performance; and (3) discrete elements of the perceptual processes can be identified, measured, and remediated by matching instruction to individual learning needs. It is hypothesized that children who have a specific learning disability in auditory or visual discrimination may not progress in school until they receive an intense individualized remedial program.[14,15] The focus on *discrimination learning* was translated into a process-oriented approach to teaching.

This model has also been referred to as *diagnostic-prescriptive* teaching, i.e., formulating instructional prescriptions based on differential diagnostic assessment results. The therapy program is designed to remediate the specific ability weakness, formulating an instructional curriculum based on the child's strengths and weaknesses.[15] Arter and Jenkins[16] combined the terms differential diagnosis and diagnostic prescriptive teaching (DDPT) as a label that encompassed a number of "process" models. Formerly a variety of labels had been used: diagnostic remedial approach, prescriptive teaching, ability and process training, and psycholinguistic training.

The field of special education has experienced a proliferation of tests and training programs based on the DD–PT strategy. Among tests used in resolving the differential diagnoses are the Peabody Picture Vocabulary Test,[17] the Purdue Perceptual Motor Survey,[18] the Benton Visual Retention Test,[19] and the Goldman–Fristoe–Woodcock Test of Auditory Discrimination.[20] One of the more popular test inventories was the Illinois Test of Psycholinguistic Abilities (ITPA),[21] Arter and Jenkins[16] suggest that the proliferation of assessment batteries reflect an "urgency" to develop effective and innovative remedial techniques because of the high cost of special education services, and often the ineffective outcome. In addition, the more global instruments used for educational assessment (IQ tests and group achievement tests) are inadequate for planning remedial instruction. Specific educational testing inventories are appealing because they differentiate special education teachers from general educators and other professionals. The former focus is directed toward process and not product. Within this fertile professional milieu, publishers capitalized on a lucrative market for providing testing and training materials touted as "cures" for perceptual deficits.

Neurophysiological, psycholinguistic, and differential diagnostic-prescriptive teaching has been criticized on theoretical and empirical grounds. Assumptions generated from this model have been challenged because of its questionable validity and failure to demonstrate improvements in academic skills. Hammill and Larsen[22] noted that if psycholinguistic training is valid, it would strengthen weak areas and result in improved classroom learning. However, if the assumption is not valid, much time, effort, and money would be needlessly expended.

The premises underlying this model are the following: (1) educationally relevant psycholinguistic, perceptual–motor, auditory, and visuoperceptual processing disabilities exist and can be appropriately isolated, measured, and remediated; (2) the learning-disabled population has a uniformly unidimensional cerebral dysfunction; (3) tests used for differential diagnosis are valid and reliable; (4) valid educational prescriptions can be developed that will remediate deficits; (5) remediation of deficits will lead to improved academic performance and school successes; and (6) prescriptions can be formulated from diagnostic profiles that will have an impact on academic achievement, with direct training in areas of weak ability. Cumulatively, these hypothetical claims serve to emphasize the inadequacies of the model and to raise questions regarding its validity.

These assumptions have been criticized because almost none of the claims made by this model is defendable. The claim that there are perceptual processing disabilities that can be appropriately isolated has been questioned. Indeed, there has been little agreement on ability labels. Hammill[23] noted that some investigators view perception as the process from stimulus reception to cognitive analysis, while others have assigned perception to nonsymbolic, nonabstract stimuli. These diversities in terminology generate confusion in communication among professionals—inter- and intradisciplinary miscommunications.

Another obstacle is the difficulty in attempting to measure these basic hypothetical constructs. Underlying abilities or potentials cannot be accurately assessed by observing responses to activities which are believed to be diagnostic, since these tasks are influenced by the variables. For example, the seemingly simple task of motor manipulation of blocks is influenced by such factors as visual perception, motoric ability, cognitive interpretation of instructions, short-term memory, meditation, rehearsal, and application. In essence, the accurate assessment of isolated abilities is basically a deceptive measurement.

It is also difficult to demonstrate that those factors that hinder the learning-disabled child from mastering basic academic skills are significantly different from characteristics noted in other deficient learners. Paradoxically, children with no discernible abnormalities may manifest serious learning deficits, whereas children identified as learning disabled may be functioning in the average range of academic achievement.

The basic hypothesis of a uniformly unidimensional cerebral dysfunction that correlates with learning and academic disabilities has not been supported. Nevertheless, for many years (1950s to the early 1970s), educational therapy for learning-disabled youngsters tended to be univocal. The child was most often enrolled in a remedial program that offered isolated interventions. Although failing to convince educationalists, research-clinicians demonstrated that the mental processing operations underlying academic achievement are variable in its clinical presentation.

Studies focusing on reading, stemming from the work of Orton, have resulted in data on the generic problem designated developmental dyslexia. This category of learning disability may include disorders in reading, spelling, mathematics, and language, or combinations of these problems. In attempting to provide a taxonomy of learning disabilities, the major focus had been on the identification of subtypes that attempt to delineate a more homogeneous grouping of impairments. These subgroups attempt to establish a diagnosis by definition of attributes, rather than a diagnosis by exclusion.

Subtype characteristics can also be used in designing a more meaningful remedial program. Efforts in delineating a classification of subtypes of learning disabilities, particularly in both general and dyslexic groups, have increased in intensity.

Using different techniques, Johnson and Myklebust[15] and Boder[24] were able to distinguish an audiophonological and visuospatial type of disability. The differentiation is established by examining the kinds of reading and spelling errors children make. Boder classified children into three groups: (1) dysphonetic disability (difficulty with symbol–sound integration), (2) dyseidetic (Gestalt-blind or word-blind) deficits (difficulty in the ability to perceive letters and whole words as a configuration), and (3) mixed dysphonetic–dyseidetic–dyslexia–alexia (combinations of 1 and 2). She suggested that there was a much higher incidence of dysphonic dyslexia in English-speaking and English-reading children.

Mattis *et al.*[25] studied 113 children and identified three distinct syndromes. These syndromes accounted for 90% of the subjects' disabilities: (1) primary language disorder, (the largest group); (2) discoordination in articulatory and graphomotor activities and (3) visuoconcentration, and visuospatial–perceptual difficulties (the smallest category).

Morrison *et al.*[26] examined memory-encoding skills in poor and good readers and concluded that "learning disabled children may have problems in information processing, perhaps in encoding, organization or retrieval skills." Satz and Fletcher[27] and Kinsbourne[28] theorized that these children may have a developmental lag. They are not classified as mentally retarded because they are processing in the same sequence as their peers, but at a much slower rate. As a result, children with developmental lags are limited in their ability to participate in age-related school tasks. Rourke[29] supported the concept of "immaturity," more particularly a lag in the maturation of the left cerebral hemisphere. He noted that these children do not "catch up" in reading ability; he therefore postulated a deficit rather than a developmental lag. Petrauskas and Rourke[30] identified three distinct subtypes of retarded readers: (1) poor concept information, moderately to severely impaired verbal fluency, word blending, and sentence memory; (2) impaired ability to sequence, poor linguistic ability, and deficits in finger recognition; and (3) deficits in visuospatial memory and verbal coding. Investigations of the deficit model suggest that these children experience difficulty in effectively acquiring and integrating information; poor linguistic abilities, rehearsal, and control processes; and memory deficiencies.

Pirozzalo[31] suggested that dyslexia could be divided into two subgroups: (1) an auditory–linguistic group with deficits in verbal ability, and (2) a group characterized by deficits in visuospatial–perceptual ability. Pirozzalo differentiated the two groups on assessment of lateralization and visuoperceptual, eye-movement latency, and patterns during reading.

The third edition of the Diagnostic and Statistical Manual of Mental Disorders (DSM III)[32] provided the following diagnostic options:

1. Attention-deficit disorder
   a. With hyperactivity
   b. Without hyperactivity
   c. Residual type

2. Developmental reading disorder
3. Developmental arithmetic disorder
4. Developmental language disorder
   a. Expressive type
   b. Receptive type
5. Developmental articulation disorder
6. Mixed specific developmental disorders
7. Atypical specific developmental disorder

The classification equates developmental reading disorder with developmental dyslexia. The descriptive diagnosis recommends that there be a 1–2-year discrepancy in reading skills, as compared with chronological age, mental age, and school experiences for children between the ages of 8–15. No guidance for deficit performance in those above or below those ages is provided. The characteristics are described in the previous research, such as difficulties in oral reading, comprehension, writing and copying ability, bizarre spelling, and language disorders. Added to the classification are behavioral problems, such as attention-deficit disorders and conduct disorders. Thus, the DSM III encompassed and formalized the specific disability of dyslexia.

Research data clearly do not support the concept that learning disabilities or reading disabilities can be attributed to a single specific anatomical dysfunction. Findings suggest a bimodal separation into left and right hemispheric specialization of function. Subgroups with verbal deficiencies appear to have reduction or inappropriate use of the left hemisphere, in contrast to those with visuospatial dysfunction who have damaged right hemispheric capacity.

Studies suggest questionable validity and an ambiguous relationship between academic achievement, differential diagnosis, and prescriptive teaching tests. Investigations of construct validity have similarly yielded mixed results. They challenge the hypotheses of Kirk and Kirk,[14] which relate responses on the Illinois Test of Psycholinguistic Abilities (ITPA) to reading disabilities, speech disorders, mental retardation, cerebral palsy and depressed socioeconomics. Overall, there is a lack of empirical support for psycholinguistic and visual–auditory proponents. Whether these abilities are crucial for academic success and require specific training has been investigated. Several review articles emphasize that psycholinguistic training is not effective. It has been concluded that sensory modality training does not merit even minimal support.

Advocates of the modality preference approach take exception to this conclusion. Unfortunately this view is similar to that of many special educators. They have ignored or are unaware of the cumulative research indicating that modality preference strategies have no positive effect.

Cerebral Laterality Studies

There is an expanding data base of the specialized, discrete functioning of the two cerebral hemispheres. Differences in right and left brain information processing seem to be offering new insights into the differences between normal and learning-disabled children. The accumulated fund of information indicates that the left hemisphere appears to be specialized for language functions: (1) Broca's area (located in the frontal lobe), producing smooth, well-articulated language; and (2) Wernicke's area (in the temporoparietal lobe), concerned with the semantic meaningful aspects of language. These specializations are a consequence of the greater effectiveness of left hemisphere in processing modes of thought, of which verbal language processing is one manifestation. The right hemisphere is believed to be more effective for pictorial, intuitive, subjective, synthetic, visuospatial, holistic manner of mediating information.

Historical Background

Gall in 1850 proposed that the human brain was an assemblage of discrete organs, each of which formed the material substrate of a specific intellectual facility or personality trait.[33] This concept initiated the pioneering studies of Broca[34] in 1863 and of Fritsch and Hitzig[35] in 1870 that provided evidence that the brain is localized for specific functions. Broca demonstrated that trauma to the left temporal region results in distruption of language far more frequently than does injury to the right temporal area. Wernicke in 1874 confirmed and extended Broca's findings, describing the kinds of aphasia that may be related to different lesion sites in the left hemisphere.[36] The early studies of Fritsch and Hitzig[35] demonstrated, by electrical stimulation of the cerebral cortex, that there is crossed cortical localization of motor control.

Historically, the left hemisphere was considered the dominant hemisphere, in terms of language and handedness, while the right was considered the "newer" or subordinate hemisphere. It was not until the studies of Jackson in 1874 that unique functions were assigned to the right (minor) hemisphere.[37] Jackson suggested that this portion of the brain served distinctive purposes in the mediation of mental activities, noting that damage to the right hemisphere was associated with loss of visuospatial perception, failure to recognize faces, and inability to recall names or to dress oneself. Piercy postulated the existence of two distinct and interacting apparatuses of the brain, one mediating "verbal conceptual" thinking, the other mediating "spatial-practical" thinking.[38]

Clinical Research

During the 1920s and 1930s, there was great interest in describing and assigning behavioral deficits to lesions in certain brain sites. By the 1940s, many theories of intelligence stressed the diversity of cognitive skills of the two hemispheres. Studies, particularly of brain-injured World War II veterans, further delineated the function of the right and left brain in their areas of specialization. As the growing body of research defined right–left hemispheric functioning, the concept of cerebral dominance was modified in favor of the notion of hemispheric specialization rather than of dominance. Research emphasis shifted to an interest in discovering how the various mental processes are distributed between the two hemispheres. Neuropsychological research progressed from observing cognitive deficits following brain damage to defining functional specialization of the two hemispheres.

Split-Brain Research

The most dramatic data in split-brain research was obtained as a result of neurosurgical attempts to control the spread of epilepsy. Split-brain surgery (commissurotomy) was originally performed on the cat by Myers and Sperry.[39] In experimental animals, each cerebral hemisphere appears to be equivalent to the other with respect to cognitive functions. Sperry and Myers observed that in cats that were monocularly trained on visual discrimination tasks interocular transfer did not occur. This finding indicated that visual learning is restricted to the trained half of the brain.

Bogen et al.[40] then proposed that the brain could be split for the purpose of controlling the interhemispheric spread of epilepsy, which proved to be largely correct. The first patient, W.J., was extensively studied both pre- and postoperatively on a series of tests devised at the California Institute of Technology. The purpose was to study each hemisphere systematically in isolation, as well as the function of the corpus callosum. In subsequent studies, W.J. and 12 other surgically "disconnected" patients were observed, providing information and direct comparisons of the behavioral and processing capacities of the segregated hemispheres.[40,41]

Despite the massive size of the sectioned neocortical system estimated to contain more than 200 million fibers cross-connecting nearly all regions of the cerebral cortex, a commissurotomy apparently causes little change in daily behavior. Sperry and co-workers[42,43] noted that a patient 2 years after a commissurotomy might pass a routine medical checkup without demonstrating evidence of having undergone the surgical procedure. Verbal reasoning, speech, calculation, established motor coordination, memory, personality, and temperament were apparently preserved, to a surprising degree. The left and right hemispheres appear to function independently as parallel, separate, fully conscious minds. Numerous studies demonstrate the superiority of the right hemisphere on nonverbal tasks, whereas the left half-brain appears to be the hemisphere of choice for verbal processing. The studies can be criticized on the basis that some compensatory reorganization of cerebral function has occurred. Additional criticisms include (1) the relatively small number of patients, (2) the variations in surgical technique, and (3) the predisposing factor of patient variability. The extensive nature of the surgery per se and the postoperative reorganization of the brain must also be considered.

In order to evaluate the results of split-brain research, a number of less invasive techniques have been used to assess lateralization of hemispheric function. However, split-brain research was an important part of the development of neuroscience and neurology.

Dichotic Listening Research

Dichotic listening and tachiscopic visual half-field research is based on the hypothesis that a stimulus presented to the hemisphere specialized for the processing of that activity will result in a performance superior to that obtained when the stimulus is presented to the opposite hemisphere. The evidence suggests that each ear has strong connections to the opposite hemisphere, with minor connections to the ipsilateral hemisphere. The auditory input is transmitted across the corpus callosum and through the minor ipsilateral and the major contralateral pathways. When both ears receive input, the ipsilateral pathway is blocked and sound is transmitted only through the contralateral pathway. Information transmitted across the corpus callosum seems to be weakened because the hemisphere is engaged with the other input. It is then possible to test ear advantage on various listening tasks.

A dichotic listening task study conducted by Kimura[44] consisted of subjects listening to different pairs of digits presented simultaneously in rapid succession through sound-isolating earphones. The right ear input was more frequently and more accurately reported than was the left ear input, suggesting that the right ear advantage was an indication of left brain dominance. This is not an unexpected finding, since the left ear message must first go to the right hemisphere before transferring to the contralateral hemisphere's auditory system. Extensions of these studies with careful selection of the stimuli have served to help clarify cerebral localization. The findings of these investigations include (1) the superiority of the left hemisphere (right ear) for language tasks, and (2) the function of the right hemisphere (left ear) for nonlanguage musical pitch perception, environmental sounds, and vocal nonspeech sounds such as coughing, laughing, and crying.

Tachistoscopic Research

In the standard lateralized tachistoscope presentation procedure, subjects fixate on a point straight ahead while a stimulus is briefly flashed either to the left or to the right of the point of fixation. The human visual system projects information seen to the right or left of a control fixation point, exclusively to the contralateral hemisphere.

In "split-brain" patients, the initial lateralization to one hemisphere or the other is possible to maintain because the connective pathways have been severed. In a normal subject, however, unless the tachistoscopic presentation is briefer than the latency of saccachic eye movements (less than 200 or 150 msec), the information will be perceived by each hemisphere. Therefore, investigations have focused on the rapidity of reaction time. The reasoning is the same as in dichotic listening tasks; i.e., one hemisphere will be able to process information more accurately and faster according to the nature of the task. These studies have confirmed the compensatory mediation of the hemispheres in processing and reacting to stimuli. The right visual field/left hemisphere reveals superiority in identifying letters and words, whereas the left visual field/right hemisphere is superior in visual spatial parallel processing (recognition of faces, depth perception, appreciation of configuration and structure of words and letters).[45]

Electroencephalographic Studies

Although dichotic listening and tachistoscopic presentation of stimuli have been productive techniques for studying hemispheric functional differences, both methods have been subject to criticism. They are not measures of cerebral activity per se. Cerebral involvement within the context of a specific cognitive activity can only be inferred. By contrast, electrical activity of the cortex can be recorded while the subject is performing a task. Changes in the patterns of activity can be used to study the loci and degree of cerebral involvement. The electroencephalogram (EEG) and average evoked potentials are the most common methods of recording EEG phenomena, in order to assess changes in asymmetry of cerebral function. Waveforms can be grouped into bands on the basis of frequency and associated amplitude. Of particular interest are α (8–12 Hz) and β (over 13 Hz) frequencies. The α rhythm characterizes relaxed wakefulness. The waves are largest over the occipitoparietal areas when the eyes are closed. If the eyes are opened or a sensory stimulus is presented, the α rhythm is "suppressed" and replaced by a β rhythm having higher frequency and lower voltages. This phenomenon has been used to identify and localize hemispheric involvement during a particular task.

The average evoked potential is a measurement of the specific changes in the electrocortical responses to external events such as auditory or visual stimuli. These event-induced electrical "peaks" are very small and virtually undectable individually. However, if the event is repeated many times and averaged by a computer, a waveform emerges. The shape and temporal characteristics of the wave depend on the modality of the stimulus, cortical location, and task. Differences in α suppression between the right and left hemispheres confirm (1) preferential left hemisphere utilization on verbal language-related tasks, and (2) right hemisphere engagement for tasks such as face recognition or for visuospatial imagery and listening to music.

There is also some indication that the degree of α suppression may be related to the intensity and efficiency at which the subject performs the tasks presented. Studies have reflected that less efficient global operation may initially activate the right hemisphere and shift quickly to the left hemisphere in proportion to the speed of task solution. Clinical research has also shown that responses to musical and rhythmical stimulation tasks are known to activate the right hemisphere but involve the left hemisphere as well. Normal, less analytical, nonmusician responses show more specific right hemisphere activation, whereas experienced, higher-level musician responses are more likely to demonstrate left hemisphere specialization. However, most EEG research confirmed what is known about brain lateralization for speech and nonlanguage stimuli.[46,47] Electroencephalographic and evoked potential (EP) studies have generally proved to be of limited use because of the large amount of information that must be analyzed to interpret brain function. These require spectral analysis, temporal summation, and statistical analysis. The sophisticated analysis of EEG by computers has opened up many new diagnostic possibilities. Of particular interest are neuroimaging techniques, brain electrical activity and mapping (BEAM), topographical EEG mapping, and sensory-evoked potentials (EP), which have extended investigations of brain function in learning-disabled children.

During the mid-1970s, Duffy et al.[48] developed a comprehensive computerized procedure to enhance the interpretive analysis capability of the EEG and EP in localizing brain function. The methodology, known as BEAM,[48,49] uses EEG data from 20 electrodes that are spectrally analyzed by means of the fast-Fourier transform (FFR) technique. Spectral analysis and temporal summation are automatically performed by computer. The amount of EEG energy in each of the frequency bands is calculated from each electrode's spectral function. A topographical plot of energy distribution in each spectral range is generated and visualized on a color graphics terminal. Shades of red are used to denote positive values and shades of blue for negative, permitting clinical interpretation of images.

The dynamic change of electrical activity over time is topographically mapped for analysis of EP data. Each of the 20 EP waveforms, created for each stimulus modality, is viewed in rapid sequence on the color graphics terminal by a process known as cartooning. The important spatial and temporal characteristics produces an animation effect that indicates EP activity of the head, localization of function, and determination of functional asymmetry.

BEAM and EP techniques provide immediate visual information about the spectral and spatiotemporal data of the brain. Mapping changes in brain electrical activity before and during performance of right/left dominance on tasks (e.g., reading or musical and rhythm discrimination) have defined localization of posterior, anterior regional activation. Duffy *et al.*[49] suggest that the posterior regions (occipital, parietal) and the anterior (frontal, temporal) parts of the brain are activated during cerebral processing. During language processing and reading tasks, electrical activity mapping suggests frontal involvement of both hemispheres. The medial frontal lobes, which were not previously recognized as being involved in the language process, now appear to be prominently and consistently involved. During silent reading, oral reading, and speaking, the medial frontal lobes are activated, as well as the traditional regions within and adjacent to Broca's area and Wernicke's area. Duffy and co-workers observed different electrophysiological activation between dyslexic boys and controls across the extensive anterior regions. These investigators suggest that dyslexia in its "pure state" may represent dysfunction across the widely distributed brain system devoted to language processing. Duffy and co-workers postulate further that the clinical overlap and the statistical association of hyperactivity and attentional deficits with dyslexia may be due to some as-yet unspecified frontal lobe dysfunction.

Regional cerebral blood flow (rCBF) studies have also confirmed the profound and global reduction of alpha during the decision-making process, indicating the general activation of the entire cerebral hemisphere. Mapping of the changes in brain electrical activity suggests that the posterior region appears to be involved primarily in the reception, recall and initial analysis of auditory stimuli. The frontal region may be engaged in higher level auditory discrimination. It appears that the more intuitive, Gestalt-like tasks involve the posterior area and that the evaluative, more critical decision-making processes are associated with the frontal, temporal, anterior portions of the brain. The latter also appears to require participation of a more global activating mechanism.

Expansion of EEG and EP analyses by the BEAM technique augments the knowledge base of physiological concomitants of dyslexia and other educationally correlated neurodevelopmental deficits. These methodologies should allow for important clinical correlations, thereby expanding information about functional asymmetry and cerebral specialization.

Computed Tomography and Nuclear Magnetic Resonance Imaging

The computed tomography (CT) and nuclear magnetic resonance (NMR) scanners[50,51] are useful in demonstrating the anatomy of the nervous system. The CT scan provides a three-dimensional reconstruction of the brain's absorption of X rays, whereas the NMR uses a high-density magnetic field to provide an analogous three-dimensional reconstruction. Positron-emission tomography (PET) is useful in mapping brain function. Substrates, such as glucose, are labeled with positron-emitting atoms; their metabolism is measured, indicating sites of functional activation. Although resolution of the PET scan image is less than that of the CT or the NMR, it is more sensitive to cerebral function. However, PET scanning is a more invasive technique and takes longer for image construction.

rCBF imaging consists of mapping changes in blood flow induced by alterations in the subject's functional state. Yarowski and Ingemar[52] developed techniques for measuring regional cerebral blood flow in an awake and functioning individual. The subject inhales an inert gas with a low-level radioactive tracer that is charted on a diagram of the brain. The resultant diagram is useful in determining which areas are most active during the performance of specific tasks. As anticipated, the mean left hemisphere blood flow increases during the performance of verbally related tasks. Right hemisphere flow is increased during performance of a picture completion task. PET study observations indicate that the greatest differences were found in posterior and anterior activity. Thus, although hemispheric differences have been observed, blood-flow studies reveal striking similarities in the pattern in both hemispheres during highly lateralized tasks such as speech. Functional mapping techniques have significantly increased the understanding of cerebral specialization. However, except for BEAM, their invasive nature limits broad applicability.

Neuroanatomical Studies: Biological Interactions

Various studies have attempted to define anatomical differences that correlate with hemispheric asymmetries. For example, in the language areas, the Sylvian fissures are usually different in shape and length; the left fissure is longer posteriorly and the adjacent temporal and parietal lobes are longer on the left side than on the right. The left planum temporale (a major part of Wernicke's speech area) is larger than the right. The pattern of folding of the cortex is different on the two sides and the surface area is typically larger on the left.

On a microscopic level, the left frontal area reveals more specific cellular architecture and patterns of connections.[53] The temporal and parietal language areas, and in some nuclei of the posterior thalamus involved in language function, exhibit similar microscopic findings.[54]

There is also documented asymmetry in right-handed and left-handed individuals. Sex differences, although harder to demonstrate, seem to suggest that female brains are more asymmetrical with larger right-sided language areas.

The same structural asymmetry observed in the adult brain exists in children. The immature brain reveals asymmetries of the planum temporale and the Sylvian fissures. Examination of fetal brains also indicate differences in the rates at which structures within the hemispheres grow. The language areas of the left hemisphere, which will increase in size in comparison to the homologous right side, appear to develop more slowly.

STUDIES OF LEARNING DISABILITIES

Studies of the performance of children with learning disabilities, particularly those with dyslexia and "normal" abilities, reveal a dichotomy of deficiencies of right/left hemispheric functioning. These studies are providing a more meaningful conceptualization of subtypes of learning dysfunction.

Learning difficulties in children involve various cognitive functions of the left and right hemisphere. It appears that neuropsychological studies may be applicable to understanding these childhood disorders. For example, it may be determined that a child is applying the "inappropriate" hemisphere to a specific task, suggesting no abnormality in either hemisphere but rather an assignment error. On the other hand, the "appropriate" hemisphere may be employed but, because of some defect in that hemisphere, performance may be poor. In such a situation, it is conceivable that the task may be reassigned to the opposite hemisphere with less than optimal results. Finally, each hemisphere may independently function normally, but optimal performance may require the combined and coordinated operation of the two hemispheres. Insufficiencies in transfer between hemispheres may be causing the learning disabilities. Zaidel[55] concluded that dysphonetic dyslexic readers, identified by Boder, represent a left hemisphere deficiency and that dyseidetic dyslexics represent either a bilateral or a right hemispheric dysfunction.

A number of techniques have been used for studying hemispheric functional asymmetry and dysfunction, such as dichotic listening, tachistoscopic display to visual halffield, and electroencephalographic and haptic studies. These studies have been used, adapted if necessary, in infants and children, in an effort to determine functional lateralization, onset and maturation, and learning disabilities. Studies of language function, form, and space perception in the visual and haptic modalities have revealed inappropriate hemispheric utilization. Witelson[56] devised tasks of dihaptic stimulation that were used in studies of dyslexic boys. The results of these studies suggested that the problem may be due to a lack of right hemisphere specialization for spatial perception resulting in bilateral representation of spatial processing. Thus, the left hemisphere is overtaxed by linguistic and spatial demands resulting in interference and impaired performance. Gordon[57] and Pirozzalo and Rayner[58] used of tachistoscopic studies to demonstrate that learning-disabled children use the right hemisphere for language- and reading-related tasks, resulting in gross inefficiencies.

In EEG studies, Kletzkin[59] noted task-related hemispheric lateralization of cognitive function in a group of academically deficient boys. There appeared to be deficits in the ability to integrate the activities of the two hemispheres, possibly due to (1) impaired or underdeveloped interhemispheric commissural pathways, and/or (2) more delayed maturation of the myelin sheath of the corpus callosum than in other children. The result is diminished efficiency of the interhemispheric coordination as the underlying cause of poor cognitive performance.

Hiscock and Kinsbourne[60] and Hynd et al.[61] attempted to explore laterality differences and their association with attention deficits. Galaburda and Kemper[62] described the CNS of dyslexics at postmortem examination. He noted that anatomically there were cerebral differences between normal and dyslexics. Galaburda and Kemper suggested that the physical differences may be causal to educational underachievement.

Geschwind and Behan[63] studied the association between sinistrality and immune disorders, which they postulated may be explained by high levels of testosterone. It was suggested that this could explain the male predominance for dyslexia and left-handedness, as well as for other illnesses occurring before and during puberty. Genetic predisposition is also being studied, as it relates to cerebral dominance, symmetry, asymmetry, and cortical connections of the brain. Torgensen[64] recommends the study of behavior and how the learning-disabled child processes information, suggesting that theories of learning disabilities must be sensitive to the neuropsychological paradigm.

APPLICATION OF THEORIES

Some critics contend that cases of neurological impairment in children are too rare to apply an educational neuroscientific mode. Research data indicates that learning difficulties may not be a consequence of "hard" or "soft" neurological impairments but a result of inappropriate use of the two specialized hemispheres. Consequently, a previously ignored learning-disabled population may not be identified. The cumulative research on the left/right brain in normal subjects clearly indicates that the two hemispheres differ in the types of stimuli they are most specialized to deal with. Therefore, it is not only the verbal or spatial mode of imparting information to children that is important but the type of organization of transformation of that information. Accrued information is meaningful when it can help the child learn. The brain, specialized within each hemisphere, as well as across the hemispheres, is a complex organ with many unexplored areas. The implications for the future are that children should be taught to classify stimuli in two ways. This can be accomplished by integrating both the analytical sequential–linguistic and the holistic visuospatial processing simultaneously. This should ultimately result in a more functional application of information, facilitating the multiple processing systems of the brain.

Previously well-respected theories of development and cognitive processes are being discarded. New contributions are expanding a body of knowledge of how the brain deals with information and its function in behavior. The contributions adding to our ability to diagnose and remediate problems, such as dyslexia and learning disabilities, have evolved from advances in neuroscience, education, and behavioral and clinical psychology. Collaboration of various disciplines should ultimately result in increased knowledge of the genesis of learning disabilities.

Several questions remain to be answered in order to appreciate the complex nature of learning disabilities. Are there critical periods during maturation, when a child is particularly vulnerable to factors that trigger learning disorders? Are there conditions in the environment that make a child more susepctible to these injuries? These questions represent the challenges for future research in learning disabilities.

A combined cognitive, behavioral, informative approach, when correlated with the fund of information evolving from neuropsychology, holds the greatest promise for the successful diagnosis and management of the learning-disabled child.

REFERENCES

1. United States Office of Education: *Better Education for the Handicapped: Annual Report, Fiscal Year 1969*. U.S. Government Printing Office, Washington, D.C., 1970.
2. U.S. Education for All Handicapped Children Act for Public Law 94-142: U.S. Office of Education. *Federal Register 42* (No. 230), 52404–52407, 1976.
3. Cruickshank, W. M.: When winter comes can spring . . . ? *Exceptional Child* **25**:3–25, 1978.
4. Cruickshank, W. M.: *Learning Disabilities. A Definitional Statement*. Unpublished manuscript. University of Michigan, Ann Arbor, 1981.
5. Orton, S. T.: *Reading, Writing and Speech Problems in Children*. Norton, New York, 1937.
6. Vandenberg, S. G.: Comparative studies of multiple factor ability measures, in Royce, JR (ed.): *Multivariate Analyses and Psychological Theory*. Academic, New York, 1973, pp. 149–202.
7. Calanchini, P. R., and Traut, S. S.: The neurology of learning disabilities, in Tarpolin, L. (ed.): *Learning Disorders in Children: Diagnosis, Medication, Education*. Little, Brown, Boston, 1971, pp. 207–251.

8. Strauss, A. A., and Lehtinen, L. E.: *Psychopathology and Education of the Brain Injured Child*. Grune & Stratton, New York, 1947.
9. Kephart, N. C.: *The Slow Learner in the Classroom*. Merrill, Columbus, Ohio, 1960.
10. Getman, G. N.: The visual motor complex in the acquisition of learning skills, in Hellmuth, J. (ed.): *Learning Disorders*, Vol. 1. Special Child Publications, Seattle, 1965, pp. 49–76.
11. Cruickshank, W. M.: *Learning Disabilities in Home, School and Community*. Syracuse University Press, Syracuse, New York, 1977.
12. Barsch, R. H.: *Enriching Perception and Cognition*, Vol. 2. Special Child Publications, Seattle, 1968.
13. Frostig, M., Lifever, D. W., and Whittlesey, J. R.: A developmental test of visual perception for evaluating normal and neurologically handicapped children. *Percept. Mot. Skills* **12**:382–394, 1961.
14. Kirk, S. A., and Kirk, W. D.: *Psycholinguistic Learning Disabilities, Diagnosis and Remediation*. University of Illinois Press, Urbana, 1976.
15. Johnson, D. L., and Myklebust, H. R.: *Learning Disabilities: Educational Principles and Practices*. Grune & Stratton, New York, 1967.
16. Arter, J. A., and Jenkins, J. R.: Differential diagnosis—prescriptive teaching: A critical appraisal. *Rev. Educ. Res.* **49**:517–555, 1979.
17. Dunn, L. M.: *Peabody Picture Vocabulary Test*. American Guidance Service, Circle Pines, Minnesota, 1959.
18. Roach, E. G., and Kephart, N. C.: *The Purdue Perceptual Motor Survey*. Merrill, Columbus, Ohio, 1966.
19. Benton, A. L.: *Benton Visual Retention Test*, rev. ed. Psychological Corporation, New York, 1955.
20. Goldman, R., Fristoe, M., and Woodcock, R. W.: *Goldman–Fristoe–Woodcock Test of Auditory Discrimination*. American Guidance Service, Circle Pines, Minnesota, 1970.
21. Kirk, S. A.: *Illinois Test of Psycholinguistic Activities. The Diagnosis of Evaluation of Psycholinguistic Disabilities*. University of Illinois Press, Urbana, 1966.
22. Hammill, D. D., and Larsen, S. C.: The effectiveness of psycholinguistic training. *Except. Child.* **41**:39–44, 1972.
23. Hammill, D. D.: Training visual perceptual processes. *J. Learning Disabilities* **5**:39–44, 1972.
24. Boder, E.: Developmental dyslexia. A diagnostic approach based on three atypical reading–spelling patterns. *Dev. Med. Child Neurol.* **15**:663–687, 1973.
25. Mattis, S., French, J. H., and Rapin, I.: Dyslexia in children and young adults: Three independent neuropsychological syndromes. *Dev. Med. Child Neurol.* **17**:150–163, 1975.
26. Morrison, F. J., Giordiani, B., and Nagy, I.: Learning disability: An informational processing analysis. *Science* **196**:77–79, 1977.
27. Satz, P., and Fletcher, J. M.: Minimal brain dysfunctions: An appraisal of research concepts and methods, in Rie, H. E., and Rie, E. D. (eds.): *Handbook of Minimal Brain Dysfunction: A Critical Review*. Wiley, New York, 1980, pp. 669–714.
28. Kinsbourne, M.: Minimal brain dysfunction as a neurodevelopmental lag. *Ann. N.Y. Acad. Sci.* **205**:268–273, 1973.
29. Rourke, B. P.: Issues in the neuropsychological assessment of children with learning disabilities. *Can. Psychol. Rev.* **18**:89–102, 1976.
30. Petrauskas, A. J., and Rourke, B. P.: Identification of subgroups of retarded readers. A neuropsychological, multivariate approach. *J. Clin. Neuropsychol.* **11**:17–37, 1979.
31. Pirozzalo, F. J.: *The neuropsychology of Developmental Reading Disorder*. Praeger, New York, 1979.
32. American Psychiatric Association: *Diagnostic and Statistical Manual of Mental Disorders (DSM III)*, 3rd ed. American Psychiatric Association, Washington, D.C., 1980.
33. Gall, J. F.: Sur les fonctions du cerveau et celles de chacune de ses parties. Balliere, Paris, 1925.
34. Broca, P.: Remarks on the seat of the faculty of articulate language, followed by and observation of aphemia, in Bonin, G. von (trans.): Some papers on the cerebral cortex. Thomas, Springfield, Illinois, 1960. Reprinted from *Bull. Soc. Anat. Paris* **6**:330–357, 1961.
35. Fritsch, G., and Hitzig, E.: On the electrical excitability of the cerebrum, in G., von Bonin (trans.): *Some Papers on the Cerebral Cortex*. Thomas, Springfield, Illinois. 1960. Reprinted from *Arch. Anat.* **37**:300–323, 1970.
36. Levy, J.: Psychobiological implications of bilateral asymmetry, in Dimond, S. J., and Beamont, J. (eds.): *Hemisphere Function in the Human Brain*. Halsted, New York, 1974, pp. 121–183.

37. Jackson, J. H.: On the nature of the duality of the brain. *Brain* **38**:80–103, 1915. Reprinted from *Med. Press Circ.*
38. Piercy, M.: Studies of the neurological basis of intellectual function, in Williams, D. (ed.): *Modern Trends in Neurology.* Butterworth, London, 1967. pp. 775–790.
39. Myers, R. E., and Sperry, R. W.: Interhemispheric communication through the corpus callosum. *Arch. Neurol. Psychiatry* **80**:298–303, 1958.
40. Bogen, J. E., Fisher, E. D., and Vogel, J. P.: Cerebral commissurotomy. A second case report. *J.A.M.A.* **194**:1328–1329, 1965.
41. Bogen, J.: The other side of the brain: The oppositional mind. *Bull. L.A. Neurol. Soc.* **34**:135–162, 1969.
42. Sperry, R. W.: Hemisphere deconnection and unity of conscious awareness. *Am. Psychol.* **23**:723–733, 1968.
43. Sperry, R. W., Gazzaniga, M. E., and Bogen, J. E.: Interhemispheric relationships: The neocortical commissures, syndrome of hemispheric disconnection, in Vinken, P. S., and Bruyn, G. W. (eds.): *Handbook of Clinical Neurology*, Vol. 4: *Disorders of Speech, Perception and Symbolic Behavior.* North-Holland, Amsterdam, 1969, pp. 273–290.
44. Kimura, D.: Cerebral dominance and the perception of verbal stimuli. *Can. J. Psychol.* **15**:156–165, 1961.
45. Rizzalatti, G., Umilta, C., and Berlucci, G.: Opposite superiorities of the right and left cerebral hemispheres in discrimination reaction time to physiognomical and alphabetical material. *Brain* **94**:431–442, 1971.
46. Galin, D., and Ornstein, R.: Lateral specialization of cognitive mode: An EEG study. *Psychophysiology* **9**:412–418, 1972.
47. Glass, A., and Butler, S. R.: Asymmetries in suppression of alpha rhythm possibly related to cerebral dominance. *Electroencephalogr. Clin. Neurophysiol.* **34**:729, 1973.
48. Duffy, F. H., Burchfield, J. L., and Sombroso, C. T.: Brain electrical activity mapping (BEAM): A method for extending the clinical utility of EEG and evoked potential data. *Ann. Neurol.* **8**:309–321, 1979.
49. Duffy, F. H., Bartels, P. H., and Burchfield, J. I.: Significance probability mapping: An aid to the topographic analysis of brain electrical analysis activity. *Electroencephalogr. Clin. Neurophysiol.* **51**:455–462, 1981.
50. Baker, H. I., Houser, O. W., Campbell, J. K., *et al.:* Computerized tomography of the head. *J.A.M.A.* **233**:1304–1308, 1975.
51. Krammer, D. M., Schneider, J. S., Rudim, A. M., *et al.:* True three dimensional nuclear magnetic resonance zeugmatographic images of a human brain. *Neuroradiology* **21**:239–244, 1981.
52. Yarowski, P. J., and Ingemar, D. H.: Symposium summary. Neuronal activity and energy metabolism. *Fed. Proc.* **40**:2342–2362, 1982.
53. Galaburda, A. M.: La région de Broca: Observations anatomiques faites un siecle après la mort de son découvreur. *Rev. Neurol. (Paris)* **136**:609, 1980.
54. Eidelberg, D., and Galaburda, A. M.: Symmetry and asymmetry in the human posterior thalamus. I. Cytoarchietectonic analyses in normal persons. *Arch. Neurol.* **39**:325–332, 1982.
55. Zaidel, A.: The split brain and half brains as models of congenital language disability, in Ludlow, C. L., and Doran Quine, M. E. (eds.): *The Neurological Basis of Language Disorders in Children: Methods and Directions for Research.* NINCDS Monograph No. 79-440. U.S. Department of Health, Education and Welfare, Bethesda, 1980, pp. 55–86.
56. Witelson, S. F.: Brain lateralization in children: Normal and dyslexic, in *Lateralization of Brain Functions.* Boerhaave Commission, Leidem, Netherlands, 1975, pp. 122–146.
57. Gordon, H. W.: The learning disabled are cognitively right. *Top. Learning Learning Disabilities* **3**:29–39, 1983.
58. Pirozzalo, F. J., and Rayner, K.: Cerebral organization and reading disability. *Neuropsychologia* **17**:485–489, 1979.
59. Kletzkin, D.: Electroencephalographic, Neurological and Psychometric Correlates of Right and Left Cerebral Hemisphere Functions in on Grade and Below Grade Elementary School Boys. Unpublished doctoral dissertation. Rutgers University, New Brunswick, New Jersey, 1980.
60. Hiscock, M., and Kinsbourne, M. Asymmetries of selective-listening and attention switching in children. *Dev. Psychol.* **16**:70–82, 1980.
61. Hynd, G. H., Obrzud, J. E., Weed, J., *et al.:* Development of cerebral dominance. Dichotic listening asymmetry in normal and learning disabled children. *J. Exp. Child Psychol.* **28**:445–454, 1979.

62. Galaburda, A. M., and Kemper, T. L.: Cytoarchitectonic abnormalities in developmental dyslexia: A case study. *Ann. Neurol.* **6**:94–100, 1979.
63. Geschwind, H., and Behan, P.: Left handedness association with immune disease, mirgraine and developmental learning disorder. *Proc. Natl. Acad. Sci. (U.S.A.)* **79**:5907, 1982.
64. Torgensen, J. K.: Learning disabilities theory: Its current state and future prospects. *J. Learning Disabilities* **19**:399–407, 1986.

8

Psychological Testing

Peter W. Zinkus

INTRODUCTION

Psychological assessment provides an opportunity for observing behavior in an objective, standardized manner. The child performs a series of standardized tasks, from which impressions are formulated on the nature of the child's abilities as well as disabilities. It is most important to recognize that psychological tests per se reveal nothing in and of themselves. Tests are sensitive only when administered by a sensitive examiner. Interpretations of the test results represents the crucial aspect in diagnosis. Adams[1] noted that children are assigned various "diagnoses" based essentially on the same behavioral observations, including hyperactivity, distractiability, poor impulse control, perceptual disorders, and reading difficulties. The examiner's particular interpretation of the test results may yield reports of seemingly contradictory terminology. This is of no surprise to professionals familiar with the field of developmental disabilities.

Peter W. Zinkus • Child Psychology Division, Le Bonheur Children's Medical Center, Memphis, Tennessee 38103.

STANDARDIZATION

Psychological testing offers a much more expedient approach to acquiring needed information, as it is impractical, or impossible, to follow a child through daily activities for several weeks in order to formulate behavioral impressions. Systemic observations can be made and presented in a standardized manner. The performances are then compared with a normative group and patterns of assets and liabilities derived. Standardized testing requires valid information on the distribution of a particular skill in a population of people. Large groups of children are tested; their performance scores provide the norms. The individual's test data are then compared with these norms. Test inventories for children must also provide a balance within normative groups, with age, socioeconomic class, and sex considered. These factors have been shown to be significant factors that influence test performance. Age, for example, is a critical factor, since many skills such as visuoperceptual abilities follow a developmental sequence. Therefore diagnostic testing for visuoperceptual development must factor for the variability of the child's age in establishing norms for adequacy of performance. Psychological tests must be both reliable and valid. Reliability is the measure of consistency of the test and its ability to produce a stable score on several testings. Validity is a concept related to whether a test actually measures what it claims to measure or how well it does its job. Validity is established by correlating test performance with an independent measurement of the variable to be evaluated. For example, a test is designed and used to predict readiness for reading. The scores would then be compared with the degree of success in learning to read. The correlation coefficient obtained by comparing the readiness test scores to reading performance provides a validity score. Validity scores in the range of 0.80–0.90 are obviously very good scores.

DIAGNOSTIC APPROACHES

A variety of approaches can be used to interpret test results; caution must be exercised if the results are to be used effectively. The approach to interpretation of test results on the basis of the test per se and in part by the inclinations of the examiner is summarized as follows:

1. *Level of performance:* This interpretation uses pre-established cutoff points, beyond which performance on the test is considered abnormal. Several tests for brain damage use this method, and a score beyond the cutoff point is assumed to result from CNS dysfunction. Although the information is accurate and correct, a major disadvantage of this approach is that the abnormal score does not contribute to the course of rehabilitation or re-education. Scores on a level of performance serve only to assist professionals in constructing and delivering an educational program. The diagnostic label is generally clouded with surplus meaning. Poor performance on a test of brain damage is often generalized by an assumption that it is one of many symptoms commonly associated with organic brain dysfunction. Unfortunately, this may close the case with a diagnosis, rather than establishing the needs and course of treatment for the child.

2. *Pathognomonic sign:* This clinical symptom approach uses what is commonly referred to as the medical model. The clinician attempts to delineate signs of pathol-

ogy, which if present indicate an underlying organic deficit. For example, a child who has an abnormal electroencephalogram (EEG) is manifesting a clinical sign of brain dysfunction. The pattern of brain waves (frequencies, amplitudes) provides information about the etiology, chronicity, and severity of the CNS abnormality. By contrast, a normal EEG provides considerably less information—The absence of positive findings on the EEG does not necessarily mean that the brain is functioning normally. Interpretations of diagnostic tests should provide information about the child's abilities, as well as detect deficits. A realistic statement regarding strengths and weaknesses is crucial to the management of the child's problem.

3. *Pattern analysis approach:* This alternative is probably the most profitable, as it involves the use of test data. The overall performance of a child is synthesized on a multitude of test variables, and this information is amalgamated into a compendium of strengths and weaknesses. This profile for a learning-disabled child would include several major variables: learning skills and deficits, intellectual abilities, perceptual problems, personality, and emotional and behavioral tendencies. The formulated register of strengths and weaknesses would be invaluable in constructing a meaningful and clearly defined program of therapeutic intervention.

A single (isolated) score, used as an indicator or predictor of a child's overall level of ability, generally provides a restricted and narrow base of information, thereby increasing the opportunities for misinterpretations. The concept of intelligence quotient (IQ) is a good example of this limited perspective of a child's abilities. IQ scores are frequently used to describe a child's level of performance, implying a ceiling on ultimate potential. Descriptive terms such as "mental retardation," "dull normal," "average," and "superior" are diagnostic categories based on the child's IQ. The IQ is neither a static phenomenon nor a stable entity; it can change over time. Of greater significance is that the IQ value, derived from a child's performance on a standardized test, is profoundly influenced by the presence of perceptual disorders, emotional factors, and a myriad of other variables.

For example, a child may show an IQ of 100 on the Wechsler Intelligence Scale for Children–Revised (WISC–R), in a number of different ways. The subtests that contribute to this IQ score may be performed in significantly different ways, indicating different patterns of strengths and weaknesses. Child A may obtain a full-scale IQ of 100 based on a verbal IQ of 80 and a performance IQ of 120, whereas child B may have an identical full-scale IQ with reversed verbal and performance IQ scores. The verbal components of the WISC–R are sensitive to auditory processing and language abilities, in contrast to the performance sections, which are sensitive to visual processing and visual motor skills. Different interpretations of the test data are necessary despite calculation of identical full-scale IQ values. IQ values per se are inadequate to categorize a child's intellectual ability, often not reflecting significant deficits in auditory or visual processing skills. In the cases cited, the values indicate that both children possess "average" intelligence but may erroneously mask a diagnostic error of significant consequence. Pattern analysis explores the performance that yielded the verbal and performance scores. For example, child B may have obtained a discrepant performance IQ because of problems in visual memory, visuospatial orientation, visuomotor abilities, or a multitude of visual-processing deficits. A much different interpretation of the test performances based on the children's ages cited in the previous example might be offered. A 5-year-old child showing the scores reported might be diagnosed differently than a 9-year-old with identical scores. Reitan and Davidson[2] indicated that the verbal and performance sections of the WISC show different sensitivities to dysfunction in the left and right hemispheres of the brain, respectively. Children aged 5 years old do not exhibit the same clear-cut relationship as do 9-year-olds. Age and developmental factors must be considered and the results interpreted with caution.

Individual test items may be critical factors in the utilization of pattern analysis. If, in response to the test question, "What must you do to make water boil?," the child responds "Eggs," significant information has been related to the examiner, raising suspicions of a particular deficit. The child's auditory sensitivity and auditory processing skills may be impaired. Numbers on test protocols are probably not as important as observing unscorable, yet significant, aspects of the child's performance. Simply indicating a "failure" to the question cite ignores a much more valuable insight into the child's overall difficulty.

THE EVALUATION PROCESS

A meaningful psychological evaluation of a child involves assessment of behaviors over a wide range of situations. A comprehensive evaluation would involve assessing the whole child—not just intelligence and achievement. The adequate documentation of historical information is a most critical component of psychological testing. The obstetrical history may reveal factors that have compromised the child's central nervous system. The age at which developmental milestones were acquired (e.g., walking and talking) should be reviewed. It is important to assess educational history, performance, and behavior in school. Additional significant factors to be reviewed include relationships with peers and siblings, severity of behavioral difficulties, and parental attitudes. These factors constitute the environment in which the child must function. As a rule, potentials cannot be fully realized in the face of major limiting factors.

The examination per se attempts to resolve questions regarding strengths and weaknesses in a child's intellectual, perceptual, emotional, and behavioral skills. A principle of psychological testing is to ensure a valid examination, attempting to achieve the child's best performance. Good rapport with the examiner is a critical factor that must be established before formal testing is initiated. Poor rapport can yield results of questionable validity despite a lengthy examination. The examiner should focus not only on test scores but on the manner of achieving those scores as well. Observations may suggest significant problems despite a score that is considered "normal." Average scores, regarded as within normal limits, may not reflect impressions that the child is capable of better performance. For example, a child with perceptual delays may not function to his full potential on the test. The examiner should select a battery of test instruments that are valid and reliable and that cover a full range of skills.

The necessity to observe and record the child's behaviors during the testing session cannot be overemphasized. Significant problems with attention span, concentration, and level of activity during the testing may provide behavioral clues about the child's ability to function in a classroom, as well as their influence on the test performance per se. A very distractible child may show a spuriously low test performance that, if taken at face value, is not a true estimate of ability. The child's reaction to frustration and ability to relate to the examiner are critical in assessing test performance and may prognosticate the success of remedial programs. A child with a poor self-concept may require months of emotional support by teacher and family before remediation programs can be initiated. Information obtained from behavioral observations during diagnostic testing may be valuable in formulating program direction.

TESTS AND APPLICATIONS

The use of psychological tests will be reviewed using a learning-disabled child as a hypothetical illustrative case. The publishers of the tests cited and additional tests of interest are included in Appendix B of this volume.

> *Case History*   John was performing poorly in the second grade. He was experiencing difficulty with reading and report cards indicated very erratic grades. John was often frustrated, had difficulty focusing attention, and often was found daydreaming. An effort to motivate John by depriving him of a recess break proved unsuccessful. The teacher recommended that John repeat the second grade.

In designing a psychoeducational test battery for John, several questions appear to require resolution: (1) What is his intellectual ability?, (2) How well is he achieving academically?, (3) Are there reading problems and, if so, how severe?, (4) Are there deficits in the processing of auditory stimuli?, (5) Are there personality, behavioral, or emotional problems?, and (6) How well is he developing in language, motor, self-help, and social skills? In addition to these six major questions several issues require review: (1) the advantages and limitations of the neuropsychological approach, and (2) available screening tests for the physician.

Intellectual Ability

Individual and group tests and special examinations for handicapped persons provide data on intelligence levels. Intelligence tests provide suggestions about learning potentials. The Wechsler Intelligence Scales were developed during the late 1940s. The Wechsler Preschool and Primary Scale of Intelligence (WPPSI) was designed for children aged 4–6½ years, the Wechsler Intelligence Scale for Children (WISC) for ages 5–15, and thr Wechsler Adult Intelligence Scale (WAIS) for ages 16 and older. A major revision of the Wechsler Intelligence Scale for Children (WISC–R) provides a more current and valid set of test items. The normative population was carefully selected to allow for important variables such as race, socioeconomic class, and rural–urban residence.

The WISC–R is divided into two major sections: verbal and performance areas. The verbal and performance areas are each composed of six subtests. A full-scale IQ is calculated from scores obtained on the verbal and performance tests, providing an index of functional intellectual level (Table I). In addition, a comparison of verbal and language skills (verbal IQ) with visually oriented skills (performance IQ) is possible. Significant differences between the verbal and performance scores (usually 15 points or more) suggest the presence of auditory or visual perceptual deficits, requiring further evaluation.

Table I. IQ Scores and Functional Classification

IQ score	Range of intellectual function
≥130	Very superior
120–129	Superior
110–119	Bright normal
90–109	Average
80–89	Dull normal
70–79	Boderline
≤69	Mentally deficient

These test scores (IQ values) should be interpreted with caution, since perceptual deficits or other learning problems may yield an IQ score that is relatively low and that fails to reflect potentials. The associated deficits may mask the fact that the child has average or above-average intelligence. Careful observation by the examiner, as well as critical analysis of the pattern of test scores and performance, is necessary to prevent a grave error of mislabeling. Individual subtests of the WISC–R are analyzed to determine the pattern of strengths and weaknesses in the verbal and performance areas. Verbal subtests measure the child's general fund of knowledge, abstract reasoning ability, comprehension, sequential memory, and vocabulary. Performance subtests yield information regarding abilities in visuomotor coordination, visual-spatial orientation, visual memory, visual sequencing, and other areas (Table II).

Another method of intellectual assessment is the Stanford-Binet Intelligence Scale; the present version represents numerous revisions of the test devised by Binet and Simon in 1916. The concept of mental age (MA) is used to summarize test performance. The MA is then compared with the chronological age (CA) to derive an IQ value:

$$IQ = \frac{MA}{CA} \times 100$$

The Stanford-Binet may be used with children as young as 2 years of age. The test is arranged by age levels, with six subtests at each age level. Intervals of 6 months are used

Table II. Subtest Included in the Verbal and Performance Areas of the WISC–R

Verbal tests	Performance tests
Information	Picture completion
Similarities	Picture arrangement
Arithmetic	Block design
Vocabulary	Object assembly
Comprehension	Coding
Digit span	Mazes

for ages 2–5 years and 1-year intervals for 6–14 years. Each interval contains subtests measuring a wide range of verbal and performance skills. Analysis of the child's test performance includes discerning patterns of strengths and weaknesses at various age levels. Poor performance on items commensurate with the CA may indicate perceptual deficits or other developmental problems. The Stanford-Binet has some limitations in that it is a highly verbally oriented test. There is also some bias favoring the white middle-class population, making its validity for low-income or disadvantaged groups questionable.

Group intelligence tests are sometimes used, particularly in the school setting. The concept of group testing evolved from a need to secure information on large numbers of children. Standardized intelligence tests such as the Lorge–Thorndike Intelligence Tests and the Otis–Lennon Mental Ability Test have been administered to millions of children, during some stage of their school career. The IQ values obtained have been used to plan teaching strategies. Although group testing is more expedient than lengthy individual evaluations, many of the variables that influence the outcome of test performance (motivation, attitude, or distraction) escape detection when group testing is performed. The child with a learning disability generally performs very poorly on a group intelligence test, displaying low IQ values. Consequently, it would be a great disservice if conclusions regarding intellectual ability and potential were to be formulated on the basis of these scores. If a child obtains a poor performance on a group test, questions arise and individual testing is indicated.

Children with obvious deficits (blindness, deafness, articulation problems, and/or motor deficits) often require testing to assess intellectual capacities. A variety of test instruments are available that compensate for particular handicaps and yield a profile of intellectual abilities. For example, the Peabody Picture Vocabulary Test does not require that the child speak; this test may be used for children with severe expressive language problems. Visually oriented tests such as the performance section of the WISC–R, the *Leiter International Performance Scale,* or the *Hiskey–Nebraska Test of Learning Aptitude* can be used for hearing-impaired children. Verbally oriented tests such as the verbal section of the WISC-R or the Kuhlman–Anderson Intelligence Test are valuable tests in evaluating children with visual handicaps.

Academic Achievement

In the diagnosis of learning disabilities it is important to identify whether there is a gap between the child's ability and actual achievement in academic areas. In the case history cited, John was not achieving in the classroom, despite a potential that appeared higher. As a general rule, academic achievement should be commensurate with intellectual levels; i.e., average intelligence suggests average educational achievement. Assessment of the disparity between competence and performance should be measured in degree of severity.

Very few children complete a school year without taking at least one of the standard group achievement tests. The Stanford Achievement Test and the Metropolitan Achievement Test are widely used instruments. Although typically lengthy to administer, these tests provide information on a wide range of academic areas, such as arithmetic, reading, and social studies. A child's performance on these group tests may be partially contingent on motivational variables. However, a learning disability may be reflected in low or inconsistent achievement levels and the mechanics of taking the test. Most teachers are cognizant that a poor performance on a group achievement test indicates the need for additional evaluation.

Individual achievement tests are much more reliable in the diagnosis of learning disorders. Reading, spelling, and math can be evaluated on an individual basis to determine the child's academic skills, as well as controlling for motivational variables. Of greater significance is the ability to assess the type of errors made in reading, spelling, and math—data that should be incorporated into the diagnostic evaluation. Examinations such as the Wide-Range Achievenent Test or the Peabody Individual Achievement Test provide information of this type. For example, the child may be required to spell from dictation. This assessment provides an opportunity to obtain a sample of handwriting and observation of fine motor skills. Letter reversals, sequencing errors, and the presence of auditory processing disturbances may similarly be detected. Problems in auditory–visual integration, (i.e., the ability to translate auditory symbols into visual symbols) may also be identified. In reading, the child may misread the word "was" as "saw," "plot" as "blot," or "bulk" as "bluk." Identification of word and letter reversals and of sequencing errors provides clues to answering the question: "Why is the child not achieving full potential?"

The reading and/or spelling grade levels define the gap between potential and performance. Wide-Range Achievement Test scores may be converted into standard scores that are generally equivalent to IQ distributions. Comparisons of IQ with achievement standard score provide evidence of a gap between competence and performance. A disparity of 2 or more years between actual grade level and reading grade level may be a diagnostic criterion for dyslexia. (The term "dyslexia" is falling into disrepute as a diagnostic entity, since it has become a catchall for all reading problems.) Performance on achievement tests should include observations of how the child approaches, organizes, and completes the tasks. The pattern of reading and spelling errors may provide useful information in designing remedial programs.

Auditory and Visual Processing

Children with average or above-average intelligence who are not achieving at a level commensurate with their intellectual ability may have significant processing deficits. These children may be experiencing difficulty in understanding various aspects of what they see or hear. Coordinating sensory–perceptual–motor activity may be a problem of such magnitude as to render normal teaching strategies of little value. Auditory and visual acuity screening frequently demonstrates an intact peripheral sensory system. The deficit appears to occur on a perceptual or central receptive level, i.e., a cortical level of understanding and interpreting visual or auditory information. It has been hypothesized that the CNS is in some way functioning improperly, thereby preventing proper analysis of the visual and/or auditory sensory–perceptual information.

Auditory Perceptual Evaluation

The verbal portion of the WISC–R may be used to understand better a child's auditory processing and receptive-expressive language skills. A low verbal IQ, discrepant from the performance IQ by more than 15 points, may suggest an auditory processing and receptive language deficit.

Individual subtests on the verbal section of the WISC-R provide information on auditory perceptual skills. Each subtest of this scale has an average score of 10; a discrepancy of 3 or more points between subtests may indicate a deficit in auditory processing. The subtests measure general comprehension, concept formation, abstract reasoning ability, arithmetic reasoning, concentration (attention), and auditory sequential memory. In addition, the examiner may observe unusual responses from a child suggestive of deficits in the ability to process auditory information.

The Illinois Test of Psycholinguistic Ability (ITPA) was developed to measure the child's ability to recognize and understand what is heard, to organize this material, and express it in a meaningful way. The subtests of the ITPA are constructed to measure understanding of auditory symbols, ability to relate orally presented concepts, verbal expressions of concepts, use of syntax and grammatic aspects of language, and utilization of sequential memory skills.[3] Performance on these subtests provides a composite psycholinguistic age (PLA) score, an overall index of the level of psycholinguistic development. The score is expressed in years and months, is easily understood, and can be integrated into a remedial program. Scaled scores for each subtest can be translated into an age score, representing the child's functional level in more specific areas of auditory processing. Comparison of the child's CA with age scores suggests the severity of the deficit in a given auditory processing or language skill. Patterns of abilities and disabilities may be used in designing remedial programs.

Visual Perceptual Evaluation

The performance section of the WISC-R may be useful in determining the presence of deficits in visual processing. A performance IQ that is low and discrepant from the verbal IQ (by more than 15 points) suggests the possibility of visual processing deficits. The six subtests that make up the performance section of the WISC–R measure various visual processing skills for which a pattern of strengths and weaknesses can be determined. The subtests measure visual sequencing ability, visual memory, figure-ground discrimination, visuospatial organization, rapid visuomotor coordination, and conceptual abilities related to visual stimuli.

The Frostig Test of Visual Perception was constructed to measure the child's developmental level in five major areas of visual perception that seem to have particular relevance to school performance. The subtests measure eye–hand coordination, figure-ground perception, form constancy, position in space, and spatial relationships. Frostig *et al.*[4] indicated that the test may be administered on a group or on an individual basis and is appropriate for children aged 3–9 years. A perceptual age level score is obtained and, when compared with child's CA, offers information regarding the degree of deficit in visual perceptual development. A perceptual quotient (PQ) may also be obtained; a median score is 100. An overall profile of the pattern of abilities and disabilities may be obtained that assists in the design of remedial strategies.

Other Tests of Visual Perceptual Skill

Many other tests are available that assess visual-processing abilities, varying in degrees of usefulness in achieving diagnostic and remedial goals. The Bender–Gestalt Test requires the child to reproduce nine geometric patterns. Comparison of the child's performance with age norms permits estimation of a developmental age in visual processing areas. Visual memory tests such as the Benton Visual Retention Test and the Graham–Kendall Memory for Designs Test may be useful in assessing memory components of visual perception in older children. The Ayres Battery of Perceptual Tests is a recent addition to the test batteries available to assess visual processing.

Reading Skills

Perhaps no other area of academic achievement has received more attention relative to learning disabilities than reading. The prevalence of reading disabilities in the school systems in the United States varies from approximately 5 to 10%. Jastak and Jastak[5] defined reading as the process of transcoding a series of visual–motor symbols into oral or suboral sequences. Elements of auditory and visual perception play a predominant role in the process of reading. In addition, intelligence, motivation, and personality are critical factors in the acquisition and enhancement of reading skills. Since many variables influence the ability to read, the design of remedial strategies requires a comprehensive reading evaluation. The most effective diagnostic reading tests investigate a variety of subskills: oral reading proficiency, listening comprehension, word analysis, phonetic analysis, and spelling.

The Gates–McKillop Reading Diagnostic Test is an individual diagnostic test useful in identifying disabled readers. In addition to the visual reading factors previously mentioned, the test measures reading elements such as word perception, letter sounds, auditory and visual blending, and spelling. The data on specific perceptual difficulties can be evaluated effectively and incorporated into remedial programs to improve reading. The Spache Diagnostic Reading Scales provide a standardized evaluation of oral and silent reading skills as well as auditory comprehension. The scales consist of word-recognition lists, 22 reading passages, and eight phonics tests. The teacher is provided with information useful in preparing remedial reading programs. The child's reading speed and potential, as well as the nature and extent of reading errors, are evaluated. In addition, a measure is obtained of the level to which a child's reading may be raised through remedial training. The professional is therefore able to assess reading problems accurately as well as establish reasonable goals for improvement.

The tests cited are examples of a wide number of reading diagnostic tests available to the diagnostician. The choice of tests should be based on their ability to measure as many variables as possible in the reading process.

Personality, Behavior, and Emotions

Children with a learning disability often develop emotional and/or behavioral reactions that can become as detrimental to learning as the learning disability itself. It is readily appreciated that a child who is frustrated in an attempt to achieve and gain recognition in the classroom may suffer debilitating effects on self-concept. A variety of behavioral manifestations such as acting-out behaviors, withdrawal, and a severe decline in school interest are often associated with poor self-esteem. Continuous failure becomes overwhelming and creates frustrations that generate anxiety, further reducing this child's chances of learning. Recognition that may be denied through normal channels of academic success may become available through misbehavior. Frequent acting-out behaviors include becoming the class clown, bully, or show-off in order to gain recognition. Personality tests generally provide a better understanding of the child's emotional difficulties and may be extremely valuable in guiding therapy for parents, teachers, and the child. These tests measure the emotional and behavioral characteristics of an individual and are generally of two major categories: personality inventories and projective tests.

Personality inventories employ self-report techniques wherein either the child or the parents indicate certain behavioral and emotional traits in response to structured questions. Such tests as the California Personality Inventory, the Early School Personality Questionnaire, Children's Personality Questionnaire offer a standardized measure of personality traits. These instruments are relatively easy to administer and provide information regarding strengths and weaknesses in the child's personality. Evaluation of test results requires special training and expertise.

In projective testing, a relatively unstructured task is presented to the child. The test stimuli are usually ambiguous, permitting the child to perceive and interpret in his own characteristic manner. In a sense, the child projects his own personality characteristics, needs, and conflicts into the test material. The most popular projective testing technique is The Rorschach Inkblot Test. Ten cards are used, each of which contains a printed inkblot. The child examines the blot and describes what he sees. Interpretation of the child's descriptions includes assessment of the location used for the response, the shape, color, and movement perceived as well as the content of the response.

The Thematic Apperception Test (TAT), in contrast to the Rorschach, is a more structured projective test. Rather than ambiguous inkblots, the TAT uses pictures of people in various situations. The child is asked to create a story to fit each picture. The child typically identifies with one of the characters of the story, revealing the conflicts, needs, and emotions present in his own life situation. Specialized versions of the TAT (more suitable for children), include the Children's Apperception Test (CAT) and the Symonds Picture Story Test. The CAT is appropriate for children aged 3–10 years. The Symonds Picture Story Test is useful for children aged 10–16 years.

Figure-drawing techniques are also used to assess personality. The Draw-a-Person test involves interpretation of the quality of a child's human figure drawing. The House–Tree–Person test requires the child to draw a house, which symbolically represents his home environment, a tree that represents his perceived life role, and a person who relates to his interpersonal relationships. Completion of the drawings is combined with an interview in an attempt to obtain insight into the child's personality. These and other projective tests must be interpreted with caution because of their highly subjective nature. In the hands of a skilled diagnostician, however, they can be of tremendous value in understanding the child's personality.

Development

Assessment of the child's development requires data on the approximate functional level in language, motor, self-help, and social areas. Developmental inventories and screening tests may provide this information. On occasion, it would be important to evaluate the child's intellectual development at an earlier age than is provided by most standardized intelligence tests. A developmental assessment may be indicated when there is a family history of mental retardation or learning disabilities, high-risk obstetrical factors, or suspicion regarding maturational delays or dysfunctions. Similarly, a more comprehensive neurodevelopmental evaluation may be required when screening reveals uneven development of comprehension, language, or fine and gross motor skills. A variety of developmental inventories and infant and preschool screening tests are available to monitor a child's development. The information may be obtained directly by observation and performing screening tests or indirectly by historical review of another's observations. The screening tests require individual administration and are generally appropriate for the first 5 years of childhood.

The Gesell Developmental Schedules measure infant development in four major areas: (1) communication skills, (2) motor behavior, (3) adaptive behavior, and (4) personal–social behavior. The child's responses to standard stimuli (e.g., toys) are noted and supplemented by information provided by the mother. Behavioral abnormalities can be measured as early as 4–6 weeks of age. The Cattell Infant Intelligence Scale is a downward extension of the Stanford–Binet and is used to measure infant development for ages 2–30 months. Mental age scores expressed as IQs may be obtained. The Bayley Scales of Infant Development are applicable from birth to 15 months and are useful in assessing mental and psychomotor development. Comparisons with norms permit measurement of developmental strengths and weaknesses as well as providing a baseline of the child's developmental progress. The Denver Developmental Screening Test (DDST) is a quick screening test for children aged 2 months to 6 years. Information regarding development in the areas of fine motor, gross motor, language, and personal–social skills is obtained through direct observation of the child as well as from information obtained from parents. Developmental delays can be identified by this screening test, which requires 10–20 min of administration time. The inventory assists in making judicial referrals for more comprehensive developmental assessments.

Developmental testing often includes structured interview techniques with the parents. Questions are asked that relate to the child's development, and a parental appraisal of the child's level of proficiency is obtained. The Vineland Social Maturity Scale consists of 117 items grouped into year levels and presented to an informant, usually a parent. Developmental progress in areas of general self-help, self-help in eating, dressing, and self-direction, communication, locomotion, and socialization is assessed. A social age (SA) and a social quotient (SQ) are obtained to provide an overall assessment of social development. Analysis of individual scales may provide information regarding areas of delayed development. The Minnesota Child Development Inventory is another standardized instrument that measures the child's development using the mother's observations. A developmental profile is obtained based on 320 statements describing the behaviors of children in the first 6 years of life. The areas evaluated include general development, gross motor, fine motor, expressive language, comprehension-conceptual, situation comprehension, self-help, and personal–social skills. Initial research on this instrument indicates a high correlation between the developmental profile and the results of extensive psychological evaluation. Caution must be exercised in checking the reliability of the informant. The inventory itself is utilized only as a supplement to interview and other testing procedures.

NEUROPSYCHOLOGICAL TESTING

A neuropsychological battery is often needed to provide a more comprehensive diagnostic evaluation. Numerous tests are currently in use that are claimed to be diagnostic of "brain damage." On the basis of an agreed-upon score, the implication is made that a child has brain damage. However, just as IQ is not a useful term to describe a pattern of strengths and weaknesses in a child, the diagnosis of brain damage offers little or no concrete information for constructing remedial strategies.

Neuropsychological assessments help define how a child processes certain types of information, comparing strengths and weaknesses of information processing by different sense modalities. The symmetry of functioning of the cerebral hemispheres is similarly compared. The data obtained are compared with expectancy level on the basis of anticipated developmental milestones of normative groups with documented lesions.

Reitan and Davidson[2] illustrated the applications of the neuropsychological testing approach to the understanding of learning disabilities. Although tests such as the Bender–Gestalt or Draw-a-Person Test may be used to demonstrate the presence of brain dysfunction, they are nonspecific in terms of localization. Neuropsychological approaches provide an assessment in the following major areas: (1) motor functions (motor speed, strength, coordination, and motor problem solving), (2) tactile–perceptual functions (tactile from recognition and localization), (3) verbal abilities, (4) visual–spatial and visual–sequential abilities, (5) immediate alertness, (6) memory, (7) concept formation and reasoning ability, (8) auditory perception–auditory discrimination, (9) speech and language, (10) personality, and (11) achievement.

The diagnosis of brain dysfunction and localization is made by comparing the relative functioning of the right and left cerebral hemispheres. For example, on tests of motor functions, performance with the dominant and nondominant hands is compared. Information is provided regarding the integrity of the contralateral cerebral hemisphere. Relative functioning within a hemisphere is also investigated. Anterior and posterior portions of the dominant cerebral hemisphere serve different functions in terms of language skills. Tests of receptive and expressive language may be compared in an effort to understand the nature of the deficit in this area. The value of such testing is that it offers a pattern of strengths and weaknesses from which proper remediation approaches may be implemented.

SCREENING TESTS FOR THE PHYSICIAN

Screening tests are available for use by the physician in practice. The physician is usually the first professional encountering a child with suspected problems in development, learning, or emotional adjustment. Pediatricians, family practitioners, and other primary health care professionals can use screening batteries such as the Denver Developmental Screening Test to obtain a clearer picture of a child's area of difficulty and make appropriate referrals. Behavioral reports are obtained from parents, teachers, and others having contact with the child. The screening battery also contains follow-up procedures to monitor the child's progress. Although this screening battery in no way takes the place of a comprehensive evaluation by psychologists, speech pathologists, and educators, it does provide a tool whereby the physician can rapidly assess areas of deficit and make appropriate referrals.

SUMMARY

The complexities of diagnostic psychological evaluation have been presented in this chapter with a twofold purpose. First, various tests that have sufficient reliability and validity to be useful in evaluating children have been examined. Many other tests are available, and it remains to the examiner's sophistication and knowledge to choose the most appropriate instruments for his purposes. The second and most important emphasis concerns a basic philosophy of the proper use of these tests. Because of the intermingling of intellectual, academic, and emotional factors, the understanding of the total child must be a priority in testing.

Although tests are useful in providing answers to various questions asked about children, without the diagnostician's thorough understanding of the multiplicity of factors that enter into child development and behavior, good tests are useless. Only by asking the proper questions can tests be administered to find the proper answers.

REFERENCES

1. Adams, J.: Clinical neuropsychology and the study of learning disorders. *Pediatr. Clin. North Am.* **20:**587–598, 1973.
2. Reitan, R. M., and Davidson, L. A.: *Clinical Neuropsychology: Current Status and Applications.* Wiley, New York, 1975.
3. Kirk, S. A., and Kirk, W. D.: *Psycholinguistic Learning Disabilities: Diagnosis and Remediation.* University of Illinois Press, Urbana, 1971.
4. Frostig, M., Maslow, P., Lefever, D. W., *et al.: The Marianne Frostig Test of Visual Perception: 1963 Standardization.* Consulting Psychologists Press, Palo Alto, 1963.
5. Jastak, J. R., and Jastak, S. R.: *The Wide Range Achievement Test.* Guidance Associates of Delaware, Wilmington, 1965.

9

Major Variations in Intelligence

Marvin I. Gottlieb

INTRODUCTION

During the past two decades, the traditional concept of comprehensive health care for children has been significantly modified, with particular emphasis on providing for the child's psychobiological, educational, and psychosocial needs. The primary care physician has been mandated increasing responsibilities in the management of developmental–behavioral problems. For the pediatrician, this expanded medical challenge requires the acquisition of skills in neurodevelopmental screening, counseling, management strat-

Marvin I. Gottlieb • Institute for Child Development, Hackensack Medical Center, and Department of Pediatrics, University of Medicine and Dentistry of New Jersey–New Jersey Medical School, Hackensack, New Jersey 07601.

egies, and child advocacy roles, for children with a variety of chronic handicapping conditions. A spirited pediatric interest for children with developmental disabilities is in part the result of (1) improved skills in prevention and management of acute pediatric problems (e.g., infection control), (2) an increasing population of children with chronic handicapping disorders, (3) federal legislation (PL 94-142) enacted to protect the rights of all handicapped children, (4) successful lobbying by various parent advocacy groups, (5) popularizing these issues by the communications media, and (6) a renewed commitment by professionals to protect and improve the quality of life for *all* children.

As a general rule, the chronic handicapping conditions of childhood share common characteristics: (1) family dynamics are often disrupted; (2) the educational system is generally stressed, often necessitating special services; (3) the potential for adult productivity is compromised; (4) there is often a superimposed behavioral complication; and (5) early identification and interventions may lessen the impact of the disability. Children with variations in intelligence—the mentally retarded and the gifted—frequently share these common sequelae, thereby qualifying for designation as "handicapping disorders." Mentally retarded *and* gifted children generally require some form of special education assistance in order to accommodate for their unique differences in learning styles. Special programming is generally necessary in order to enhance potentials for psychoeducational achievement as well as to promote good self-concept.

INTELLIGENCE

The concept of intelligence is mercurial in nature, often clouded by (1) confusions in terminology, (2) discipline-oriented classification schemas, (3) varying methods of assessment and data interpretation, (4) heterogenicity of population samples, and (5) poor practical application of psychoeducational data to life situations. Paradoxically, variations in intelligence constitute a major diagnostic/management challenge for pediatric health care professionals. Frequently pediatricians are expected to provide either value judgments or documentations of a preschooler's cognitive skills and potentials, or both. The "norms" of intelligence and methods of evaluation are reviewed in Chapter 8. The present chapter focuses on two deviations in intellectual development: below average intelligence (mental retardation) and very superior intelligence (giftedness). Although representing divergent extremes of intelligence, mental retardation and very superior intelligence share similarities in their ultimate impact on child, family, educational system, and community. Each represents a significant clinical challenge for the primary health care provider, particularly in the early identification and management of preschool age children.

Intelligence per se is generally regarded as a hypothetical construct; its quantification is valuable as a possible marker in understanding and predicting adaptive behaviors. Unfortunately, there are a myriad of psychological, educational, and social interpretations of the nature of intelligence, many of which are contradictory. No single definition of intelligence has enjoyed universal or lasting acceptance.[1] It is generally agreed that IQ and intelligence are *not* synonymous, although they are often used interchangeably. The IQ score is only an estimate of an individual's rate of intellectual development as compared with the average rate for same-age peers. Erickson notes that an IQ score of 100 indicates

Table I. Intelligence Classification Based on IQ Scores

WISC-R		Stanford-Binet		Cattell	
IQ Score	Definition	IQ Score	Definition	IQ Score	Definition
>130	Very superior	140–170	Very superior	≥122	Markedly above average
120–129	Superior	120–139	Superior	112–122	Appreciably above average
110–119	High average	110–119	High average	108–112	High average
90–109	Average	90–110	Average	92–108	Average
80–89	Low average	80–90	Low average	88–92	Low average
70–79	Borderline[a]	70–79	Borderline defective	88–88	Appreciably below average
55–69	Mild retardation	30–70	Mentally defective	50–78	Markedly below average
40–54	Moderate retardation				
25–39	Severe retardation				
<24	Profound retardation				

[a]Category deleted in revised classification by the American Association of Mental Deficiency.

that the subject's rate of intellectual development is exactly the same as the average rate for age mates.[2] For practical purposes, results of intelligence tests have been used to identify variations from the average and to predict the need for special education interventions. Although these tests are not perfect, they do serve (within limits) to subgroup children into major categories of expected educational/social/psychological behaviors. The subgroups delineated by IQ scores suggest a spectrum of anticipated cognitive and adaptive abilities (see Appendix). This chapter focuses primarily on children whose potential can be categorized in the major groupings of mental retardation and very superior intelligence, representing significant variations from average intellectual abilities (Table I).

MENTAL RETARDATION

Historical Background

Several texts[3,4] provide a concise historical background on mental retardation, noting that the earliest medical writings can be traced to the beginning of the seventeenth century. Paracelsus (1603) wrote about the futility of treating cretins who were mental defectives; subsequently, Platter (1656) described cretinism in greater detail and "their innate simple-mindedness." Medical management of mental retardation was first reported by Guggenbuhl (1816–1863) in his attempt to treat cretinism. Little (1843) noted the association between neonatal brain damage and mental retardation. Several years later, Down (1866) described and differentiated mongolism and its associated mental retardation. In 1887, Sachs characterized the features of amaurotic familial idiocy. Toward the end of the nineteenth and early twentieth centuries, Weisman (Germany), Mendel (Austria), and Goddard (United States) popularized the significance of heredity as causative factors. Subsequently, encephalitis, faulty metabolism, rubella during gestation, and erythroblastosis were associated with mental retardation. In 1801, Itard (1774–1838) reported on his attempts to educate "the wild boy of Aveyron." Itard's special education for his mentally defective patient were unsuccessful by his standards; i.e., the child was still retarded. Seguin (1812–1880), a physician–pupil of Itard, stressed education of the mentally retarded by utilizing sensorimotor drills and exercises. Seguin's writings contain some of the earliest descriptions of Down syndrome and fetal alcohol syndrome. Montessori (1869–1952), the Italian physician, further advanced the movement for providing educational opportunities for mentally retarded children by expanding on the techniques of Itard and Sequin.

The psychological evaluation of children at various levels of intellectual development was first attempted by Galton in 1883. Cattell (1893) in the United States made similar attempts. It was not until 1905, when Binet, a French psychologist, and Simon, a French physician, designed an examination for comparing a child's mental level with his actual age, the Binet–Simon intelligence test. The Binet–Simon test represented a break from subjective classification of mental retardation and became the basis for other psychological examinations designed to provide IQ scores.

During the past half-century, several significant achievements have contributed to our appreciation of the etiology, diagnosis, and management of mental retardation. Gesell (1888–1961) systematically documented aspects of infant and early childhood development. The discovery by Levine of the Rh antigen led to the development of RhoGam and the prevention of mental retardation associated with kernicterus. The landmark discovery by Lejeune (1959) in defining the chromosomal abnormality in Down syndrome opened a new arena of medical technology and investigation. A host of genetic and chromosomal disorders have been identified that may be associated with mental retardation (e.g., trisomy 18 syndrome, Klinefelter syndrome). Most recently, the fragile X syndrome has been delineated, which similarly has been linked with cognitive disorders.[5] Possibly the greatest contribution was made by President John F. Kennedy, who made mental retardation an issue of medical and public concern. From this intervention originated a new positive philosophical approach to understanding and managing mental retardation as a chronic handicapping disorder.

Terminology

It was not until 1961 that the American Association of Mental Deficiency (AAMD) proposed a definition of mental retardation that was generally accepted by most disciplines. Mental retardation refers to "significantly subaverage general intellectual functioning which manifests itself during the development period and is characterized by inadequacy in adaptive behavior."[6]

Subaverage intellectual functioning refers to an intelligence quotient below 70, i.e., performance that is greater than two or more standard deviations (>2 SD) below the population mean group involved. The definition suggests that the problem originates during the developmental period, generally regarded as between birth and 16 years of age—more accurately from the instant of conception to 18 years. The AAMD definition measures the expression of mental retardation by impaired adaptive behavior, i.e. impaired maturation, learning, and/or social adjustment. Deviations in the anticipated patterns of maturation (sequential development of gross and fine motor skills, language, personal social skills, and personality) are more obvious markers in children with moderate, severe or profound mental retardation. Difficulties in learning (the capacity to acquire new information) and social adjustment (ability to adapt within the community to activities of adult life at work and within the home) may be the first manifestations of intellectual subnormalcy in individuals with borderline or mild mental retardation. Children with borderline or mild retardation may only manifest subtle motor and language delays.

In essence, for an individual to be designated as "mentally retarded" three criteria must be fulfilled:

(1) an IQ score at least 2 standard deviations below the mean, (2) manifested before 18 years of age, and (3) accompanied by impairments in adaptive behavior.[4]

Incidence

The incidence of mental retardation has been roughly calculated based on IQ scores ≥2 SD below the norm, i.e., about 3% of the population. This can be generalized as approximately six million or more persons (more than 130,000 persons born annually so involved). Approximately 0.1% of annual births will be so severely involved that they will not be able to care for their daily living needs, 0.3% will remain below the mental age of 7 years, and the remaining 3.0% are individuals with mental retardation who will require special training and assistance in order to acquire limited job skills and a measure of independence. It has been estimated that approximately $12 billion is the total annual expenditure for services for the mentally retarded.[7] The severity of mental retardation cannot be measured solely on the basis of incidence or financial impact but must take into account the pervasive stress on family, educational system, and community.

Classification

Virtually all classification systems for mental retardation depend on the IQ score as an index of measurement. It must be emphasized, however, that the IQ is not the only criterion to be used in assessing an individual's level of retardation. Factors such as social adaptability and emotional control are significant factors that may influence the overall evaluation of the patient. The AAMD classification defines four levels of mental retardation that are correlated with levels of IQ (Table II). Grades of mental retardation (mild, moderate, severe, profound) are delineated by the number of standard deviations of the IQ from the mean. Intelligence tests use the statistical concept of a standard deviation for each age level tested. This method is used to compare each child with an age-mate peer. Generally the IQ of a retarded child is stable over time, with variability depending on test instrument bias or improper administration of test materials.

For the primary care physician, the developmental quotient provides a good clinical index of the child's functional ability:

$$\text{Developmental quotient} = \frac{\text{mental age}}{\text{chronological age}} \times 100$$

or

$$(DQ = MA/CA \times 100)$$

Table II. Levels of Retardation: Associated Terminologies and Potentials

IQ range	Standard deviations below mean	Educational terminology	Psychological terminology	Prototype	Academic grade-level potential	Usual time of diagnosis
84–70	1	Slow learner	Borderline[a]	May not be diagnosed except as a "slow learner"	May complete schooling with assistance	Increasing academic difficulties
69–55	2 and 3	Educable	Mild	Socioeconomically deprived	Fourth to sixth grade	Kindergarten or first grade; when confronted with academics
54–40	3 and 4	Trainable	Moderate	Organic MR (e.g., trisomy 21)	Can be taught survival words and self-help, vocational and social skills	Early childhood; delayed development as a preschooler
39–25 25	4	Subtrainable	Severe; <25: profound	Organic; severe CNS injury or syndromy	Need aid in self-help	Infancy and early childhood

[a]Category deleted in revised classification by American Association of Mental Deficiency. Adapted in part from Accardo and Capute.[4]

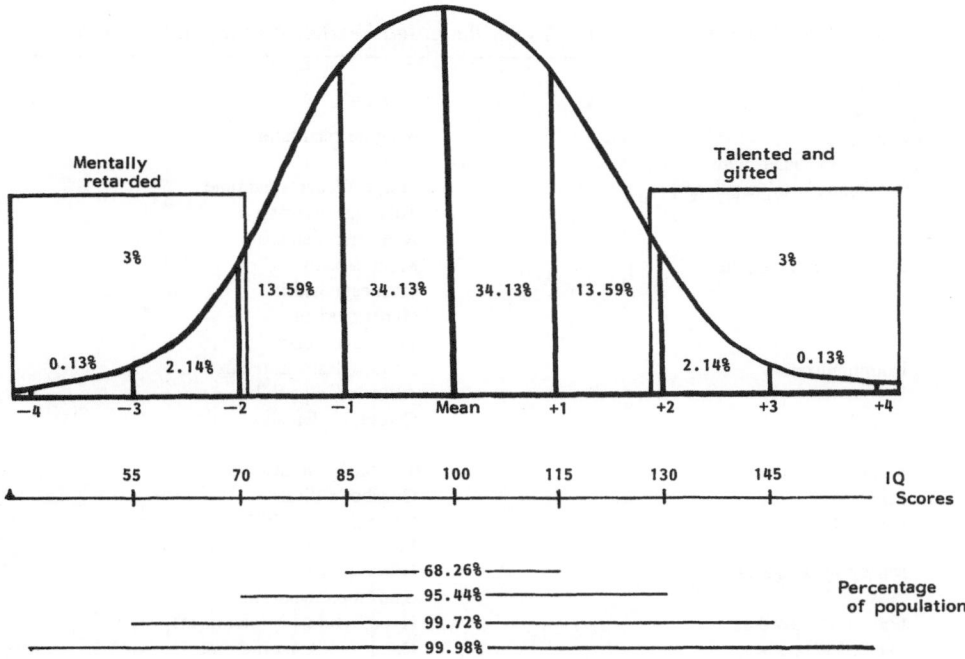

Figure 1. The theoretical distribution of intelligence, based on IQ scores. (Adapted from Magrab and Johnston[10]).

A meaningful classification of mental retardation requires an assessment of potential level of function, i.e., a schema designed to prognosticate educational, vocational and social abilities (Table II).

The theoretical distribution of IQ scores is generally depicted as a standard bell curve (Fig. 1). The actual distribution reveals a "two group" theory of mental retardation. In reality, five-sixths of the retarded population fall into the classification of "mild," located on the tail end of the predicted normal distribution, whereas only one-sixth have IQs below 55 and occupy their own distribution curve. The "mild" (five-sixths of the population) are composed primarily of socioeconomic, cultural, or familial retardates; one-sixth of the population have the highest incidence of organic pathologies.[4]

Etiology

A variety of factors have been associated with mental retardation, occuring before, during, or after birth. Table III summarizes some of the factors which can interfere with brain development during its most vulnerable period of maximal growth. As a rule, gross abnormalities of the brain are associated with the more severe levels of mental retardation. However, the brain's adaptive capacity to make use of alternate pathways limits the ability to make absolute prognostications regarding ultimate function. As Accardo and Capute[4] summarized:

Table III. High-Risk Factors Associated with Increased Incidence of Mental Retardation

Prenatal factors	
Genetic factors	
Nonspecific	Familial retardation
Specific, associated with	
Cutaneous manifestations	Sturge-Weber syndrome
	Tuberous sclerosis
	Neurofibromatosis
Craniofacial anomalies	Microcephaly
	Craniosynostosis
	Hypertelorism
	Apert syndrome
Isoimmunization	Erythroblastosis fetalis
	ABO incompatibility
CNS degenerative disease	Cerebral sclerosis
Metabolic disorders	Tay-Sachs disease
Lipids	Gaucher's disease
Amino acids	Phenylalanine (PKU)
	Maple syrup urine disease
Mucopolysaccharide	Hurler's syndrome
	Sanfilippo syndrome
Endocrine disorders	Hypothyroidism (cretinism)
Skeletal anomalies	Dandy-Walker syndrome
	Arnold-Chiari deformity
Specific chromosomal anomalies	
Autosomes	Down syndrome (trisomy 21)
	Trisomy 18 syndrome
	Trisomy 13–15 syndrome
	Cri-du-chat syndrome
Sex chromosomes	Klinefelter syndrome (XXY)
	XXX syndrome
	XYY syndrome
	Fragile X syndrome
Infections during pregnancy (maternal and fetal)	Rubella
	Chickenpox
	Syphilis
	Toxoplasmosis
	Cytomegalic inclusion virus
Maternal anoxia during pregnancy	Anesthesia for surgery (others)
Obstetrical complications	Toxemia of pregnancy
	Gestational bleeding
	Polyhydramnios
Maternal intoxications	Alcohol embryopathy
	Drug addiction
	Medications (known and unknown)
Maternal metabolic/endocrine disorders	Hypothyroidism
	Diabetes mellitus
	Maternal PKU
Maternal vascular disorders	Hypertension
	Cardiovascular disorders
	Renal disorders

Table III. (Continued)

Miscellaneous high-risk factors	Advanced maternal age (>40)
	Radiation exposure
	Nutritional deficiences
	Excess smoking?
	New growths
Perinatal factors	
Presentation	Breech
Labor	Prolonged
	Precipitate
Cord	Prolapsed
	Nuchal
	Knotted
Placenta	Placenta previa
	Abruptio placenta
	Infarction
Fetus	Prematurity (<34 weeks)
	Low birth weight for gestational age
	Fetal–placental transfusion
	Fetal–fetal tranfusion
Newborn	Anomalies
	Birth injuries
	Endocrine
	Infections
	Intoxications
	Neonatal anoxia
	New growths
	Nutritional
	Seizures
	Trauma
	Vascular
Postnatal factors	
Infections	Encephalitis
	Meningitis
	Meningoencephalitis
	Cerebral abscesses
	Postinfection hydrocephalus
Encephalopathies	Environmental contaminations (lead, mercury)
	Postimmunization
Craniocerebral trauma and cerebrovasular accidents	Closed and open head injuries
	Aneurysms
Cerebral anoxia	Chemicals
	Physical
	Infections
	Seizures
Pseudoretardation	Psychiatric problems
	Socioeconomic deprivation
Miscellaneous	Nutritional disorders
	Metabolic/endocrine problems
	Severe dehydration
	New growths

The capacity of the organism to adapt to brain injury makes the neurologic examination of the newborn infant (and the child under 2 years of age) a poor predictor of developmental outcome; the fact that moderate to severe brain damage does contribute significantly to the incidence of retardation allows for the positive correlations found between newborn evaluations and later outcome.

The major organic adverse conditions associated with mental retardation include genetic and chromosomal abnormalities, asphyxia, CNS trauma, infections of the nervous system, toxins, malnutrition, and metabolic disorders. Low birth weight (prematurity or small for gestational age) has a high correlation with mental retardation. Infections *in utero,* such as rubella, toxoplasmosis, herpes, and cytomegalovirus can adversely affect the developing brain. Autosomal abnormalities (e.g., trisomies 13, 18, and 21; deletion of short arm of chromosome 5) are almost always associated with mental retardation; a less striking tendency is noted in sex chromosome abnormalities (Turner syndrome). So-cioeconomic and cultural factors may be similarly associated with organic deficits or exist singly as an etiological precipitant of mental retardation.

Mental retardation is associated with more than 200 known medical entities, includ-ing genetic/chromosomal disorders, infections during pregnancy, accidental poisonings and injuries, metabolic disorders, and CNS infections. Mental retardation is generally a multifactorial disorder in which numerous variables depress intellectual potential (e.g., cerebral palsy, deafness, language impairment). The mentally retarded are at significant risk for concomitant developmental disabilities.[4] Approxmately two-thirds of handi-capped children present with more than one handicap (one-third have one handicap, one-third have two handicaps, and one-third have three or more handicaps). As Accardo and Capute[4] indicate, "the more severe the retardation, the greater the probability of an associated disability" (i.e., prevalence of other disabilities associated with mental retar-dation includes hearing loss 3%, visual loss 1%, cerebral palsy 10%, epilepsy 4%, and psychiatric disorders 40%). As the authors point out, the prevalence of mental retardation associated with each disability can be approximated if one starts from epidemiological studies of their disabilities, i.e., 15% of deaf, 23% of blind, 50% of cerebral palsied, 15% of epileptics, and 12% with psychiatric disorders.

Diagnosis: Role of the Physician

Federal legislation during the 1970s reflected an attitudinal change by society in their concern for the mentally retarded. The rights of the mentally retarded were acknowledged in the Education for All Handicapped Children Act of 1975 (P.L. 94-142) and in the Rehabilitation Comprehensive Services and Developmental Disabilities Amendment of 1978 (PL 95-602). The legislation focused on education and support services for the handicapped, with an ultimate goal in promoting near normal functioning and enhancing independence. In addition to legislation, there has been an increasing pressure on physi-cians to assume a leadership role in the coordination of medical, educational and psycho-logical care for children with developmental disabilities. The mandate implies an active responsibility in the early identification of developmental disabilities and the initiation of appropriate medical, educational, and psychological services. The dictum of "the earlier the diagnosis, the better the prognosis" does not differentiate acute from chronic pediatric disorders. As the first professional to serve infants and children, the primary care physician is charged with a significant responsibility in the initial identification and management of infants and young children with developmental disabilities or any other potential chronic handicapping conditions.

The delineation of mental retardation is in part dependent on the age of the child and the severity of the retardation. For example, a 3-year-old with mild mental retardation may be a formidable diagnostic challange, generally unnoticed as retarded by the casual observer. However, the child may indeed be slower to walk, talk, and feed himself than most children. On the other hand, a 3-year-old with severe retardation would more likely exhibit marked delays in motor, language, and personal–social skills (see Appendix).

The neurodevelopmental assessment of children of all ages and the early identification of mental retardation will generally require (1) a comprehensive history, (2) a complete physical and neurological examination, (3) appropriate laboratory studies, (4) developmental screenings, and (5) judicious referral to supporting professionals.[8]

A comprehensive history is critical in defining high-risk factors which may be associated with an increased incidence of mental retardation (Table III). These factors are generally associated with a higher incidence of CNS pathologies. In addition to delineating high-risk markers (e.g., obstetrical complications, neonatal disorders), the history may document evidence of maturational lags and/or dysfunctions. Frequently the parents (or grandparents) recognize that there is something wrong with the child. "Wrong" may pertain to a lag in one or more areas of development.

The physical and neurological examinations are important in defining evidence of organic impairment, including handicaps that simulate mental retardation (e.g., the pseudoretardation of deafness). It has been noted that "facial appearance often provides a clue to specific diagnosis in the mentally retarded child" (e.g., trisomies 13, 18, and 21; congenital hypothyroidism, fetal alcohol syndrome, Rubenstein-Taybi syndrome).[9] Examination of head size (microcephaly), the skin (hypopigmented macules of tuberous sclerosis), eyes (cataracts of congential rubella), and the skeletal system (polysyndactyly of Apert syndrome) all may provide diagnostic clues.

The neurological examination may provide direct evidence of CNS injury, which is associated with mental retardation. Laboratory studies are often diagnostic, such as abnormal metabolic screening, chromosomal abnormalities, computer-assisted tomography (CAT) scan findings. In clinical practice, a variety of neurodevelopmental screening inventories are available for defining the child's range of functioning abilities (see Chapters 8 and 21). The Denver Developmental Screening Test, The Lexington Developmental Screening Test, and others provide information regarding an infant's or preschooler's abilities in motor, language, personal–social, and cognitive skills (see Chapter 21). Many of these inventories compare favorably with the Bayley Scales of Infant Development and the Stanford–Binet Intelligence Scales. More global delays, in contrast to isolated areas of delay, may arouse suspicions of mental retardation. Screening inventories serve to identify children who appear to function below age level expectancy but are not designed to provide IQ scores or a definitive diagnosis.

The data accrued from these screening interventions may serve not only to initiate referrals but to provide the basis for *judicious* referrals. The definition of strengths and weaknesses (the developmental–behavioral profile) may suggest the need for one or more specific professional assistance, such as a psychologist, speech–language clinician, or learning disability consultant. The definition of suspected mental retardation may necessitate the coordination of an interdisciplinary evaluation. The multidisciplinary approach is often required in order to provide a more accurate differentiation of various levels of ability (intellectual, educational, behavioral control). The diagnostic data are important in ultimately designing a management program as well as helping to formulate a meaningful prognosis.

Management

The role of the physician in the direct treatment of mental retardation is limited; management is generally psychoeducational. Special medical interventions for the mentally retarded may include the use of adjunctive medications (anticonvulsants, psychotropic agents), surgical procedures (myelomeningocele, craniostenosis, cerebral palsy), and psychiatric consultations.[10]

The physician, however, may participate in a variety of indirect interventions for the mentally retarded, such as the judicious selection and coordination of a multidisciplinary management team (psychologist, speech pathologist, special educator). Periodic assessment and follow-up services for the patient are similarly often initiated, arranged, and reviewed by the primary care physician.

The physician frequently serves as the primary counselor for the parents. The psychological supports often involve reviewing issues of education, medical care and family problems. Legal and ethical issues are similarly discussed (e.g., sterilization, guardianship, institutional care). The physician is expected to participate in these discussions because of his more protracted and closer relationship with the family (often providing care for other family members).

The physician is probably the most important advocate for children with chronic handicapping disorders. Interventions by physicians at a public (community) level have particular meaning in helping secure needed services for children with developmental disabilities. A meaningful advocacy role requires familiarity with the legal rights of the developmentally disabled and their families (Table IV).

It must be emphasized that the primary care physician should provide for the mentally retarded child's general health and for any condition that may contribute to the mental retardation. The management of acute medical situations accompanies the responsibilities of the long-term care of the child afflicted with a chronic handicapping disorder. New expertise in neurodevelopmental screening, interdisciplinary management, parent/child/professional counseling, and active advocacy are the expected skills of physicians providing comprehensive health care for children with mental retardation.

A major management goal for children with mental retardation is the enhancement of skills to promote maximal independence as an adolescent and adult. This challenge is a primary focus of special education intervention. The mildly retarded child had been stereotypically grouped in the "educable class," a traditional self-contained program. The educable class frequently failed to recognize the individual differences and needs of the child. The mildly retarded child may have educational needs similar to those of normal children, unless there are associated specific learning, cognitive, or behavioral problems. The rate of learning is slower and the level of achievement is approximately at the fifth- or

Table IV. Levels of Medical Management of Children with Mental Retardation

Primary medical care
1. Traditional preventive medicine and acute pediatric care
2. Investigation of primary factors contributing to mental retardation
3. Assessment of secondary contributing factors (e.g., hearing loss)
4. Coordination of multidisciplinary management team
5. Periodic neurodevelopmental assessments
6. Interventions to enhance self-concept and promote social adaptation/independence
7. Counseling supports for family members

Long-term medical care
1. Maintenance of good health care practices
2. Health and sex education for child and family
3. Follow-up services to monitor intellectual, educational, and psychosocial development
4. Coordination of multidisciplinary services and recommendations for modifications based on re-evaluations
5. Ongoing counseling services for child and family (e.g., medical needs, legal rights)
6. Parent and child education programs

Coordination of health needs
1. Interfacing with members of the multidisciplinary team (improve intraprofessional communications)
2. Coordination of medical, psychological, educational and social services in perspective of the child's changing needs
3. Community advocacy roles (support parent organizations and efforts to obtain community services)
4. Maintenance of parent support system and long-range planning

sixth-grade level. The current educational philosophy is to mainstream the mildly retarded child, providing an individualized educational program supplemented with special services and resource room activities. The ultimate goal is to provide an academic program until early or midadolescence, when the emphasis will refocus on vocational training. For the mildly retarded child who is unable to accomplish these goals successfully, alternate strategies must be programmed.

The educational focus is significantly different for the moderately and severely retarded child, formerly grouped in a "trainable class." In general, mainstreaming does not appear to be a viable educational strategy, and self-contained classrooms are required. The emphasis of the program (based on degree of retardation) is designed to promote (1) acquisition of primary reading skills, (2) improved verbal communication, (3) personal-social skills (e.g., toileting, hygiene), and (4) health and sex education. Needless to say, independent function is a basic goal.

The profoundly retarded child is generally not included in the broad schema of educational interventions. The programs are designed primarily to provide sensory and social stimulation. In each of these educational categories, the teacher and physician should interface to provide a comprehensive program that will jointly address the medical, educational, and psychosocial needs of the child. The educational environment is an ideal geographic and professional milieu in which to provide a support system for parents and family members. Ideally, support groups can be a cooperative effort of school personnel and primary care physicians.

VERY SUPERIOR INTELLIGENCE: THE "GIFTED" CHILD

Historical Background

Interest in gifted children dates back to antiquity. Indeed, Plato recommended searching for and preparing these children for leadership roles. This philosophy suggested that giftedness was not limited to royalty and aristocracy. However, the curiosities reported by Lewis Terman,[11] during this century, mark the "modern" interests and investigations into the nature of children with very superior intelligence. After completing his standardization of the Stanford–Binet Intelligence Test, Terman began the first systematic study of the gifted. His goal was to define the medical, psychological, and social characteristics of gifted children. Terman's subjects were required to have an IQ of 140 or above, placing them in the top 1% of their age mates in school. The selection process had numerous built-in biases, however, the selected group of children were compared with control group averages. Terman followed the children for more than 30 years, publishing five volumes on their lives at various ages.[11] Terman's studies disputed the common myths about the gifted, suggesting that the gifted are superior in all developmental parameters. Until the 1960s high IQ scores were related synonymously with giftedness. Currently, identification of the gifted is multidimensional; involving assessment of potential for achievement, behavior, and educational needs. In essence, the concept of giftedness gradually changed during the post-Terman era, emphasizing that academic potential was not synonymous with giftedness unless it yielded "socially productive contributions." Renzulli[12] popularized the concept of a continuum of giftedness; i.e., one could be gifted in certain areas and not in others and at certain times and not at other times.

Terminology

Professionals assumed increasing roles in advocacy when the myth was dispelled that giftedness automatically ensured educational, psychological, and social success. The concept of giftedness evolved to include areas other than academic achievement, and "talent" was incorporated into the philosophical construct. There was a concomitant recognition that IQ was not the sole criterion for designating giftedness. From these new perspectives, a more universally accepted definition of giftedness was proposed by the Marland Report in 1972[13]:

> Gifted and talented children are those identified by professionally qualified persons who, by virtue of outstanding abilities, are capable of high performance. These are children who require differentiated educational programs and/or services beyond those normally provided by the regular school program in order to realize their contribution to self and society.

> Children capable of high performance include those with demonstrated achievement and/or potential ability in any of the following areas, singly or in combination:
> (1) general intellectual ability
> (2) specific academic aptitude
> (3) creative or productive thinking
> (4) leadership ability
> (5) visual and performing arts
> (6) psychomotor ability

The work of Torrance, Taylor, Barron, and others modified perceptions of the nature of giftedness to include *creativity*. Creativity has been viewed as a necessary ingredient of intellectual giftedness and as a kind of giftedness. Renzulli[12] recommended a new definition of giftedness that he proposed would be more useful to school practitioners—an operational definition:

> Giftedness consists of an interaction among three basic clusters of human traits—these clusters being *above-average general abilities, high levels of task commitment,* and *high levels of creativity.* Gifted and talented children are those possessing or capable of developing this composite set of traits and applying them to any potentially valuable area of human performance. Children who manifest or are capable of developing an interaction among these clusters require a wide variety of educational opportunities and services that are not ordinarily provided through regular instructional programs.

As with mental retardation or intelligence in general, there is no universally applicable definition of giftedness because the descriptions include a heterogeneous population of children. As Passow notes[14]:

> The gifted and talented come in a tremendous variety of shapes, forms and sizes. Some gifted youngsters are only slightly above average with respect to the criteria applied while others are so unusual as to be extremely rare; some individuals are gifted/talented in a single area, while others seem to be unusually able in practically any area. Some individuals who seem to have outstanding ability have relatively little motivation or interest in developing that potential while others are both highly talented and highly motivated. Some are high achievers and quick absorbers of information, while others utilize knowledge in new and different ways. Some are basically consumers of knowledge while others are potentially outstanding producers as well as consumers. Some are especially precocious manifesting unusual potential at early ages while others are "late bloomers" and do not show unusual potential or performance until much later. There are cultural differences with respect to which talent areas are more likely to be rewarded and, consequently, which will be nurtured.

For purposes of this discussion, the focus is on children with gifted intellectual ability. The trials and tribulations of the talented child are beyond the scope of this review. (*Talent* implies an inborn ability in a special field that is capable of being cultivated and is often, but not necessarily, associated with superior intelligence.)

Myths and Misinformation

Throughout the ages, intellectually gifted children have been shrouded in an atmosphere bordering on the "mystical." A host of myths and misinformation have clouded perceptions of their physical, academic, psychosocial, and vocational abilities and needs. The myriad of misperceptions concerning gifted children relate to their educational, psychosocial, and physical attributes. The more popular misconceptions suggest that *"They will succeed without help"*; *"They are socially isolated by their own choice"*; *"Gifted children are eccentric"*; *"We educate gifted children at the expense of others"*; and *"Their giftedness will be revealed spontaneously."* As Gallagher[15] notes "Persistent myths about gifted individuals exist despite an increasing volume of scientific refutation." Unfortunately even during this generation of "sophistication," many of these misperceptions still persist, perhaps even at a professional level.

Four common myths have been specifically attributed to intellectually gifted children:

1. They are generally weaklings, physically inferior, or "eggheads."
2. They are usually loners, eccentric, and socially backward.
3. They all turn out to be successful in academics and vocations, regardless of special interventions.
4. They walk a very fine line between genius, instability, and insanity.

Research data, from longitudinal studies of gifted children, do not support these mythical hypotheses. In regard to physical development, gifted children are of at least average height, weight, and physical appearance. Terman's gifted children appeared to be more mature physiologically and superior in height, weight, and muscular strength.[11] Indeed, much of the research has shown that the stereotyped concept of a weakling physical stature of the gifted child is simply not true, perhaps with the exception of an increased incidence of poorer eyesight.[16] The health records of gifted children appear to be better than those of the average population, because they (and their parents) understand the need for good physical health. As a group, gifted children may be more attentive to good health practices.

In exploring myths concerning eccentric and socially backward behaviors, once again studies suggest that this is an inappropriate concept. Gifted children appear to be socially well adjusted and are generally more sensitive to human interactions. They are often leaders among their peer group. Gallagher[17] notes that "There is little or no question about the general social status of high-IQ elementary school children. It is high." There appears to be a positive correlation between IQ scores and popularity.

In regard to the concept that all gifted children are successful, some partial truths exist. Although most gifted children are successful in school (advancing to college graduate studies) and hold professional jobs, some commit crimes, are poorly adjusted, and may be unemployed. High IQ in isolation does not ensure success in all areas of development. Gifted children are subject to the myriad of variables that may compromise success (e.g., physical and emotional disorders, learning disabilities).

Perhaps the most ludicrous of the myths is that gifted children border on insanity. The mental image of the "mad scientist of the movies" perpetuates the myth that the very bright vacillate between genius, emotional instability, and insanity. In reality, gifted children appear to have better than average mental health records, with a less than average incidence of suicide and hospitalization for mental illness. As Gallagher[17] commented:

> Many of the personal problems of gifted children stem from the same general sources as those of average-ability children. Since there is a tendency for the high-IQ children to be a little better off in family stability and physical health, they are less likely to have problems than is the average child. This does not mean, however, that one cannot find gifted youngsters who are in a great deal of emotional trouble and in need of a good deal of special help and assistance.

Gifted children with IQs in the 130–150 range do not appear to have major personality problems, but children who are highly gifted (IQs greater than 180) may have a tendency toward underachievement, peer isolation, and suicide.[18]

Characteristics of Gifted Children

The profile of gifted children is a cumulative construct of various longitudinal studies of educational and social behaviors (e.g., see Terman's studies,[11] the Gulbenkian Project[16]). In general, it is possible to subgroup this profile into several major characteristic categories[16–20]:

General intellectual ability and cognitive skills
  1. Formulates abstractions and shows advanced comprehension
  2. Processes information in complex ways
  3. Observant and analytical
  4. Curious, enthused by new ideas
  5. Capacity to hypothesize
  6. Rapid acquisition of knowledge
  7. Accelerated and flexible thought processes
  8. High level of verbal ability and advanced language development
  9. Ability to generate original ideas and solutions
  10. Capacity for appreciating diverse relationships

Specific academic ability
  1. Excellent memorization skills
  2. Advanced comprehension
  3. Rapid learning of basic knowledge
  4. Reads widely in areas of interest
  5. High academic successes in interest areas
  6. Enthusiastic pursuits in interest areas
  7. May not be advanced in all academic areas

Creative thinking
  1. Independent thinker
  2. Originality in oral and written modalities
  3. Creative and inventive
  4. Particularly challenged by creative tasks
  5. Ability to improvise, develop novel alternatives, and problem-solve

Mental characteristics
  1. Mature expression of thoughts; mental processes "beyond their years"
  2. Early interest in definitions and meanings of words
  3. Particular interest in encyclopedias and dictionaries
  4. Reading self-taught at an early age (before school)
  5. Desire to acquire accurate information

Visual performing art skills
  1. Excellent sense of spatial relationships
  2. Fine ability to express moods and feelings
  3. Good motor coordination
  4. Originality, not content with copying
  5. Creative expression

Personality traits
1. Generally above-average stability
2. Usually cheerful, honest, faithful
3. May be argumentative, bold, and overconfident
4. Occasionally perceived as lazy, impatient, and loquacious
5. Good sense of humor

Psychomotor skills
1. Challenged by difficult athletic activities
2. Enjoys participation in athletics
3. Generally good gross motor coordination
4. Good manipulative skills
5. Enthusiastic and high energy levels

Leadership abilities
1. Assumes responsibilities
2. High expectations for self and others
3. Forsees consequences and implications of decisions
4. Good judgment
5. Excellent organizational skills
6. Generally well liked by peers
7. Self-confident

Gifted children do not appear to demonstrate significant deviations from the average population in physical development. If socioeconomic factors are equated in the analysis, differences between the groups are less significant. Comparisons in cognitive development do suggest major differences, however. Gifted children appear to speak earlier than children with average intelligence, and there is apparently a relationship between language complexity and later higher IQ. Early reading acquisition is also an apparent marker of potential superior intellectual ability (nearly 50% of Terman's gifted children were reading before they entered first grade). Only the very highly gifted (IQ above 180) appeared to have personality and emotional problems. The average gifted child may "run the gamut of personality, styles, from outgoing to retiring, from self-confident and assertive to feeling inferior."[18] Needless to say, the profile of the gifted child represents a heterogeneous amalgamation of characteristics, influenced by the variables of genetic templates, socioeconomic factors, and other psychobiological and psychosocial influences.

Identification: Role of the Physician

The expanded role for physicians in neurodevelopmental assessment has traditionally focused on early identification of children with developmental delays and dysfunctions. Although the task is somewhat more challenging, attempts at identification of the gifted child (preschooler) is no less a responsibility of the primary care physician. Brink[21] provided useful developmental guidelines for identification of the gifted preschool child that can be realistically applied in an office setting. The physician and office personnel should be observant, during office contacts, for some of the more characteristic behaviors:

1. Uses advanced vocabulary, beyond chronological age
2. Discusses experiences in detail
3. Interjects sense of humor in general conversation
4. Uses (and comprehends) abstract concepts
5. Has ability to master new skills without the necessity for repetition or drilling
6. Shows evidence of early physical maturation
7. Displays sensitivity about feelings of others
8. Has good attention span and task perseverance
9. Is curious and frequently asks "why"
10. Has some understanding of number concepts
11. Observes and comments on relationships

Brink[21] tabulated developmental guidelines showing norms for comparisons with precocious achievement. The tabulation is so constructed that if a child is about 30% more advanced than the average in most items of a section (e.g., general motor ability, fine motor ability, cognitive language), the child might be suspected of being gifted or talented.

Identification of the gifted preschool child requires that the physician investigate the diagnostic possibilities, similar to the protocol for delineation of any developmental disability, including (1) comprehensive history to document sequential development and the maturational timetables, (2) physical and neurological examinations, (3) neurodevelopmental screening with one or more testing inventories (e.g., Denver Developmental Screening Test, Bayley Scales of Infant Development, Gesell Developmental Schedules), and (4) judicious referrals to clarify suspicions of suspected intellectual giftedness or talent.

The pediatrician is the child's most significant and influential advocate and should be prepared to recognize and document "giftedness," as early as possible. The physician is expected to render traditional health care services and must provide constructive input in the supervision of the child's educational, emotional, and social development. The expanded role for the physician serving children with potentially chronic handicapping disorders requires active interfacing with the educational system, coordination of professional services, and counseling with the family. The gifted child is not an exception to this general rule of delivering quality health care service.[22]

The very bright child is too often identified relatively late in childhood, or worse ignored. Not infrequently, the gifted child might first be diagnosed as a "behavioral problem." The child's development may be jeopardized by a misunderstanding and a rigid adult environment. Persistent myths may engender a host of biases that must be overcome in order to nurture a healthy emotional and social development. In this effort, the physician may have a critical role as the gifted child's most significant professional advocate. The physician may be designated as the coordinator of interdisciplinary efforts as well as counselor for family and professionals. Indeed the physician may be the key to the gifted child's successful utilization of intellectual potential.[22]

Management

Interest in gifted education was enhanced by public reaction to the launching of the Russian satellite, Sputnik. The interest focused on assisting the development of enrich-

Table V. Educational Models for Gifted Children[a]

Type	Program design	Advantages	Disadvantages
Ability grouping	Special school Special classes Pullout programs Summer workshops Flexible grouping	Opportunity to work at level of ability Program designed to meet needs of child Learning experience is continuous	Need specially trained teachers Program often not individualized Student may not be gifted in all subjects Exaggeration of feelings of difference Expensive
Acceleration	Early school entrance Grade "skipping" Move through the material at an ac- celerated rate Less time to com- plete school	Used in any school Enter careers earlier; more productivity Educational costs are lowered Less boredom Social/emotional adjustments are high	Bias of teachers, admin- istrators, and parents Possible social disruptions Law does not permit early entrance
Enrichment	Addition of areas of learning not nor- mally in curriculum	Children are not separated Less expensive than ability grouping	Used in a traditional classroom Teachers may not be spe- cially trained Poor program coordination

[a]Adapted from: Clark.[23]

ment and accelerated educational and scientific programs for gifted children. During the 1960s, this impetus was somewhat dampened by the refocus of social energies toward the socially disadvantaged. A resurgence of concern for the gifted was observed during the 1970s and 1980s. As Schechter[18] commented,

> School systems have been able to reconcile a concern for the socially disadvantaged child with an interest in gifted children. In addition, most states now have laws that mandate the identification and evaluation of gifted children, and many states have statutes mandating programming.

The confusions and controversies in criteria for "selection of gifted children" has been discussed. The type of educational approach for gifted children has similarly gener-ated concern and controversy. Three major educational models have been proposed: (1) ability grouping, (2) acceleration, and (3) enrichment programming (Table V).[23] Each of these methods has advantages and disadvantages. Acceleration is probably the most common practice for children who are highly intellectually gifted. Enrichment programs allow for children to be placed in special resource programs for all or part of the day. The basic educational issue of self-contained or mainstreaming for children with special needs has not been resolved for gifted children. The heterogeneous nature of the gifted child suggests that no single educational recommendation can meet the needs of all children with very superior intelligence. As with other children requiring special educational services, an individualized approach should be considered, recognizing the intellectual, psychological, social, physical, and economic variables that constitute the profiles of gifted children. Similarly, it is critical to provide gifted children with teachers who have had specialized training in this area of education.

Special Issues of Gifted Children

Learning-Disabled and Handicapped Gifted Children

By definition, the learning-disabled gifted child represents an apparent contradiction of terms, a paradox, in which a handicap neutralizes or masks a "gift." The accepted definition of "gifted and talented" has been presented. In order to appreciate this special group of learning-disabled gifted children, an additional definition is necessary:

> Children with specific learning disabilities exhibit a disorder in one or more of the basic psychological processes involved in understanding or using spoken or written language. These may be manifested in disorders of listening, thinking, talking, reading, writing, spelling and arithmetic. They include conditions which have been referred to as perceptual handicaps, brain injury, minimal brain dysfunction, dyslexia, developmental aphasia, etc. They do not include learning problems which are due primarily to visual, hearing or motor handicaps, to mental retardation, emotional disturbance or to environmental disadvantage.[24]

There are approximately 45 million school-age children in the United States, and 1.5 million would be classified as gifted/talented. It is further estimated that there are 120,000–180,000 gifted but handicapped children in American public schools. Mauser[25] recognized this dilemma:

> In essence, individuals with disabilities who are gifted constitute a minority group within a minority group. The types of disabilities experienced by the group are quite diverse and as such require the knowledge, commitment and experience of every conceivable talent within the field of regular education and special education for maximum progress and adjustment.

The gifted/handicapped child will generally require some form of special education intervention, in order to accommodate for the handicap (e.g., learning disability, neuromotor dysfunction, communication disorder). Unfortunately, the special programming usually focuses solely on the handicap and tends to ignore the giftedness. Whitmore[26] suggested that gifted/handicapped children are often overlooked because of (1) stereotypical expectations that gifted children will excel in all areas of development, (2) developmental delay in any one area is expected to result in some delay in cognitive development, and (3) inability is perceived as lack of opportunity to evidence superior mental abilities.

The gifted but learning-impaired child may surface as an underachiever or perform in the range of marginal to average. As each academic year passes, there may be a widening of the disparity between potential and performance. As a consequence of delayed identification, a "point of educational no return" is reached; i.e., rehabilitation may not be as productive as desired. Prevention of the psychoeducational wastage of a gifted learning-disabled child begins with the early recognition of the giftedness. In a temporal framework, the giftedness is usually manifested long before the disordered learning.[27]

Daniels[28] subgrouped gifted children into four major categories: (1) *gifted achievers* (gifted with no learning, reading, or language disability), (2) *gifted nonachievers* (gifted, with no learning, reading or language disability but not performing at their potential academic level), (3) *gifted pseudoachievers* (gifted with a learning disability, but functioning at grade level), and (4) *gifted/learning disabled* (gifted, with a learning disability, but not succeeding either at grade level or level of academic potential). Daniels noted that

The pseudoachievers are missed because they do not appear as failures. Their scores on achievement tests tend to approach the mean of the grade, so no alert is sounded. The gifted/learning disabled usually demonstrate their disabilities early in school and the dysfunction is treated, often as an isolated factor. When such a program is inaugurated, the giftedness often goes undetected.

The gifted/handicapped child is both a diagnostic and management challenge for parents, physicians, and concerned professionals. Understanding the clinical manifestations and impact of giftedness and of the handicap (individually) is a prerequisite for appreciating their effects in combination.

Minority Gifted Children

Socioeconomically disadvantaged children in the United States (black, Indian, or Oriental) are exposed to sociocultural deprivation, overcrowded living conditions, and traditional hazards associated with poverty. Nevertheless, it must be emphasized that highly gifted children exist among socioeconomically deprived minority groups. Gifted children may represent a threat and source of anxiety to their parents, who may "put down the child's performance or to retaliate aggressively because the parent feels the child is challenging his or her authority."[19] The gifted child in a suppressing, nonsupportive family may become depressed, as emotional supports are lacking. Lack of emotional support for the gifted child may be directly proportional to the economic and social pressures that are common in minority families. The home atmosphere and support is a significant factor directing the development of a gifted child. Financial constraints (limiting intellectual and social stimulation), parental background (lack of an education and relatively poor educationally oriented motivations), and a pervasive aura of hopelessness may adversely affect the development of a highly gifted child in a minority setting.

The gifted child in a minority group may be similarly penalized by an "unappreciative" educational milieu. The minority child may not be expected to be gifted, indeed may be perceived in an even more negative atmosphere of potential intellectual ability. Once identified there may be an apathy in securing special services for the minority gifted. Frasier[19] commented that "minority gifted children are found in all areas and are more like the gifted children in the general population than they are like their nongifted peers in their own minority group." Frasier further noted from past research that "the recognition of minority gifted children may be suppressed because many of them come from impoverished backgrounds, but traditional testing procedures will identify disadvantaged minority children who are gifted." It should be recognized that minority gifted children may be so different from their neighborhood peers that particular psychological stresses are generated.[20]

Webb et al.[20] noted that "existing services to the gifted and talented do not reach significant numbers of people, particularly the handicapped, minorities, or other disadvantaged people. In minority groups the social and educational environments have "every configuration calculated to stifle potential talent."[13] The educational environment may not be flexible enough to enhance potential of the gifted minority child. The verbal emphasis in early grades may be a particular difficulty (or suppressing influence) for minority children whose language and verbal concepts may be deviant from that of the school environment. Identification of the minority gifted may be similarly much more difficult because of the problems associated with group testing.

Parents, teachers, and concerned professionals must abandon stereotyped misconceptions about gifted minority children. A primary objective is to recognize that these children *are* capable of achieving and that the educational environment must meaningfully support this belief. The home and educational environments should provide positive reenforcement and bolstering of the child's self-esteem. "The challenge is for educators and parents to mobilize their efforts in the promotion of achievement."[19]

In essence, the failure to identify learning-disabled, handicapped, or minority gifted children represents a loss of a national resource.[27] The impact of unintentional or willful neglect of these children is measured for society in the loss of valuable potential and compromised productivity. For the individual child who is so abused, the "bottom line" may be reflected in loss of self-esteem, poor self-confidence, and deviant behavior.[29]

SUMMARY

Mental retardation and intellectual giftedness, although representing divergent extremes of intelligence, share common concerns: (1) early identification and initiation of psychoeducational services may be directly correlated with more favorable academic, psychological, and social successes; (2) special education resources are generally required to enhance learning and social potentials; (3) poor management practices may result in behavioral complications (ranging from elitism to poor self-concept); and (4) parent support systems are usually required to promote sound family dynamics and meaningful advocacy roles.[29,30]

The pediatrician has multifaceted responsibilities in providing services for mentally retarded and gifted children: (1) provides neurodevelopmental screening during the preschool period for early identification; (2) undertakes judicious selection and coordination of a multidisciplinary team when variations in intelligence are suspected; (3) contributes a medical profile to the construct of an individual educational program (IEP); (4) promotes good health practices; (5) provides counseling, support, and advocacy services for child and family; and (6) ensures adequate follow-up evaluation to monitor periodically the effectiveness of management services.

The child with a variation in intelligence (mental retardation or intellectual giftedness) represents a complex psychobiological, educational and social challenge for the health care provider. The professional's level of concern, expertise, and dedication is ultimately reflected in the timeliness and quality of services secured for the child. The final common pathway for meaningful professional interventions is enhanced *quality* of life for the mentally retarded or gifted child.

REFERENCES

1. Brown, J. S., and Zinkus, P. W.: Screening techniques for early intervention, in Gottlieb, M. I., Zinkus, P. W., and Bradford, L. J. (eds.): *Current Issues in Developmental Pediatrics: The Learning Disabled Child*. Grune & Stratton, New York, 1979, pp. 315–342.
2. Erickson, M. T.: Psychological assessment methods, in Gabel, S., and Erickson, M. T. (eds.): *Child Development and Developmental Disabilities*. Little, Brown, Boston, 1980, pp. 203–222.

3. Levinson, A., and Bigler, J. A. (eds.): *Mental Retardation in Infants and Children*. Year Book, Chicago, 1960.
4. Accardo, P. J., and Capute A. J. (eds.): *The Pediatrician and the Developmentally Delayed Child*. University Park Press, Baltimore, 1979.
5. Hagerman, R. J., McBogg, P., and Hagerman, P. J.: The fragile X Syndrome: History, diagnosis and treatment. *J. Dev. Behav. Pediatr.* **4**:122–130, 1983.
6. Grossman, H. J.: *Manual on Terminology and Classification in Mental Retardation*. Special Publication No. 2. American Association on Mental Deficiency, Washington, D.C., 1973.
7. Cohen, H. J.: Introduction, Mental retardation. *Pediatr. Ann.* **11**:424, 1982.
8. Pearson, P. H.: The physician's role in diagnosis and management of the mentally retarded. *Pediatr. Clin. North Am.* **15**:835–859, 1968.
9. Herskowitz, J., and Rosman, N. P. (eds.): *Pediatrics, Neurology and Psychiatry—Common Ground*. Macmillan, New York, 1982.
10. Magrab, P. R., and Johnston, R. B.: Mental retardation, in Gabel, S., and Erickson, M. T. (eds.): *Child Development and Developmental Disabilities*. Little, Brown, Boston, 1980, pp. 241–257.
11. Terman, L. M.: *Genetic Studies of Genius. Vol. 1: Mental and Physical Trails of a Thousand Gifted Children*. Stanford University Press, Stanford, California, 1925.
12. Renzulli, J. S.: What makes giftedness? Reexamining a definition. *Phi Delta Kappan* **60**:180–184, 261, 1978.
13. Marland, S., Jr.: *Education of the Gifted and Talented*. Report to the Congress of the United States by the U.S. Commissioner of Education. U.S. Government Printing Office, Washington, D. C., 1972.
14. Passow, A. H.: The nature of giftedness and talent. *Gifted Child Qt.* **25**:5–10, 1981.
15. Gallagher, J. J.: Gifted children: Enhancing their development, in Frankenberg, W. K. (ed.): *Children Are Different, Behavioral Development*, Ross Laboratories, Columbus, Ohio, 1984, pp. 1–9.
16. Freeman, J.: *Gifted Children*, University Park Press, Baltimore, 1979.
17. Gallagher, J. J.: *Teaching the Gifted Child*, 2nd ed. Allyn & Bacon, Boston, 1975.
18. Schecter, N. L.: The gifted child, in Levine, M. D., Carey, W. B., Crocker, A. C., and Gross, R. T. (eds.): *Developmental–Behavioral Pediatrics*. W. B. Saunders, Philadelphia, 1983.
19. Miller, B. S., and Price, M.: *The Gifted Child, the Family and the Community*. Walker, New York, 1981.
20. Webb, J. T., Meckstroth, E. A., and Tolan, S. S.: *Guiding the Gifted Child*, Ohio Psychology Publishing Co., Columbus, Ohio, 1982.
21. Brink, R. E.: The gifted preschool child. *Pediatr. Nursing* **8**:299–303, 1982.
22. Gottlieb, M. I.: *The Gifted Child—Advantaged or Handicapped? A Pediatrician's Challenge*, Round Table. American Academy of Pediatrics Annual Meeting, New York City, October 1982.
23. Clark, B.: *Growing Up Gifted*. Charles E. Merrill, Columbus, Ohio, 1979.
24. United States Office of Education, National Advisory Committee on Handicapped Children. Children with Specific Learning Disabilities Act of 1969.
25. Mauser, A. J.: Programming strategies for pupils with disabilities who are gifted. *Rehab. Lit.* **42**:270–275, 1981.
26. Whitmore, J. R.: Gifted children with handicapping conditions: A new frontier. *Exceptional Child.* **48**:106–114, 1981.
27. Gottlieb, M. I.: *Gifted learning-disabled children: Loss of a national resource*. Presented at Conference on Learning Failure: An Interdisciplinary Approach to the Learning-Disabled Child, Boston University School of Medicine, Boston, October 1983 (abst).
28. Daniels, P. R.: *Teaching the Gifted/Learning Disabled Child*. Aspen Systems, Rockville, Maryland, 1983.
29. Gottlieb, M. I., and Williams, J. E.: Self-concept in the latency period and adolescence. *Feelings Med. Signif.* **24**:23–26, 1982.
30. Gottlieb, M. I., and Zinkus, P. W.: Educational health and development: The learning-disabled child, in Hughes, J. G., and Griffith, J. G. (eds.): *Synopsis of Pediatrics* C. V. Mosby, St. Louis, 1984, pp. 36–60.

Speech and Language Disorders

III

Speech and Language Disorders

10

Neurological Correlates of Speech

Emily A. Tobey and Donald L. Rampp

Disorders of speech and language in children are a major management concern for the primary care physician and parents. Delays, disorders, and dysfunctions of communication skills constitute some of the most frequent reasons for referral to the developmental pediatrician and/or interdisciplinary diagnostic centers. The next several chapters review issues of speech and language disorders in childhood from various perspectives. This chapter highlights recent neurological findings related to the control of speech skills.

The chapter focuses on the peripheral events coordinated by the brain when language is used via speech production. Under most ordinary circumstances, adult speakers may be conscious of what they intend to say. They are cognizant of their search for appropriate words to express their intention, and perhaps the feelings that underlie what they intend to say. However, adults are rarely conscious of planning and executing speech gestures, per se. Only under circumstances of novelty (e.g., learning a new language or attempting to pronounce new words) is an adult conscious of the processes necessary for producing and coordinating speech events. Under these conditions, adults may experience the complexity that faces children learning to talk.

Emily A. Tobey and Donald L. Rampp • Department of Communication Disorders, Louisiana State University Medical Center, New Orleans, Louisiana 70112.

CORTICAL PARTICIPATION IN SPEECH AND LANGUAGE

Cortical participation in speech and language usually is discussed along two dimensions: hemisphere side and specific cortical site. The left hemisphere is generally considered the dominant or major controller for speech and language in most right- and left-handed individuals.[1,2] The right hemisphere appears to be dominant in only a few left-handed individuals.[2−6] Support for a left-hemisphere dominance for speech and language is found in a variety of studies using dichotic listening,[1] intracarotid sodium Amytal perfusions,[7] callosal sections,[8] or electrical stimulation mapping[2,9,10] Cortical lesions of the left hemisphere appear to impair various speech and language skills selectively, particularly if the lesion is located in either Broca's or Wernicke's areas.[11]

Areas involved in speech–language skills have been determined primarily by correlating disrupted performance with a particular cortical site encompassed by the lesion. Several studies suggested that lesions in the anterior left hemisphere limit or restrict central control operations used to organize and execute speech acts. Analyses of speech errors demonstrated that phoneme selection as well as articulatory implementation was disrupted.[12] Production errors were often misarticulations[13−17] and frequently represented the substitutions of one phoneme for another.[14,18,19] Examination of these substitutions revealed the anticipation of later portions of the utterance and suggested inappropriate serial organization prior to the execution (or implementation) of sequentially ordered neuromuscular representations.[12,13] By contrast, serial organization may remain intact, while processes encoding phonological units appeared disrupted.[14] In this type of disruption, there appeared to be a reduced capacity to program both the positioning of speech musculature for phoneme production and to sequence muscle movements properly for the reproduction of words.[20] Poor execution of complex motor sequences (including speech) has been commonly observed in patients who failed to demonstrate concomitant weakness,[20] deficiencies in understanding,[20,21] incoordination,[21,22] sensory losses,[22] or ataxia.[23] Patients with left-hemisphere lesions also appeared to demonstrate some intact residual function by producing error-free utterances in combination with errors of serial organization and neuromuscular articulatory representations. The presence of correct and erroneous productions suggested that total disruptions to speech rarely occurred; rather, the neurological system for speech appeared reduced in such a way that it produced intermittent errors.

Mapping cortical sites by electrical stimulation is a technique that has a number of advantages, including assessing the contributions of nonlesioned cortex and providing a finer resolution than lesion mapping.[2,4,9,10] Cortical stimulation of the left hemisphere suggests that the motor speech area (Broca's area) in the posterior inferior frontal lobe, immediately in front of the facial motor cortex, may be smaller than traditionally believed.[19] Moreover, this particular site appears to play at least some role in higher-level perceptual processing because more than 50% of the sites stimulated in this area affect phonemic identification.[10] Combinations and sequences of orofacial movement patterns are affected over a broad range of cortical sites encompassing the frontal, temporal, or parietal perisylvian areas, although imitation of similar repeated orofacial movement patterns remains intact.[4,10]

Different roles for the frontal and temporal–parietal lobes in short-term memory also are observed. It appears that the perisylvian area has a major role in sequencing motor gestures necessary for speech and decoding phonemes, whereas surrounding temporal and parietal areas are involved in short-term memory. Reading and naming appear to fall within the interface between the perisylvian (motor sequencing) and surrounding frontal, parietal, and temporal regions concerned with short-term memory.[4,10,24,25]

Right hemisphere participation in speech–language tasks is extensively studied in individuals with congenital corpus callosum agenesis or following callosum sections (see Chapter 7). The right hemisphere appears to contribute a role in nonverbal, non-mathematical, and nonsequential tasks.[8,26] Right hemisphere participation is evident in such activities as reading faces, discriminating and recalling shapes, determining whole objects from parts, and distinguishing between musical chords.[26] Relatively recent reports suggest that right hemisphere injuries may cause difficulty in modulating prosody and speaking rate.[27,28] Other central nervous system (CNS) sites also appear to contribute to speech and language control. Changes in speaking rate may follow stimulation of the lateral portions of either side of the thalamus.[29,30] Anomia or short-term memory deficits appear following left thalamic stimulation.[31,32]

DEVELOPMENTAL FACTORS INFLUENCING CORTICAL PARTICIPATION

Extensive central and peripheral nervous system changes occur during the first year of life and influence the development of different postural and movement patterns. The CNS of a neonate differs from an adult in several general ways: (1) the commissures connecting the two hemispheres in the neonate are not fully developed,[33,34] (2) myelination of the cerebral commissures begins during the third month and continues through the seventh year,[35] (3) only sparse axonal–dentritic branching to cortical association areas is apparent in the neonate,[35,36] and (4) marked growth in the middle and anterior sections of the cerebral neocortex is reported after the first year.[37] The neonate can thus theoretically be thought of as functionally split-brained.[33,38]

Most behaviors of the infant appear mediated by subcortical structures, since cortical cell myelination and dendritic branching in the neonate is not complete.[36,37] Sensorimotor development during the first year appears to include the myelination of upper motor neuron (corticospinal and corticobulbar) and post-thalamic (auditory and somatosensory) pathways.[39–41] During this period, myelination of the corpus striatum and middle cerebellar peduncle also occurs.[41] Myelination of these pathways generally is not complete in most children until near the second year.

Only a few neural functioning systems responsible for reflexive behavior, such as sucking, breathing, and swallowing, appear intact in the infant.[37,42,43] Rapid development of corticospinal and corticobulbar tracts during the first year as well as post-thalamic somatosensory pathways begin to form the hard wiring necessary for inhibiting many of the primitive reflexes observed in the infant. Innervation of the facial nerve to the lips appears complete in the infant but innervation to other muscles of expression does not appear until later.[39,41] Full innervation of the respiratory system does not appear complete until around 8 months.[38] During these rapid neural changes, the larynx and nasopharynx also begin to separate and become more adultlike in form.

DEVELOPMENTAL FACTORS AFFECTING THE VOCAL TRACT

The repertoire of neonatal vocalizations is heavily influenced by the relationships of peripheral anatomical structures in the vocal tract. The infant's peripheral vocal tract differs significantly from an adult vocal tract, resembling that of other nonhuman primates.[44,45] The vocal tract of the human adult consists of three cavities—pharyngeal, oral, and nasal—whereas the infant's vocal tract basically consists of only two cavities— oral and nasal. The lack of a pharyngeal cavity in infants occurs because the larynx is high with the epiglottis located around the first cervical vertebra and the inferior border of the cricoid cartilage located at the fourth cervical vertebra.[44,45] The epiglottis and inferior border of the cricoid cartilage are located around the third and sixth cervical vertebrae, respectively, in the adult.[45] The anterior wall of the suprapharyngeal area can be observed in the infant.

Oral and nasal cavity relationships also differ. In the infant, the soft palate lies relatively parallel to the hard palate and is capable of approximating the epiglottis.[44] Epiglottic action may close off either the oral cavity during quiet breathing of the larynx during feeding. Epiglottic and soft palate approximation is precluded in the adult vocal tract because of the relatively low position of the epiglottis, and the suprapharyngeal area serves as a common pathway for both air and food in the adult. In the infant, the oral cavity is primarily occupied with the tongue, which usually rests on the lower lip.[44,45] It is important to note that developmentally most infants are compulsive nose-breathers, because of the combination of a relatively narrow oral cavity, in conjunction with soft palate and epiglottic approximation. It is not until these structures begin to separate that some children become chronic mouth breathers.

The mandible and tongue also do not appear capable of independent actions in the neonate.[46,47] The tongue is unable to elevate for sounds made in either the anterior or posterior portion of the oral cavity,[47] movements critical for the formation of many vowels and consonants. Independent action of the tongue and lips from the mandible is only observed in limited situations, notably the presence of a smile following tactile stimulation.[46]

RESPIRATION FOR QUIET BREATHING VERSUS SPEECH

Respiration plays a major role in speech because all English sounds are produced on the exhaled airstream.[48-50] The airstream, itself, may be modulated by the phonatory processes mediated at the larynx and further shaped by changing the configuration of the vocal tract by moving the velum, tongue, lips, and mandible. Changes in inhalation and exhalation patterns are necessary for producing speech.

Inhalation for speech differs from the inspiration associated with quiet breathing in three major ways: (1) a speaker assumes voluntary control over breathing patterns during speech, (2) speakers are able to anticipate the respiratory needs for speech, and (3) inspiration for speech is quicker and composes less of the total respiratory cycle than does quiet breathing. Voluntary control permits the speaker to adjust the volume and airflow to accomplish a number of different types of speech acts such as singing, acting, or yelling.[48-50] A greater volume change will occur if the speaker anticipates that he will need more energy for either a loud or a long sentence.[49] In addition, inhalation occupies approximately 40% of the entire respiratory cycle during quiet breathing; however, it occupies only about 10% of the entire cycle during speaking.[49,50]

During quiet breathing, elasticity, thoracic torque, and gravity appear to have major roles in changing the volume–pressure relationships.[50] However, the speaker must maintain a constant pressure in order to hold a single note (as in the case of the singer) or to sustain a vowel (as commonly used in laryngological evaluations). These conditions require the speaker to pair the passive recoil of the rib cage–lung coupling with active muscle contractions. Active muscle participation during expiration allows the speaker to more carefully control the outflow of air and the reduction in thoracic volume. You can demonstrate for yourself the need for expiratory control by a three-step procedure. First, take a deep breath, open your glottis, and then relax your thoracic muscles. Note how rapidly the air flows out and imagine how much you might be able to say on that air (particularly if you were upset or angry).[50] It obviously is not an efficient way to control the exhalation you need for speech. Thus, inspiratory and expiratory muscles appear coactivated to assist the speaker in efficiently controlling the airflow.[49,50]

Respiratory patterns for the neonate and infant differ in a number of respects from older speakers.[51] Higher respiratory rates (measured in breaths per minute) are noted for infants of different ages during quiet breathing and crying activities. For example, 1-month-old infants are reported to average 87 breaths/min during quiet breathing and 50 breaths/min during crying behavior; a 6-month-old infant averages 61 and 31 breaths/min for quiet breathing and crying, respectively. By the end of the first year, the child is averaging 42 and 23 breaths/min for quiet breathing and crying activities. These data suggest that the decrease in breaths per minute observed during crying behavior actually reflects a faster inhalation period and a longer exhalation period; a pattern similar to that observed in the adult speech act. Respiration in the neonate appears to be largely controlled by the diaphragm muscle activity until about 6 months of age, when the infant's posture changes and sitting is observed.[47,51] Posture adjustments, accompanied by developing corticospinal connections, allow the infant to increase lung volume by diaphragm and rib cage adjustments.

Central controllers for respiration appear to lie in the dorsal and ventral respiratory neurons located in the midbrain of the CNS.[52] These neurons appear responsive to hydrogen concentrations carried through blood carbon dioxide or bicarbonate levels. From a peripheral standpoint, the carotid bodies and aortic bodies appear responsive to changes in partial pressures of oxygen, carbon dioxide, and hydrogen. Information from these receptors is then channeled to the CNS via the cranial nerves IX and X.[52] It is not clear how these processes are modified for voluntary speech acts.

PHONATORY PROCESSES IN SPEECH VERSUS QUIET BREATHING

During quiet breathing, the major laryngeal muscle activity is observed in the posterior cricoarytenoid which abducts (opens) the vocal folds to provide a large glottal opening for airflow.[48,50–54] However, all English vowels and most consonants require the vocal folds to be in an adducted (closed, midline) position. Rotation of the arytenoid cartilages by the interarytenoid and lateral cricoarytenoid muscles bring the vocal folds to a midline position.[53,54] Midline positioning of the vocal folds impedes airflow until air pressure below the folds is greater than that above the vocal folds.[55] Air pressure will continue to build, eventually pushing open the vocal folds and permitting a puff of air to escape. The elastic properties of the vocal folds, in conjunction with Bernoulli's effect, draw the vocal folds back to a midline position and the cycle continues.[55]

One way to illustrate the basic principles underlying the laryngeal processes of voiced sounds is to produce a "Bronx cheer" or a "raspberry."[50] In order to produce this sound, muscle activity is required to approximate the lips. Vibration of the lips occurs as the air pressure in the oral cavity behind the lips becomes greater than the air pressure in front of the lips. The lips are vibrated as the air pushes through and separates the lips. Elastic properties and Bernoulli's effect return the lips to a closed position and the cycle continues. Precise muscle action, in conjunction with the aerodynamics of exhaled air, is necessary; it may be illustrated by trying to produce the sound when the lips are slightly open, very tense, or very loose. No sound is generated under these conditions.

Voiced sounds, thus, require vibrations of the vocal folds. Apparently, the only muscle activities involved in the vibrations are associated with moving the folds to a midline position and adjusting the relative tenseness of the folds, themselves.[53,54] The actual vibrations are produced by coordinated aerodynamics and elasticity effects.[55] Voiced sound is maintained when air pressure below the vocal folds is greater than the pressure above. Voicing is effected by any condition that changes the mass of the vocal folds, the muscles responsible for bringing the folds to a midline position, or the tight seal necessary to build air pressure below the folds.

Frequency of laryngeal vibration is usually referred to as fundamental frequency. The psychological impression of that frequency is commonly referred to as pitch. Frequency of vibration is influenced by several factors: (1) frequency differences across different speakers, and (2) frequency differences produced by a given speaker. Frequency differences across different speakers are related to differences in the size of anatomical structures.[48,50] Adult males, for example, have larger vocal folds than adult female speakers or children. The more massive vocal folds of the adult male vibrate at a lower frequency and are perceived as a lower pitch. Children tend to have very high-pitched voices because their vocal folds are less massive and shorter. Frequency differences within a given speaker are primarily controlled by the muscle activity of the cricothyroid, which tilts the thyroid cartilage forward relative to the cricoid cartilage.[53,54] This action lengthens the vocal folds; the perception of the physiological activity is that the pitch is higher. Manipulations of fundamental frequency are used by speakers to change their stress or intonation in order to (1) express emotions, (2) distinguish between questions and declarative sentences, and (3) indicate the relative importance of words.[48,50] Meanings of sentences may be altered in identical sentences simply by changing the stress on one word versus another (i.e., "I *want* that", versus "I want *that*" versus "*I* want that"). Stress and intonation changes may be aided by intensity and duration changes, as well. For example, the stress differences between the noun "produce" and the verb "produce" may be mediated by either a relative change in syllable duration (stressed syllables are usually longer), an increase in intensity (stressed syllables are usually louder), fundamental frequency changes, or a combination of these factors.[48,50]

A number of consonant sounds are voiceless, i.e., without laryngeal vibrations. The laryngeal configuration for these sounds is similar to that used for quiet breathing: the posterior cricoarytenoid muscle activity moves the arytenoid cartilages and separates the vocal folds.[53,54] The reciprocal action of the posterior cricoarytenoid muscle versus the lateral cricoarytenoid and the interarytenoid muscles is a critical factor involved in voiced–voiceless contrasts.[53,54] A lack of reciprocity in these laryngeal muscles is observed in many persons who stutter; i.e., these individuals appear to coactivate the three muscles.[56] Coactivation of these muscles resembles a spasmlike movement as the vocal folds attempt to open and close simultaneously. Many people who stutter tend to have difficulty in producing the voiced–voiceless contrasts involved in ongoing speech. The neonate's larynx is located high in the neck and appears to be initially capable of relatively gross laryngeal actions.[44,45,57] It is not until the infant approaches 9 months to 1 year of age that he is capable of routine, consistent, voiced–voiceless contrasts and finer manipulation of fundamental frequency associated with intonation and stress.[44,47] Additional laryngeal control occurs around the end of the first year, when the child produces the gross pitch contrast associated with squealing and growling. Improved coordination between respiratory and laryngeal activity is also observed during this period as children become more proficient at yelling.

Neural control of the intrinsic muscles of the larynx is carried via two branches of cranial nerve X.[57] The cricothyroid muscle, primarily responsible for frequency modulations within a given speaker, is innervated by the superior laryngeal branch of the vagus, while the remaining intrinsic laryngeal muscles are innervated by the recurrent laryngeal branch. Thus, damage to either branch of the vagus may adversely effect laryngeal contributions to speech production.

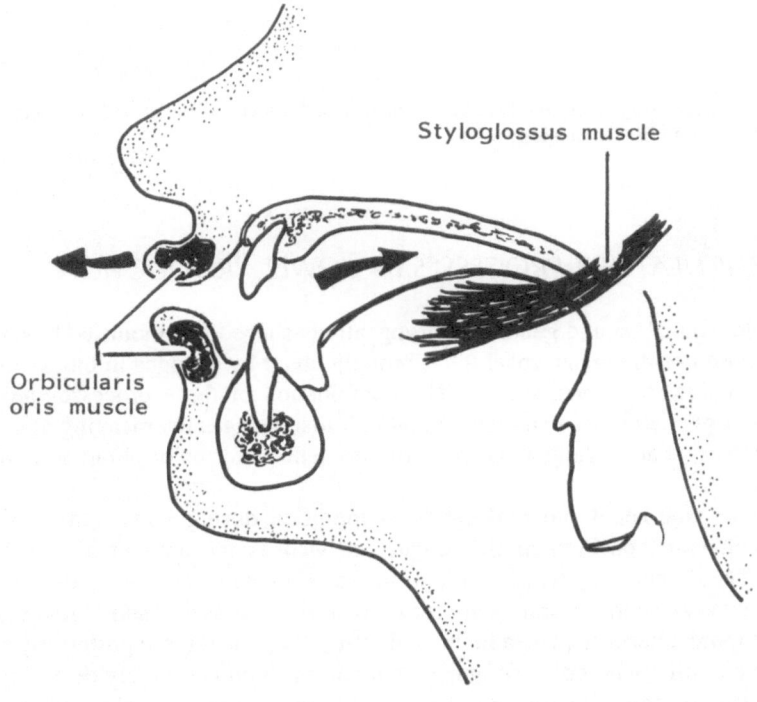

/u/

Figure 1 Activation of the styloglossus muscle pulls the tongue in an upward and posterior direction This action is used for sounds such as /u/, /k/, and /g/ (Adapted from Borden and Harris [58])

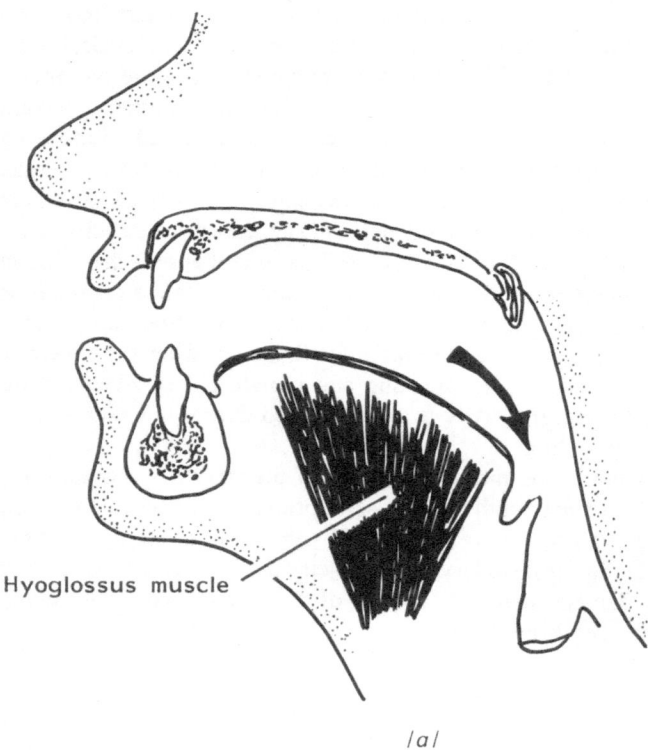

/a/

Figure 2. Activation of the hyoglossus muscle pulls the tongue in a downward direction and is used for sounds such as /a/. (Adapted from Borden and Harris.[58])

ARTICULATORY PROCESSES IN VOWEL PRODUCTION

An audible "buzz" sound generated laryngeally is shaped and modified by changes in the configuration of the upper vocal tract, brought about by changes in the position of the velum, mandible, lips, and tongue. The combination of these processes produces speech sounds or phonemes (the smallest sound unit that changes the meaning of a word, e.g., "bat" versus "cat"). English consists of two general forms of phonemes, vowels and consonants.

The relative volume of the oral cavity is modified during vowel production by altering the height and position of the tongue, as well as the amount of mandibular opening.[48,50] The tongue may be placed high in the oral cavity for vowels like /i/ as in "heed" or relatively low in the oral cavity for vowels like /ae/ as in "had." Likewise the tongue may be more anteriorly placed in the oral cavity for /i/ and more posteriorly placed for /u/ as in the word "who'ed." Tongue height and position are largely determined by the action of the extrinsic tongue musculature. Figure 1 illustrates the action of the styloglossus muscle, which pulls the tongue upward in the posterior portion of the oral

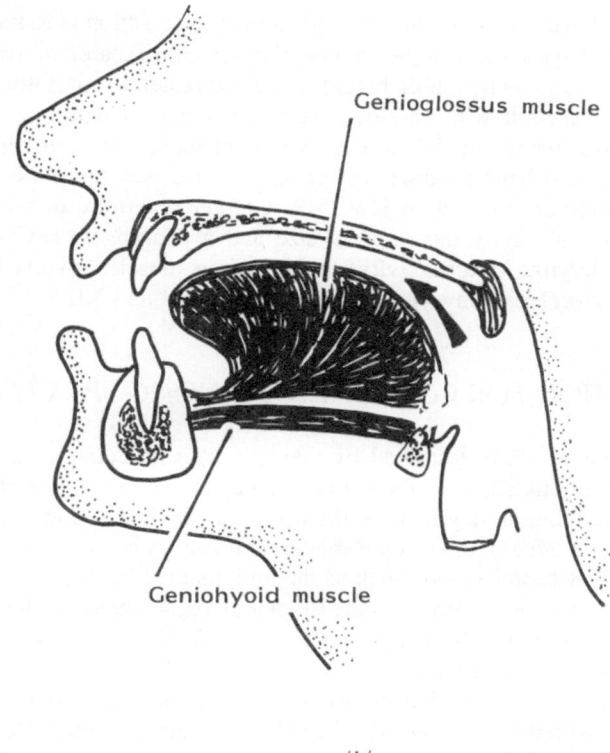

/i/

Figure 3. Activation of the genioglossus muscle pulls the tongue in an upward and anterior direction. This action is used for sounds such as /i/, /t/, and /d/. (Adapted from Borden and Harris.[58])

cavity. This muscle has a major role in producing the vowel /u/ and in placing the tongue in position for consonant sounds such as /k/ and /g/. Figure 2 illustrates the hyoglossus muscle which is responsible for depressing the tongue in the oral cavity for sounds, such as the vowel in the word, "saw." Figure 3 illustrates the effects of the genioglossus muscle, which elevates and pulls the tongue forward for vowels such as /i/ in the word "heed" or /I/ in the word "hid."

Mandibular height also has a role in vowel production. The mandible is in a more closed position for the vowel /i/ as in the word "heed" than in the vowel /ae/ as in the word, "had." Although the masseter, temporalis, and medial pterygoid are traditionally classified as mandibular elevators and the anterior belly of the diagastric and inferior lateral pterygoid muscles as mandibular depressors, these particular muscular relationships appear to hold only for nonspeech maneuvers like chewing.[55,56]

Several studies investigating the electromyographic (EMG) patterns of mandibular muscles during speaking indicate that the medial pterygoid and superior lateral pterygoid muscles act in relationship to one another in order to elevate the mandible during speech events.[59,60] Conversely, the inferior lateral pterygoid and anterior belly of the digastric muscles act to lower the mandible.[61] Thus, a reciprocal action is found during speech for the inferior and superior lateral pterygoids.[62] Adults are capable of independently manipulating their tongue and mandible height. An exaggerated form of this independence may be viewed in the adult who continues speaking while clenching a pipe between their teeth;[63] however, the mandible and tongue are not capable of acting independently in the neonate. Instead, infants produce vowel-like sounds that resemble mid and low-front vowels by simple dropping their jaw.[64,65] A larger repertoire of vowels appears in the infant as their oral cavity increases in size and a pharyngeal cavity is formed by the descent of the larynx. Motor activity for the various muscles involved in the articulatory processes for vowels is conveyed via cranial nerves V and XII.[44,50]

ARTICULATION FOR CONSONANTS DURING SPEECH PRODUCTION

Consonants are best described by their place of articulation, the manner in which they divert the air stream, and whether or not they are voiced or voiceless.[48,50] As Figure 3 indicates, articulation may involve the lips only (bilabial sounds such as /b/, /p/, and /m/), the upper teeth and lower lip (labial-dental sounds such as /f/ and /v/), the tongue and teeth (lingual-dental sounds such as the initial sound in "the" and the final sound in "teeth"), the tongue and alveolar ridge (lingua-alveolar sounds such as /t/, /d/, and /n/), the tongue and hard palate (linguapalatal sounds such as /r/ and /l/) or the tongue and soft palate (linguavelar sounds such as /k/, /g/, and /ng/).

Consonant production also involves manipulating the airflow in several different ways. Plosive, stop consonants /b,d,g,k,p,t/ are produced by completely blocking airflow for a brief period and then suddenly releasing the constriction. Constriction of the airflow can occur at the lips (/b/, /p/), the alveolar ridge (/d/, /t/), or the velum (/k/, /g/). A second type of constriction is used for producing fricative consonants (/f/, /v/, /s/, /z/, /sh/, /zh/, /th/). In these sounds, the airflow is constricted only enough to make the air turbulent but, as in the case of the stop consonants, this may occur in different places in the vocal tract. For example, airflow is constricted at a labial location for /f/ and /v/ but at a lingua-alveolar position for /s/ and /z/. Another class of consonants, affricatives, represent the combination of plosive and frication events. Such combinations are the foundation for the sounds /tʃ/, as in the word "church," and /dʒ/ as in the final sound in the word "judge." In these cases, the speaker must constrict the vocal tract for a brief period of time and then slightly adjust their tongue position to make the airflow turbulent.

Two consonants, /l/ and /r/, are produced by fairly complex peripheral manipulations. Two variations of /l/ commonly occur: a light /l/, which occurs before voiced sounds (as in the word "lamp"), and a dark /l/, which occurs after voiced sounds (as in the word "gal"). The light /l/ is made with the tongue blade in a forward position touching the alveolar ridge, whereas the dark /l/ is generally produced with the body of the tongue approximating the velum. Many variations in tongue position and movement patterns are used to produce /r/. Two of the most common patterns are a glidelike pattern that appears when an /r/ occurs before a vowel (as in the word "red"), and a vowel-like /r/ will occur when the /r/ preceeds another consonant (as in the word "bird"). In many parts of the country, the sound /r/ is dropped all together and replaced with a vowel-like production (a dialectical variation sometimes found in the northeastern portions of the

United States). The consonants /w/ and /y/ are usually described as semivowels. In this case, the consonants are produced by changing the vocal tract to resemble a vowel-like position and moving rapidly to the position of the next vowel in the word.

An additional method of diverting the airflow involves the nasal cavity. In these sounds (/m/, /n/, /ng/), the velum is lowered and air is allowed to divert through the nasal cavity while changing the articulatory relationships in the oral cavity. The place of articulation for these three consonants is similar to that of the stop consonants /b, d, g/. In English, only these three consonants divert air through the nasal cavity. The remainder of the consonants and vowels depend on adequate closure of the velopharyngeal port. Warren[66] defines velopharyngeal competency as the ability to "stop down" the port to 20 mm^2 or less. Measurements not withstanding, closure of the port apparently depends on the dynamic activity of many muscles. Several investigators (cf. ref. 67) report that the lateral pharyngeal walls move medially, the posterior pharyngeal walls (at the level of the first cervical vertebra) move forward, and the velum is "stretched" upward and backward to close off the port. The lateral pharyngeal wall appears displaced by contraction of the levator veli palatini and the superior pharyngeal constrictor muscles. The velum apparently is reconfigured by the actions of the palatopharyngeus muscle, which pulls down and back, and the levator veli palatini, which pulls it up and back. Such actions combine for a net vector force of an upward and backward movement. Velopharyngeal closure is not a static event either during speaking or from a developmental standpoint: it is continually changing and responding to the downward and forward growth of the facial skeleton, the downward and backward growth of the pharynx, the advance and retreat of the adenoid masses, the continual dropping away of the hard palate and velum from the cranial base, and the increase in angulation between the hard palate and velum.

The ability to achieve accurate consonant and vowel production pivots around the proper balance and dynamic interaction of the oral, pharyngeal, and palatal musculature. Innervation patterns for the muscles involved in the production of oral consonants have been briefly reviewed. Here, we shall briefly highlight the innervation patterns involved in the pharyngeal and palatal area. Motor activity of the muscles, themselves, are derived from cranial nerves (V, IX, X, and XI). The trigeminal, or fifth cranial, nerve, innervates the tensor veli palatini[68] and tensor tympani muscles.[68] The levator veli palatini, musculus uvulae, palatoglossus, and palatopharyngeus muscles are activated by the accessory or eleventh cranial nerve.[69] More recently, however, it has been suggested that the levator veli palatini muscle may be modulated by the facial (seventh cranial) nerve.[70] The pharyngeal muscles are dependent on a plexus of nerves (the pharyngeal plexus) which is composed of branches from the glossopharyngeal (IX), vagus (X), and spinal accessory (XI) nerves.

SUMMARY

This chapter highlights the neurological control of speech and reviews the physiological processes underlying speaking acts. From a developmental standpoint, it should be clear that children must learn to approximate anatomical structures, to provide these approximations in a variety of locations in the vocal tract, and to manipulate airflow systematically. The learning procedure must take place while drastic remodeling of the vocal tract and widespread neural linkages are occurring. Moreover, the child must learn to reorganize and adapt a number of physiological processes, such as respiration, for speaking. Thus, it is possible that a speech and/or language problem may develop if (1) the vocal tract is remodeled abnormally; (2) cortical and neural linkages fail to occur; (3) respiration cannot be modified for speech; (4) laryngeal structures fail to provide the manipulations necessary for pitch, stress, intonation, and voicing contrasts; and (5) the articulators in the oral and nasal cavities fail to divert the air stream properly.

REFERENCES

1. Berlin, C. I.: Hemispheric asymmetry in auditory tasks, in Hardard, S., Doty, R., Goldstein, L., Jaymes, J., and Krauthaner, G. (ed): *Lateralization in the Nervous System*, Academic, New York, 1977, pp. 127–136
2. Penfield, W., and Roberts, L.: *Speech and Brain Mechanisms*. Princeton University Press, Princeton, New Jersey, 1959.
3. Lenneberg, E.: *The Biological Foundations of Learning*. Wiley, New York, 1967.
4. Ojemann, G., and Mateer, C.: Human language cortex: Localization of memory, syntax, and sequential motor-phoneme identification systems. *Science* 205:1401–1403, 1979.
5. Kimura, D.: Cerebral dominance for speech, in Tower, D. (ed): *The Nervous System*, Vol. 3: *Human Communication and Its Disorders*. Raven, New York, 1975, pp. 91–104.
6. Luria, A.: *Traumatic Aphasia*. Mouton, The Hague, 1970.
7. Rasmussen, R., and Milner, B.: The role of early left brain injury in determining lateralization of cerebral speech functions. *Ann. N. Y. Acad. Sci.* 299:355–369, 1977.
8. Sedtis, J., Volpe, B., and Wilson, D.: Variability in right hemisphere language function after callosal section: Evidence for a continuum of generative capability. *J. Neurosci.* 1:323–331, 1981.
9. Ojemann, G.: *Epilepsy: A Window to Brain Mechanisms*. Raven, New York, 1980.
10. Ojemann, G.: Brain organization for language from the perspective of electrical stimulation mapping. *Behav. Brain Sci.* 2:189–230, 1983.
11. Buckingham, H., Jr.: Neuropsychological models of language, in Lass, N. J., McReynolds, L., Northern, J., and Yoder, D. (eds): *Speech, Language, and Hearing*, Vol. 1: *Normal Processes*. Saunders, Philadelphia, 1982, pp. 183–195.
12. Blumstein, S., Cooper, W., Goodglass, H., *et al.*: Production deficits in aphasia: A voice–onset time analysis. *Brain Language* 2:153–170, 1980.
13. Fry, D.: Phonemic substitutions in an aphasic patient. *Language Speech* 2:52–61, 1959.
14. Shankweiler, D., and Harris, K.: An experimental approach to the problem of articulation in aphasia. *Cortex* 2:277–292, 1962.
15. Johns, D., and Darley, F.: Phonemic variability in apraxia of speech. *J. Speech Hear. Res.* 13:556–583, 1970.
16. Deal, J., and Darley, F.: Effect on phoneme duration control of three utterance-length conditions in an apractic patient. *J. Speech Hear. Res.* 15:639–653, 1972.
17. Trost, E., and Canter, G.: Apraxia of speech in patients with Broca's aphasia: A study of phoneme production, accuracy, and error patterns. *Brain Language* 1:63–79, 1974.
18. Blumstein, S.: *A Phonological Investigation of Aphasic Speech*. Mouton, The Hague, 1973.
19. Martin, A.: An investigation of phonological impairment in aphasia. Part II: Distinctive feature analysis of phonemic communication errors in aphasia. *Cortex* 10:317–328, 1974.
20. Darley, F., Aronson, A., and Brown, J.: *Motor Speech Disorders*. W. B. Saunders, Philadelphia, 1975.
21. Geshwin, N.: The apraxias: Neural mechanisms of disorders of learned movements. *Am. Sci.* 63:188–95, 1975.
22. Carpenter, M.: *Human Neuroanatomy*, 7th ed. Williams & Wilkins, Baltimore, 1976.
23. Chusid, J.: *Correlative Neuroanatomy and Functional Neurology*, 16th ed. Lange, Los Altos, California, 1976.
24. Ojemann, G.: Individual variability in cortical localization of language. *J. Neurosurg.* 50:164–169, 1979.

25. Ojemann, G., and Dodrill, C.: Predicting post-operative language and memory deficits after dominant hemisphere anterior temporal lobectomy by intraoperative stimulation mapping. *Am. Assoc. Neurol. Surg.* **23:**76–77, 1981.

26. Sperry, R.: Some effects of disconnecting the cerebral hemispheres. *Science* **217:**1223–1226, 1982.

27. Ross, R.: The aprosodias: Functional-anatomic organization of the affective components of language in the right hemisphere. *Neurology (N.Y.)* **38:**561–569, 1981.

28. Tobey, E.: Motor speech adaptation: An acoustic study of temporal and spectral response patterns following focal cortical injury. Unpublished dissertation, City University of New York, 1981.

29. Guiot, G., Herzog, E., Rondot, P., *et al.:* Arrest or acceleration of speech evoked by thalamic stimulation in the course of stereotaxic procedures for Parkinsonism. *Brain* **84:**363–379, 1961.

30. Ramanurti, B.: Stimulation response in the diencephalon. *Neurology (N.Y.)* **15:**123–126, 1967.

31. Toth, S.: Effect of electrical stimulation of subcortical sites on speech and consciousness, in Somjen, C. (ed): *Neurophysiology Studies in Man,* Excerpta Medica, Amsterdam, 1972, pp. 221–245.

32. Ojemann, G., and Fedio, P.: The effects of stimulation of human thalamus and parietal and temporal white matter on short-term memory. *J. Neurosurg.* **29:**51–59, 1968.

33. Gazzaniga, M. S.: *The Bisected Brain.* Appleton, New York, 1970.

34. Trevarthen, C.: The development of cerebral mechanisms for language, in Kirk, W. (ed): *Neuropsychology of Language, Reading, and Spelling.* Academic, New York, 1983, pp. 45–76.

35. Milner, E.: CNS maturation and language acquisition, in Whitaker, H. and Whitacker, H. (eds): *Studies in Neurolinguistics,* Vol. 1. Academic, New York, 1976, pp. 172–183.

36. Woodruff, D.: Brain electrical activity and behavior relationships over the life span, in Baltes, P. (ed.): *Life-Span Development and Behavior,* Vol. I. Academic, New York, 1978, pp. 63–70.

37. Wyke, B.: The neurological basis of movement—A developmental review, in Holt, K. (ed): *Movement and Child Development.* Heinemann, London, 1975, pp. 142–151.

38. Kent, R.: Sensorimotor aspects of speech development, in Astin, R., Alberts, J., Peterson, M. (eds): *Sensory and Perceptual Development: Influences of Genetic and Experiential Factors.* Academic, New York, 1983, pp. 87–98.

39. Conel, J.: *The Postnatal Development of the Human Cerebral Cortex.* Vol. II: *The Cortex of the One Month Infant.* Harvard University Press, Cambridge, Massachusetts. 1941.

40. Conel, J.: *The Postnatal Development of the Human Cerebral Cortex,* Vol. II: *The Cortex of the Three Month Infant.* Harvard University Press, Cambridge, Massachusetts, 1947.

41. Yakovlev, P.: Morphological criteria of growth and maturation of the nervous system in man, in Kolb, L., Masland, R., Cooke, R. (eds): *Mental Retardation.* Research Nervous Mental Disease, Bethesda, Maryland, 1962, pp. 54–63.

42. Taft, L., and Cohen, H.: Neonatal and infant reflexology, in Hellmuth, J. (ed): *Exceptional Infant,* Vol. I: *The Normal Infant.* Special Child Publications, Seattle, Washington, 1967, pp. 128–134.

43. Capute, A., Accardo, P., Vining, E., *et al.: Primitive Reflex Profile.* Monographs in Developmental Pediatrics, Vol. I. University Park Press, Baltimore, 1978.

44. Bosma, J. F.: Anatomic and physiologic development of the speech apparatus, in Tower, D. (ed): *The Nervous System,* Vol. III: *Human Communication and Its Disorders.* Raven, New York, 1965, pp. 1345–1361.

45. Liberman, P. *On the Origins of Language: An Introduction to the Evolution of Human Language.* Macmillan, New York, 1975.

46. Weiffenbach, J., and Thach, B.: Elicited tongue movements: touch and tests in the newborn human, in Bosma, J. (ed): *Oral Sensation and Perception: Development in the Fetus and Infant.* DHEW Report (NIH) no. 73-546. National Institutes of Health, Washington, D. C., 1973, pp. 7–17.

47. Netsell, R.: The acquisition of speech motor control: A perspective with direction for research, in Stark, R. (ed): *Language Behavior in Infancy and Early Childhood.* Santa Barbara Press, Santa Barbara, California, 1979, pp. 111–123.

48. Denes, P., and Pinson, E.: *The Speech Chain.* Anchor Press/Doubleday, Garden City, New York, 1963.

49. Hixon, T.: Respiratory function in speech, in Minifie, F., Hixon, T., and Williams, F. (eds): *Normal Aspects of Speech, Hearing, and Language.* Prentice-Hall, Englewood Cliffs, New Jersey, 1973, pp. 73–127.

50. Borden, F., and Harris, K.: *The Speech Science Primer: Physiology, Acoustics and Perception of Speech.* Williams & Wilkins, Baltimore, 1980.

51. Wilder, C., and Bacon, R.: Respiratory patterns in infant cry. *Human Commun.* **3**:18–34, 1974.
52. Levitzky, M.: *Pulmonary Physiology.* McGraw-Hill, New York, 1982.
53. Faaborg-Andersen, K.: Electromyographic investigation of intrinsic laryngeal muscles in humans. *Acta Physiol. Scand.* **41**:1–148, 1957.
54. Hirose, H., and Gay, T.: The activity of the intrinsic laryngeal muscles in voicing control. *Phonetica* **25**:140–164, 1972.
55. Van den Berg, J.: Direct and indirect determination of the mean subglottic pressure. *Folia Phoniatr.* **8**:1–24, 1956.
56. Freeman, F., and Ushijima, T.: Laryngeal muscle activity during stuttering. *J. Speech Hear. Res.* **21**:538–562, 1978.
57. Negus, V.: *The Comparative Anatomy and Physiology of the Larynx.* Hafner, New York, 1962.
58. Borden, G., and Harris, K.: *Speech Science Primer: Physiology, Acoustics, and Perception of Speech*, 2nd ed. Williams & Wilkins, Baltimore, 1984.
59. Carlsoo, S.: Nervous coordination and mechanical function of the mandibular elevators. *Acta Odont. Scand.* **4** (Suppl. 11):1–226, 1952.
60. Hickey, J., Stacy, R., and Rinear, L.: Electromyographic studies of mandibular muscles in basic jaw movements. *J. Prosth. Dent.* **7**:565–570, 1957.
61. Sussman, H., MacNeilage, P., and Hanson, R.: Labial and mandibular dynamics during the production of bilabial consonants: Preliminary observations. *J. Speech Hear. Res.* **16**:397–420, 1973.
62. Tuller, B., Harris, K., and Gross, R.: Electromyographic study of the jaw muscles during speech. *Status Report on Speech Research SR59/60*, Haskins Laboratories, New Haven, Connecticut, 1979, pp. 83–102.
63. MacNeilage, P.: Motor control of serial ordering on speech. *Psychol. Rev.* **77**:182–196, 1970.
64. Stark, R., and Nathanson, S.: Spontaneous cry in the newborn infant: Sounds and facial gestures, in Bosma, J. (ed): *Oral Sensation and Perception: Development in the Fetus and Infant*, U.S. Government Printing Office, Bethesda, Maryland, 1974.
65. Oller, D., Wiemar, L., Doyle, W., *et al.*: Infant babbling and speech. *J. Child Lang.* **3**:1–11, 1976.
66. Warren, D.: Velopharyngeal orifice size and upper pharyngeal pressure-flow patterns in normal speech. *Plast. Reconstr. Surg.* **33**:148–152, 1964.
67. Rampp, D., Pannbacker, M., and Kinnebrew, M.: *Velopharyngeal Incompetency.* Modern Education, Tulsa, Oklahoma, 1984.
68. Rich, A.: The innervation of the tensor veli palatini and levator veli palatini muscles. *Bull. Johns Hopkins Hosp.* **31**:305–310, 1930.
69. Dickson, D.: Anatomy of the normal velopharyngeal mechanism. *Clin. Plast. Surg.* **9**:280–291, 1975.
70. Ibuki, K.: The course of facial nerve innervation for the levator veli palatine muscle. *Cleft Palate J.* **15**:209–214, 1978.

11

Receptive and Expressive Language Disorders

Rachel E. Stark

INTRODUCTION

It has been suggested that delay or difficulty in acquiring language milestones in early childhood may be the most reliable indication of developmental disorders of all kinds. These deficits may provide more reliable predictors than motor delays, visuoperceptual or attentional deficits, or any other signs of high-risk status. Why should delay in language acquisition be of greater significance than any other developmental delays? It may be that language acquisition is one of the most complex of all developmental processes. Acquisi-

Rachel E. Stark • Department of Neurology, John F. Kennedy Institute, Johns Hopkins University School of Medicine, Baltimore, Maryland 21205.

tion of both receptive and expressive language may depend on the integrity of many different mechanisms and also on the establishment of smooth interactions among these mechanisms. Thus, if any one is impaired or if they are not properly integrated, language delay may result and may provide the first indication of disorder.

· If so, it would seem quite surprising that delay in language acquisition has not been employed more effectively than it has for the detection of developmental problems in young children. In the recent past, the consensus among pediatricians has been that most forms of language delay in young children are temporary in nature. The probability was considered to be high that any given child aged 2–3 years who was not yet speaking would show rapid recovery in the later preschool years and would become indistinguishable in this respect from his peers.

Large surveys of language development in preschool children would appear to support the recovery point of view, at least in part. Language milestones show a wide range in age of attainment among children who eventually show normal language abilities.[1] Many potentially normal children are much slower than average in producing first words and phrases. It is possible that delays with respect to any one of the mechanisms subserving language may have a disproportionate effect on its acquisiton in the earlier preschool years. As soon as a certain threshold level is reached with respect to more slowly developing mechanisms, however, it may be that the necessary integration of abilities is effected promptly and that acceleration in language growth results. Thus, while the processes of language acquisition may be particularly sensitive to developmental delays or deficits, this very sensitivity may lead to overidentification of children at risk for a severe and persisting communication disorder.

This chapter is concerned with the classification of language disorders in young children. A number of explanatory models for language disorders will be considered, each yielding a different classification scheme. Most recent models take account of both comprehension (reception) and production (expression) of language. Both aspects tend to be affected in language-disordered children, but the disorder may be primarily one of reception or one of expression. The antecedents of each may be quite varied in character. Information about such antecedents may enable us to become better able to recognize children at risk for severe and persisting language disorders and to differentiate them from children who show relatively mild, remitting delays in language acquisition.

IDENTIFICATION OF LANGUAGE DISORDERS IN CHILDREN

In approaching the problem of identification, many investigators differentiate speech disorders, that is, disorders in the ability to plan and execute the oral movements required for speech articulation, from language disorders. Speech disorders may be present, for example, in the case of the structural anomalies found in children with cleft lip and palate, together with normal comprehension of spoken language and the ability to produce grammatical forms in an age-appropriate manner. Speech and language disorders are quite likely, however, to co-occur in children.

Disorders of reading and writing are frequently found in school-age language-disordered children. At the same time, some forms of learning disability in the areas of reading and writing do not appear to be related to language disorders. Learning problems are discussed in other chapters.

At least 3% of preschool children are significantly delayed in language acquisition. Many more may be delayed by at least one year and yet have a normal potential for language. Identification of language disorders in young children is not, therefore, a simple matter in the preschool years when, as we have seen, variability in rate of acquisition of language even among normal children is great. Approaches that have been employed for the purpose of identification include reliance on parent report or on the judgments of teachers and clinicians, and the use of standardized tests and measurements, including standardized intelligence tests.

Each approach has disadvantages. Parent reports are not always reliable, even in the preschool years. Also, many children who are quite properly considered by clinicians to be language delayed in the preschool years overcome this delay and manifest normal language and learning ability in the later school years.

The development and use of standardized tests and measurements are frequently based on an assumption of a normal underlying distribution of linguistic or of cognitive abilities. Children with severe and persisting language problems may form an entirely separate group unrelated to a normal distribution. In most cases, however, language impairment has to be defined in terms of an arbitrary cutoff score, for example, two standard deviations from a given mean score. Follow-up studies suggest that the scores of children identified in this manner as language impaired may place the child in a low normal category at one time and in a language-impaired category at another.[2] In addition, there are many different language tests, each one purporting to measure a different aspect of language. There is no accepted method for combining scores on these tests in order to derive an overall language score. A language scale, comparable to an IQ scale, has not yet been developed. In addition, for some aspects of language (e.g., those concerned with the social, communicative use of language), standardized scales or measurement procedures are unavailable.

A conservative approach to the identification of language disorders at the present time would be to take into account the reports of parents and teachers and the judgments of clinicians. These judgments should subsequently be evaluated in relationship to a child's scores on a comprehensive battery of speech and language tests and also to the results of careful observation procedures.[3]

NATURE OF LANGUAGE DISORDERS IN CHILDREN

Language disorders in children may be defined strictly in terms of an impairment in acquisition of the forms of language; i.e., they may manifest themselves primarily as a delay (or disorder) in the acquisition of linguistic units and structures.[4] The units are the phonemes or sounds of speech, word units, and phrases and sentences. Sequences of these units are governed by grammatical rule systems that specify the manner in which sounds may be combined in words, and words may be combined and modified in the larger linguistic units of phrases and sentences.

Alternatively, language disorders may be defined in terms of a dissociation between the child's ability to produce language forms and his ability to use them meaningfully in everyday communicative contexts. Some forms of dissociation, e.g., the dissociation of linguistic form and content of language, may relate to severe cognitive deficits or thought disorder; others, e.g., dissociation of linguistic form and the social uses of language, may relate to significant social or emotional disorders affecting communication. Thus, in assessing a language disorder it is important to consider the child's intelligence, mental processes, and social communicative abilities as well as linguistic abilities.[5]

Medical Classification

The possible manifestations of language disorder may be considered in relationship to presumed etiology. According to the traditional medical model, mental retardation, hearing loss, emotional and behavior disorders, and neurological deficits or lesions may be primary causes of language disorders.

1. *Mental retardation:* There are many different forms of mental retardation, and many different etiological agents or environmental causes may be involved (e.g., lead poisoning, neurodegenerative lipid and other diseases, encephalitis, and sociocultural deprivation). Although it is true that mentally retarded children are, by definition, likely to be delayed in acquisition of language, they are also more likely to present unusual or deviant patterns of language acquisition than are children in the normal range in nonverbal intelligence. It may be useful to consider receptive and expressive language disorders in children in relationship to the etiologies of mental retardation, but mental retardation per se can no longer be considered a single cause of language disorders in children.

2. *Hearing loss:* Hearing loss in children is associated with delay in the acquisition of speech and language forms. Although such factors as intelligence and socioeconomic status of the family must be taken into account, there is believed to be a significant association between the nature and extent of hearing loss and the extent of language delay in hearing-impaired children. Hearing loss, even that found in young children with recurrent otitis media, reduces significantly the frequency of exposure of the affected child to the language spoken in his environment. Thus, the comprehension of linguistic forms may be noticeably delayed even when the hearing loss is relatively mild. In addition, the child will have difficulty in acquiring language production in proportion to the extent of his hearing impairment. The severely hearing-impaired child may be socially isolated and may become depressed or emotionally frustrated as a result of this impairment. Also, in some children, hearing impairment may be associated with damage to the central as well as to the peripheral auditory system. In these cases, cognitive and/or social abilities are also likely to be affected and more profound or complex language disorders may be present than in the case of peripheral hearing loss alone.

3. *Emotional and behavioral disorders:* Emotional and behavioral disorders are thought to follow as a consequence of language disorder in some children. In others, however, the emotional/behavioral problem may be a primary one and may also be of such severity that social communicative abilities are impaired. Children affected by these disorders do not exhibit normal social awareness or the ability to interact normally with others in comprehension or production. They do not learn important communication skills such as the taking of turns, repairing of conversational breakdown, or asking for clarification. The comprehension and production of linguistic forms in relationship to these communicative abilities may also be impaired. Nonverbal communication or the use of sign language may be more successful for some communicatively impaired children than the use of spoken language. In children with less severe behavioral disturbances, e.g.,

those presenting hyperactivity and impulsivity, linguistic forms may be acquired to some extent. However, they may not be used in the regulation of behavior, in listening, or in the development of learning strategies.

4. *Neurological deficits or lesions:* Neurological deficits have been associated with language disorders of all types. Neurological deficits may be associated with different forms of mental retardation, central auditory disorders, emotional and behavioral disorders, and speech motor disorders. They may be developmental in nature or acquired. Lesions to, or dysgenesis of, cerebral structures in the left hemisphere are most commonly thought to be associated with language disorders in children. For some more global language disorders, however, massive bilateral lesions may be a necessary antecedent. A lack of the normal asymmetries affecting both the left posterior and right anterior portions of cerebral cortex has been implicated in dyslexia[6] and may also be present in some language-impaired children. It has been suggested that both the right and left hemispheres have potential for the development of language. Left hemisphere dominance for language is presumed to be related to its earlier maturation in infancy. Studies of children in whom right or left hemispherectomies have been performed very early in life because of severe central nervous system malformation, before language is acquired, suggest that an undamaged right hemisphere, although capable of acquiring language, may not be as successful with respect to certain analysis and synthesis capabilities as an undamaged left hemisphere.[7] It has been pointed out that the takeover of language functions by an undamaged right hemisphere may be accomplished at the expense of development of spatial and other related nonverbal abilities.

It has been found that infantile right hemiplegia (and therefore presumed left hemisphere lesion) is associated with delay in acquisition of linguistic rule systems more frequently than infantile left hemiplegia. It has also been shown, however, that if a damaged left hemisphere continues to function, in adults or in children, the right and left hemispheres may interact in controlling language functions in a poorly integrated and defective manner.

5. *Specific language impairment:* Benton[8] described a developmental language disorder in children, referred to as developmental dysphasia[9] and as a specific language impairment or deficit.[3] This language disorder is defined by exclusion, i.e., as unrelated to hearing loss or history of middle ear problems, to mental retardation, or to emotional or behavioral disorder. Benton suggested that the disorder may be related to neurological deficit. In a relatively recent study, however, Stark and Tallal[3] did not find many specifically language-impaired children to be frankly neurologically impaired. Specifically language-imparied (SLI) children make up approximately 50% of children identified as language impaired in the early school years. Their language deficits may range from mild to severe.

Objections have been raised that children classified in each subgroup proposed in the medical model do not present patterns of perceptual and motor deficits or of receptive or expressive linguistic deficits by which they can be reliably identified.[10,11]

Rosenthal *et al.*[11] attempted to differentiate subgroups of language-impaired children originally classified in a traditional manner. Cluster analyses were applied to 32 variables that were routinely included in their evaluation for this purpose. These included medical history variables (e.g., history of prenatal and perinatal insult and EEG abnormalities), psychological and social variables, and speech motor variables. Rosenthal and colleagues first classified 82 children from their case load on an *a priori* basis as mentally retarded, severely hearing impaired, neurologically impaired/aphasic, oral apraxic, dysarthric, autistic, and delayed in maturation. It was expected that these same groupings would be recovered in the cluster analyses. Instead, only two clusters were formed, one comprising mentally retarded and autistic children, the other comprising all others, i.e., the children with severe hearing impairment, aphasia, oral motor problems, and maturational lag. Discriminant function analyses were carried out in order to determine which of the 32 evaluation variables best discriminated the two major groups identified by the cluster analyses. The only basis on which the investigators were able to differentiate these two groups was that of general performance on tests of intelligence and performance on individual subtests from scales for measuring intelligence. The two groups in other words were not differentiated on the basis of such variables as laterality, delayed motor development, or performance on tests of auditory discrimination.

The lack of correspondence between patterns of perceptual and motor deficits or medical history variables and proposed etiology has caused some investigators to question the value of the medical model. This lack of correspondence may reflect the influence of multiple etiological factors and interactions among them in most language-impaired children. These factors may be capable of producing many different forms of language disorder.

Behavioral Classification

Attempts have also been made to classify language disorders in children on the basis of patterns of linguistic deficits.[10,12] Variables considered in these attempts at classification were measures of comprehension (reception of language) formulation (language expression) and repetition. The patterns described relate to phonological disorders (disorders in production and perception of the sounds of speech and in the use of the rule systems that specify possible sound combinations in any given language); semantic disorders (disorders of recognition and production of words in relationship to their meaning); and syntactic disorders (disorders in reception or production in the use of the rules describing grammatical relationships among words and ways in which sentences may be changed, e.g., to form questions, commands, or negative statements).

Aram and Nation[10] employed a set of standard speech and language tests, as well as some nonstandard adaptations of these tests, in developing their classification scheme. They were able to delineate six different patterns of deficit among 47 children aged 3–7 years on the basis of these procedures. Subsequent studies suggested that longitudinal outcomes at 9 years of age varied across these six subgroups. The patterns of linguistic deficits were not however, related to any of the nonlinguistic measures obtained (socioeconomic status, age, sex, race, intelligence, and speech mechanism adequacy), with the exception of age. No data are provided, however, with respect to the range of IQ scores or of the ratings of adequacy of oral movements among the subjects of this study.

Rapin and Allen[12] based their classification primarily on linguistic analyses of videotaped samples of naturally occurring language production. These samples were obtained from 35 preschool language-disordered children. The investigators also took into account aspects of the child's medical history and patterns of social interaction shown by the child. Some of their data are longitudinal in nature, others cross-sectional. The aim of these investigators was to group language-impared children under tentative syndromes on the basis of their linguistic deficits. Their ultimate goal was to understand the pathogenesis of the symptoms peculiar to these syndromes.

There is some overlap in the classification systems proposed in these two studies. Both groups described the following: (1) severe classic expressive language problems in children with relative sparing of comprehension (in both studies there were some subgroups within this general category, the most important of these being verbal apraxia); (2) severe comprehension deficits with higher expressive abilities; (3) severe deficits in both receptive and expressive language; and (4) superior speech sound and sentence repetition ability with difficulty in both comprehension and formulation. Rapin and Allen[12] suggested that there may be deficient word comprehension as well as inappropriate use of spoken language in communicative contexts in some of the children in this category. Both studies indicated that comprehension, formulation, and repetition may be differentially affected. Both groups of investigators point out that patterns of linguistic deficit are not fixed but may change markedly with age.

This approach to classification has received some support in terms of localization of malfunction from a recent study of regional cerebral blood flow (rCBF). Specifically, Lou et al.[13] reported abnormally reduced rCBF bilaterally in 13 dysphasic and/or attentional deficit-disordered (ADD) children aged 6½–15 years. The regions of hypoperfusion were both cortical and subcortical. They were different for different types of language disorder. Children with verbal dyspraxia (and severe expressive language disorder) showed this anomaly in anterior perisylvian regions. Children with more global language disorders (severe deficits in both receptive and expressive language) had both anterior and posterior perisylvian hypoperfusion, whereas the one subject who had a severe receptive deficit (verbal agnosia) had bilateral posterior perisylvian hypoperfusion involving cortical areas as well as subcortical but normal perfusion in the left anterior perisylvian region.

The behavioral–linguistic model may also lack explanatory value in certain cases, however. Some disorders of reception of language, for example, are not primarily linguistic in nature but relate at least in part to a severe cognitive deficit or to a profound social or interpersonal disorder. Quite different types of neurological impairment could be involved in such cases. Disorders that are and are not primarily linguistic in nature are discussed separately in relationship to production and comprehension.

DISORDERS OF LANGUAGE PRODUCTION

Classification in terms of disorders that are primarily of receptive or of expressive language receive greatest emphasis in this chapter. There are probably many gradations of disability with respect to both expressive and receptive language. However, consideration of the most extreme cases is often instructive and may contribute most to the understanding of language disorders in general.

Expressive language disorders in children may occur with relative sparing of language comprehension. These disorders may be linguistic in nature, that is, they may take the form of difficulty in encoding of spoken language at the phonetic, semantic, and/or syntactic level. Alternatively, expressive language disorders (1) may take the form of disruption in social communication, i.e., they may be manifested as a witholding of speech in certain situations; or (2) may reveal a more primary thought disorder.

Disorders of Linguistic Formulation

MacNeilage et al.[14] described severe and persisting difficulties in swallowing, chewing, and speaking in a 17-year-old woman. Examination of this young woman yielded considerable evidence of damage to central mechanisms (of transmission and processing) of somesthetic sensory perception. Stereognosis, sensitivity to painful stimuli, tactile localization, and two-point discrimination on the surface of the body were all impaired, although light touch, temperature, and position sense and taste appeared normal. The patient was ambulatory and could perform gross hand and arm movements. She was incapable, however, of executing the motor commands for finer movements differentiated in time and space of the type required for speech production. Her speech was unintelligible to all but her immediate family members. Speech perception abilities were grossly intact, and she was not mentally retarded. Intelligence, as measured by the Wechsler Bellevue Scale, was in the dull normal range (full-scale IQ 90), and she had succeeded quite well in academic studies in a regular public school. However, verbal IQ was 83 and her performance IQ 99. The 16-point difference between verbal and performance IQ suggested the presence of a mild language disorder, probably expressive in nature, in addition to her speech motor disorder.

Lenneberg[15] also described a 4-year-old child who was totally incapable of speech and who had difficulty in producing any vocalization. He was said to have congenital anarthria, although the speech motor disorder was not accompanied by chewing or swallowing difficulties. He was also described as having normal or near-normal comprehension of language. Performance on comprehension tests at 8 years indicated a knowledge of grammatical rules and structure as well as of lexical items, i.e., of the key words in a sentence. The child had normal or borderline intelligence and had learned to read satisfactorily.

The term *verbal apraxia* is sometimes applied to speech motor problems associated with expressive language disorder. The term implies a difficulty in formulating a motor plan for speaking similar to that found in a classic Broca aphasia in adults. Speech is slow and labored and sometimes telegraphic in nature; i.e., only the key or content words are produced and function words such as "in," "to," "the," or "and" are omitted.

Children with severe expressive language problems tend to avoid speaking except in highly familiar situations, and produce shorter utterances than children of the same age and/or cognitive level who do not show any language disorder. They may produce series of single words or, like the Broca aphasic, may omit small function words. It may be that, even in less severe cases, a primary difficulty in mastering speech motor skills retards the development of higher-level expressive-linguistic abilities. Alternatively, the same underlying deficits or lesions may result in impairment of both speech motor abilities and language production. These disorders may be primarily phonological in nature; i.e., the primary deficit may be in the speech sound system, both receptively and expressively.

Case History B. T., at 10 years, 8 months, had a history of a severe expressive language disorder, difficulty in learning in school, and behavioral problems relating to dependency and frustration over his difficulty in speaking. Pregnancy and delivery were unremarkable. Birth weight was 9 lbs. Motor milestones were somewhat delayed, and the child was still considered poorly coordinated at the time of the evaluation. Language milestones had been delayed to a greater extent than motor milestones, however. B.T. was still babbling at 2 years of age. He did not produce his first words, which he combined with gestures, until 3 years of age, and he did not combine words into longer units until he was 5–6 years of age. Speech therapy services had been provided on two occasions but without success. The family lived in a rural community. The parents had no known history of language disorder but the father could not read or write. Three siblings had normal language and were doing quite well in school. A paternal second cousin was mute and mentally retarded.

At the time of an interdisciplinary evaluation, B.T. had normal hearing and was functioning at a borderline level in nonverbal intelligence. His performance IQ on the WISC–R was 82. However, performance in reading, writing, and arithmetic were all at the first-grade level. B.T. had been placed in a class for the educably mentally retarded. Neurological evaluation indicated no abnormalities. On neurodevelopmental evaluation, B.T. showed a number of significant "soft" signs. He could sustain unipedal stance only very briefly. Choreiform movements upon arm extension, impaired sequencing of finger opposition movements with mirroring on the opposite hand, and dysdiadochokinesis were noted. The impairment of sequencing of hand and finger movements was greatest on the left side. In addition, identification of two fingers in response to simultaneous touches and left–right orientation were impaired. B.T. used short sentences only (mean of three to four words) with immature language forms, e.g., "me go." His expressive language skills were at a 3-year level. He was moderately unintelligible.

Language comprehension was considerably less impaired. Single-word comprehension was at an 8-year level. Performance on sentence comprehension tests ranged from 5½ years to 7 years, depending on the amount of contextual information provided.

It was further determined that B.T. had considerable difficulty in sequencing voluntary nonspeech oral movements in spite of the presence of completely normal patterns of chewing, swallowing, and sucking. Sequencing of speech movements in nonsense syllable production was impaired in rate and accuracy, even for those syllables that could be produced correctly in isolation.

It was concluded that this child had a severe developmental verbal dyspraxia and an auditory processing disorder. In fact, his speech motor dysfunction and speech sound discrimination problems may have been symptoms of a single underlying phonological disorder. Disruption or maldevelopment of those structures of the left hemisphere in which both sequencing of non speech oral movement and consonant sound discrimination appear to be represented might be capable of producing an expressive language disorder of this severity.[16]

In some children with severe expressive language disorders, the extent of oral motor dysfunction, if present, is not sufficient to account for the severity of the expressive language disorder. Some of these children have a history of oral motor apraxia that has shown remission, but with persistence of an expressive language disorder. These children may be able to repeat words and phrases that they cannot produce spontaneously in communicative contexts, as was true of B.T. after treatment. They may produce unusual grammatical forms, such as "The baby is cry" (for "The baby cries" or "is crying"), in communicative situations that cannot be explained as an immature expression typical of a·

much younger child. The semantic (word meaning) content of these expressions is not, however, bizarre or incomprehensible.

Expressive Language and Thought Disorders

Atypical expressive language may also be related primarily to a thought disorder. Affected children may produce idiosyncratic or bizarre expressions that are unusual in grammatical form but are even more strikingly aberrant in semantic content.

When symptoms of this kind are encountered, it is important to make sure that a profound receptive language deficit is not present as well. Some children with superior facility in expression but severely depressed word comprehension may produce unusual utterances, because (1) they do not know the true meanings of the words that they have learned or (2) they produce statements which seem to reflect loose associations but which may be based upon a sequence of actual events that is poorly explained.[17]

> *Case History*   W.C., at 6 years, was reportedly delayed in language milestones and showed a marked attentional deficit in school and lack of ability to establish social contacts with her peers. She had engaged in ritualistic behaviors during the preschool years and had shown difficulty in adapting to stress and novel situations. W.C. was echolalic on occasion and showed some gaze aversion. Her father, a successful professional, had by report shown similar difficulties in childhood.
>
> At 4 years of age, W.C. was found to have normal hearing. A receptive language disorder was diagnosed because her responses to questions were often bizarre. For example, when asked what she liked to watch on television, W.C. responded "Because so many, I like to talk with 60 minutes, 40, 2 and 3." When asked how old she was, W.C. responded "My three, two, three fingers is one." Her responses on receptive language tests where she was not required to make a verbal response did not support a diagnosis of receptive language disorder primarily.
>
> At 5 years of age, her IQ was 69, on the Stanford Binet Test of Intelligence. Her language abilities were said to range from 2 years, 0 months to 5 years, 3 months. Her expressive language was said to have remained odd and idiosyncratic. At 6 years, a marked improvement in all areas was reported. Her IQ on the Stanford Binet Test of Intelligence was 97. Language abilities still showed a wide scatter (range: 3 years, 1 month to 8 years, 4 months). The child's poorest abilities were in language production, characterized by "rambling" and "lack of logical coherence." W.C. also had difficulty following directions and in regulating her attention in the classroom. She was more socially responsive than before but had difficulty in dealing with academic failure or with teasing by her classmates.
>
> Her conversation with adults was relatively coherent, but her telling of stories was still marked by unusual word use and loose associations. Examples are:
> 1. Conversation (Note: the adult's turns in the conversation are underlined): <u>Tell me what you're going to do at your party.</u> /Maybe my mama might share some party hats but I don't think she has some. She has to go to the shopping center and get some./ <u>Some party hats?</u> /Yeah/ <u>So, you're going to have party hats for your friends? What else are you going to do at your birthday party?</u> /Party napkins and party plates. And my mama has some strawberry ice cream and some koolaid./ <u>Are you going to have a cake?</u> /Well I better think so but I think my mama might make me a special treat when

it's my birthday in January./ Well, what kind of cake would you like your mother to make you? /Maybe chocolate./ Is chocolate your favorite? /Yeah/ How many candles would be on your birthday cake this time. /One, two, three, four, five, six, seven./ Seven? You're getting pretty old aren't you? Are you going to be seven years old?/ No, I'm going to be six years old in January when it's my birthday. / That's what I thought. But you want seven candles on your cake? One extra one? /Extra, and my candles are going to be pink./ Pink candles? /Pink candles. I don't think I have enough but I'll try to find seven of them.

2. Story telling: You want to find another story to tell me about? /Yeah. I'll find another story. It just has to look really nice and strange, but if you can't read it, I'll try to help you say the words. We've already read this one. Dancing man, dancing man, dancing man, you're so wonderful. You are dancing so nice I can't believe it. Why are you dancing, you're so much telled? I'm not goint to see—I'm going to see that dancing again. Let me see that dancing, that dancing has to keep dancing. How do you know my dancing is wonderful? Why are you locked in that dangerous cage? You ought to be ashivered of yourself. I didn't know but I couldn't be locked. Get out of there you stupid rabbit. We're waitin for the dance to come. O.K./O.K. snitched his hand on the stick and scratched his head with the other. He snitched up and down like a jumping jack and this mouse was playing the horns and this mouse was playing a badget. And they made lots and lots of loudest and loud noisy dance with joy and all of a sudden he danced and he looked at the dance and the dance was all his fault. He danced for just a nice week. Why is these two muts under in jail? I don't know. It's the policeman, he said. Why that does it. I hate to be locked in this truck. His claws opened the door and it was snitched open and they made the dance and they lived happily ever after.

A diagnosis of mild remitting autism was made when W.C. was 6 years old. The prognosis was considered good.

Expressive Language and Social/Communicative Disorders

Expressive language disorders in children may take the form of selective or elective mutism. In such children, the language disorder is thought to be related primarily to social withdrawal or to a pathological fear of speaking in some or all social situations. Children with these relatively uncommon forms of expressive language disorder are capable of speech production in some situations but appear to withhold speech in others. Their language comprehension is commensurate with their cognitive abilities.

It may be difficult, however, to distinguish elective mutism from a higher level speech motor disorder or linguistic-expressive disorder. The disorder usually manifests itself when a child first enters school. It may also be precipitated by some other traumatic event. It is thought to be associated with an unsatisfactory mother/child relationship, either one in which the child is criticized for his speech attempts or one in which there is a very strong attachment or symbiosis between the mother and child. The child may have a speech articulation deficit or more primary expressive language delay. The refusal to speak in some situations may represent a useful adaptation on the part of the child to demands he is unable to meet, strong avoidance behavior and/or manipulative behavior. This disorder is not readily amenable to intervention.

DISORDERS OF LANGUAGE COMPREHENSION

Receptive language disorders in children may occur with relative sparing of linguistic production. Disorders that are primarily receptive are frequently misdiagnosed by pediatricians and other professionals because of the common assumption that receptive language abilities must always precede expressive language abilities in the developmental sequence. When sophisticated language-production capabilities are observed, it may be erroneously concluded, on the basis of the above assumption, that receptive language abilities are intact.

"Pure" receptive language disorders may be linguistic in nature, that is, they may take the form of difficulty in decoding speech at all linguistic levels (phonetic, semantic or syntactic). This type of receptive language impairment appears to be associated with auditory disorders. Other types of receptive language disorders may reflect either profound cognitive or social/communicative deficits, or both. The child with these latter types of disorders may repeat words and sentences accurately but with a total lack of comprehension.

Auditory Disorders

Hearing loss and other auditory disorders that are acquired in childhood (e.g., complication of encephalitis, meningitis, and other CNS diseases or a hereditary hearing loss of late onset) may affect the child's linguistic system in proportion to the age of onset of the disorder. The child aged 3–6 years in whom speaking and listening abilities are not yet fully acquired may gradually lose expressive language as well as receptive language abilities after the onset of severe hearing impairment or severe central auditory disorder. By contrast, the child aged 6–12 years in whom speaking and listening skills are beginning to be automatic or overlearned in some respects will show a loss of comprehension of spoken language but may maintain expressive language abilities and show only mild deterioration in the accuracy of speech production.

Children with congenital or early acquired (prelingual) hearing impairment or central auditory disorders do not perceive speech normally and have difficulty in comprehending language. They may also have great difficulty in acquiring expressive language even if their speech motor system is intact. Auditory motor linkages cannot readily be established because of the severely reduced auditory language input.

It is assumed in the case of severe central auditory disorders (i.e., where peripheral hearing is normal but auditory stimuli are responded to in an inconsistent and aberrant manner) that extensive bilateral damage to the central auditory system must be present. If the lesion were unilateral, presumably the intact auditory cortex and subcortical structures on the unaffected side would be able to take over the functions proper to the affected side.

One such disorder is verbal auditory agnosia, described by Rapin et al.[18] A characteristic feature of this disorder is the presence of bilateral paroxysmal discharges in EEG records obtained from the temporal areas even though seizures do not always occur. Rapin and co-workers presented a series of such cases. They reported that the onset may be observed in later childhood, after a period of normal language development. It may be accompanied by a marked regression in all language abilities. Comprehension difficulties are noted first and are usually so severe that peripheral hearing loss may be suspected.

EEG patterns may later return to normal. The language deficit may then show some remission. However, the illness which gives rise to the bitemporal discharges may be chronic, e.g., a viral encephalitis, and the symptoms described may persist for years. Remission, if present, may be attributable to language intervention or to the increasing maturity of the child.

Case History   This disorder is illustrated quite well in the case of a 5-year-old boy, S.W. This child was the product of an adolescent pregnancy complicated by toxemia and preeclampsia. His birth weight was 8 pounds. 11 ounces. His early developmental history was normal. S.W. was an active child, and at the age of 3½ years he was toilet trained, exhibited appropriate self-care skills, knew the names of colors, could count to 10 by rote, and was speaking in short sentences. There was a family history of learning disability and, more strikingly, of kidney disease.

At the age of 3 years, the grandmother observed that S.W. was not hearing properly. Over the next 6 months, his responses to speech became increasingly inconsistent. Sometimes he appeared reluctant to respond or gave totally irrelevant responses to questions. Subsequently his expressive language began to deteriorate. At first it was noticed that S.W. was leaving out function words and that his speech was becoming slurred. By the time he was 5 years old, his language production was limited to single words. Gradually even this form of output disappeared, however, and S.W. produced only babbling, typical of a 9-month-old, together with a few single words such as "no" and "mom." He communicated chiefly through gesture.

Various syndromes were considered. An attempt was made to rule out hearing loss, especially since S.W. had a history of recurrent otitis media, but the results of hearing evaluation were at first inconsistent and inconclusive. The possibility of elective mutism was considered. This hypothesis was rejected, however, on the grounds that S.W. vocalized freely in many play situations but gave no indication that he could elect to use speech in any particular context. The possibility of childhood psychosis was also considered. S.W. was referred for psychotherapy because of behavioral problems and his habit of "tuning out the world." At 5 years of age he became hyperactive and showed frustration and rage at times. S.W. attempted to throw himself out of a moving vehicle on one such occasion. It was observed, however, that S.W. did not show any autistic behaviors, such as lack of eye contact, or stereotyped ritualistic or self-stimulatory activities.

S.W. was finally admitted to a tertiary care center to rule out a neurodegenerative disorder and to study his profound communication disorder. The neurodevelopmental examination revealed essentially normal motor and tactile sensory functioning. Optic discs and fundi were normal. Psychological evaluation suggested low normal intellectual functioning. S.W.'s performance IQ on the WPPSI was 86. The results of a computed tomography (CT) scan of the skull did not indicate structural CNS lesion.

Behavioral tests in audiological evaluation again yielded inconsistent results. S.W. showed awareness to pure tone stimuli at 85–90-dB hearing level in the left ear and to 105 dB only in the right ear, although it was difficult to obtain repeatable pure-tone responses. It was also observed that a head turn could be elicited quite reliably in response to his own name spoken at a normal conversational level.

Tympanometry suggested reduced mobility of the ossicular chain. Acoustical reflexes were not elicited. Bilateral middle ear dysfunction was suggested. Auditory evoked potential testing was then carried out. The results suggested normal peripheral auditory sensitivity in the left ear and a mild hearing impairment in the right ear. Consistent cortical responses at 500 Hz and at 3000 Hz were also obtained when click signals were presented to the left ear. Presentation of the same signals to the right ear did not yield consistent cortical responses. A central auditory disorder could certainly not be ruled out on the basis of these results.

EEG examination revealed copious spikes consistently lateralized to the left and showing a maximum in the left posterior temporal region. Shortly after the EEG results were obtained, S.W. began to have seizures. These were characterized by staring, lip smacking, eye blinking, mouthing movements, and occasional automatic scratching of the right leg. They lasted for approximately 5 sec.

A diagnosis of epileptic aphasia syndrome was made. The child was put on medication for his seizures. The prognosis for recovery of speech and language skills was guarded.

Cognitive Semantic Disorders

In other groups of children, profound disorders of language comprehension are related to a lack of understanding of the nature of events or activities and much less to a purely linguistic or grammatical deficit. In these groups of children, auditory processing disorders may or may not be present. In some, the ability to repeat words and phrases, i.e., to establish auditory—motor linkages, appears to be intact or at least superior to their comprehension of simple utterances. For example, echolalia may be present in an acute or a mitigated form. In other children, long and even quite complex utterances may be used spontaneously and in a manner that suggests loose associations at least between the content of the utterances and an ongoing familiar event or activity. These utterances may be at least semiappropriate to the situational context. The child may fail completely, however, to understand novel statements or direct questions about these same events or about activities that have formed the topic of the conversation.

Case History   This moderately retarded adolescent had an IQ in the low 40s and was reported to be highly verbal throughout childhood.[17] Performance IQ was significantly lower than verbal IQ. She showed echolalia in the early school years and later became an incessant talker. It was reported that, in later childhood, her utterances were often irrelevant, and she was referred to as "hyperlinguistic." She lived at home with her family, whose members were all highly educated, until she was 15 years old. At 18 years, she was able to produce long, complex, and well-formed utterances. She showed a grasp of pronominalization, complex verbs, passive constructions, and other complex grammatical forms. These were all used productively, i.e., in novel utterances and in formulating and expressing ideas, not merely in an echoic fashion.

By contrast, this child was not proficient in receptive language. She did not always understand constructions that she was capable of using in her own spoken language. She had a poor understanding of the meaning of certain types of words. For example, she did not have a grasp of number concepts or of temporal relationships. She did not understand quantifiers such as "one" or "none", nor did she understand adverbial words such as "yesterday" and "tomorrow." Her performance on some tests of comprehension was at a 2–3-year level in spite of her apparently higher-level comprehension in informal conversation. She often seemed generally aware of what was being asked of her and could provide an appropriate if not completely accurate response.

This child's reception of language was at the level of her performance IQ. Her expressive abilities were much higher and became a source of confusion to educators and other professionals, who tend to view linguistic sophistication as being highly correlated with academic competence.

It is noteworthy that she was reported as showing signs of emotional disturbance at the time of puberty. Yamada[17] states "M. had to be hospitalized due to what were termed 'psychotic' behaviors. Her preoccupation with certain themes (e.g., death, vomiting), an increase in her unresponsiveness and in her excessive, seemingly free associative speech, and a decrease in her self-help skills, resulted in a diagnosis of schizophrenia. While the appropriateness of this diagnosis is debatable, it is important to note that the psychotic behaviors were viewed as secondary not primary to M's retardation."

Less severe forms of the "hyperlinguistic" receptive language disorder may be found in hydrocephalic children. The affected children are highly verbal but have difficulty with number concepts and nonverbal classification tasks. Verbal IQ is significantly higher than performance IQ. Dennis et al.[19] suggested that a posterior cerebral lesion may be present in such children.

MIXED PRODUCTION/COMPREHENSION DISORDERS

Mixed receptive/expressive language disorders in children are probably encountered more frequently than either expressive or receptive language disorders alone. Here we will deal primarily with those that are most profound. Such disorders may be primarily linguistic in nature or they may involve either cognitive or social/interactive systems primarily, or a combination of both. Examples of the former are provided by the child with severe to profound congenital hearing impairment or the child with a severe phonological–syntactic disorder. Examples of the latter may be provided by the autistic child or by the child who is retarded but who has in addition a social/communicative disorder of greater severity than would be predicted on the basis of his nonverbal intelligence. Differential diagnosis may present a challenging problem in these children.

Phonological/Syntactic (Global) Disorders

de Ajuriaguerra and colleagues[20] described a child with severe global dysphasia, i.e., a severe phonological–syntactic disorder with semantic (word finding and word meaning) difficulties as well. This child, at 8 years, 10 months, used a telegraphic style of speech, frequently placing the key element of a message at the beginning of a sentence even when this order violated grammatical rules. In comprehension, he showed difficulty in perception, analysis, and retention of verbal materials. He would attempt to form a synthesis or bolistic percept from those linguistic elements he did retain, often showing only partial understanding or at worst complete misunderstanding of what was said to him. Speech was poorly articulated and partly unintelligible. He stuttered for a time when he had difficulty in expressing himself. Reading and spelling were impaired and the child's attempts to restate the material he had read in his own words were poorly structured and revealed lack of comprehension of the text.

This child was followed until he was 12 years, 9 months of age. Although reported to be of normal nonverbal intelligence at 8 years, 10 months, he had difficulty with seration of elements in both time and space. He retained a concrete mode of reasoning and trial and error approaches to the solution of problems. He made some advances with age in production and comprehension of language, which remained deficient; however, academically he was 3 years below grade level at the age of 12 years, 9 months.

de Ajuriaguerra and co-workers concluded that language was developed as a relatively isolated system of verbal stereotypes that could be coordinated with psychological constructs only when these were at a concrete level. The verbal stereotypes, they believed, led to a relatively rigid approach to problem solving and tended to disorganize his thinking. He did not acquire a logical referent system that would allow him to separate himself from the concrete; his strategies continued to be controlled by immediacy and impulsivity. In this account, therefore, impaired cognitive development is considered secondary to language disorder and not a primary deficit, as in the "hyperlinguistic" child described earlier. This difference reflects the difficulty in neurodevelopmental disorders in general of separating out causative and neurodevelopmental effects.

Autism

Autistic children are thought to manifest both cognitive and linguistic deficits. A few are of normal nonverbal intelligence. Lockyer and Rutter[21] contrasted a group of such autistic children with a group of "dysphasic" children, matched with the autistic group in age, sex, and performance IQ. The autistic children were identified on the basis of such characteristics as lack of eye contact, limited group play, and ritualistic activities. Both groups had shown delayed development of language and inconsistent responses to sounds in early childhood. Many had been suspected of deafness. However, several language characteristics differentiated the two groups. These were pronoun reversal (e.g., "You" for "I"); echolalia; stereotyped utterances; lack of social communication, even by gesture; and lack of understanding of gestures, which were found among the autistic children, and disorders of articulation which were predominantly present in the dysphasic children. Lockyer and Rutter[21] concluded that the autistic children's receptive language deficit was more severe than that of the dysphasic children, and that their language output was more deviant, even bizarre. Unlike the dysphasic children, the autistic children were also impaired in social or pragmatic aspects of spoken language, and gesture.

The receptive language deficit in the above group of autistic children appears to be unlike that of the so-called hyperlinguistic child. These autistic children presumably did not have difficulty with object concepts, number concepts or nonverbal classification. Instead, they appear to have had a profound social emotional deficit. Possibly they were quite unable to establish interpersonal contacts and thus to abstract meaning from signs or symbols produced by the people who cared for them. Their deficits in coding, extracting, and organizing of incoming information may be peculiar to information presented in interpersonal contexts.

Milder Mixed Deficits

Mixed receptive/expressive language disorders that are less severe may be manifested by children with dysphasia or specific language impairment (SLI). Stark and

Tallal[3], in attempting to identify a group of school-age SLI children, examined 132 children aged 4–8½ years. These children had already been identified as language impaired by teachers and speech/language pathologists and were receiving educational and speech/language intervention for their language problems. Of these 132 children, three were hearing impaired, 50 were mild to moderately retarded, and 33 were no longer significantly language impaired. Only one child was found to be frankly neurologically impaired.

In the 39 SLI children in the Stark–Tallal study, expressive language scores were impaired to a significantly greater extent (mean expressive language age 54.6 months) than receptive language scores (mean receptive language age 64.4 months). However, some of the children showed relatively more severe deficits in expressive language than in receptive language, whereas others did not.

Expressive language abilities in SLI children appear to be highly correlated with speech articulation variables (e.g., number of errors on a speech articulation test).* In children with expressive language disorder in the Stark–Tallal study, error scores on a test of articulation were found to correlate highly with performance on tests of expressive syntax, both those involving formal test responses and those involving spontaneous speech sampling. These same children were found to be significantly poorer than normal children in their performance tests of word formulation, i.e., in a confrontation naming task and in tests of word fluency. Expressive language abilities in SLI children did not, however, appear to be highly correlated with performance on experimental tests of consonant–vowel syllable discrimination.

The belief that expressive language is much more severely affected than receptive language in SLI children may derive from the observation that these children show good language comprehension in unstructured conversations. Their nonverbal cognitive abilities are, by definition, within the normal range. Thus, they may have difficulty in analyzing linguistic structure in order to derive precise meanings. When the topic of discussion is familiar to them, however, they are well able to use their knowledge of words and of simple, linguistic structures, together with cognitive strategies, for the purposes of language comprehension. When their language comprehension is more rigorously tested, their difficulty with greater sentence length and complexity becomes apparent. This difficulty is of particular significance in the classroom, where instructions are frequently complex and are given without preparatory explanation or contextual support.

Because the effects of hearing impairment and of central auditory disorders may be profound, and because SLI children do manifest receptive language impairment in difficult listening situations, it is often assumed that, in SLI children, auditory disorders must be present and must have a primary causal role in relationship to the language disorder.[9] It has been pointed out, however, that if linguistic stimuli are used to assess auditory perceptual abilities, then the scores obtained may simply reflect the language disorder itself.

In the Stark–Tallal study of SLI children, computer-generated nonsense syllables were presented to normal and SLI children in identification, sequencing, and serial memory tasks. The SLI children performed at a significantly lower level than the normal

---

*In addition, it has been observed that speech articulation-disordered children who function within the normal range in expressive language are nevertheless likely to perform at a slightly lower level in expressive language abilities than are normal-speaking children matched with them in age and overall intelligence.

children in almost every one of these tasks. Their difficulties might well be interpreted as reflecting rate processing deficits, i.e., difficulty in identifying, sequencing, and remembering stimuli that incorporate brief-duration events or changes or that are presented in rapid sequence.

The scores obtained by the children on these tasks, and also on others that employed tonal stimuli instead of nonsense syllables, were highly correlated with their receptive linguistic abilities. Receptive language abilities were also quite highly correlated with certain neurodevelopmental variables, but not at all with speech motor variables. Receptive language and both auditory perceptual and speech motor abilities were found to be highly correlated with one another in the normal control group children. The above patterns of correlation might suggest that auditory perceptual and speech motor abilities are less well integrated in SLI than in normal children.

It is still not possible, however, to infer a causal relationship between auditory processing deficits and receptive language disorders in SLI children. Some children with normal language have been found to have difficulty with speech perception tests. For example, it has been shown that auditory processing deficits, in particular those related to attentional deficits and failure on vigilance tasks may be present in hyperactive children who do not have a language disorder. Instead, the children's performance on both auditory processing tasks and on tests of receptive language may reflect an underlying deficit or disability which affects both in common. It is unlikely that this deficit will be found in the peripheral auditory system. Rather, it is likely to be a higher-level processing or perceptual learning disorder that is implicated.

It may also be important to point out that level of expressive language in the SLI children studied by Stark and Tallal was not highly correlated with their scores on tests of speech perception. Thus it seems unlikely that an auditory disorder is a primary one in relation to expressive language.

The suggestion has been made that the language deficits found in SLI children may be related to subtle cognitive deficits rather than to more peripheral disorders of auditory processing or speech motor planning. However, SLI children were found by Stark et al.[2] to show no greater variability in performance on nonverbal subtests of the Wechsler Intelligence Scales than did normal children with whom they were matched in performance IQ.

It will be recalled that the receptive language disorder in SLI children is a linguistic disorder. Specifically, these children have difficulty in comprehending questions or in following commands of increasing length and complexity, especially when they do not have any idea as to what the content of the question or command will be. When they do know the content, or when the situational context is familiar, they are able to take advantage of contextual clues (e.g., gestures, direction of gaze of the conversational partner immediately preceding events) or of linguistic redundancy (repetition or use of constructions in which the same information is encoded in two different ways). In the absence of such aids, SLI children are able to comprehend ideas and concepts up to the level of their grammatical comprehension only. However, it is of interest that both receptive linguistic and auditory processing abilities appear to improve with increasing age in SLI children.[2] So, too, does their performance on tests of speech sound articulation and of consonant-vowel syllable discrimination.

It has been suggested that SLI children may be delayed in their acquisition of language abilities as compared with their visual spatial reasoning abilities, but that they are not neurologically impaired. A neurodevelopmental evaluation was carried out with the children in the Stark–Tallal study in order to find out whether they manifested a generalizeed maturational lag in all motor and sensory abilities. Thirty-three of the SLI children, aged 5–8½ years, were able to undergo this neurodevelopmental examination. Their performance was compared with that of a control group of 37 children who were developing language normally. The language impaired children manifested a variety of neurological soft signs suggesting neurodevelopmental delay.[21] These signs included reduced rate of performance of movement sequences, difficulty in processing dichaptic stimuli, and longer than normal duration of involuntary movements (when the child was asked to maintain a fixed posture of hand and arm). Accuracy of movement, presence of overflow movements, and balance and straight-line walking were not significantly different in the normal and language-impaired children.

As a result of these findings, delayed maturation of the central nervous system in the SLI children was suspected. The bilateral nature of the neurodevelopmental deficits found in the language-impaired children suggested that the cortical influences on language performance were not confined to the left hemisphere. It was not clear, however, whether these minor neurological deficits were related causally to the specific language disorder or whether they reflected a more global, unrelated CNS involvement.

SUMMARY

Receptive and expressive language impairments in children may provide an early indication of a variety of developmental problems. Milder delays in language acquisition tend to disappear with increasing age. This observation has led physicians to treat delay in language acquisition with a general disregard. Unfortunately, there is at present insufficient information about the precursors of language to permit the developmental psychologist or the speech-language pathologist to estimate the extent or severity of language delay in young nonspeaking children. The antecedents of language impairment in children are not sufficiently well understood. It is surmised that speech perception, speech production and social and cognitive abilities must all be important to language acquisition as must be development of social communication abilities.

Attempts to classify language disorders in older children might provide suggestions as to those processes that are important for language acquisition. Information of this kind cannot, however, be recovered from the traditional medical model of classification. This model does not show a meaningful relationship to the patterns of perceptual and motor deficits encountered in language-impaired children nor does it predict the patterns of linguistic deficits that can be identified in subgroups of language-impaired children. On the other hand, neither the patterns of perceptual and motor deficits nor the patterns of linguistic deficits in children have yet been studied in sufficient detail to permit detailed evaluation of such relationships. An additional problem arises from the fact that the nature of language problems in children appears to change with age.

In future studies of language-impaired children it will be important to measure perceptual and motor abilities with greater precision. Measurement of these abilities and of linguistic abilities also should be based on a theoretical model of normal language processes and of their development in young children. Studies of language-impaired children may also profit from the experience of investigators concerned with adult aphasia. Some of the procedures employed in studying acquired language disorders in adults may be usefully applied to the study of both developmental and acquired language disorders in children. These procedures should include CT scan and EEG studies, whenever feasible, as well as behavioral measures.

An improved understanding of receptive and expressive language disorders in children is important to the design of intervention. Although it may not be possible to alter deficits in the basic neurological processes subserving language, it may be possible in many cases to teach the child compensatory strategies and thus to facilitate his educational progress. This approach will help the child realize his potential for intellectual and social development more fully than if appropriate well-designed treatment were not provided.

REFERENCES

1. Morley, M.: *Development and Disorders of Speech in Children.* Williams & Wilkins, Baltimore, 1965.
2. Stark, R. E., Bernstein, L. E., Condino, R., *et al.:* Four-year follow-up of language delayed children. *Ann. Dyslexia* **34:**49–68, 1983.
3. Stark, R. E., and Tallal, P.: Selection of children with specific language impairments. *J. Speech Hear Dis.* **46:**114–122, 1981.
4. Ludlow, C.: Children's language disorders: Recent research advances. *Ann. Neurol.* **7:**497–507, 1980.
5. Bloom, L., and Lahey, M.: *Language Development and Language Disorders.* Wiley, New York, 1978.
6. Galaburda, A. M., Kemper, T. L., LeMay, M., *et al.:* Right-left asymmetries in the brain. *Science* **199:**852–856, 1978.
7. Dennis, M., and Whitaker, H. A.: Hemisphere equipotentiality and language acquisition, in Segalowitz, S. J., and Gruber, F. A. (eds.): *Language Development and Neurological Theory.* Academic, New York, 1977, pp. 93–106.
8. Benton, A L.: Developmental aphasia and brain damage. *Cortex* **1:**40–52, 1964.
9. Tallal, P., and Piercy, M.: Developmental aphasia: Rate of auditory processing and selective impairment of consonant perception. *Neuropsychologia* **12:**83–94.
10. Aram, D. M., and Nation, J. E.: Patterns of language behavior in children with developmental language disorders. *J. Speech Hear. Res.* **18:**229–241, 1975.
11. Rosenthal, W., Eisenson, J., and Luckan, J.: A statistical test of the validity of diagnostic categories used in childhood language disorders: Implications for assessment procedures. *Papers and Reports in Child Language Development.* Stanford University Press, Palo Alto, California, 1972.
12. Rapin, I., and Allen, D.: Developmental language disorders: Nosologic considerations. In V. Kirk (ed.): *Neuropsychology of Language, Reading, and Spelling.* Academic, New York, 1983.
13. Lou, H. C., Henriksen, L., and Bruhn, P.: Focal cerebral hypoperfusion in children with dysplasia and/or attention deficit disorder. *Arch. Neurol.* **41:**825–829, 1984.
14. MacNeilage, P. F., Rootes, T. P., and Chase, R. A.: Speech production and perception in a patient with severe impairment of somesthetic perception and motor control. *J. Speech Hear. Res.* **10:**449–467, 1967.
15. Lenneberg, E.: Understanding language without ability to speak. *J. Abnorm. Soc. Psychol.* **65:**419–425, 1962.
16. Ojemann, A., and Mateer, C.: Human language cortex: Localization of memory, syntax, and sequential motor-phoneme identification systems. *Science* **205:**1401–1403, 1979.
17. Yamada, J.: Evidence for the independence of language and cognition: Case study of a "hyperlinguistic" retarded adolescent. *UCLA Working Papers in Cognitive Linguistics,* Vol. 3, 1981.
18. Rapin, I., Mattis, S., and Rowan, A. J., *et al.:* Verbal auditory agnosia in children. *Dev. Med. Child Neurol.* **19:**197–207, 1977.
19. Dennis, M., Fitz, C. R., Netley, C. T., *et al.:* The intelligence of hydrocephalic children. *Arch. Neurol.* **38:**607–615, 1981.

20. de Ajuriaguerra, J., Jaeggi, A., Cjuignard, F., *et al.:* The development and prognosis of dysphasia in children. In D. M. Morehead and A. E. Morehead (eds.): *Normal and Deficient Child Language.* University Park Press, Baltimore, 1976.
21. Lockyer, L., and Rutter, M.: A five- to fifteen-year follow up of infant psychosis: 4 Patterns of cognitive ability. *Br. J. Social Clin. Psychol.* **9:**152–163, 1970.
22. Johnston, R. B., Stark, R. E., Mellits, E. D., *et al.:* Neurological status of language-impaired and normal children. *Ann. Neurol.* **10:**159–163, 1981.

Overview of Articulation and Fluency Disorders

Sylvia M. Davis and Donald L. Rampp

Articulation and fluency disorders represent major categories of communication disorders. Although specific behavioral characteristics associated with articulation disorders are different from fluency disorders, commonalities exist in that both can (1) interfere with effective communication, (2) be manifested in the early years of development, and (3) cause frustrations and anxieties. Early identification and management are critical for remediation of articulation and fluency disorders. Articulation disorders comprise the large majority (65.5%) of patients seen by speech pathologists. Fluency disorders, however, represent only 3.2%.[1]

Sylvia M. Davis and Donald L. Rampp • Department of Communication Disorders, Louisiana State University Medical Center, New Orleans, Louisiana 70112.

ARTICULATION

Traditionally, articulation refers to the speaking process. It involves vocal tract movement for sound production, with accuracy in placement of the articulators, timing, direction of movement, force extended, speed of response, and neural integration. The interactions between various parameters involved in speech production, such as resonance, phonation, respiration, and prosody, are of primary concern.[2] More recently, emphasis has focused on the role of the speaking process in language; speech and the articulation of speech are considered within the framework of linguistic rule systems.[3]

Normal Aspects of Speech Sound Production

Speech may be defined as an arbitrary symbol system that relates meanings with sounds. These arbitrary but designated symbols comprise the individual components of language. Although language may be communicated by speaking, writing, or signing, speech has special importance. During the normal course of development, speech is the primary, first-learned modality for language users. The major components of the speech mechanism include (1) the respiratory system, (2) the larynx, and (3) the vocal cavities and articulatory mechanism.

The production of audible sounds depends on the ability to inhale a quantity of air into the lungs and to exhale it in a gradual, controlled manner. Speech sounds are formed by interrupting, constricting, diverting, and modulating the air stream as it passes through the larynx, pharynx, and the oral and nasal cavities. The major function of the respiratory system in speech is to propel air into the larynx and the oral and nasal cavities.

The respiratory system and larynx work synchronously to provide the upper airway with two major types of airflow: (1) a series of air pulses created by the action of vibrating vocal folds for production of voiced sounds, and (2) a continuous airflow that can be used to generate noise energy in the vocal tract for voiceless sounds. The vocal folds are adaptable to differences in length, thickness, stiffness, and medial compression. This adaptability allows for interactions between the vocal folds and the air pressure from the lungs, which provides variations in pitch, loudness, and tone quality. Phonation is the process of voice production.

The acoustical dimensions of phonations are controlled in large part by the makeup and control of the vocal cavities and the articulators. The vocal tract or upper airway is the site of speech articulation. Most movements required to form the various sounds of speech take place in the oral cavity. The size and shape of the oral cavity can be altered greatly by the actions of the articulators: tongue, lips, mandible, and velopharynx. Velar elevation is important in the production of most consonant sounds and all vowel sounds.

The nervous system translates the message to be communicated into a pattern of signals that are transmitted to the various muscles of the speech mechanism. The movement of muscles required for the production of a specific sound (or series of sounds) must be coordinated in order for contact to occur at the right time and in the proper sequence. If the timing of a muscle contraction is off by just a few milliseconds, a misarticulation will result.

Classification of Speech Sounds

Speech production has been analyzed from several approaches, including (1) *phonology,* the study of the rules that govern how sounds are put together to form words; (2) *acoustic phonetics,* the study of the relationship between the acoustic signal and the articulation of speech; (3) *articulatory phonetics,* the study of how individual sounds are made by the articulators; and (4) *speech perception,* the study of how decisions regarding phonetics are made from the acoustical signal. A common characteristic of each of these approaches is that of distinctive features.

The concept of distinctive feature classification describes meaningful sound attributes, i.e., attributes applied to phones, individual speech sounds. This provides a description of phonetic features for classifying speech sounds, relative to a set of standardized sounds. This classification, in turn, leads to a description of the phonemes of the language. Phonemes represent a group or family of closely related speech sounds, all of which have the same distinctive acoustical characteristics. Each phoneme represents the shortest arbitrary unit of sound in a given language that can be recognized as being distinct from other sounds in the language. In English, these elements include the presence or absence of voicing and contrasts in the place and manner of articulation.

There are 45–50 phonemes used in the three main dialects of English spoken in the United States,[4] grouped into categories of consonants and vowels. Consonants are generally distinguished from one another on the basis of presence or absence of (1) voicing (vocal fold vibration–voiced /d/, and no vocal fold vibration–voiceless /t/); (2) place of articulation; and (3) the manner in which the sound is produced.

Manner of articulation is described according to the acoustic properties of the way in which air is emitted for speech sounds produced. Bilabial /b/ is classified as a stop because the air is stopped completely and then released. Fricatives, such as /s/ and /z/ are made with a narrow constriction, creating a noisy sound. Affricates, such as /ch/ and /g/ (as in "gin"), are combinations of stop and fricative segments. In the production of these sounds, there is a period of complete closure followed by a brief fricative segment. Nasal sounds are produced with nasal resonance (/n/, /m/, and /ng/). The lateral /l/ is produced with the air coming out over the sides of the tongue. Sounds with a glide (semivowel) manner of production are characterized by a gradual change in articulatory shape. Example of glides are /w/ and /j/, as in "yellow."

All vowels are voiced, and all vowels are produced through an open passage out of the mouth. For the production of all vowels, the velum is raised to prevent air from escaping through the nose; there are no nasal vowels in English. The vowels serve as the nuclei of syllables and are categorized with respect to tongue position (front, central, back, mid, and low), lip position (rounded and unrounded), and degree of tension (tense–long and lax–short). Closely related to vowels are diphthongs, which are produced with an open vocal tract; they serve as the nuclei for syllables. Dipthongs are formed with an articulation involving a progressive change in vocal tract shape during production of the sound.

Although there are several distinctive feature classification systems, the basic concept is to classify sounds according to a set of binary features, designed to describe the phonemes in all languages of the world. The features included in Table I exemplify this

Table I. Classification of Consonants and Vowels[a]

Phonetic symbol and keyword	Place of articulation/ cavity feature[b]	Manner of articulation	Voicing	Distinctive features other than place, manner, voice
		Consonants		
/m/ (man)	Bilabial	Nasal	+	Anterior
/b/ (bat)	Bilabial	Stop	+	Anterior/consonantal
/p/ (pot)	Bilabial	Stop	−	Anterior/consonantal
/w/ (water)	Labial/velar	Glide (semivowel)	+	Rounded/high/back
/ʌʌ/ (which)	Labial/velar	Glide (semivowel)	−	Rounded/high/back
/v/ (vote)	Labiodental	Fricative	+	Consonantal/continuant/strident/anterior
/f/ (fair)	Labiodental	Fricative	−	Consonantal/continuant/strident/anterior
/ð/ (that)	Linguadental	Fricative	+	Consonantal/coronal/anterior/continuant
/θ/ (thin)	Linguadental	Fricative	−	Consonantal/continuant/coronal/anterior
/d/ (did)	Linguadental	Stop	+	Consonantal/coronal/anterior
/t/ (to)	Linguadental	Stop	−	Consonantal/coronal/anterior
/z/ (zap)	Lingua-alveolar	Fricative	+	Consonantal/continuant/strident/coronal/anterior
/s/ (sew)	Lingua-alveolar	Fricative	−	Consonantal/continuant/strident/coronal/anterior
/n/ (no)	Lingua-alveolar	Nasal	+	Consonantal/anterior
/l/ (like)	Lingua-alveolar	Lateral	+	Vocalic/consonantal/continuant/coronal/anterior
/ʒ/ (rouge)	Linguapalatal	Fricative	+	Consonantal/continuant/strident/coronal/high
/ʃ/ (show)	Linguapalatal	Fricative	−	Consonantal/continuant/strident/coronal/high/back
/dʒ/ (judge)	Linguapalatal	Affricate	+	Consonantal/strident/coronal/high

	Place of articulation	Manner		Features
/tʃ/ (chair)	Linguapalatal	Affricate	−	Consonantal/strident/coronal/high
/r/ (row)	Linguapalatal	Rhotic (semivowel)	+	Consonantal/vocalic/continuant/coronal
/j/ (yellow)	Linguapalatal	Glide (semivowel)	+	
/g/ (go)	Linguavelar	Stop	+	Consonantal/high/back
/k/ (kite)	Linguavelar	Stop	−	Consonantal/high/back
/ŋ/ (ring)	Linguavelar	Nasal	+	Consonantal
/h/ (who)	Glottal (laryngeal)	Fricative	−	Low
		Vowels		
/i/ (feet)	High/front	Tense	+	Vocalic/unrounded
/I/ (him)	High/front	Lax	+	Unrounded
/e/ (tape)	Mid/front	Tense	+	Vocalic/unrounded
/u/ (boot)	High/back	Lax	+	Vocalic/rounded
/ʊ/ (look)	High/back	Lax	+	Rounded
/o/ (vote)	Mid/back	Tense	+	Vocalic/rounded
/ɛ/ (met)	Mid/front	Lax	+	Unrounded
/ɔ/ (taught)	Mid/back	Tense	+	Vocalic/rounded
/a/ (Tom)	Low/back	Tense	+	Vocalic/unrounded
/æ/ (cat)	Low/front	Lax	+	Vocalic/unrounded
/ɜ/ (perk)	Mid/central	Tense	+	Unrounded
/ɚ/ (other)	Mid/central	Lax	+	Unrounded
/ə/ (again)	Mid/central	Lax	+	Unrounded
/ʌ/ (cup)	Mid/central	Lax	+	Vocalic/unrounded

aThis table represents the classification of most consonants and the major vowels of English. The classification provided does not reflect all features. For a complete feature system applied in detail, one should consult Chomsky and Halle.[45]
bPlace of articulation: for consonants; cavity feature: for vowels.

type of classification system. Because distinctive features have an intended linguistic function, they may not always be relevant in the study of articulation disorders.[5]

Developmental Norms

Speech production is a very precise and practiced motor skill. The development of speech production requires changes in vocal tract anatomy, motor control of the articulators and the use of the articulators and the larynx to produce intelligible speech. Changes in infant sound production and the acoustical quality of these productions are dictated by anatomical development, maturation of neuromotor control, and the relationship between movement of the articulators and sounds produced. Anatomical relationships of the vocal tract change during infancy and childhood; as a result, certain patterns of sounds will be produced at different ages. These pattern variations include acoustical differences, such as resonance, loudness, and pitch differences, as well as differences in manner and place of sound production. Adult and infant sounds resonate differently because the infant's vocal tract is shorter, the pharynx is shorter and wider than it is long, the mouth is flatter, and the tongue more nearly fills the mouth. Motor activities of the articulators are also different because of differences in the relative locations of the articulators, which cause the muscles of the mouth and pharynx to function differently.

Oller[6] outlined the nonreflexive stages of vocalization of the child during the first year of life. Anatomical changes occurring in consonance with these stages were addressed by Kent.[7] These stages should be considered as a general sequence of development; i.e., ages assigned to each stage are approximations, and considerable overlap may occur between stages.

Phonation Stage

The period from birth to 1 month is the phonation stage. Reflexive vocalization such as hunger cries, discomfort sounds, or sounds associated with vegetative activities are produced. In addition, some nonreflexive sounds are produced during the phonation stage.[6] The most frequent of these, nasalized vowels, have been termed quasiresonant nuclei; these sounds are produced with normal phonation. There is no systematic contrast between opening and closing of the vocal tract as required for the production of a fully resonant sound. Anatomically, nasal breathing and nasalized vocalizations occur because of the engagement of the larynx and nasopharynx. The tongue, which nearly fills the oral cavity, has mostly back-and-forth motions.[7]

Gooing Stage

The gooing stage occurs during the period from 2 to 3 months. The vocalizations produced during this period consist of nasalized vowels and approximations of the consonants /k/ and /g/. Although these vocalizations are not systematically associated with full resonant vowels, they are repetitive and produced regularly.

Expansion Stage

The period from 4 to 6 months has been identified as the expansion stage, during which several types of vocalizations occur regularly. Predominant vocalizations consist of fully resonant nuclei described as repetitive vowel-like elements (/a/), labial closures (fricatives), bilabials, and/or labiolingual trills.[8] Phonetic development in this stage has been classified in categories of normal vowels, raspberry sounds, squealing, growling, yelling, and marginal babble.[6,7] The infant's increased ability to separate the oral and nasal cavities allows for the production of nonnasal vowels. Raspberry (labial) sounds can be produced because the infant can build the necessary oral air pressure required when the larynx becomes disengaged from the nasopharynx. It has been postulated that contrast in vocal pitch, as heard in squealing and growling, is heightened because descent of the larynx into the neck makes the vocal folds more vulnerable to the forces of supralaryngeal muscles. Better coordination of the respiratory system and larynx permits a loud voice. Thus, yelling seems to represent a systematic manipulation of vocal amplitude, which is common at this stage.

Marginal Babbling Stage

The production of marginal babble occurs later in the expansion stage, between 5 and 6 months. Marginal babbling consists of sequences of fully resonant vowels alternating with closures of the vocal tract. The difference between the infant's vocalizations at this stage and mature phonologically well-formed verbalizations is found in the timing characteristics. The vocalizations produced do not include the vocalic transitions characteristic of adult speech. Vocalic transitions in marginal babble are either too slow or they are shaky and/or intermittent.[8] In addition to the irregularity of timing among syllables, there is a lack of syllable reduplication.[5] Anatomically, the alteration of full opening and closing of the vocal tract is enhanced by the larynx–nasopharynx disengagement.

Canonical Babbling Stage

The canonical babbling stage (reduplicated babbling) occurs between 7 and 10 months of age. These vocalizations are characterized by reduplication of syllables such as /da-da-da/ or –ma-ma-ma/. These are more speechlike than previous vocalizations and are often labeled by parents as the infant's first words. Although these vocalizations probably are not meaningful in the beginning, they do contain vocalic transitions that conform to timing constraints of mature language. Furthermore, it has been suggested that during the early stages of babbling, sound elements produced may be similar across linguistic communities. Intonation patterns during the reduplicated babbling stage are more like those of adults. That is, infants produce rising inflection for questions and falling inflection for declarative sentences.

Variegated Babbling Stage

The final stage outlined by Oller,[6] variegated babbling, occurs between 11 and 12 months of age. Initially different vowels and consonants emerge in the infant's reduplicated babbling. Different consonant and vowel elements are vocalized within a series of utterances. Variegated and reduplicated babbling are easily distinguished, and the former usually occurs after the onset of words.[5]

Deviances in speech sound production may be detected before a child begins to use meaningful first words. Physicians and parents, who are concerned about a child's level of sound development, usually attend more to the child's use of sound in speech. Considerable differences occur among normal children relative to the exact ages at which specific speech sounds are accurately produced. It is more appropriate to consider age ranges for the normal acquisitions of a given speech sound, with some children acquiring the sound earlier than others.

Linguistic Stage

When a child begins to use words, usually between the ages of 10 and 13 months, it is inferred that he has passed from the prelinguistic to the linguistic stage of speech–language development. A variety of research methodologies have been employed in investigating speech sound production across various stages of language development. Typically, subjects in these studies are required to name or imitate pictures spontaneously or to engage in conversational speech. A phonemic inventory based on analyzed data, usually serves as the means for reporting the data. There is some disagreement among investigators regarding the criterion, or accuracy level of production, for considering a speech sound mastered or acquired. Wellman et al.[10] analyzed the responses of 204 children aged 2–6 years to picture stimuli and questions. The speech sounds elicited were classified as consonants, consonant clusters, vowels, and diphthongs. These investigators report the earliest ages at which various phonemes in the initial, medial, and final word positions and consonant clusters were produced correctly by 75% of the subject population.

The ability of 140 children between approximately 2 and 8 years of age to articulate consonant sounds in single words was examined. Objects, pictures, and questions were used as stimuli. The criterion for mastery of production was 100% of the subject population. Templin[12] administered a 176-item articulation test to 480 children aged 3–8 years, matched for age and sex. The criterion for sound mastery was considered the point at which 75% of the children at a given age level produced it correctly, in all three word positions. Certain groups of sounds with similar features are acquired at earlier ages than others. Nasals, stops, and glides are acquired before fricatives and affricates and consonant clusters. Prather et al.[13] reported on 147 children, grouped into seven age levels between 2 and 4 years. Results were reported in terms of a range extending from the earliest ages at which 75% produced each of the consonant phonemes in the initial and final positions of words to the age at which 90% of the children were producing the sound. A primary difference between the findings of this study and findings of earlier studies is consistently earlier age levels for phoneme production. This difference may be accounted for by the criterion of mastery of production. It should be noted, however, that the sequence of phoneme development is quite similar across all four studies.

The concept of considering age ranges when establishing norms for speech sound development is preferable to encapsulating absolute numbers. The process of phoneme development is characterized by considerable variability. It is easier to understand this developmental process in terms of definable ranges.

ETIOLOGIES OF ARTICULATORY DISORDERS

Traditionally, articulatory disorders have been addressed in a binary fashion, i.e., organic and nonorganic (functional) etiologies. The lack of specificity of the term functional and the more recent emphasis on the role of phonology in the linguistic process support a trend to consider organic etiologies and phonological disorders that stem from a language base.[3]

Organic Factors

Although an organic deficit may not affect articulatory production, certain organic deficits have been shown to precipitate articulatory disorders. Major organic deficits that have a high probablility of interfering with articulation include hearing impairment, structural anomalies and neuromotor pathologies.

Hearing Impairment

The integrity of the auditory mechanism is probably the most important variable influencing the normal development of speech–language function.[14] Interference within the auditory system (hearing impairment), renders the individual unable to perceive certain sounds that are audible to others. As a consequence, he may perceive the speech signal in a distorted fashion. The effect on the process of speech production can be correlated with the severity and age of onset of the hearing loss. The relationship suggests that the more normal a person's hearing, the more natural speech is likely to be.[15] If a severe loss is present from birth, the acquisition of language (including articulatory abilities, sentence structure, meaning, and rules for using language) will be seriously hindered. For individuals who have suffered a serious hearing loss after speech–language skills have been acquired, articulatory abilities are retained for a time. Eventually this skill deteriorates, even when amplification is provided.

Hearing loss has been associated with various types of errors across both consonants and vowels, including omissions, substitutions, distortions, and errors of addition.[16] In addition to articulatory disorders, evidenced by persons who are hearing impaired, disorders of voicing (a tendency to devoice consonants) and disorders of resonance (nasal emission) have been observed.[17]

Structural Anomalies

Structural anomalies, which can affect the proficiency of articulatory abilities, may be either congenital (cleft lip and/or cleft palate) or acquired (trauma or a disease process). The nature and severity of the articulation disorder depend on the severity of the anomaly and the effectiveness of medical intervention. The most common structural anomaly is cleft lip and cleft palate. Two categories of communication disorders have been associated in patients with cleft palate[18]: (1) organic factors, which are "diagnosable structural abnormalities that when changed by physical management result in a direct measurable improvement in speech behavior"; and (2) functional factors, which are "all other presumed causes that are not directly treatable by physical management". Of primary concern in the management of cleft palate is velopharyngeal sufficiency. Physical limitations prohibiting velopharyngeal closure will result in nasal production of consonants and vowels. These deviations can usually be corrected by surgical intervention, followed by speech therapy. Enlarged adenoids may compensate for a short or partially immobile velum and assist in velopharyngeal closure. Tonsilectomy and/or adenoidectomy at a young age may result in hypernasality requiring further surgical procedures.

Anomalies of the lips and tongue generally do not interfere with the accuracy of speech production. Compensatory actions for these anomalies usually results in acoustically acceptable speech production.[19] Deviations in dentition (particularly missing front teeth) may also produce difficulty with articulating certain consonants.[20]

Oral structural deviations may produce speech problems, however, the precise nature of the relationship between certain structural deficits and articulatory skills remains obscure. As a result, there is a reluctance to attribute deviations in the production of articulation to structural variations in the mouth and nose, unless the deviation is extreme or compensatory movements are impossible to make.[21]

Dysarthrias and Apraxias

Speech production is controlled by the nervous system. Damage that impairs motor programming for speech production (muscle strength, speed of movement, range of movement, accuracy of movement, and muscle tone) will affect motor speech production. The more common neuropathologies of speech affecting articulation are the dysarthrias and the apraxias.

Dysarthrias are characterized by a paralysis, weakness, or incoordination of the speech musculature; resulting from localized injuries to the nervous system, toxic or metabolic disorders, neurodegenerative disorders, vascular lesions of the brain, various inflammatory processes, and brain tumors.[22]

The production of imprecise consonants, resulting in reduced intelligibility, is the most significant characteristic of dysarthric speech. Other synonyms used to describe dysarthric speech include: slurred speech, thick speech, labored production, and verebral palsied speech. Disturbances in respiration, phonation, resonance, and prosody have been described in association with dysarthrias.

Apraxia refers to a motor speech disorder that differs from dysarthria. Apraxia is characterized by an impairment in the motor programming for speech production, in the absence of paralysis, weakness, or incoordination of the speech musculature. Apraxia of speech, or verbal apraxia, has been differentiated from oral apraxia.[23] Verbal apraxia is characterized by variable articulation errors in a slow and effortfull speech flow, reflecting trial and error groupings in an attempt to program for the accurate articulatory postures. Oral apraxia is characterized by the difficulty in performing volitional oral nonspeech tasks, such as protruding the tongue on command. The apraxias often, but do not always, coexist.

Nonorganic Factors

The decline in the popularity of the term functional articulation disorders is due to the inability of investigators to definitively define the term, "functional." The disorder has been redefined in linguistic terms as a *phonological disorder*. Children identified as having phonological disorders generally have no noticeable organic reason for their speech being abnormal, but produce phonemic errors in the production of meaningful speech. These children can plan and execute selected articulatory movements and are not reported to produce phonetic errors; i.e., they may not produce a sound correctly in the flow of speech or in certain words but may use that sound as a substitute for another one. These children would be identified as having a language disorder of a phonological type, rather than having a functional articulation disorder.

Unlike the traditional descriptions of articulatory deviations (omissions, substitutions, and distortions), phonologic disorders are described in terms of specific rules operating within these categories. These rules are postulated to follow a logical sequence of development. Ingram[3] described several phonological processes, including the following:

Syllable structure processes: include (1) deletion of final consonants (sto for stop); (2) deletion of unstressed syllables in which some part of adult words with more than one syllable is lost ("mato" for "tomato"); (3) reduplication, in which the child repeats the syllable of the word ("baba" for "bottle"); and (4) the reduction of clusters ("dek" for "desk")
Assimilation processes: describe the ways in which a sound is influenced by another sound in the word and account for certain types of sound substitutions and distortions
Substitution processes: represent and attempt to explain how one sound is replaced by another, without regard to neighboring sounds; examples would include stopping ("dare" for "safe," fronting (production of /k/ for /g/), and deletion ("un" for "sun").

Related Variables

Other variables related to articulatory proficiency include socioeconomic status, variations in the dialect form used, intelligence level, and educational achievement. Although socioeconomic status does not appear to contribute to the presence of an articulation disorder, greater numbers of children from low socioeconomic environments show evidence of misarticulations.[21] This may be due, in part, to differences in the language systems of persons from low socioeconomic environments and those upper socioeconomic groups. In fact, this difference may be attributable to dialectical variation.

Evidence relative to intelligence level indicates that the articulation abilities of children with reduced IQs is significantly poorer than the articulation of children with normal and higher IQs.[21] At least a portion of this difference, between persons with higher IQ and those with lower IQ, might be accounted for in differences of fine motor control needed for accurate speech production. It should be noted, however, that the correlation between IQ level and articulatory development, although positive, is low. This suggests that IQ level is more of a *prerequisite for,* rather than a guarantee of average articulatory development.

GUIDELINES FOR REFERRAL

When considering referral of a child for assessment and possible management of an articulatory disorder, the physician should evaluate (1) the parents' report and pertinent questionnaires, and (2) the intelligibility and resulting communicative effectiveness of the child's verbalizations. Intelligibility refers to the ability to be understood by an average listener. This variable is influenced by rate, fluency, voice quality, intensity, and articulation. Percentages of intelligibility at various ages across the period of speech development have been outlined.[25] Percentages of intelligibility at various ages across the period of speech development have been outlined.[24] The intelligibility of a child's speech should be at the 100% level by age 5 years and at the 90% level by 3 years. Intelligibility of the 2-year-old child should be at approximately the 65% level and that of 18-month-olds should be intelligible at least 25% of the time.

Specifically, a speech–language referral should be made under the following conditions:

1. The mother reports that family members have difficulty understanding the child's attempts at communication.
2. The child does not vocalize, other than crying during the first 12 months.
3. The child does not produce meaningful speech by the age of 18 months.
4. The child does not produce speech sounds when he reaches the upper age ranges.
5. The child is still unintelligible by the age of 30 months.
6. Obvious organic anomalies exist.
7. The child continues to misarticulate sounds that should have been mastered at his chronological age.

FLUENCY DISORDERS: STUTTERING AND CLUTTERING

Disorders of fluency have existed throughout recorded history. The concentrated study of fluency disorders has been conducted for many years by people from various professional disciplines. However, questions regarding definitions, etiologies, and treatment remain unanswered.[25] A review of the literature reveals the following statements which are accepted as "facts" about the two major types of fluency disorders: stuttering and cluttering[26–30]:

1. Stuttering is found among people from all parts of the world.
2. Stuttering usually begins in childhood before the age of six years.
3. The incidence of stuttering is higher in the male population.
4. The incidence of stuttering is higher in twins.
5. Stuttering does have a familial incidence pattern.
6. The development of stuttering is cyclical with periods of remission and exacerbation.
7. A significant number of people experience a spontaneous remission of stuttering.
8. Stuttering changes in severity and form with increasing age.
9. Advanced stutterers are aware of their speech difference and experience fear and frustration because of it. They also avoid certain situations, words, and sounds.
10. Stuttering cannot be explained by cultural factors alone.
11. Stuttering behavior does not occur during choral reading.
12. Stuttering behavior does not occur during singing.

This list is not intended to be all-inclusive but rather is intended to serve as background information for the discussion to follow. The incidence of stuttering is higher than that of cluttering, therefore the main focus of this discussion will revolve around the former. Stuttering is more prevalent in the preschool years with an incidence of approximately 4%, which declines thereafter to approximately 1% of the general population.

Definitions

Fluency cannot be defined with any degree of scientific accuracy because the variables of fluency have not been analyzed systematically.[31] The most characteristic properties of fluency are smooth intraunit and interunit transitions that occur at sound, syllable, phrase, and sentence sequencing levels of verbal production. Although this description of fluency would seem to be adequate, it is, in fact, too simplistic, because there are acceptable forms of nontransition speech behaviors. For example, words may be repeated for emphasis or at the listener's request, pauses of varying lengths occurring at certain frequency levels may be considered appropriate, and a variety of interjections, hesitations, and other fluency disruptors may be considered normal behaviors; i.e., they may not interfere significantly with the speech-transition process.

In the absence of a positive precise definition of fluency, an accepted definition of nonfluency has still to be derived. The consistent universal features of stuttering have not been identified adequately as yet; however, there is legitimate reason to believe that these universal features do exist, "if for no other reason than that for centuries people have been able to identify stuttering."[29] Existing definitions of stuttering can be grouped into five categories: (1) definitions based on avoidance behaviors; (2) perceptual–judgmental definitions based on listener reactions; (3) experimental–theoretical definitions based on independent variables that control stuttering behavior; (4) definitions based on hypothetical variables, such as stuttering being an indication of the presence of an identifiable problem; and (5) definitions based on the "moment" of stuttering, during which time some nonspecific behaviors occur.[31] Rather than pursue the definition of stuttering through one or more of these categories (which at best depends on nonspecific behaviors dictated by theoretical preference), specific speech features will serve as the criteria for the identification of stuttering.[29,31]

Stuttering may be defined as a particular type of speech dysfluency marked by (1) repetitions of sounds, syllables, words, or phrases; (2) prolongations; (3) interjections; (4) hesitations; and (5) revisions and incomplete phrases. Of the dimensions of repetitions, the two most obvious are length or frequency and amount of effort involved. Repetitions of initial sounds, when the sound is repeated no more than two times at a regular rate (b-b-baby), would not be as serious as three or more sound repetitions at a hurried, irregular rate (b-b-b-b-baby) or a repetition with the additions of a schwa vowel occurring with the initial sound (ba-ba-ba-baby). Syllabic repetitions when the initial syllable is repeated only once (pe-people) would be questionably identified as stuttering, whereas repeated (pe-pe-pe-people) would not. Should any of the repetitions be accompanied by either audible or visual signs of undue effort, the repetition would be considered stuttering behavior. The features of frequency and effort also would determine the significance of whole word and phrase repetitions. As a general rule, repetitions would not be considered stuttering behavior if (1) the occurrence rate were nine or fewer per 100 words uttered, (2) the repetition was not accompanied by struggle, and (3) the schwa vowel was not perceived by the listener.

Prolongations are a sign of struggle behavior and a definite danger signal.[27] The traditional definition of prolongation is the extension of a sound for an abnormal duration as in weeeeeeeent. There are also visual cues of undue effort in the initiation of sound production that would mark abnormal behavior.

Interjections are considered to be sound-filled pauses that occur in the flow of connected speech. Examples are sounds such as ''uh,'' ''um,'' ''mmm''; words such as ''well,'' ''okay,'' and ''and''; or phrases (lemme see, excuse me). Interjections occur in almost everyone's speech and can be considered normal or stuttered speech behavior. Wingate[28] delineated subtypes of interjection behaviors. Normal interjected speech behaviors would be those that are voluntary, meditative, circumstantial, and do not occur at a high rate. Abnormal interjections are identified as those that assume proportions of elemental prolongations (ummmmm) and repetitions (uh-uh-uh). Also included in this delineation is a description of verbal features that are longer interjections used by the stutterer as a ''starter'' device with which to begin a stuttered word.

Hesitations and the term ''pauses'' refer to silent intervals of unspecified length or character in the flow of speech. Hesitations occur in everyone's speech. The frequency of their occurrence varies among individuals and within the speech of the same individual, from time to time. Wingate[28] classified three types of normal hesitation behaviors: voluntary, circumstantial, and meditative. He described involuntary hesitations as abnormal speech behaviors denoted by the terms block, blockings, or silent prolongations. The unique character of involuntary hesitations may be signified by visual cues, in which silence is broken by excessive loudness, prolongation, or repetition and/or by the occurrence of the silent interval in unusual places.

Revisions (I rent–went) and incomplete phrases (I brought–she found) represent changes in wording, pronunciation, grammatical structure, or the content of the message. These fluency irregularities are observed in all speakers and are generally accepted as normal dysfluencies. However, stutterers report using revisions or not completing a speech utterance in order to avoid experiencing the speech difficulty. Although these avoidance behaviors are not considered stuttering by the stutterer or the listener, when used in this fashion, revisions and incomplete phrases are considered verbal features of stuttering behavior.

Accessory features that reflect the stutterer's efforts to produce fluent speech are referred to more commonly as secondary characteristics. These characteristics may not be observable in the very young stuttering child. They appear to develop initially as starter devices, to aid in the production of fluent speech. They become habitual in the speaking process and noneffective for enhancing fluency. These features typify struggle behaviors in confirmed stutterers. Accessory features of speech-related movements are characterized by exaggerated movements of the peripheral speech mechanism, which occur concurrently with stuttering. These inappropriate movements might include lip-pursing, tongue protrusion, teeth-clenching, and/or an open mouth posture. They are localized in the mouth area and may or may not be consistent with movements required for the sound being attempted.

Ancillary body movement include other kinds of inappropriate bodily activities that accompany stuttering behavior. These movements might include eye blinking, head jerking, head turning, clenching the fists, facial grimacing, foot stomping and the like. Accessory movements that appear across verbal features might include certain types of word and phrase repetitions of more than one syllable or certain kinds of interjections, or both. The major characteristics that signal these features are that (1) they appear at inappropriate points within the context of the message; (2) the repetitive behavior is more pronounced, and (3) they are representative of struggle behavior.

Etiological Considerations

Theoretical approaches regarding the etiology and development of stuttering behavior can be considered under the classifications of neurotic theories, organic theories, and learning theories. Although there is no conclusive proof to support any of these theoretical classifications, the present authors are biased toward some type of organic origin.

Neurotic Theories

The proponents of neurotic theories view stuttering as a basic personality disturbance that can be manifested in several ways. Stuttering has been postulated to be the overt behavior satisfying anal or oral erotic needs and/or repressed hostility. The stutterer has been described as presenting a basic neurotic personality; that is, the individual experiences unpleasant feelings, is unable to accept and/or understand those feelings, and establishes stuttering behaviors that symbolize the original unpleasant feelings. Therefore, the moment of stuttering has been viewed as representing a conflict between the urge to speak and the urge to be silent. In other words, stuttering can be viewed as the unconscious need to repress speech.[30,32–34]

Following this line of reasoning, it would seem that stuttering should be but one symptom of a neurotic conflict, that also should be evident in disturbed interpersonal relationships and in other neurotic symptoms. Research has shown, however, that stuttering behavior does not cluster with other behavior problems.[35] In this regard, stuttering differs from other emotional disorders in children. Furthermore, stutterers and parents of children who stutter do not evidence more neurotic symptoms than do nonstuttering children or their parents.[36] Although there is no conclusive proof that would support neurotic theories as the etiologic component of stuttering behavior, this view will retain some popularity. Perhaps this is true because of the flexibility with which these viewpoints can be interpreted. If the stutterer is assessed as having personal problems, it may be assumed that stuttering represents a manifestation of those problems. On the other hand, if the stutterer is assessed as being normal and well adjusted, the stuttering may be interpreted as being the solution to inner conflicts.[28]

Organic Theories

Organic theories that attempt to explain stuttering behavior can be classified under the general heading of breakdown theories.[25] Currently, most theories that regard stuttering behavior as a breakdown of the speech function under some type of pressure reflect the view that organic or constitutional factors are involved in its etiology. The reasoning behind this belief is not difficult to envision, as there was a period in the history of modern thinking with regard to stuttering when many believed that a child's speech might begin to deteriorate in the presence of environmental stress. A child's speech might deteriorate as a result of the impact of shock, fright, illness, or injury. Even today, these expressions may be heard occasionally, with terms such as "fright" or "shock" being replaced with "emotional pressures" or "insecurity." However, it is not clear why the vast majority of children suffering from a serious illness or sustain some type of injury do not stutter as a result. In addition, most children with emotional difficulties do not experience significant fluency problems. Those who ascribe to an organic theory of stuttering sidestep this difficulty claiming that some have a weakness in the area of speech that causes them to react to stresses by stuttering.

From this dysphemic viewpoint, the stutterer is believed to be inherently different from the nonstutterer. The child is believed to be predisposed to stutter, and this predisposition is believed to be the result of a constitutional difference. Such theories have adopted the assumption that a fluency disorder may be a joint product of an hereditary predisposition and precipitating factors within the environment. Sheehan and Costley[28] presented strong evidence regarding the role of heredity in fluency disorders, suggesting that the high familial incidence of stuttering might be interpreted as either a genetic or a cultural factor. They further argue, however, that stuttering is difficult to explain solely on the basis of cultural learning or sociopsychological factors. They also point out that stuttering exists in peoples all over the world, with consistent incidence and prevalence figures across various populations. The dysphemic point of view has been approached in many different ways, and several different theories have evolved.

The theory of cerebral dominance proposes that a conflict exists between the two halves of the cerebrum for control of the activity of the speech organs. Travis[36] hypothesized that because of right and left halves of the tongue, jaw, and other midline speech structures receive their motor nerve impulses from separate sources in the two cerebral hemispheres, smooth fluent speech results when nerve impulses are accurately synchronized. It was further hypothesized that one cerebral hemisphere is domiant over the other for the purpose of timing nerve impulses. If dominance is not established, each hemisphere would tend to function independently. This would result in poorly synchronized nerve impulses for the control of the speech musculature and a predisposition for the breakdown of speech behavior. This theory related handedness to stuttering. Children who are ambidextrous were regarded as lacking a safe margin of cerebral dominance. Those who adhered to this theory enforced strict unilaterality in all the stutterer's activities. Although Travis[36] acknowledged the futility of shifting handedness in the management of stuttering, he has not disavowed the cerebral dominance theory as an explanation of the underlying basis of stuttering.

The biochemical theory regarding stuttering adheres to the concept that the basic difference between stutterers and nonstutterers rests in metabolic factors and tissue chemistry. "The speech interruptions are 'triggered' by social and emotional pressures, but the stutterer's neurophysiological mechanism for speech is rendered vulnerable to the disruptive effects of such pressures, by a biochemical imbalance."[25] Results of research projects attempting to prove this theory have not provided conclusive evidence that this is the cause of stuttering behavior.

Another theory of the nature of stuttering is that those who evidence the problem have a *defective monitoring system* for sequential speech. Support for this organic etiologic consideration has grown out of cybernetic theory of behavior and physiological control which interprets activity and learning as self-regulated processes. Activity patterns are analyzed and described as feedback control mechanisms that are self-regulating closed-loop processes that control patterned, organized behavior such as speech. Research has indicated that fluency breaks, similar to stuttering, can be produced in normal speakers by altering the auditory feedback of their speech output, whereas, a marked reduction in stuttering can be achieved by the same process. It has been postulated that the basic disturbance in normal speakers (when auditory feedback is altered) creates a temporal disruption in the programming of motor sequences. The subsequent changes in speech behavior may be considered to be secondary reactions to the basic experience. This would seem to suggest that stuttering behavior results from a breakdown or malfunction in the closed-loop system for speech production. Subsequent research analyzing the effectiveness of stuttering management under conditions of delayed auditory feedback and biofeedback conditions provides further support for this or at least a related organic etiology.[37]

Learning Theories

Most of the current thinking about stuttering reflects the influence of learning theory. Learning plays some part in determining the patterns of behavior exhibited by advanced stutterers. The different varieties of stuttering reactions, the changes that occur as the disorder develops, the role of situational verbal factors in its precipitation all testify to the influence of learning. In an analogous vein, it is agreed that there is a biological predisposition to learn language. The language learned however, and the proficiency with which it is acquired is determined by learning experiences. In application to fluency disorders, learning theories have been addressed across operant conditioning, classical conditioning, avoidance conditioning, vicarious conditioning (which is the process of being conditioned by watching someone else's reactions when learning a behavior), and electrical conditioning, which represents any combination of the learning theories.[38] Concepts about stuttering within the frameworks of these learning theories can be grouped into two basic categories: those that view stuttering as a unitary phenomenon but rather as the interaction of at least two distinct behavioral phenomena.

The avoidance conditioning learning theories are not unlike neurotic theories in that stuttering is explained as being the result of the conflict between the opposing drives to speak and not to speak. Sheehan[39] has termed this conflict as an approach-avoidance conflict in which the motivational drives subserving both approach and avoidance are simultaneously aroused. The source of the original conflict has not been specified clearly. However, possible origins were projected to be explained through learned speech anxieties and/or unconscious personality factors that were not specified.

Operant and classical conditioning models consider interactions among behavioral phenomena. Shames and Sherrick's[40] explanation of stuttering through the operant model suggests that initial disruptions in fluency are normal nonfluencies that constitute a natural occurrence in children's speech. These initial nonfluencies are encouraged through some schedule of positive reinforcement; i.e., the child may receive more attention from parents when the fluency breakdowns occur. During this period, the child is learning to control the occurrence of the nonfluencies. As the dysfluencies increase, the parent or significant other in the child's environment will begin to react to these speech interruptions in a disapproving manner, which can be considered as punishment. The disapproval of disfluencies creates a negative self-reaction on the part of the child, which results in struggle behavior accompanying the breaks in the flow of speech. According to the operant model, it is at this point that the behavior can be termed stuttering.

Unlike the operant conditioning model, the classical conditioning model that applied to stuttering does not assume that the original nonfluencies represent normal behavior.[41] Rather, it assumes that the original disfluencies are not normal and are accompanied by cognitive and motor disorganization associated with negative emotional arousal. These original fluency breaks consist of disorganized forms of previously integrated behaviors. The fluency failures and negative emotions are then identified by the child as occurring in the presence of specific situational stimuli. These can be any stimulus complex in which fluency failure occurs. The range of stimuli to which negative emotion and fluency failures is then extended by the child.

DEVELOPMENT OF FLUENCY DISORDERS

In the absence of a specified etiology of stuttering behavior, it is critical to understand its developmental aspects. This is necessary so that it may be identified correctly in the beginning stages (or phases) when intervention to correct the problem can be instituted most effectively and efficiently. In attempts to describe stuttering development, several classification systems have been devised over the years. The concept of stages of stuttering development was originally addressed by Bluemel[42] and refined by Van Riper.[43] Phrases of development described by Bloodstein[25] were an attempt to further refine the characteristics outlined in the stages of development. Tracks of development were devised by Van Riper,[26] incorporating the concepts of stages and phases of development across four etiologic origins. Although there have been accounts of a sudden onset of stuttering characteristics following a physiological or psychological trauma (track III), or associated with significant emotional disturbances (track IV), the majority of individuals who stutter will follow one of two courses of development.[26]

Following one course of development designated as track I by Van Riper, dysfluencies first appear after a history of fluent speech, between the ages of 30 and 50 months. One of the most important characteristics of this course of development is that the dysfluent behavior is cyclical in nature. During this incipient phase of stuttering development, the child may evidence characteristics of more advanced forms of stuttering one day and simple syllabic repetitions the next day or even quite normal speech. Children following this course of development will experience more complete remissions for longer periods of time than those of the other groups. In general, the course of development progresses from easy, effortless repetitions that occur on the first word spoken with the same even rate as normal speech. The number of repetitions will average from three to no more than five per word. As the disorder develops, the rate of the repetitions become unevenly paced and there may be the appearance of the schaw vowel. Further development is marked by the emergence of prolongations that occur occasionally at first and then become gradually more predominant. Prolongations are followed by surges of tension and associated struggle behaviors indicative of a higher level of awareness on the part of the child. As the awareness level heightens and struggle behaviors become more pronounced, the child begins to develop fears. Fears are evidenced for certain words, specific situations, and/or specific speech sounds. Because of these fears, the child develops avoidance behaviors such as the use of synonyms or stallers.

Development within track II differs from track I in that dysfluencies appear from the time children first begin to produce word combinations. Most of the children in this category evidence delayed speech and language development and had no previous history of normal fluency. For these children, the onset of stuttering begins with the onset of connected speech. The syllable repetitions evidenced by these children are hurried and irregular from the beginning. As the disorder develops, there are more silent gaps and hesitations than in track I. These children also evidence more false starts, revisions, interjections, and changes in the direction of the topic of conversation. These children have more articulation errors and for the most part their sounds are disorganized. These children rarely show prolongations and fixations. If fears are developed, they will probably remain at the situation level; thus struggle and avoidance behaviors will be apparent less often. Overall, at the culmination of this developmental course stuttering characteristics will not be as pronounced as those in track I.

For children who would be classified as track III or IV stutterers, the initial speech characteristics would be more advanced than for the first two tracks. Consequently, indication of the stuttering behaviors would be accomplished more easily. In addition, the onset of stuttering would occur after several years of fluent speech.

IDENTIFICATION OF STUTTERING BEHAVIOR

The importance of making an accurate and early diagnosis of the incipient stutterer cannot be overemphasized because meaningful intervention can prevent the disorder from developing into more advanced stages. The observation of certain speech behaviors and accompanying parent reports should aid the physician in determining when to make a referral to a speech–language pathologist. Adams[44] delineated guidelines to be used when incipient stuttering is suspected by the parent or physician. The frequency of the dysfluencies per 100 words spoken should be 10 or more. The type of dysfluencies would include part-word repetitions with at least three unit repetitions per utterance, the presence of audible–silent prolongations, and a preponderance of broken words. These children will also evidence frequent difficulty in initiating and/or sustaining airflow for speech. The dysfluencies will be longer in duration, more effortful, and more pronounced.

Parental concerns as to whether a child is beginning to stutter should not be dismissed easily because parents are usually reliable reporters of deviant behaviors. Experience indicates that the usual length of time for a medical visit is not sufficient time to observe the child who may have the characteristics discussed. It normally requires approximately 90 min or 2 hr of diagnostic time to elicit enough of a speech sample to make the determination that the child is an incipient stutterer. However, parental reports and brief observation of the child should provide enough evidence to support the need for referral for further testing. In addition, if the child is in a period of remission when the speech–language evaluation is completed, the speech–language pathologist should schedule a reevaluation if the dysfluent behavior reappears.

SUMMARY

This chapter represents an overview of articulation and fluency disorders, with a focus on presenting basic information for the physician, to aid in diagnosis and referral. Articulation disorders make up the largest single category of communication disorders; this chapter emphasizes the classification of speech sounds, development norms, etiological (both organic and nonorganic) related variables, and guidelines for referral.

Fluency disorders are a low-incidence disorder but probably have received more research attention than any other single speech disorder. This is directly related to the fact that the etiology remains elusive. The emphasis here has been to present an overview of the problem with definition, etiological considerations with discussion of the three major theories of causation, developmental factors, and ways to identify fluency disorders. The general guidelines found in this chapter should provide the necessary information for referral. Whereas some children may "grow out of it," the state of the art is that we are as yet unable to predict and identify children who will or will not. If doubt exists, the authors suggest that referral to a certified professional speech–language pathologist be recommended.

REFERENCES

1. Neal, W. R.: Speech pathology services in secondary schools. *Language, speech and hearing services in the schools.* 7:6–16, 1976.
2. Sommers, R. K., and Kane, A.: Nature and remediation of functional articulation problems in Dickson, S. (ed.): *Communication Disorders: Remedial Principles and Practices.* Scott Foresman, Illinois, 1974, pp. 105–187.
3. Ingram, D.: *Phonological Disability in Children.* American Elsevier, New York, 1976.
4. Darley, F., and Spriestersbach, D.: *Diagnostic methods in Speech Pathology,* 2nd ed. Harper & Row, New York, 1978.
5. Bernthal, J., and Bankson, N.: *Articulation Disorders.* Prentice-Hall, Englewood Cliffs, New Jersey, 1981.
6. Oller, D. K.: Infant vocalizations and the development of speech. *J. Allied Health Behav. Sci.* 1:523–549. 1978.
7. Kent, R. D.: Articulatory and acoustic perspectives on speech development in Reilly, A. P. (ed): *The Communication Game.* Johnson and Johnson, Somerville, New Jersey, 1980, pp. 38–48.
8. Oller, D. K.: Infant vocalizations: A linguistic and speech scientific perspective. *Miniseminar at the Convention of the American Speech and Hearing Association,* Houston, 1976.
9. Sander, E. K.: When are speech sounds learned? *J. Speech Hearing Disorders* 37:55–61, 1972.
10. Wellman, B. L., Case, I. M., Mengert, I. G., *et al.: Speech Sounds of Young Children.* University of Iowa studies in child welfare, No. 5. University of Iowa Press, Iowa City, 1931.
11. Poole, E.: Genetic development of articulation of consonant sounds in speech. *Elem. Engl. Rev.* 11:159–161, 1934.
12. Templin, M. C.: *Certain Language Skills in Children.* Institute of child welfare monograph series, No. 26. University of Minnesota Press, Minneapolis, 1957.
13. Prather, E. D., Hedrick, D. L., and Kearn, C.: Articulation development in children aged two to four years. *J. Speech Hearing Disorders* 40:179–191, 1975.
14. Davis, S. M.: Audition and speech perception in Schiefelbush, R. (ed): *Bases of Language Intervention.* University Park Press, Baltimore, 1978, pp. 43–66.
15. Ling, D.: *Speech and the Hearing Impaired Child: Theory and Practice.* A. G. Bell, Washington, D. C., 1976.
16. Davis, H., and Silverman, R.: *Hearing and Deafness.* Holt, Rinehart and Winston, New York, 1970.

17. Hudgins, C., and Numbers, F.: An investigation of the intelligibility of the speech of the deaf. *Genet. Psychol. Monogr.* **25**:289–392, 1942.
18. Bzoch, K. R.: Etiological actors related to cleft palate speech, in Bzoch, K. R. (ed.): *Communicative Disorders Related to Cleft Lip and Palate.* Little, Brown, Boston, 1979, pp. 67–76.
19. Bloomer, H., and Hawk, A.: Speech considerations/speech disorders association with ablative surgery of the face, mouth and pharynx—Ablative approaches to learning. ASHA report #8: Orofacial anomalies. ASHA, Washington, D. C., 1973.
20. Bankson, N., and Byrne, M.: The relationship between missing teeth and selected consonant sounds. *J. Speech Hearing Disorders* **24**:341–348, 1962.
21. Irwin, J. V.: Articulation, in Weston, A. J. (ed.): *Communicative Disorders: An Appraisal.* Charles C Thomas, Springfield, Illinois, 1972, pp. 161–198.
22. Peacher, W.: The etiology and differential diagnosis of dysarthria. *J. Speech Hearing Disorders* **15**:252–265, 1950.
23. Winitz, H.: *Articulatory Acquisition and Behavior.* Prentice-Hall, Englewood Cliffs, New Jersey, 1969.
24. King, R., and Berger, K.: *Diagnostic Assessment and Counseling Techniques for Speech Pathologists and Audiologists.* Stanwix, Pittsburgh, 1971.
25. Bloodstein, O.: Stuttering. *J. Speech Hearing Disorders* **42**:148–151, 1979.
26. Van Riper, C.: The nature of stuttering. Prentice-Hall, Englewood Cliffs, New Jersey, 1971.
27. Sheehan, J. G., and Costly, M. S.: A reexamination of the role of heredity in stuttering. *J. Speech Hearing Disorders* **42**:148–151, 1977.
28. Wingate, M.: *Stuttering Theory and Treatment.* Wiley, New York, 1976.
29. Hedge, M. N.: Fluency and fluency disorders: Their definition, measurement and modification. *J. Fluency Disorders* **3**:51–71, 1978.
30. Glauber, I. P.: The psychoanalysis of stuttering, in Eisenson, J. (ed.): *Stuttering: A Symposium,* Harper & Row, New York, 1958, pp. 172–180.
31. Freund, H.: *Psychopathology and the Problems of Stuttering.* Charles C Thomas, Springfield, Illinois, 1966.
32. Travis, L. E.: The unspeakable feelings of people with special reference to stuttering, in Travis, L. E. (ed.): *Handbook of Speech Pathology.* Appleton-Century-Crofts, East Norwalk, Connecticut, 1957, pp. 916–946.
33. Glow, R. A., and Glow, P. H.: Non-syndromic behavior problems in children, in Tiller, J. W., and Martin, P. R. (eds.): *Behavioral Medicine: Proceedings of the Geigy Psychiatric Symposium.* Geigy, Melbourne, 1980, pp. 916–946.
34. Andrews, G., Craig, G., Feyer, A. M., *et al.*: Stuttering: A review of research findings and theories circa 1982. *J. Speech Hearing Disorders* **48**:226–279, 1978.
35. Travis, L. E.: Neuropsychological dominance in Travis, L. E., *Speech Pathology,* D. Appleton, New York, 1931; reprinted in *J. Speech Hearing Disorders* **43**:275–279, 1979.
36. Travis, L. E.: The cerebral dominance theory of stuttering: 1931–1978. *J. Speech Hearing Disorders* **43**:278–281, 1978.
37. Davis, S. M., and Drichta, C. E.: Biofeedback theory and application to speech pathology, in Lass, N. (ed.): *Speech and Language Advances in Basic Research and Practice.* Academic, New York, 1980, pp. 283–308.
38. Starkweather, C. W.: Eclectic learning theory and stuttering therapy. Communicative disorders in audio. *J. Contin. Ed.* **2**(8), 1977.
39. Sheehan, J.: Conflict theory and avoidance reduction therapy in Eisenson, J. (ed.): *Stuttering: A second symposium.* Harper & Row, New York, 1975, pp. 125–142.
40. Shames, G. N., and Sherrick, C. E., Jr.: A discussion of nonfluency and stuttering as operant behavior. *J. Speech Hearing Disorders* **28**:3–18, 1963.
41. Brutten, E. J., and Shoemaker, D.: *The Modification of Stuttering.* Prentice-Hall, Englewood Cliffs, New Jersey, 1967.
42. Bluemel, C. S.: *Stammering and Allied Disorders.* Macmillan, New York, 1975.
43. Van Riper, C.: *Speech Correction: Principles and Methods,* 3rd ed. Prentice-Hall, Englewood Cliffs, New Jersey, 1954.
44. Adams, M. R.: The young stutterer: Diagnosis, treatment and assessment of progress. *Semin. Speech Language Hearing* **1**:289–299, 1980.
45. Chumsky, N., and Halle, M.: *The Sound Pattern of English,* Harper & Row, New York, 1968.

Behavioral/Psychiatric Aspects of Children with Speech and Language Disorders

Lorian Baker and Dennis P. Cantwell

INTRODUCTION

Impairments in the development of speech or language are relatively common in children. The National Institute of Neurological Diseases and Strokes (NINDS)[1] estimates that there are more than two million children in the United States with such disorders. Prevalence estimates for childhood speech and language disorders vary from study to study according to the region of the country being sampled, the procedures and personnel used to identify disorders, and the age range of the children being sampled. However, the consensus of epidemiological studies suggests that as many as 15% of children may at some time show disorders of speech development and that as many as 6% may show disorders of language development.[2-7] This means that, throughout his career, the pediatrician is likely to encounter a considerable number of children with speech or language difficulties. Schwartz and Murphy[8] calculated that the "average" pediatrician in the United States sees at *least* one such child each week.

Lorian Baker and Dennis P. Cantwell • UCLA Neuropsychiatric Institute, Los Angeles, California 90024.

These children pose a complex diagnostic problem for the pediatrician, because (1) there are no simple laboratory tests for identifying communication disorders, and (2) there is a wide range of "normal" linguistic development and of disordered development. Complicating this issue further is the fact that children with speech and language problems are especially likely to have other problems that may be developmental, social, emotional, or behavioral in nature. Our study of 600 children presenting to a community speech clinic revealed other (nonlinguistic) developmental disorders in 21% of the sample and emotional or behavioral disorders in 50% of the sample. A review of the literature[9] on speech- and language-disordered children has revealed associated symptoms, including: destructiveness, disobedience, tantrums, hyperactivity, aggressiveness, excitability, immaturity, withdrawal, shyness, excessive worry, nightmares, enuresis, encopresis, and learning problems. Many of these symptoms are frequently reported to the physician as primary or presenting complaints.[10–14]

In this chapter, our aim is to clarify for the pediatrician some of the complex issues regarding speech- and language-disordered children (1) outlining the more common types of childhood speech and language dysfunctions, (2) describing the demographic "profiles" of the children who most frequently present these disorders, and (3) noting the developmental and psychiatric disorders most frequently associated with these various childhood speech and language disorders from the literature and our own data. In addition, we present some theoretical discussion about possible causes of secondary developmental and psychiatric problems in children with speech or language dysfunctions. Finally, we review treatment recommendations for these children, in the light of new data suggesting which children seem most at risk for serious secondary difficulties.

CLASSIFICATION OF SPEECH AND LANGUAGE DISORDERS

The state of the art does not yet have a single model of communication that can satisfactorily account for normal and abnormal language development. A number of different classification systems have been proposed on the basis of etiological or neurological frameworks. These classifications present serious difficulties when dealing with disorders of totally unknown origins or with disorders having "mixed" features that cannot be clearly fitted into a single diagnostic category. These difficult etiological issues are avoided here; instead, we use a descriptive approach that simply enumerates the major types of linguistic disorders which have clinical significance. These are listed in Table I.

Table I. General Classification of Speech and Language Disorders

Pure speech disorders
    Voice disorders
    Articulation disorders
    Fluency disorders
Pure language disorders
    Expressive grammatical disorders
    Receptive grammatical disorders
    Auditory processing disorders
    Pragmatic (language-use) disorders
Mixed speech and language disorders

PROFILES OF CHILDREN WITH SPEECH AND LANGUAGE DISORDERS

Data from the Literature

The literature on the adjustment and demographics of children with different types of speech and language disorders is summarized in the following sections. Although much of this literature is flawed, many of the findings are significant. Readers should be aware, however, of the more common methodological flaws that have occurred in many of the studies on speech- and language-disordered children. These include (1) the use of psychological techniques that lack validity or reliability (early studies using projective tests are particularly guilty of this), (2) assessment bias, (3) too small sample size, and (4) confounding of variables (such as concluding that speakers suffer from pervasive anxiety, when in fact their manifested anxiety may be specific only to a test-taking situation).

Children with Pure Speech Disorders

There are a paucity of demographic data on children with pure speech disorders. The literature suggests that 7% of children have voice problems[15] and that 1% of children have fluency problems.[16] Most voice disorders are associated with organic problems in the larynx, oral cavity (especially palate), nasal cavity, or ears and tend to be present in preschool-age children. Voice disorders that are not associated with organic problems[15] appear to be most commonly found in older children of latency age or adolescence, although there is little "hard" data on this topic.

By contrast, children with disorders of speech fluency tend to present as preschoolers or at the elementary school age level. In fact, speech dysfluency lasting for a few months and spontaneously remitting before age 6 is not considered by most to be a true speech problem.[17] Nonetheless, onset of "true" stuttering after the age of 9 years is quite rare. Stutterers tend to be boys, and the male-to-female ratio increases with advancing age of the child. No associations have been found between speech dysfluencies and family structure variables,[18] although some studies suggest an association between stuttering in older children and excessive parental concern over the child's speech.[19]

Articulation disorders are the most common type of speech disorder found in children. The articulation-disordered child is usually a preschool-aged boy (articulation impairments are three times more common in boys than in girls and four times more common in preschool-age children than in school-age children). There is a less significant tendency for articulation-impaired children to have lower intelligence levels, to come from lower social class homes, and to come from larger families.[20]

The psychiatric and developmental features of children with pure speech impairments are presented in Table II. There does not appear to be a clear association between voice disorders and psychiatric or developmental disorders. However, there are too few studies for any firm conclusions to be drawn. More work has been done on the adjustment of children who stutter, and it is clear that these children have more anxiety and worries than do nonstutterers, at least in a testing or verbal situation. The evidence also suggests that stutterers, at least in the early primary school-age group, may have more language disorders and more attention problems than nonstutterers. The literature reveals that children with articulation disorders also appear to have more psychiatric problems than do children with normal speech. Peer relationship problems, poor self-image, and depression

Table II. Adjustment in Children with Pure Speech Disorders

Reference	Subjects	Methodology	Findings
	Voice-disordered groups		
Muma et al.[21]	High school students with either hoarse, harsh, breathy, or nasal vocal quality; compared with normals	Minnesota Multiphasic Personality Inventory (MMPI); peer evaluations	No differences were found between the voice-disordered students and the controls. No relationships were found between the different voice qualities and personality profiles.
Wilson and Lamb[22]	Children with vocal nodules; compared with age, sex, and IQ-matched normals	Rorschach	More adjustment difficulties were found in the voice-disordered children, although no consistent personality and types were found.
Lolley[23]	Children aged 5–11; compared with normals	School achievement records; Devereux School Behavior Rating Scale	No differences were found between the voice-disorderd children and normals in educational achievement or in most school behaviors. Voice-disordered children showed more problems in "comprehension" on the Devereux Scale
	Stutterers		
Moller[24]	Predelinquents, and "adjusted" boys	Rorschach	The stutterers were found to be more maladjusted than the delinquent boys. Problems found in the stutterers included less self-awareness, poorer interpersonal relationships, and greater anxiety.

Williams[25]	At 4th-, 6th- and 8th-grade levels compared with nonstutterers from the same classes	Iowa Tests of Basic Skills	At lower grade levels, stutterers appeared to be academically retarded, particularly in language skills such as vocabulary and reading. At older ages, performance of stutterers was not significantly different.
Varbiro and Engelmayer[26]	In 3rd through 8th grade, compared with nonstutterers from the same classes	Thematic Apperception Test; California Achievement Test; projective drawings; case histories	Stutterers showed more situational fears as well as more family histories marked by psychiatric problems.
Prins[27]	8–21 years old; compared with controls with other communication disorders	California Test of Personality	Indications of personality maladjustment were found to be more common in controls than in the stutterers. There were no correlations between severity of stuttering and personality maladjustment.
Bubenickova[28]	School age; compared with nonstutterers from same classes	Examination of school records	School achievement was not significantly different between stutterers and nonstutterers, but stutterers showed more fears and negative attitudes.
Riley and Riley[29]	Ages 3–11	Examination of case records	Attention problems, including distractibility, low tolerance for frustration, inability to concentrate, and perseveration were found in 36% of the children.

(continued)

Table II. (Continued)

Reference	Subjects	Methodology	Findings
Solomon[11]	Articulation-disordered groups First-graders compared with matched normals	Interviews with mothers	The articulation-impaired children had significantly more problems in overall adjustment, peer relationships, and sleeping; they had fears, anxieties, and tension.
Sherrill[30]	As compared with classmates	Self-perception questionnaire, peer questionnaire, teacher questionnaire	Functionally articulation-impaired children are not perceived differently from normals overall. However, more severely impaired children are less well accepted than are less severely impaired children.
Broad and Bar[31]	As compared with stutterers and hearing-impaired children	Bender Visual Motor Gestalt Test, Children's Apperception Test, test of human figure drawing	"Underlying psychological conflicts" were found in all three groups of children.
Garbee[32]	As compared with normal adolescents	Dignan Ego Identity Scale	Articulation-impaired adolescents were not found to be different from normals.
Sheridan and Peckham[33]	At 7 years	Bristol Social Adjustment Guide School Reports	Approximately one-half of the severely articulation-impaired children were socially maladjusted. Educational problems were present in all the children.

Rousey[34]	General	Interviews with the children	Articulation-impaired children (with no organic impairments) are always psychiatrically disordered. The type of psychiatric disorder is associated with the type of articulation disorder.
Barrett and Hoops[35]	First-graders; two subgroups are compared: those with normal speech in third grade and those without	Index of Adjustment and Values Test	Articulation-impaired children who do not recover have poorer self-images than do spontaneous remitters.
Ferry et al.[36]	Those with organic involvement (children and adults, mixed)	Not described	"Almost all" the organically articulation-impaired patients had some associated psychiatric problems. Tantrums and depression were particularly common.
Sheridan and Peckham[37]	At 11 years	Bristol Social Adjustment Guide School Reports	Educational problems and social adjustment problems are common in 11-year-old children who had severe articulation problems at age 7.
Calnan and Richardson[38]	Or stuttering children compared with normals	School records	Speech-disordered children had poorer achievement than normals.
Sheridan and Peckham[39]	At 16 years	School reports	Various adjustment problems as well as educational problems are common in 16-year-old children who had severe articulation problems at age 7 years.

Table III. Adjustment in Children with Language Disorders[*]

Reference	Subjects	Methodology	Findings
Wing[41]	Autistic, receptive aphasic, expressive aphasic, hearing-impaired, visually impaired, and Down syndrome children	Parental ratings	The two groups of aphasics showed many behavioral problems in common with the autistic children. The children with receptive language disorder had more behavioral problems than did the children whose language disorder was purely expressive.
Griffiths[42]	Children with "delayed development of speech and language attributable to minimal cerebral dysfunction"	Interviews with children, parents, teachers, and speech therapists	More than one-half of the language-disordered children had learning problems; approximately one-half had poor emotional adjustment; and approximately one-fourth had social development problems.
Caceres[12]	Children with expressive language disorders	Case records	Psychiatric disorders, either extreme inhibition or extreme hyperactivity, were present in 84% of the sample.
Garvey and Gordon[43]	Children with "delayed development of speech" (expressive language deficits)	School records	Problems with behavior and learning were common at follow-up for both children whose language was impaired and for children whose language was normal.
Morley[44]	Children with receptive and expressive developmental aphasia	Case records	Generally, a "reasonably normal picture" of emotional development was found. Reports of tantrums, frustrations and hyperactivity were not uncommon, however.

Study	Subjects	Method	Findings
Petrie[45]	Children with receptive language disorder	Bristol Social Adjustment Guide	Withdrawal, depression, or shyness present in all the language-disordered children.
Affolter et al.[46]	Language-disordered children compared with normals	Battery of auditory and visual perceptual tests and observations during testing	Behavior, particularly attention span, was the feature that most significantly distinguished the language-disordered children.
De Ajuriaguerra et al.[47]	Receptive and expressive adolescent dysphasics	Case reports	At follow-up, social development was the area in which the least gains had been made.
Stevenson and Richman[48]	3-year-olds with expressive language defects	Behavior Screening Questionnaire	Approximately one-half of the language-disordered children had marked behavioral problems. Most common problems reported included overactivity and problems with eating, family relationships, discipline, and development.
Fundudis et al.[49]	Children who had expressive language deficits at 3 years of age	Rutter teacher rating scale, Junior Eysenck Personality Inventory, parent interview, interview of child by psychologist and psychiatrist	At age 7 years, one-fifth of the group was found to be pathologically deviant (extremely abnormal). In the remaining children, behavioral and emotional problems were found, on all measures, to be extremely common.
Aram and Nation[50]	Children who had language disorder at preschool age	Parent and teacher reports	At follow-up 4 years later, almost one-half of the children were having serious achievement problems.

are problems found in articulation-disordered children. Children with severe articulation impairment also have higher frequencies of learning difficulties.

Children with Language Disorders

Relatively little is known about the distribution of language disorders in children. Although some children exhibit pure expressive grammatical disorders and others manifest auditory processing disorders in isolation, most of the language disorders listed in Table I are found in combination with each other and with speech disorders. Language disorders appear to be most prevalent in preschool-aged and elementary-school-aged children and are more common in boys than in girls.[40]

The literature on psychiatric adjustment and developmental status of children with language disorders is presented in Table III. There appears to be a clear consensus that these children exhibit psychiatric and developmental disorders. Learning problems and behavioral disorders are most frequently reported for these children. There is evidence, however, that in a number of language-disordered children these psychiatric and developmental disorders occur in extreme forms.

Data from Current Research

Although a review of the literature indicates that children with speech and language problems are at risk for developmental and psychiatric disorders, the small and often biased samples of children in most studies limit the scope of the findings. We were unable to find a single study that evaluated large numbers of children having a wide spectrum of speech or language disorders and who were representative of the general population of speech- and language-impaired children. We take this opportunity to report data from our research that involves just such a study.

This study involved examining all children who presented to a large community speech and hearing clinic located in the greater Los Angeles area between March 1977 and April 1980. Since this clinic serves a broad social class distribution, and since the refusal rate for participation in the study was very low (less than 2%), we hypothesize that the children are representative of the general population of speech- and language-disordered children.

The psychiatric methodology in this study utilized information from various sources, including (1) a semistructured interview with the parents covering all aspects of the child's behavior and development, (2) a semistructured interview with the child, and (3) rating scales from both the child's parents and his teacher or teachers. In addition, a developmental neurological examination, educational achievement tests (the Wide Range Achievement Test and the Gray Oral Reading Test), intelligence tests, and standardized speech and language tests were administered to all children capable of completing them. The speech and language test battery included the Goldman–Fristoe Test of Articulation, the Carrow Test of Auditory Comprehension of Language, and the Illinois Test of Psycholinguistic Abilities, as well as an analysis of a sample of free speech. In addition to psychiatric diagnoses of specific clinical psychiatric syndromes utilizing DSM III criteria and descriptions of speech and language functioning, ratings were made of developmental disorders, biological complicating factors, and psychosocial stressors found for each

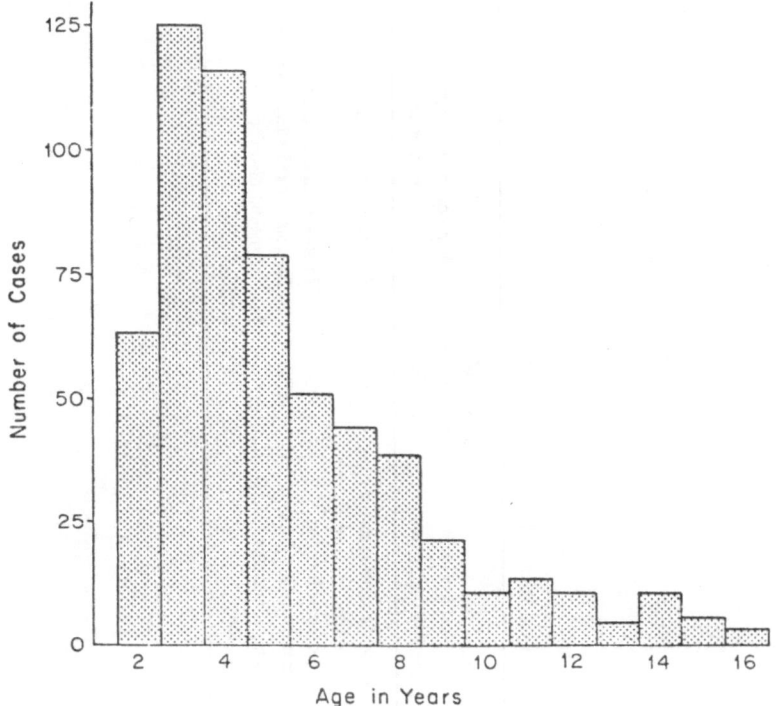

Figure 1 Age distribution of cases presenting for initial speech evaluation

child The methodology of this study has been described in greater detail elsewhere,[51] should the reader have further questions

Over a 3-year period, 600 children were assessed in this study The children ranged in age from 2 to 16 years, with the average age being 5 years, 10 months Most of the children were below the age of 6 years (Fig 1)

Four hundred thirteen of the children were boys and 187 were girls

Children with Pure Speech Disorders

Approximately one-third of the children in the study (a total of 203 children) were found to have pure speech disorders These children were typically male (67%) and had an average age of 6 years, 4 months Approximately one-third of this group had some psychiatric disorder, according to DSM III criteria The occurrence of developmental disorders was relatively low in the children with pure speech disorders, with fewer than 10% having developmental disorders The profiles of the children with pure speech disorders produced from the data from this study are presented in Table IV

Among the children with pure speech disorders, most had disorders involving *artic-ulation* There were 172 children in this category, ranging in age from 2 through 16 years of age, with an average age of 6 years, 1 month Of these articulation-impaired children,

Table IV. Profiles of Children with Speech Disorders

Speech disorder	Average age	Sex	Rate of psychiatric illness	Most common psychiatric problems	Rate of developmental disorders	Most common developmental disorders
Voice disorder (only)	9 years, 4 months	100% males	38%	No single most common problem	25%	No single most common problem
Fluency disorder (only)	6 years, 11 months	82% males	41%	Adjustment disorders	9%	No single most common problem
Articulation disorder	6 years, 1 months	64% males	30%	Attention-deficit disorders; adjustment disorder	8%	Enuresis, mixed specific developmental disorder

25 had only a lisp; 24 had impaired articulation clearly associated with organic abnormalities and the remaining 148 had articulation impairments involving speech sounds other than sibilants and not being clearly associated with organic abnormalities. The articulation-impaired children were typically males, with 30% showing psychiatric disorder and 8% having developmental disorders. The most frequently occurring psychiatric disorders were attention-deficit disorder (characterized by developmentally inappropriate inattention, impulsivity, and hyperactivity) and adjustment disorders (characterized by maladaptive reactions to identifiable psychosocial stressors such as changes in family structure, moves, or beginning school).

Among the children with pure speech disorders whose articulation was normal, eight were found to have a voice disorder, and 22 were noted to have a fluency disorder. Both groups of children tended to be older than the pure speech-disordered children whose articulation was abnormal. The voice-disordered children averaged 9 years, 4 months of age, and the fluency-disordered children averaged 6 years, 11 months of age. The incidence of psychiatric illness in both groups of children was approximately 40%. The fluency-disordered children revealed a higher prevalence of adjustment disorders than of other disorders. The voice-disordered children manifested a variety of psychiatric problems, with none more common than others. Developmental disorders appeared to be more common in the voice-disordered children than in the fluency-disordered children, but no particular developmental disorder was more common in either of these groups.

Children with Language Disorders

Approximately two-thirds of the 600 children seen had some type of language impairment. These language-disordered children fell into two fairly different subgroups: a smaller group of older children with pure language disorders, and a larger group of younger children with mixed disorders involving both speech and language.

There were 45 children with pure language disorders. These children were typically males; the average age was 8 years, 10 months. The children with pure language disorders fell into three subgroups of approximately equal size: (1) receptive language disorders, (2) expressive language disorders but normal reception, and (3) auditory processing disorders and normal expression and reception. The profiles from the data on children with pure language disorder are presented in Table V.

It should be noted that children with receptive deficits tended to be younger (averaging 8 years, 1 month of age), whereas the children with auditory processing disorders and normal expression and reception tended to be older (averaging 10 years, 1 month of age). The children with expressive deficits and normal reception averaged 8 years, 10 months of age.

Children with pure language disorders involving receptive deficits were the only subgroup of speech- and language-disordered children seen who were not predominately males. In this subgroup, the ratio was three females for every two males; the rate of psychiatric illness was especially high at 81%. Attention-deficit disorder and adjustment disorder were the two most common psychiatric illnesses found in the group, although several other types of disorders were present. Approximately 20% of these receptively impaired children showed developmental disorders, the most commonly occurring of which was mixed specific developmental disorder.

Table V. Profiles of Children with Language Disorders

Type of language disorder	Average age	Sex	Rate of psychiatric illness	Most common psychiatric problems	Rate of developmental disorders	Most common developmental problems
Pure language disorder involving receptive deficit	8 years, 1 month	44%	81%	Attention-deficit disorder; adjustment disorder	19%	Mixed specific developmental disorder
Pure language disorder involving expressive deficit (receptive language normal)	8 years, 10 months	85%	77%	Attention-deficit disorder, depression	38%	Enuresis
Pure language disorder (involving auditory processing only)	10 years, 1 month	75%	56%	Depression	38%	Encopresis, developmental reading disorder; mixed specific developmental disorder
Receptive language disorder with associated speech disorder	5 years, 0 months	69%	63%	Attention-deficit disorder, oppositional disorder	36%	Mixed specific developmental disorder–coordination disorder, enuresis
Expressive language disorder with associated speech disorder and normal reception	4 years, 8 months	73%	49%	Attention-deficit disorder, depression; adjustment disorder	10%	Coordination disorder
Auditory processing disorder with associated speech disorder (normal expressions reception)	7 years, 6 months	61%	61%	Attention-deficit disorder; overanxious disorder	28%	Coordination disorder, enuresis

Children with pure language disorders involving expressive deficits and normal reception were predominately males, who had a psychiatric illness rate of 77%. Attention-deficit disorder and depression were the more frequently occurring forms of psychiatric illness found in these children. Thirty-eight percent of this group had developmental disorders, of which enuresis was the most common type.

Older children who had pure language disorder involving auditory processing dysfunctions, which did not affect expressive or receptive grammar, presented with lower rates of psychiatric illness than did the children in the two other pure language-disorder groups. Approximately 50% of these children had a psychiatric illness, however, most commonly some form of depressive disorder. Thirty-eight percent of these children had developmental disorder, with encopresis, developmental reading disorder, and mixed specific developmental disorder all being equally common.

Most of the children with language disorders had disorders of speech as well. We saw 352 such children in this study. The children were younger (averaging 5 years, 0 months), predominatly males (70%), and approximately 50% had psychiatric illnesses. The profiles of the children with mixed speech and language disorders are presented in Table V.

The children with mixed speech and language disorders fell into three distinct groups. The largest group, consisting of 221 children, demonstrated impairment of receptive language. These children averaged 5 years, 0 months of age, and were primarily males (69%). Sixty-three percent of these children had psychiatric disorders, the most common forms of which were attention-deficit disorder and oppositional disorder. Approximately one-third of these children had developmental disorders with mixed specific developmental disorder, coordination disorder, and enuresis equally common.

Another large group of children with mixed speech and language disorders showed impairments of expressive language with normal reception. There were 113 of these children in the study, 73% of whom were males. These children were the youngest of the language-disordered subgroup of children, with a mean age of 4 years, 8 months. Almost 50% of the children manifested psychiatric illnesses, the most common forms of which were attention-deficit disorder, depression, or adjustment disorder. Developmental disorders were less common in these children, affecting only 10% of the group. Coordination disorder was the most commonly occurring form of developmental disorder.

A small group of children were found to have combined auditory processing disorders and speech disorders, but whose receptive and expressive language tested within normal limits. These children were the oldest of the mixed speech- and language-disordered groups, averaging 7 years, 6 months of age. These children were most frequently males with psychiatric disorders consisting of either attention-deficit disorder or overanxious disorder. Twenty-eight percent of these children had developmental disorders, with either coordination disorder or enuresis being the most common forms.

CORRELATES AND CAUSES OF PSYCHIATRIC AND DEVELOPMENTAL DISORDERS IN CHILDREN WITH SPEECH AND LANGUAGE DISORDERS

The data presented from our study of 600 speech- or language-disordered children confirms conclusions derived from the literature review, i.e., children with speech or language disorders are at risk for the development of psychiatric and developmental disorders. The data indicate that psychiatric disorder is a more common associated problem than is developmental disorder and that there are no unique psychiatric or developmental syndromes found in children with speech and language disorders. The data also suggest that children with language disorders have more psychiatric and developmental disorders than do children with pure speech disorders. Furthermore, children with pure language disorders have more psychiatric and developmental disorders than do children with mixed speech and language disorders. Although no unique psychiatric or developmental syndromes were associated with the speech- and language-disordered children studied, several types of psychiatric and developmental disorders were found to occur with greater frequency than other disorders. The more frequently occurring psychiatric and developmental disorders included attention-deficit disorder, adjustment disorder, depressive disorders, anxiety disorders, enuresis, encopresis, coordination disorder, and mixed specific developmental disorder.

All of the available data suggest that at least 50% of speech- and language-disordered children have some type of clinical psychiatric disorder. This means, however, that approximately 50% of speech- and language-disordered children do *not* have any associated psychiatric problems. Comparisons were made of those children, from the 600 cases who did not have associated psychiatric disorder with those children who did have associated psychiatric disorders. This represented an attempt to isolate any factors that might make a speech- and language-disordered child more susceptible to psychiatric illness.

Among the 600 children from a community speech clinic, 298 children did not exhibit psychiatric illness (the "well" children), and 302 children had some diagnosable psychiatric illness according to DSM III criteria (the "ill" children). The sex distribution in the well and ill children was not significantly different (67% males in the well group and 71% males in the ill group). However, the age distribution revealed a significant ($p = 0.02$) difference in the direction of the well children, who were slightly younger. The mean age of the well children was 5 years, 6 months (standard deviation: 2 years, 10 months), and the mean age of the ill children was 6 years, 0 months (standard deviation: 2 years, 11 months).

There were no significant demographic differences between the two groups of children. Maternal and paternal ages, occupation, educational level, race, and religion were essentially the same in both groups of children. Similarly, the prevalence of past medical problems including pregnancy and birth complications was about the same. Handedness was the same for both groups of children. The age of attaining nonlanguage developmental milestones, such as sitting, crawling, standing, and walking, was also the same in the two groups of children.

The factors that distinguished the well children from the ill children are presented in Table VI. It can be seen that these factors are predominantly linguistic in nature: The speech group that the children belonged to, the presence of a language comprehension deficit, the presence of an expressive language deficit, the verbal intelligence level, and the age of onset of speech and first use of sentences were all significantly different between the well and ill groups of children. In addition, some environmental and demographic factors distinguished the two groups, including amount of psychosocial stress, family intactness, performance intelligence levels, and presence of neurological examination abnormalities.

Table VI. Factors Significantly Distinguishing Psychiatrically Well versus Psychiatrically Ill Children

Group	Well (%)	Ill (%)	Test	p
Speech and language groupings			χ^2	0.0001
Pure speech disorder	47	21		
Speech and language disorder	49	68		
Pure language disorder	4	11		
Language comprehension			χ^2	0.0001
Normal	72	50		
Mild disorder	2	4		
Mild to moderate	9	17		
Moderate	12	18		
Moderate to severe	4	6		
Severe	1	5		
Expressive language			χ^2	0.0001
Normal	51	28		
Mild	4	4		
Mild to moderate	15	24		
Moderate	19	27		
Moderate to severe	6	10		
Severe	5	7		
Speech			χ^2	0.0013
Normal	4	11		
Disordered	96	89		
Nonlanguage developmental disorders			χ^2	0.0013
None	84	73		
Any	16	27		
Psychosocial stressors			χ^2	0.0001
None	50	21		
Any	50	79		
Number of psychosocial stressors			χ^2	0.0001
1	29	27		
2	15	29		
3	6	23		
Neurological examination			χ^2	0.001
No abnormalities	72	64		
Any abnormalities	28	36		
Biological parents intact	83	68	χ^2	0.001
Age of first words (mean)	16.8 months	19.5 months	t-test	0.003
Age of first sentence (mean)	26.8 months	30.8 months	t-test	0.001
Performance intelligence (mean)	108.2	101.9	t-test	0.003

The fact that linguistic variables were among the most critical factors in distinguishing psychiatrically well children from psychiatrically ill children raises the question of what mechanisms are responsible for the association between psychiatric disorder and speech or language disorder. Three hypotheses have been proposed: (1) psychiatric disorder causes speech and language disorder, (2) psychiatric disorder is associated with

Table VII. Indirect Causes of Psychiatric Disorder in Speech- and Language-
Impaired Children[a]

Problem	Well group (%)	Ill group (%)
Trouble establishing social contacts and keeping friends		
Lacks friends[b]	12	29
Poor relationships with friends[b]	14	34
Solitary[b]	7	20
Poor relationship with mother[b]	15	32
Poor relationship with father[b]	15	29
Trouble achieving control over environment		
Frequent temper outbursts[c]	26	39
Frequent fights with peers[d]	10	31
Frequent fights with parents or other adults[b]	2	12
In trouble at school for behavior[d]	7	26
Angry affect[d]	4	12
Discordant home environment[d]	7	22
Poor self-image		
Thinks not likable[c]	6	22
Miscellaneous phobias and fears[c]	25	39
Learning difficulties		
Learning problem at school[b]	26	55

[a]Data from a study of 600 children, evidence from child interviews
[b]χ^2 test, $p < 0.001$
[c]χ^2 test, $p < 0.01$
[d]χ^2 test, $p < 0.0001$

speech and language disorder due to common antecedents, and (3) speech and language disorders lead to psychiatric disorder indirectly through increased environmental difficulties.

Concerning the first hypothesis, Rutter[52] points out that psychiatric disorders such as infantile autism, intellectual retardation, elective mutism, and schizophrenia are characterized by marked linguistic abnormalities. Rutter suggests that these linguistic impairments are caused by the psychiatric disorders. Our study of 600 children, however, shows that these disorders are extremely rare, and that most speech- and language-disordered children revealed other types of psychiatric disorders such as attention deficit, depression, adjustment reaction, and anxiety. It appears that in the majority of speech- and language-disordered children, it is unlikely that psychiatric disorder was the cause of the language disorder.

The second hypothesis, suggesting that some common underlying factor accounts for both the linguistic disorder and the psychiatric disorder, was not supported by our data. The factors that have been hypothesized[9] as ''causing'' both psychiatric disorder and language disorder include brain damage, low social class, intellectual retardation, and hearing impairment. In our study, the prevalence of known brain damage in the speech- and language-disordered children was rare. There was slightly more neurological dysfunction in the psychiatrically ill children, but more than one-half showed no neurological abnormalities. There were no differences between the well and ill children in other indications of possible brain damage, such as birth or pregnancy complications or ages at which any nonlinguistic developmental milestones were reached. The social class distribution (as measured by maternal and paternal occupation and education) was not significantly different between the well and ill children. While the ill children showed slightly lower intelligence scores than the well children, most of the children in both groups had normal or above-normal intelligence scores. Hearing impairment was not significantly different in prevalence in either the well or ill groups. Thus, in our large-scale study of linguistically impaired children, the factors previously proposed as common antecedents to both psychiatric and linguistic malfunction are generally not significant and, when significant, they are relevant to only a small number of children.

The findings from our study tend to support the third hypothesis. It appears that psychiatric disorder is an indirect result of having a speech or language disorder. Children "need" language for many different purposes[53] (1) to establish social contacts and for maintaining friendships, (2) to achieve some control over the environment, (3) to establish a positive self image, and (4) to develop concepts and for learning. If children are unable to achieve these factors, there is a great risk of emotional and behavioral problems developing. There was considerable evidence of problems in all the above areas. Some of this evidence is presented in Table VII. It should be noted that all these problems are significantly more common in the psychiatrically ill children than in the psychiatrically well children.

SIGNIFICANCE

The data demonstrating a very close association between childhood communication problems and psychiatric disorder emphasized the extreme importance of early diagnosis and treatment for any child with speech or language difficulties. Treatment for speech and language disorders is indicated at the preschool-age level for a number of reasons: (1) this is the optimal period for language acquisition, (2) children may respond better to speech and language therapy at this time, and (3) it may be possible to remediate linguistic problems before the gap between the language-impaired child's functional level and the functional level of his chronologically aged peers widens. Furthermore, and more important, with early language therapy, it may be possible to prevent the social, environmental, and learning problems associated with emotional and behavioral impairments.

Table VIII suggests a plan for the clinical management of children with speech and language disorders. The need for the pediatrician to be aware at all stages of management of the psychiatric and educational implications of speech or language disorder is emphasized.

When screening children for speech or language disorders, the pediatrician should be particularly vigilant with males below 6 years of age. Generally maternal concerns about speech and language development, for the most part, are extremely well founded. Any complaints of this nature should be taken very seriously. Children who deserve special scrutiny include those with (1) a family history of language or learning disabilities; (2) a history of a very deprived background; (3) evidences of neurological, motor, or oral mechanism abnormalities; (4) learning problems in school or other developmental problems; and (5) attention/concentration problems or other emotional difficulties.

Table VIII. Plan for Clinical Management of Children with Speech and Language Disorders

1. Screen all children for possible speech/language problems, keeping in mind profiles of children most commonly affected.
2. Obtain a detailed baseline history of functioning in linguistic, educational, psychological, and medical areas.
3. Refer for assessment by interdisciplinary specialists (speech/language pathologist, special education consultant, psychologist or psychiatrist).
4. Initiate multipronged treatment (alleviate environmental/medical causes, begin formal speech/language therapy, provide parental counseling).
5. Monitor progress closely, watching for development of secondary problems.

In order to manage these children adequately, a detailed history of the child's functioning in all areas is necessary. A comprehensive description of the child's linguistic functioning should be obtained. Does the child have trouble being understood? Does the child have trouble understanding others? Are there evidences of difficulty with oral movements, such as chewing or blowing? Is the child embarrassed about his speech? Is the child teased about his speech? Does the child have limited grammatical expressions? If the child is of school age, it is important to determine whether there is any history of learning problems. It is useful to try to find a precise description of what the learning problems might involve. Is there a problem with following instructions? Can the child remember instructions? Does the child have a problem with completing assignments? The medical history should include any available information about oral mechanism or hearing problems, as well as ages of reaching linguistic and motor milestones. The psychiatric history should include (1) a description of the child's relationships with peers and family, (2) an evaluation of how the child functions under conditions of frustration, and (3) whether there are any signs of depression such as appetite or sleep changes.

Referral for detailed assessment by a speech/language pathologist is indicated for any child with suggestion or history of speech/language problems. An adequate evaluation will have results from standardized testing and will provide an assessment of functioning (expressed as an age-level score or as a percentile score) in articulation skills, expressive grammatical development, receptive grammatical development, and, for older children, auditory processing skills. For children with a history of learning difficulties or emotional problems, referral to an educational specialist or to a child psychologist or psychiatrist may also be helpful.

Treatment of children with speech and language problems will often involve a multimodality approach. Medical considerations, such as treatment of oral deformities or hearing impairment, should take first priority. Speech or language therapy is usually of second priority, and other interdisciplinary methods such as educational tutoring and psychiatric or psychological therapy should be considered shortly after the initiation of speech/language therapy. Progress in treatment should be monitored carefully, and consideration should be given to factors that might be hampering progress in treatment. Factors such as inability to concentrate well, achievement anxiety, and lack of motivation can be treated with appropriate interventions if necessary. In cases in which parental achievement pressures are too high, parental counseling may be necessary.

REFERENCES

1. NINDS: *Human Communication and Its Disorders: An Overview.* Monograph No. 10. National Institute of Neurological Diseases and Stroke, Department of Health, Education and Welfare, Bethesda, 1972.
2. Elliot, L.: Epidemiology of hearing impairment and other communicative disorders. *Adv. Neurol.* **19**:399–420, 1978.
3. Milisen, R.: The incidence of speech disorders, in Travis, L. (ed.): *Handbook of Speech Pathology and Audiology.* Prentice-Hall, Englewood Cliffs, New Jersey, 1971, pp. 619–634.
4. Sheridan, M. D.: Children of 7 years with marked speech defects. *Br. J. Disord. Commun.* **8**:9–16, 1973.
5. Randall, D., Reynell, J., and Curiven, M.: A study of language development in a sample of three-year-old children. *Br. J. Disord. Commun.* **9**:3–16, 1974.
6. Stevenson, J., and Richman, N.: The prevalence of language delay in a population of three-year-old children and its association with general retardation. *Dev. Med. Child Neurol.* **18**:431–441, 1976.
7. Tuomi, S., and Ivanoff, P.: Incidence of speech and hearing disorders among kindergarteners and grade one children. *Spec. Educ. Can.* **51**(4):5–8, 1977.
8. Schwartz, A. H., and Murphy, M. W.: Cues for screening language disorders in preschool children. *Pediatrics* **55**:717–722, 1975.
9. Cantwell, D. P., and Baker, L.: Psychiatric disorder in children with speech and language retardation: A critical review. *Arch. Gen. Psychiatry* **34**:583–591, 1977.
10. Fitzsimons, R.: Developmental, psychosocial and educational factors in children with nonorganic articulation problems. *Child Dev.* **29**:481–489, 1958.
11. Solomon, A. E.: Personality and behavior patterns of children with functional defects of articulation. *Child Dev.* **32**:731–737, 1961.
12. Caceres, V. A.: Retardo del Lenguaju Verbal. *Rev. Neuropsiquiatria* **34**:(3):210–226, 1971.
13. Ingram, T. T. S.: A description and classification of the common disorders of speech in children. *Arch. Dis. Child.* **34**:444, 1959.
14. Baker, L., Cantwell, D. P., and Mattison, R. E.: Behavior problems in children with pure speech disorders and in children with combined speech and language disorder. *J. Abnorm. Child Psychol.* **8**(2):245–56, 1980.
15. Wilson, D. L.: *Voice Problems of Children,* 2nd ed. Williams & Wilkins, Baltimore, 1979.
16. Silver, L. B.: Speech disorders, in Kaplan, H. Freedman, A., and Sadock, B. (eds.): *Comprehensive Textbook of Psychiatry,* Vol. III. Williams & Wilkins, Baltimore, 1980, pp. 2579–2585.
17. Bloodstein, L.: *Speech Pathology: An Introduction.* Houghton-Mifflin, Boston, 1979.
18. Gladstien, K. L., Seider, R. A., and Kidd, K. K.: Analysis of the sibship patterns of stutterers. *J. Speech Hear. Res.* **24**:460–462, 1981.
19. Cooper, E. B.: The development of a stuttering chronicity prediction checklist: A preliminary report. *J. Speech Hear. Res.* **38**:215–223, 1973.
20. Winitz, H.: *Articulatory Acquisition and Behavior.* Prentice-Hall, Englewood Cliffs, New Jersey, 1969.
21. Muma, J. D., Laeder, R. L., and Webb, C. E.: Adolescent voice quality aberrations: Personality and social status. *J. Speech Hear. Res.* **11**:576–582, 1968.
22. Wilson, F. B., and Lamb, M. M.: Comparison of personality characteristics of children with and without vocal nodules based on Rorschach protocol interpretation. *Acta Symbol.* **5**:43–55, 1974.
23. Lolley, T. L.: An Investigation of the Relationship of Voice Disorders to Classroom Behavior & Educational Achievement. Doctoral thesis, University of Maryland, 1975.
24. Moller, H.: Stuttering, Predelinquent and Adjusted Boys. A Comparative Analysis of Personality Characteristics as Measured by the WISC and the Rorschach Test. Doctoral thesis, Boston University, 1960.
25. Williams, C. E.: Early diagnosis of deafness and its relation to speech in deaf, maladjusted children. *Dev. Med. Child Neurol.* **11**:777–782, 1969.
26. Varbiro, K., and Englemayer, A.: Traumatic fear experience as an etiological factor in the formation of stuttering. *Magy. Szichologian Szemle* **29**:223–238, 1972.
27. Prins, D.: Personality, stuttering, severity and age. *J. Speech Hear. Res.* **15**:148–154, 1972.
28. Bubenickova, M.: The stuttering child's relation to school. *Psychol. Patopsychol. Diet.* **12**:535–545, 1977.
29. Riley, B., and Riley, J.: A component model for diagnosing and treating children who stutter. *J. Fluency Dis.* **4**:279–294, 1979.

30. Sherrill, D. D.: Peer, teacher and self-perceptions of children with severe functional articulation disorders. *Diss. Abst. Int.* **28:**507–508, 1967.

31. Broad, R. D., and Bar, A.: Personality correlates of communication disorders as revealed by projective assessment and verbal expressions. *Folia Phoniatr. (Basel)* **25:**405–415, 1973.

32. Garbee, F. E.: Ego Identity in Adolescent Males with Articulatory Disorders. Doctoral dissertation, Claremont College, Claremont, California, 1973.

33. Sheridan, M. D., and Peckham, C. S.: Hearing and speech at seven. *Spec. Educ.* **62**(2):16–20, 1973.

34. Rousey, C. L.: *Psychiatric Assessment by Speech and Hearing Behavior.* Thomas, Springfield, Illinois, 1974.

35. Barrett, C. J., and Hoops, H. R.: The relationship between self-concept and the remission of articulatory errors. *Lang. Speech Hear. Serv. Schools* **2:**67–70, 1974.

36. Ferry, P. C., Hall, S. M., and Hicks, J. L.: Dilapidated speech: Developmental verbal dyspraxia. *Dev. Med. Child Neurol.* **17:**749–756, 1975.

37. Sheridan, M. D., and Peckham, C.: Follow-up at 11 years of children who had marked speech defects at 7 years. *Child Care Health Dev.* **113:**157–166, 1975.

38. Calnan, M., and Richardson, K.: Speech problems among children in a national survey—associations with reading, general ability, mathematics and syntactic maturity. *Educ. Stud.* **3:**55–66, 1977.

39. Sheridan, M. D., and Peckham, C. S.: Follow-up to the years of school children who had marked speech defects at 7 years. *Child Care Health Dev.* **43:**145–157, 1978.

40. Baker, L., and Cantwell, D.: Developmental language disorder, in Kaplan, H. (ed.): *Comprehensive Textbook of Psychiatry,* 3rd ed. Balt. Williams & Wilkins, Baltimore, 1980, pp. 2561–2570.

41. Wing, L.: The handicaps of autistic children: A comparative study. *J. Child Psychol. Psychiatry* **10:**1–40, 1969.

42. Griffiths, C. P. S.: A follow-up study of children with disorders of speech. *Br. J. Disord. Commun.* **4:**46–56, 1969.

43. Garvey, M., and Gordon, N.: A follow-up study of children with disorders of speech development. *Br. J. Disord. Commun.* **8:**17–28, 1973.

44. Morley, M.: Receptive/expressive developmental aphasia. *Br. J. Disord. Commun.* **8:**47–53, 1973.

45. Petrie, I.: Characteristics and progress of a group of language disordered children with severe receptive difficulties. *Br. J. Disord. Commun.* **10:**123–133, 1975.

46. Affolter, F., Brubaker, R., and Bischofberger, W.: Comparative studies between normal and language disturbed children based on performance profiles. *Acta Otolaryngol.* **32:**323, 1974.

47. De Ajuriaguerra, J., Jaeggi, A., Guignard, F., et al.: The development and prognosis of dysphasia in children, in Morehead, D. (ed.): *Normal and Deficient Child Language.* University Park Press, Baltimore, 1976, pp. 345–385.

48. Stevenson, J., and Richman, N.: Behavior language and development in three-year-old children. *J. Autism Child Schiz.* **8:**299–313, 1978.

49. Fundudis, T., Kolvin, I., and Garside, R. F.: A follow-up of speech retarded children, in Hersov, L. (ed.): *Language Disorders in Childhood,* book supplement to *J. Child Psychol. Psychiatry* **2:**97–113, 1980.

50. Aram, D. M., and Nation, J. E.: Preschool language disorders and subsequent language and academic difficulties. *J. Commun. Dis.* **13:**159–170, 1980.

51. Cantwell, D. P., Baker, L., and Mattison, R.: Prevalence, type and correlates of psychiatric disorder in 200 children with communication disorder. *J. Dev. Behav. Pediatr.* **2:**131–136, 1981.

52. Rutter, M.: Psychiatric causes of language retardation, in Rutter, M. (ed.): *The Child with Delayed Speech.* Heinemann, London, 1972, pp. 147–160.

53. Baker, L., and Cantwell, D. P.: Language acquisition, cognitive development and emotional disorder in childhood, in Nelson, K. D. (ed.): *Children's Language,* Vol. 31. Erlbaum, Hillsdale, New Jersey, 1982, pp. 286–321.

IV

Behavioral Disorders

Common Behavioral Disorders of Childhood

Abby L. Wasserman

INTRODUCTION

Like physical growth and development, behavior develops in stages. What is considered normal at one age may be quite abnormal for another developmental phase, and some behavioral disorders are age specific. The problems that prompt parents to seek the physician's help range from the truly pathological to those that are normal or that can be

Abby L. Wasserman • Division of Psychiatry and Psychology, St. Jude Children's Research Hospital, Memphis, Tennessee 38101.

changed by simple manipulations of the environment. Some of these problems may also reflect variations in the child's temperament, an area that has received considerable study in recent years.

Temperament determines how the child will interact with the environment and how well he will cope with the various stresses of growing up. Thomas *et al.*[1] outlined nine qualities that make up temperament in children:

1. *Activity level:* How motoric is the child?
2. *Rhythmicity:* How predictable is the child's sleep–wake cycle, eating, and elimination?
3. *Approach or withdrawal:* How does the child react to a new situation?
4. *Adaptability:* How quickly and easily is the child able to adapt this behavior to changes in the environment?
5. *Intensity of reaction:* What is the amount of energy the child expends in expressing moods?
6. *Threshold of responsiveness:* What is the stimulus intensity necessary to evoke a response in the child?
7. *Quality of mood:* Is the child normally pleasant and joyful or unpleasant and negative?
8. *Distractibility:* How much stimulation is necessary to make the child change or modify ongoing behavior?
9. *Attention span and persistency:* How long will the child pursue a given activity and continue to persevere in the face of obstacles?

Even during the first few months of life, children differ markedly in these features, which influence their environment and the parental responses they receive. Carey[2] classified infants into difficult, intermediate, and easy babies. Difficult infants tend to remain difficult with increasing age. However, extremely difficult and the extremely easy infants tend to move toward the average.[3] Parents will have more problems managing a child whose temperament differs from their own, regardless of whether the child is perceived as a difficult or an easy child. For example, the parent who is extremely active and energetic will have just as much trouble with a slow and methodical child as will the quiet, more passive parent with a very active child.

Some behavioral disorders are age specific, such as breathholding spells or school avoidance, whereas others span all of infancy and childhood, such as problems with eating or sleeping. This chapter looks at behavior by age group, realizing that some of the problems described will be found in more than one group. Suggestions as to how to handle the various behavioral problems described are based on the "average" child in a fairly typical environment and may therefore not be entirely appropriate for the severely disturbed child or a child in an extremely chaotic environment.

INFANCY

Many infant behaviors that are normal variants are taken personally by the parents, who need reassurance that their baby is showing normal behavior. This is especially true for the first child. An example is, the mother who touches the baby's cheek to get him to turn toward the breast or bottle—when the baby turns in response to the rooting reflex, the mother might interpret this behavior as defiance or lack of love. Explaining this to the mother can help avert future problems in the mother–child interaction.

Crying

A universal behavior of infants that causes much parental distress is crying. Crying is the young baby's only form of communication. It is the caretaker's responsibility to interpret the crying and relieve or remove its source, if possible. Problems arise when the caretaker, usually the mother, feels ineffectual because the crying continues despite her efforts, and a thorough physical examination shows no physical abnormality to account for the crying. Parents should be told that they won't "spoil" their babies by picking them up and comforting them when they cry.[4] Bell and Ainsworth[5] showed that when mothers responded to their babies' cries quickly and frequently during the first 6 months of life, the babies cried less during their second 6 months.

Some common parental techniques that have been used over the years to quiet the crying baby include warm water bottle under the baby's abdomen; pacifier; rocking the child; singing or playing music; cuddling; rides in the car, carriage, or stroller; placing the baby in an infant seat on top of an operating washer or dryer (making sure the child is secure and not left alone)[6]; and walking around with the child in a soft carrier worn on the front of the parent's body.

If none of these approaches works, the parents should allow the child to "cry it out" without feeling guilty. Most babies will fall asleep within an hour. An exception is colic, a benign, self-limited phenomenon. Wessel's[7] definition of colic is the one most doctors use today: He describes infants who are "otherwise healthy and well-fed, who have paroxysms of irritability, fussing, or crying lasting for a total of more than three hours a day and occurring on more than three days in any one week." The incidence of colic ranges from 7 to 36%.[8] Colic usually starts about 2 weeks of age and ends by 12 to 16 weeks. The crying is usually confined to the evening hours. Medication is sometimes used in treating colic, yet its benefit has not been proven in double blind studies.[9] Reassurance that the child is healthy and that the colic will end, and support of the parents are probably the best treatment measures.

Eating Disorders

The Committee on Nutrition of the American Academy of Pediatrics[10] describes three overlapping stages of infant feeding: the nursing period, the transitional period, and a modified adult period. Each stage has its own associated problems which should be dealt with before problems at mealtime become ingrained in the family functioning.

Breastfeeding is gaining advocates as the advantages for both the mother and infant are identified.[11–16] Yet there are still problems that may discourage some mothers from continuing breastfeeding. The first few weeks of nursing are extremely tiring for the new mother. Her nipples and/or breasts may be painful. As the child gets older, the mother may feel tied down since everything she does must revolve around the baby's need for food. Moreover, some fathers may feel left out because they can't feed their baby; others may not want to "share" their wife's breasts, or see breastfeeding as detracting from their wife's sexuality. The father's feelings may cause problems within the marital relationship, which may be long-term if the mother and child form an alliance against the father (not a psychologically healthy outcome). The primary physician should ask about marital problems and try to help resolve them as soon as possible.

The mother needs support, encouragement, and reassurance. Teaching the mother how to express her milk for later use or letting her know that use of supplemental bottles with formula are not detrimental will give her more freedom and will also allow the father to take an active part in feeding the infant. Besides the doctor or nurse helping the new mother with breastfeeding, the LaLeche League,* a support group for nursing mothers, is a good referral source.

Some mothers may feel guilty when unable, or choosing not, to breastfeed. These mothers need to know that the infant formulas are very nutritious and that if they hold their babies during feedings, they are giving their babies the same psychological advantages as those of a breastfed baby.

The transition period starts when solid food is introduced into the baby's diet, ideally when the baby is 5 to 6 months old. Illingsworth and Lester[17] believe that if solid food is not introduced by the time the average child is 6–7 months old, a "critical period" will be missed and feeding difficulties will ensue wih the child refusing to chew or vomiting when solids are given. Fomon *et al.*[18] are concerned about the introduction of beikost (foods other than milk or formula) before 5 months of age because the neuromuscular development at this age is too immature to allow the baby to indicate when he wants to eat and when he does not. This practice then becomes a type of forced feeding that can lead to overfeeding and in turn to obesity. Right from the beginning, infants should be allowed to stop eating at the earliest indication that they are full so as to learn not to overeat, avoiding all the long-term physical and emotional problems with which overweight children are confronted.

At about 8–12 months of age, self-feeding begins. Some parents have problems with the messiness of self-feeding. Besides eating the food, children are interested in its texture, smell, color, and so forth. Some parents may punish their child for playing with the food, when in fact this is normal behavior. Parents generally accept this stage more readily if they are forewarned and are told to put something around the highchair to protect the floor and to put a large bib on the child. It may be suggested to mothers to bathe their baby after eating rather than before. The more relaxed parents are at mealtimes, the less the child will use this time as a means of manipulating the family.

Food preferences also begin about this time. If a child refuses a type of food, the parents can offer it later. If a child continues to refuse a particular food, it may be best to plan meals avoiding that food. Parent-child altercations about food at this stage can be the start of life-long "who-is-in-control" problems.

The modified adult period usually begins after the first year. Most of the child's nutrients now come from table food, and the use of a spoon is usually mastered by 16 months of age.

Weaning from the bottle should also be in progress. Some children cling to their bottles for security. This is no problem if the child uses the bottle at mealtime or snack

---

*LaLeche League International, 9616 Minneapolis Avenue, Franklin Park, Illinois 60131; (312) 455-7730.

time on occasion. However, the child should never be allowed to drink from a bottle kept in the crib or to walk around with a bottle, sucking on it intermittently. Use of the bottle as a pacifier must be avoided. Milk caries[19] or iron deficiency anemia[20] may ensue from a diet largely composed of milk. Some mothers may actually discourage the child from weaning because of an unconscious wish to have the child remain a baby.[21] If the primary physician is unable to deal with this type of mother, professional counseling is indicated because the problem of infantilization will only get worse as time goes on.

LeBel and Zuckerman[21] outline some very practical suggestions for trying to prevent feeding problems:

1. Parental and sibling example are important in showing the child how to select food and to eat properly.
2. Parents should try not to nag, threaten, yell, or force-feed the child.
3. Parents should try to let children older than 9 months feed themselves as much as possible.
4. Parents should give the child small portions, which the child can finish.
5. Parents should allow the child some choice among equally nutritious foods.
6. Parents should praise children when they do well.
7. Parents should not be too rigid about certain foods; there are always substitute foods that will offer the needed nutrients.
8. Discipline should be consistent and short.
9. Meals should have a predetermined length. If everyone is finished and the child is still eating, the food should be removed, and the child is not allowed anything to eat until the next meal.
10. Desserts and snacks should be given only if the child has finished the meal. ("Junk food" should be discouraged for all children of any age.)
11. Parents should not insist that children clean their plates. (An exception would be an older child who has been warned that he has taken too much food and should put some back in the serving bowl, but refuses to do so.)
12. Use a highchair, as feeding on laps presents too many problems.
13. General approach to meals and feeding should be as consistent as possible.

Sleeping Disorders

The major sleep disorders at this age are getting the baby to go to sleep and stay asleep. By the time the infant is 3 months old, there should be wakefulness in the daytime and nighttime sleep.[22] Settling (sleeping from midnight to 5:00 A.M. for at least 4 weeks) occurs in 70% of infants by 3 months of age, in 83% by 6 months, and in 90% by 9 months. However, 50% of those who have settled begin to wake up during the night during the second half of the first year.[23]

Feeding and rocking will usually put the infant to sleep. As children become more mobile and inquisitive, however, they see sleep as an obstacle to be fought. Also, during the normal negativistic period ("terrible twos") children will make bedtime an issue just because the parents want them to go to bed.

Parents need to be forewarned about these bedtime problems. The child should be put in his crib, and the parents should leave the room. The child may cry, hoping for mother or father to return, but if the child knows that they will not return, he is more likely to go to sleep or to play quietly until he falls asleep. During this time rituals (e.g., storytelling, singing, cuddling) may have to be added to ease the transition from wakefulness to sleep. Parents must be warned not to overdo the rituals, as they will start taking longer and longer each night. Long afternoon naps can also cause bedtime problems.

Children awaken during the night for many reasons that are easily rectified: an itch, an erupting tooth, being too hot or too cold, hunger, noise, or too much light or darkness. However, other sources of night awakening relate more to rearing practices. Schmitt[24] describes trained night feeding and trained night crying as reasons for night awakening. Trained night feeding denotes a prolonged need for middle-of-the-night feeding (95% of infants can do without the 2 A.M. feeding by 4 months of age). This problem can be dealt with by giving a feeding right before the child is put to bed. A pacifier may help if the child is not hungry but just needs more sucking.

Trained night crying is seen in infants older than 4 months of age who continue to awaken during the night after they have given up their middle-of-the night feeding. Anders[25] found that 84% of 9-month-old infants awakened one or more times during the night for periods of 1–36 minutes (average 9 min); some cried, whereas others went back to sleep without crying. How the parents handle night waking with crying will influence whether this behavior becomes habitual. Obviously, if the child is in pain, has stuffed nasal passages, or has had a bowel movement, the situation should be rectified; the child should then be put back into his crib, and the parents should leave the room. If the parents give their children a lot of attention or bring them into their bed, the secondary gain will cause the behavior to persist. If nothing is bothering the child, the parents should just let him cry himself back to sleep. Many sleep related problems can be averted if parents are taught that there is no set amount of sleep a child of any age must have. Some children need more sleep and others less sleep than the average. A child who wakes up easily in the morning and does not appear sleepy during the day is getting sufficient sleep.

Breathholding

Seeing a child cry, hold his breath during expiration, turn blue, and possibly have convulsive movements is extremely frightening for parents. According to Lombroso and Lerman,[28] almost 5% of their large sample of children had breathholding spells, which they separated into the more common cyanotic type and the less common pallid type. Most spells had their onset between the ages of 6 and 18 months. Epilepsy and mental deficiency were unrelated to the attacks. A high familial incidence of breathholding was found. The major differential diagnosis of breathholding spells is epilepsy; differentiating factors are outlined in Table I.

Parents should be told that breathholding spells are essentially innocuous. Parents usually realize that frustration and anger typically precipitate the episodes and they need support in not reinforcing this behavior. As long as the child is protected from hurting himself, the parents should ignore these episodes and not allow the child to manipulate them in this way.

Head Banging

Head banging is a rhythmical motor habit characterized by repeated striking of the head against a solid object. The reported incidence of head banging varies from 3.3 to

Table I. Differential between Breathholding Spells and Epilepsy[a]

	Severe breathholding spells	Epilepsy
Precipitating factor	Always present	Usually not apparent in younger children
Crying	Almost always present before onset of convulsion	Not usually present
Cyanosis	Always occurs before loss of consciousness if cyanotic type; does not occur if pallid type	When present occasionally occurs at onset of seizure, but usually after attack has been in progress (prolonged seizure)
Opisthotonos	Usually present	Rarely occurs
EEG	Almost always normal	Usually abnormal, but may be normal

[a]Adapted from Livingston.[27]

15.2%.[28] Two studies[29,30] agreed on the following characteristics: (1) head banging typically begins at about 8 months of age and usually stops before age 4, (2) the male-to-female ratio is approximately 3 : 1, (3) most head bangers have previously displayed other rhythmical habits, (4) head banging usually takes place at bedtime but may also be seen when the child is upset or irritable.

The parents must be reassured that the child will outgrow this symptom and that no brain injury will occur. Music or a metronome[31] set to the rhythm of the head banging can be helpful. Kravitz et al.[29] believe that in severe chronic (beyond 3 years) cases of head banging, a neurological and psychiatric evaluation is indicated. In some such cases, they have had some success with various sedatives and tranquilizing drugs. If the child has other self-stimulative behaviors besides head banging (e.g., twirling, hand flapping) and/or difficulty in relating to the environment, pervasive developmental disorders including infantile autism, language difficulties, and mental retardation must be ruled out.

TODDLERS AND PRESCHOOLERS: 2–4 YEARS OLD

Temper Tantrums

Temper tantrums are very common in children between 1 and 4 years of age. Tantrums often start when children are denied something or do not get their way. Illness, fatigue, and hunger can also cause increased irritability. Children with delayed language development often have tantrums when they cannot make themselves understood. These outbursts of rage may also be an imitation of someone else in the household.

Honig[32] suggested that tantrums occur in the more active, outgoing, aggressive child, especially when there is a clash between the child's wants and those of the parents or when the child needs to obtain attention. Insecure children have an increased propensity toward tantrums. Parental attitudes and behavior such as overindulgence, excessive strictness, overprotectiveness, inconsistency, or unreasonable expectations can foster temper tantrums.

The best treatment is to decrease opportunities for the child to resort to temper tantrums. Child-proofing the environment enables children to explore without the parents constantly warning them of dangers. Toys and tasks that are age appropriate decrease frustration, which can lead to tantrums. If the child is doing something the parents do not want him to do, distracting him is preferable to just saying "no."

Bakwin and Bakwin[33] believe that the outbursts should be treated calmly and casually. Parents should be consistent and understanding and should not attempt to reason with the child during a tantrum.

If the tantrum is ignored and the child derives no benefit from it, there is less chance that it will be repeated. Children who see that their actions benefit them, that they get what they want through the tantrums, will probably persist in the behavior. Children must be protected from hurting themselves or someone else during a temper tantrum and may have to be removed to a safer place before being left alone to vent their anger. Parents can be reassured that violent temper tantrums are usually outgrown, and other forms of behavior are used to show anger and frustration as the child matures.

Thumb and Finger Sucking

All infants suck on their fingers, thumbs, hands, and even toes. The infant finding out about himself and about the world around him uses his mouth as one of the means to explore and to incorporate information. Sucking provides a feeling of security for the infant and a release from tension, supplements the oral gratification of feeding, and also promotes jaw and facial development.[34]

As the baby develops, other ways of learning and obtaining gratification become available. Thumb and finger sucking usually decrease and have stopped by the time the child reaches school age. Most children have ceased thumb sucking by about 3.8 years, although 2% will continue beyond age 13 despite the effects of peer pressure.[35]

Whether thumb sucking is a means of relieving anxiety for the child or is simply a habit is not well defined. It is probable that the behavior serves both functions, depending on the circumstances. While watching TV or drifting off to sleep, thumb sucking may be just a habitual response; when the child is being punished or is sick, it is probably a means of helping relieve the stress.

Parents should be reassured that thumb and finger sucking is normal and that probably no intervention is necessary before 4–6 years of age. Where there are no other behavioral problems, most children beyond age 4 can stop thumb sucking by being encouraged to use more age appropriate ways of handling stress and through behavior-management techniques.[36] Several dental appliances make thumb sucking so difficult that the child will stop. However, one wonders whether in some children the subsequent problems related to the child's inability to release anxiety may be more severe than the thumb sucking itself, especially if it served as a means of relieving tension for the child.

Sleeping Disorders

In children older than 2 years of age, physiological measures recorded during sleep have assumed adult forms, although the sleep stage proportions have not achieved adult ratios.[22] As in infancy, the major problems with sleep are getting the child to sleep and to stay asleep.

It is not in the child's best interest (or the parent's) to allow the child to be disruptive at bedtime. Bad bedtime habits will plague the parents for the remainder of childhood unless they gain control over the situation at this age. Parents need to set firm limits for the child. Bedtime need not be unpleasant. The parents can establish a rule that only after the child is in bed will they read a story, listen to a record, or sing a song.

Bedtime fears (e.g., of the dark, of nighttime intruders, shadows on the wall) begin at this age and may continue through to adolescence. Moving to a new house or sleeping in a strange room while visiting are both very disturbing to some children. Children need to know that their parents understand their fears and are there to protect them. A night light is usually of benefit. Sometimes just talking to the child about his/her fears and anxieties helps resolve them and enables the child to sleep. If the fears seem unconsolable, one of the parents might sit on a chair near the door so that the child can see him or her. The parent should not converse with the child but should rather read, sew, and so on until the child falls asleep.

Sleep disturbances such as nocturnal enuresis, nightmares, night terrors, sleepwalking, and sleeptalking begin during the preschool years. Excluding nightmares, these conditions are classified as non-rapid eye movement (NREM) dyssomnias[22] and are associated with emergence from stage 3–4 NREM sleep. A child may experience two or more of these disorders at different times. Often there is a positive family history. The disorders are paroxysmal, characterized by nonresponsiveness to the environment, the child's actions appear automatic, and there is retrograde amnesia for the episode.[37]

Night terrors and nightmares must be differentiated, as their treatment and course differ. Table II compares these two phenomena on several variables. In night terrors, the child suddenly sits up and screams. The child is unconsolable and cannot be awakened. There is increased autonomic discharge with tachycardia and tachypnea. These episodes, which can last for 10–20 min, disturb the parents more than the child, who does not remember anything the following morning. If these attacks are severe or frequent, diazepam[38] or imipramine[39] may be tried; dosage depends on the age of the child. Diazepam reduced night terrors by 80% in adults.

Nightmares are vividly recalled if they awaken the child; most are remembered the next day. Some children become so frightened by the experience that they have trouble falling asleep. Parents should be sympathetic; the child should be told that nightmares are imaginary and cannot hurt them.

Although sleepwalking and sleeptalking occur primarily in the school age child, they

Table II. Comparison of Nightmares and Night Terrors

	Nightmares	Night terrors
Stage of sleep	REM	Stage 3–4 NREM
Amount of anxiety	++	+++
Amount of autonomic discharge	+	+++
Amount of motility	+	+++
Amount of vocalization	±	+++
Amnesia	No	Yes
Ability to be awakened	Easy	Difficult

are occasionally seen in preschoolers. Guillenault and Anders[37] estimate that 15% of all children between the ages of 5 and 12 have walked in their sleep at least once. The episode may last 15–30+ minutes if actual walking occurs rather than just sitting up in bed. Parents must protect the child from hurting himself. Sleeptalkers usually mumble and make little sense. Purposeful speech and walking during sleeptime, unlike the NREM syndromes, suggest psychological disorders, for which a more intensive evaluation is in order.

Sibling Rivalry: Birth of New Baby

Sibling rivalry is easier to control with careful preparation than to have to deal with a child who hates his new sibling. Careful preparation of the child for the new arrival helps keep jealousy and feelings of being displaced to a minimum.

If the older child is still in the nursery or the crib that will be used for the new baby, the child's room should be changed and the child should be put into a regular bed before being told about the new baby. Making the transition from crib to a "big person's bed" and out of the nursery into another "special bedroom reserved for a big boy or girl" are important events in the child's life. If the child feels that these moves are being made for the baby, he will be resentful and less accepting of the changes. If a fuss is made about how big the child is getting and how he needs a big room with a big bed, the child will feel positive about the moves. Allowing the child to help pick out a new bed or to help decide on the color of the new room adds to the excitement and acceptance of the changes and of growing up.

It is better for the parents not to ask whether the child wants a new baby. The child may say "no!" The child should be told that mommy and daddy have decided to have another baby, someone for the older child to play with when the baby gets older. It is important to explain that newborn babies are unable to do anything except eat, sleep, cry, and mess their diapers, lest the child be disappointed in the new "playmate." The parents should not promise a brother or a sister unless they actually know the sex of the fetus. It is much better for them to reply, "I know that you would like a baby brother (sister), but we won't know what it is until it is born."

The older child should be an integral part of the preparations for the new baby. The child can be given the opportunity to make the choice in such things as the color of a jumpsuit or may even be given the opportunity to buy a gift for the new baby.

Arrangements should be made in advance for taking care of the child while the mother is in the hospital. If a close relative or familiar babysitter is not available, the person who will care for the child should be introduced to the child and the child's routine in advance so that they can get to know each other well. The child's daily routine should be kept as constant as possible after the baby's arrival. If the child is already in a day-care situation, this should be continued even if the mother plans to be home. If the child asks to stay home, however, probably wondering what mother does at home when he is at the day care center, the child should be allowed to stay home to see what is going on. Usually, after a few boring days at home the child decides that it is more fun to go to day care, where his friends are.

Many hospitals are now allowing children to visit their mothers and to see the new arrival in the nursery. This is an excellent idea in helping the other children feel a part of the event. Also, the anxiety related to separation from mother and worrying about mother is relieved when the child can actually see her. When it is time to bring the new baby home, it is nice if there is a present for the older child from the baby. A doll that looks like a newborn is a nice idea, as the older child can do with the doll what the mother is doing for the infant (e.g., bathe, feed, change diaper). If a doll is an inappropriate gift, something the child desires as a present from the new arrival is a way of lessening the threat of the baby as seen by the older child.

The older child should be included in the baby's care. He can get the needed diaper, or hold the bottle if he wants to. Parents should not use the child as an errand boy, because the child will feel that he is being used and will resent it. If the child desires, he should be allowed to hold the new baby. If the parents worry whether the child can support the infant properly, the infant can be laid on a pillow in the child's arms.

If the mother is breastfeeding, the older child may ask whether he can taste the milk. If the mother is too embarrased to let the older child suck at her breast, she can hand-express some milk onto a spoon or into a cup so that the older child can taste the milk. One taste usually satisfies the older child that his regular food tastes better than the baby's milk.

It is good for the parents to relate that they remember when the older child did such and such like the new baby, but how much better they like him grown up. It is even a nice idea to get out the baby pictures of the older child to show him what he was like as an infant. Yet the parents must give positive reinforcement to the older child for being older and for growing up; otherwise, the child will resent the baby and will regress to babyish behavior (e.g., wetting his pants, babyish talk). If regression does occur, the parents should not become overly concerned but should tell the older child how much they like him the way he is and to give him extra privileges or things to do (i.e., go to the movies or out to eat)—things only "big kids" can do.

Physical aggression against the new baby cannot be allowed. The child can be encouraged to take out his aggression on a doll or a punching bag. A jog around the neighborhood with father is another way of dealing with negative feelings. If the child feels neglected and unimportant, he may become quiet and withdrawn. The parents should sit down and help him express his feelings. Making sure the older child has some time alone with at least one parent on a regular basis is highly recommended. While the baby is napping is a good time to give the older child some special attention.

As the children get older, bickering and fighting with each other become more prominent. The parents have to understand that this is normal behavior; and unless one child is injuring the other, the parents should allow the children to resolve their own conflicts. Taking sides is one way the parents can increase sibling rivalry.

SCHOOL-AGE CHILDREN: 5–12 YEARS OLD

This portion of a child's life is when the child starts to learn the skills that will sustain him from now on. Erickson[40] calls this psychosocial stage *industry versus inferiority*. In other words, if the child learns how to read, write, and how to do basic mathematics he has the basic tools for most careers. The greatest danger for a child in this stage is that he will feel inferior to his peers rather than competent. Many behavioral problems seen during this age are a result of this conflict within the child regarding his self-perception.

Problems with Toileting

Enuresis and encopresis are fairly frequent behavioral problems brought to the attention of the physician. Enuresis is the discharge of urine, and encopresis is the discharge of feces in places not considered proper for elimination. There are both primary and secondary enuresis and encopresis. Primary enuresis/encopresis refers to a child who has never gained bladder/bowel control either during the day (diurnal) or at night (nocturnal); whereas secondary enuresis/encopresis occurs in a child who had control for a period (4–6 months) and then started wetting/soiling again.

Enuresis

According to McLaine,[41] the incidence of enuresis is about 19% of the children between the ages of 4 and 5 and decreases with increasing age (8% at age 8 and 5% at age 10). About 1–2% of adolescents remain enuretic. Enuresis is seen more often in boys and in children with a positive family history. Enuresis is primary in about 75% of the cases. About 80% of enuretic children have nocturnal enuresis alone; 5% have diurnal enuresis alone, and 15% have both nocturnal and diurnal enuresis. About 15% of the enuretic children also have encopresis. Leventhal[42] writes that secondary enuresis occurs commonly in school-age children; 5–20% of children who were dry at age 5 relapse before the age of 11 years. Diurnal enuresis, especially if it is secondary, is considered a more serious problem than nocturnal enuresis, and psychological factors should be considered.

After age 6 years, about 15% per year of enuretic children spontaneously stop wetting, supporting developmental or neuromaturational delay as a major etiological factor in enuresis. Starfield[43] found that enuretic children had a significantly smaller volume of urine per voiding than their nonenuretic siblings, pointing to a functionally small bladder capacity in enuresis. Furthermore, enuretic children have daytime urgency and frequency which goes along with the smaller bladder capacity.

After all organic causes for the enuresis have been eliminated, the question of treatment arises. First, the child must be told that bedwetting is a fairly common problem, and then he should be asked if he wants help in trying to stop the bedwetting. Unless the child takes an active interest, no form of treatment will be effective. The major treatment methods include behavior modification, conditioning, bladder training, medication, and counseling.

Behavior modification can involve either positive or negative reinforcement; the former is usually more successful. Putting a star or stickers on the calendar to signify nights when the bed is kept dry is very encouraging to children. Moreover, most children will try very hard to stay dry if they are also working for small prizes (e.g., a pack of gum, barrettes, matchbox car) for keeping dry. The number of dry nights needed for each subsequent prize should be increased. The older child (8 years and up) should also take responsibility for taking the wet sheets off the bed, letting the bed air out, putting the sheets and wet pajamas in the laundry room, and washing himself off before dressing. These chores may be seen by some children as punishment, but they must be told that if they wish to go to sleep in a clean bed they need to accept some responsibility for helping with this chore.

In conditioning, another approach to behavior modification, an alarm awakens the child when he/she wets the bed. The initial aim of this treatment is to awaken the child as soon as urination begins; the ultimate goal is to have the child awaken before voiding. The alarm system works best in children over 7 years of age and probably should not be used in children under 5 years of age.

Bladder training or stretching is a way of increasing the functional capacity of the bladder. The child is told to drink as much as possible during the day and to hold his urine for increasing lengths of time, up to a maximum of 30–40 min. Once a day the child should hold his urine as long as possible; the voided urine should then be measured. With bladder capacities above 240–360 ml, bedwetting may stop.

Imipramine hydrochloride has been shown to be effective in helping children stop bedwetting.[41] Its mechanism of action is unknown, although there has been much speculation. The major drawback to this approach is that once the imipramine is stopped, a large percentage of children start wetting again. For occasional or short-term use (e.g., overnight camp, staying overnight at a friend's), imipramine may be the treatment of choice. The dosage is 1–3 mg/kg about ½ hr before bedtime. The side effects are mostly due to the anticholinergic properties: irritability, dry mouth, sleep disturbances, constipation, tachycardia, orthostatic hypotension, urinary retention, and blurred vision.

Counseling is usually provided in conjunction with the above mentioned treatments. It includes telling the child that he is normal and that a lot of children his age wet their beds. If the parents were bedwetters, the child can be told this and will usually feel better about himself. Hypnosis may be used as an adjunct to counseling. If serious psychopathology is suspected, referral to an appropriate person for evaluation and therapy is indicated.

Encopresis

The incidence of encopresis is approximately 1.5%, with a male-to-female ratio of 6:1.[36] Encopresis may or may not be associated with constipation. If constipation is present, prolonged retention of stool leads to impaction, rectal distention, loss of bowel tone, and, finally, functional megacolon. The large amount of stool in the rectum produces a partially dilated anal sphincter with subsequent intermittent leakage of liquid stool and mucus flowing around the impaction.

Evaluation involves a complete history, including psychosocial factors and physical examination. A plain film of the abdomen may be obtained to assess degree of stool retention and the existence of functional megacolon.

Treatment includes emptying the colon of any retained stool, keeping the stools soft, and training the child in regular bowel habits. If encopresis in which stools of normal caliber are passed without evidence of constipation, a behavioral approach is recommended, such as using the star chart for positive reinforcement. In the case of chronic impaction with stool withholding and overflow soiling, many different approaches have been used in dealing with this problem and the reader is referred to Levine,[44] Gabel,[45] or Whitington[56] for treatment protocols. Encopresis has a fairly high relapse rate. If significant resistance is met in the child or family regarding treatment, or if psychosocial problems appear to be at the root of the problem, referral to a psychiatrist is in order.

Aggressive Behavior

The aggressive behaviors which are of most concern at this age are cruelty to animals, fire setting, and fighting/bullying. All are serious; cruelty to animals and fire setting require consultation with a specialist as well as immediate therapy.

Cruelty to animals is often associated with other signs of poor control over aggressive impulses. In Felthous's study,[46] men who as boys had tortured dogs were more aggressive against people than those who had tortured cats. Also, those who actually killed the animals were more aggressive against humans than were those who did not. This behavior is usually seen in boys who come from unstable homes with aggressive role models. Absent father figures, either from alcoholism or separation, may have a role in both cruelty to animals and fire setting.

Children are fascinated by fires and will light matches and watch them burn or set paper on fire in an ashtray or sink. Usually these small fires are easily extinguished and are not serious. Lewis and Yarnell[47] described the school-age fire setters they saw as average or below average in intelligence; 15% were enuretic, and many had a history of other antisocial acts. Yarnell[48] wrote that fire setting in the latency-age child is an aggressive act directed at a family member in order to accomplish a desired end such as punishing a parent for disapproving of the child. Vandersall and Wiener's[49] population of fire setters came from homes with significant amounts of parental psychopathology. Fire setting was usually only one of many behavioral problems manifested by these children. A sense of exclusion, loneliness, and unfulfilled dependency needs was prominent. The one consistent factor in all the incidents was a temporary breakdown of the child's impulse controls. Bakwin and Bakwin[50] list these four motivations for fire setting in preadolescents: vengeance, compensatory behavior for feelings of guilt, resentment against home or school, and identification with firemen. Professional therapy is indicated for all children who set serious fires.

Most children who pick fights and bully other children have poor self-esteem. Since they tend to choose smaller or younger opponents, they usually win the fights, which increases their self-concept. Although one occasionally sees a very aggressive girl, most of this behavior is seen in boys. Children who resort to fighting usually come from families where physical assault is a means of communication; child abuse should be considered and looked for. In some cases, the families are so chaotic that there are no limits on the child; the fighting is a call for help, a plea for structure. Moreover, the bully is usually an unhappy and lonely child; other children are reluctant to play with him, and neighborhood children are usually warned by their parents to stay away from him. Constant fighting is a sign of deeper problems. If the primary physician is unable to find out what is bothering the child, the child and his family should be referred for professional counseling.

Antisocial Behavior

Most children will do some lying, stealing, or running away at some point during their childhood. This is usually only an occasional occurrence. The children use these behaviors to test the limits of their environment. Parents bring these behaviors to the attention of their doctor when they become chronic, out of control, and disruptive to the child and/or functioning of the family.

Lying

Children below the age of 5 are not able reliably to separate fact from fiction. They make mistakes in their choice of words, and they enjoy exaggerating. Although this may lead to untruthfulness, their goal is not to deceive. Parents should be told that their preschooler is not lying when he makes up fantastic stories. This is a normal part of development. The parents need only help the child see the difference between reality and fantasy. The understanding of truthfulness is generally attained by age 6 or 7 years.

Bakwin and Bakwin[50] enumerate the different types of lies children tell. Imitative lies are those in which the child copies a parent who may exaggerate or color events to make a story more interesting to others. The child realizes that things did not happen that way as they are being described, yet is not mature enough to understand "artistic license." When a parent tells a "white lie," the child will recognize that it is not the truth and may then feel that lying is right. An offshoot of this category is the lie of exaggeration, bragging. This type of lying may get children in trouble with their friends but otherwise is not serious. As with all lying, however, children have to be told that they should only tell the truth.

Children usually lie to escape punishment. If one truly suspects a child of wrongdoing, it is better not to ask the child if he did something wrong since the temptation to lie is too great for most children. Rather, the parents should confront the child with the error and punish if necessary. If a child tries to lie about something the parents are sure he did, he should be punished for the lie as well as for the act.

Children should not be asked to make promises, since most do not understand this concept. In this way, children are not put in the position of being thought of as liars when they do not keep their promises.

Lying can be a means of getting attention. In families where the children do not get much attention, some resort to misbehaviors for which they know that they will be punished. These children feel that even negative attention is better than no attention.

Revenge is another motive for lying. Children will lie to "get even" with parents, siblings, and others. They will make up stories to get other people, or even themselves, into trouble. The child derives a feeling of importance when his lie is believed. Very often vengeful feelings arise in response to overly authoritative parents. Lies are also used to avoid compliance with a request or to deliberately provoke another person. These are called antagonistic lies.

Children frequently lie in order to win admiration and praise. Sometimes the lies are excuses for failure or are substitutions for what the child is unable to do. The parents need to accept the child for what the child is, not for what they want the child to be. Also, the child has to accept himself and his limitations. This is an area in which the primary physician can prevent a lot of future problems by being attuned to parents' tendencies to push children beyond their capabilities and to the child's failure to accept himself. When children lie chronically, an effort should be made to try to find out why the child lies. Psychiatric help may be necessary if the lying cannot be controlled. The pathological liar of adolescence and adulthood began as a child telling falsehoods.

Stealing

Stealing is a common behavior of childhood and usually is innocuous. Children younger than 6 years do not understand the concept of property rights. Children raised in crowded environments who have little privacy also have trouble learning this concept. Other children may have been taught to share their belongings and expect others to share with them, to the point of taking others' possessions without asking, which can be interpreted as stealing but which the child would consider only borrowing.

School-age children who knowingly steal usually do so for three reasons: to bribe other children, to possess the stolen article, or to express negative feelings toward their parents.[50] A child who steals to bribe other children usually feels inadequate in some way and may have been teased by other children for some reason or other. The bribes are the child's way of trying to gain peer acceptance. Some children succeed in bribing their way to popularity, as children like to receive gifts and will be friendly toward a child who gives them gifts. These children need help in realizing that bribery is not a good way to obtain friends and that whatever defect they see in themselves is either correctable or should be accepted. The child needs to know that he is an important person regardless of his imperfections.

Stealing as an outlet for vengeful feelings is done mainly to annoy the parents. The child may feel that he has not been treated fairly by his parents. The parents may be too authoritative, making the child account for everything he does and, in fact, may not be fair to the child. Children who revolt in whatever fashion against an overly authoritative parent may grow up to disregard authority and law enforcement. Such parents need help in understanding the difference between legitimate and excessive limits on their children.

No matter what the reason behind the stealing, children have to know that stealing is wrong and will not be tolerated. They must be taught that stealing is not only acquiring an object but also depriving someone else of it. The child's possessions should not be disturbed without his permission (except if taken away as a punishment), and the child should be expected not to bother other people's possessions. The reason for the stealing should be explored and corrected if possible. The stolen object should be returned by the child with an apology or, if return is not possible, the owner should be reimbursed by the child from his own money, if possible. Moreover, the parents should look at their own behavior and see whether they are giving a covert message to their children that stealing is all right (e.g., cheating on income taxes, bringing home goods from work).

Running Away

The most frequent reason for running away is anger or resentment toward the parents or some other dissatisfaction with the home. Most runaways are adolescents, but this behavior is occasionally seen in a school-age child or preadolescent. Usually they do not go far and will return when hungry, tired, or cold. The parents should show an understanding of why they think the child felt the need to run away. If the problem can be corrected, it should be.

Child abuse and/or sexual abuse should be suspected in the chronic runaway. If things are really bad at home, these children may be better in foster placement or in a boarding school. However, if the children feel that problems can only be solved by running away, they may resort to running away no matter where they are; more intensive work with such children is indicated.

Fears

All normal children have fears at some point in their development. Fears can range from the stranger anxiety seen in the infant to the jitters experienced before the first date. Most fears are outgrown in the normal course of development. A few children, however, experience fears of such magnitude or severity that they are brought to the attention of the physician.

Lapouse and Monk[51] found that what the child feared was dependent on the age of the child as was the number of fears. Younger children feared loud noises, lightning, strangers, and unfamiliar objects. Fears of specific animals peaked at 4 years of age. Older children feared the dark, death, being ridiculed, examinations, imaginary creatures, and robbers. The younger children had more fears. Berecz's[52] excellent review article cited a number of studies showing an increase of fears at about 11 years of age. Although no reason was given, one wonders whether developing sexuality or entrance into junior high school might be involved.

According to the work of Angelino et al.,[53] the content of the child's fear differs according to the family's socioeconomic status. The poorer children had more fears of the supernatural, mysterious events, parental quarrels, examinations, noise, and punishment. Children of a higher socioeconomic class feared car accidents, juvenile delinquency, and school accidents. The fear of darkness was observed equally in all social classes.

Pozanski[54] noted that children with excessive fears tended to have the onset of their fears associated with a definite historical event. Most of the children who were excessively fearful seemed to have more than the usual amount of anxiety before the onset of the excessive fears, and a mild situational stress precipitated a more open display of fears and anxiety. She was also able to loosely divide the fears into three categories: fears of abandonment, fears of mutilation, and sexualized fears. Most of the children expressed more than one category of fear and 75% had a marked increase in fearful behavior at night.

What can be done about the fear, or whether anything needs to be done, is dependent on the child's stage of development and whether the fears are interfering with the functioning of the child and/or his family. The young child clinging to mother when a stranger is present is engaging in normal behavior; this behavior is abnormal in the older school-age child. Nothing beyond some words of comfort may need to be given to the urban child with a fear of snakes, whereas the southern rural child who refuses to leave the home because of a fear of snakes needs more aggressive intervention.

The treatment methods that have dominated the literature are psychoanalysis and behavioral techniques. Most methods involve having the child confront the feared object or situation and then learn how to cope with it.

Shirley[55] advises that handicapping fears should be considered with understanding and sympathy. He advocates encouraging the child to talk about the fears. Sometimes the fear is due to misinformation; when this is corrected, the fear disappears. When fears are persistent, severe, or affect the child's development, however, referral to a mental health professional is indicated.

SUMMARY

In concluding this chapter it should be emphasized that common behavioral problems of childhood are so designated *because* they are common. Most children will at one time or other manifest some of the behaviors discussed in this chapter. The behaviors are usually not problems in themselves, but how the parents interpret them and how the behaviors affect the child and his relationship with his family, school, and friends are significant. The physician cannot evaluate these behaviors without also asking about these other aspects. If guidance from the primary physician is ineffectual in eliminating the behavior or helping the child and parents understand the behavior, then referral to someone who is trained in this area (e.g., psychiatrist, psychologist, social worker, guidance counselor) is indicated.

REFERENCES

1. Thomas, A., Chess, S., and Birch, H. G.: *Temperament and Behavior Disorders in Children.* New York University Press, New York, 1968.
2. Carey, W. B.: Clinical applications of infant temperament measurements. *J. Pediatr.* **81:**823–828, 1972.
3. Carey, W. B., and McDevitt, S. C.: Stability and changes in individual temperament diagnoses from infancy to early childhood. *J. Am. Acad. Child. Psychiatry* **17:**331–337, 1978.
4. Brazelton, T. B.: Crying in infancy. *Pediatrics* **29:**579–588, 1962.
5. Bell, S. M., and Ainsworth, M.: Infant crying and maternal responsiveness. *Child Dev.* **43:**1171–1190, 1972.
6. Garretson, J. F.: Paroxysmal crying and colic in infants, in Block, R. W., and Rash, F. C. (eds.): *Handbook of Behavioral Pediatrics,* Yearbook Medical, Chicago, 1981, pp. 70–75.
7. Wessell, M. A., Cobb, J. C., Jackson, E. B., *et al.*: Paroxysmal fussing in infancy, sometimes called colic. *Pediatrics* 14:421–435, 1954.
8. Zuckerman, B. S.: Crying and colic, in Gabel, S. (ed.): *Behavioral Problems in Childhood: A Primary Care Approach.* Grune & Stratton, New York, 1981, pp. 167–180.
9. O'Donovan, J. C., and Bradstock, A. S.: The failure of conventional drug therapy in the management of infantile colic. *Am. J. Dis. Child.* **133:**999–1001, 1979.
10. American Academy of Pediatrics Committee on Nutrition: On the feeding of supplemental foods to infants. *Pediatrics* **65:**1178–1181, 1980.
11. Berger, L. R.: Factors influencing breastfeeding. *J. Cont. Ed. Pediatr.* **20:**13–29, 1978.
12. Newton, N., and Newton, M.: Psychologic aspects of lactation. *N. Engl. J. Med.* **277:**1179–1188, 1967.
13. American Academy of Pediatrics Committee on Nutrition: Nutrition and lactation. *Pediatrics* **68:**435–441, 1981.
14. Jelliffe, D. B., and Jelliffe, E. F. D.: "Breast is best": Modern meanings. *N. Engl. J. Med.* **297:**912–915, 1977.
15. Nichols, B. L., and Nichols, V. N.: Lactation, in Barness, L. (ed.): *Advances in Pediatrics,* Vol. 26. Yearbook Medical, Chicago, 1979, pp. 137–161.
16. Kemberling, S. R. Supporting breast-feeding. *Pediatrics* **63:**60–63, 1979.
17. Illingsworth, R. S., and Lister, M. B.: The critical or sensitive period, with special reference to certain feeding problems in infants and children. *J. Pediatr.* **65:**839–848, 1964.
18. Fomon, S. J., Filer, L. J., Anderson, T. A., *et al.*: Recommendations for feeding normal infants. *Pediatrics* **63:**52–59, 1979.
19. Nowak, A. J.: Pediatric dentistry: Part I—The pre-eruption and eruption periods (birth to 36 months). *J. Cont. Ed. Pediatr.* **21:**11–22, 1979.
20. Dallman, P. R.: Nutritional anemias, in Rudolph, A.M. (ed.): *Pediatrics.* 17th ed. Appleton-Century-Crofts, East Norwalk, Connecticut, 1982,
21. LeBel, J., and Zuckerman, B. S.: Feeding problems, obesity, in Gabel, S. (ed.): *Behavioral Problems in Childhood, a Primary Care Approach.* Grune & Stratton, New York, 1981, pp. 181–194.

22 Anders, T F and Weinstein, P Sleep and its disorders in infants and children A review *Pediatrics* **50:**312–324, 1972
23 Moore, T , and Ucko, C Night waking in early infancy Part I *Arch Dis Child* **33:**333–342, 1957
24 Schmitt, B Infants who do not sleep through the night *J Dev Behav Pediat* **2:**20–23, 1981
25 Anders, T F Night waking in infants during the first year of life *Pediatrics* **63:**860–864, 1979
26 Lombroso, C T , and Lerman, P Breath-holding spells (cyanotic and pallid infantile syncope) *Pediatrics* **39:**563–581, 1967
27 Livingston, S Breath-holding spells in children. differentiation from epileptic attacks *J A M A* **212:**2231–2235, 1970
28 Sallustro, F , and Atwell, C W Body rocking, head banging, and head rolling in normal children *J Pediat* **93:**704–708, 1978
29 Kravitz, H , Rosenthal, V , Teplitz, A , et al A study of head banging in infants and children *Dis Nerv Svst* **21:**203–208, 1960
30 deLissovoy, V Head banging in early childhood *Child Dev* **33:**43–56, 1962
31 Lourie, R S The role of rhythmic patterns in childhood *Am J Psychiatry* **105:**653–660, 1949
32 Honig, T Temper tantrums *Curr Prob Pediatr* **5:**77–78, 1975
33 Bakwin, H , and Bakwin, R M *Behavior Disorders in Children* 4th ed WB Saunders, Philadelphia, 1972
34 Honig T Thumb-sucking and finger-sucking *Curr Prob Pediatr* **5:**78–79, 1975
35 Block, R W , and Rash, F C *Handbook of Behavioral Pediatrics* Yearbook Medical, Chicago, 1981
36 Telzrow, R W Habit patterns, in Gabel, S (ed) *Behavioral Problems in Childhood A Primary Care Approach* Grune & Stratton, New York, 1981, pp 307–315
37 Guilleminault, C , and Anders, T F Sleep disorders in children *Adv Pediatr* **22:**151–174, 1976
38 Fisher, C , Kahn, E , and Edwards, A A psychophysiological study of nightmares and night terrors, the suppression of stage 4 night terrors with diazepam *Arch Gen Psychiatry* **28:**252–259, 1973
39 Pesikoff, R B , and Davis, P C Treatment of pavornocturnus and somnambulism in children *Am J Psychiatry* **128:**778–781, 1971
40 Erickson, E H *Childhood and Society*, 2nd ed Norton, New York, 1963
41 McLain, L G Childhood enuresis, in Gluck, L (ed) *Current Problems in Pediatrics* Yearbook Medical, Chicago, 1979 pp 1–36
42 Leventhal, J M Enuresis, in Gabel, S (ed) *Behavioral Problems in Childhood* Grune & Stratton, New York, 1981, 195–211
43 Starfield, B Functional bladder capacity in enuretic and non-enuretic children *J Pediat* **70:**777–781, 1967
44 Levine, M D Encopresis Its potentiation, evaluation and alleviation *Pediatr Clin North Am* **29:**315–330, 1982
45 Gabel, S Fecal soiling, chronic constipation and encopresis, in Gabel, S (ed) *Behavioral Problems in Childhood A Primary Care Approach* New York, Grune & Stratton, 1981, pp 213–228
46 Felthous, A R Aggression against cats, dogs and people *Child Psychol Hum Dev* **10:**169–177, 1979
47 Lewis, N D C , and Yarnell, H Pathological fire setting (pyromania) Nervous and Mental Disease Monographs, 82, 1951
48 Yarnell, H Fire setting in children *Am J Orthopsychiatry* **10:**262–286, 1940
49 Vandersall, T A , and Wiener, J M Children who set fires *Arch Gen Psychiatry* **22:**63–71 1970
50 Bakwin, H , and Bakwin, R M Lying, stealing, running away, fire setting, homicide, antisocial personality, in Bakwin, H , and Bakwin, R M (eds) *Behavior Disorders in Children* 4th ed W B Saunders, Philadelphia, 1972, pp 586–601
51 Lapouse, R , and Monk, M Fears and worries in a representative sample of children *Am J Orthopsychiatry* **29:**803–818, 1959
52 Berecz, J M Phobias of childhood Etiology and treatment *Psychol Bull* **70:**694–720, 1968
53 Angelino, H , Dollins, J , and Mech, E Trends in the "fears and worries" of school children as related to socioeconomic status and age *J Genet Psychol* **89:**263–275, 1956
54 Pozanski, E D Children with excessive fears *Am J Orthopsychiatry* **43:**428–438, 1973
55 Shirley, H F *Pediatric Psychiatry* Harvard University Press, Cambridge, Massachusetts, 1963

Emotional Disorders of Childhood

William C. Adamson

INTRODUCTION: SELF-CONCEPT

The nature and acceptance of the sense of ''self'' as a psychological concept and mental construct have gone through many metamorphoses. Cohen[1] observed that from Aristotle's

William C. Adamson • Department of Mental Health Sciences, Hahnemann University, Philadelphia, Pennsylvania 19102.

de Anima through the metapsychology of Descartes, "the self was the locus of feelings, initiatives, and passions." He then commented that "after falling into disrepute in certain circles, the concept of the self has recently been resurrected in psychoanalysis, invigorated by the new type of observations which clinical inquiry provides."

Kohut's[2] monograph provided the stimulus for re-examining the meaning and place of the self in the development of both clinical theory and personality issues. A brief historical account is outlined in the following section. First, however, the term should be defined within the context of current usage. According to colloquial meaning, Webster's Dictionary[3] defines the noun "self" as "one's individual person or the subject of individual consciousness."

Beres[4] wrote that the term "self" is a multifaceted abstraction that is difficult to define. It is generally used with the addition of a prefix or suffix such as self-concept, self-esteem, or self-awareness. He also suggested the following distinction between the terms "self" and "ego": *self* to indicate a complex of subjective experiences and functions; *ego* to designate certain functions which are grouped together in conflict and adaptation.

Historical Perspective on Self and Object Theory

In his prologue to the volume *The Evolving Self,* Kegan[5] outlined several psychological traditions that have focused on personality development and on issues related to the "self," the "person," and the "ego." Table I is a compilation of the theorists most closely associated with each psychological tradition and the title of their major work.

Evaluation of the Self-concept Theories

Freud began with his ambitious project for a scientific psychology in 1895. He was seeking a quantitative approach for understanding and elaborating on the nature of psychic functioning, which he called "a kind of economics of nerve force." In 1915 he offered a metapsychological theory of instincts and their vicissitudes, focusing more on the intrapsychic topographical structures of the conscious and unconscious mind. His 1923 paper on "The Ego and the Id" laid the foundation for the development of ego psychology that was to follow; here he used the German form *das ich* to mean "one's own person." In critiquing the psychoanalytic theories of the self, Ticho[6] observed that Freud continued to use the German *ich* in three ways: "first, to signify the individual (as a person); second, as part of the psychic structure; and third, as the experiencing, subjective self."

William James[7] is generally identified as the earliest "self" psychologist. In 1890 he developed an "I—me" dichotomy: the "self-as-knower" and the "self-that-is-known." Damon and Hart[8] wrote an excellent review on James's theory focused on self-understanding, which they view as the cognitive basis for self-conception. Within this frame of reference, the self as a cognitive concept is analyzed in its diverse components (see Table II). Damon and Hart then summarize the empirical studies of self-understanding in infants, children, and adolescents. Their findings and commentary have been used as background in the discussion of self-concept in this chapter.

The tradition of theorizing about the self in social psychology goes back to Mead's *Mind, Self, and Society.*[9] Rogers's clinical application of a self-psychology in his client-centered therapy[10] also had an impact on thinking about the self. The recent interest in the

Table I. Historical Perspectives in Self–Object Theory

Author	Year	Titles
Psychoanalytic Psychology		
Freud	1895	*Project for a Scientific Psychology*
	1914	*On Narcissism*
	1923	*The Ego and the Id*
Neopsychoanalytic Ego Psychology		
A. Freud	1936	*Ego and the Mechanisms of Defense*
Hartman	1939	*Ego Psychology and the Problem of Adaptation*
Schilder	1950	*The Image and the Appearance of the Human Body*
Erikson	1950	*Childhood and Society*
G. Klein	1966	*Perspectives to Change in Psychoanalytic Theory*
Kris	1975	*Selected Papers of Ernst Kris*
Loevinger	1976	*Ego Development*
Neopsychoanalytic Object Relations Theory		
Rank	1936	*Truth and Reality*
	1941	*Beyond Psychology*
Jacobson	1964	*The Self and the Object World*
Sandler and Rosenblatt	1962	*The Concept of the Representational World*
Lichtenstein	1963	*The Dilemma of Human Identity: Notes on Self-transformation, Self-objectivation, and Metamorphosis*
Winnicott	1965	*The Maturational Process and the Facilitating Environment*
Mahler and Furor	1968	*On Human Symbiosis and the Vicissitudes of Individuation*
Schafer	1968	*Aspects of Internalization*
Guntrip	1968	*Schizoid Phenomena, Object Relations, and the Self*
Kohut	1971	*The Analysis of the Self*
	1977	*The Restoration of the Self*
Kernberg	1976	*Object Relations: Theory and Clincial Psychoanalysis*
Tolpin	1971	*On the Beginnings of a Chohesive Self*
Gedo and Goldberg	1973	*Models of the Mind: A Psychoanalytic Theory*
Lichtenberg	1975	*The Development of the Sense of Self*
Existential–Phenomenological Psychology		
Lecky	1945	*Self-consistency*
Rogers	1951	*Client Centered Therapy*
Maslow	1954	*Motivation and Personality*
May *et al.*	1958	*Existence: A New Dimension in Psychiatry and Psychology*
Binswanger	1963	*Being-in-the-World*
Angyal	1965	*Neurosis and Treatment: A Holistic Theory*
Constructive–Developmental Psychology		
Baldwin	1906	*Social and Ethical Interpretation in Mental Development*
Mead	1934	*Mind, Self, and Society*
Piaget	1936	*The Origins of Intelligence in Children*
Dewey	1938	*Experience and Education*
Kohlberg	1968	*Stage and Sequence: The Cognitive Developmental Approach to Socialization*
Kegan	1979	*The Evolving Self: A Process Concept for Ego Psychology*
Selman	1981	*The Growth of Interpersonal Understanding: Developmental and Clinical Analyses*
Kegan	1982	*The Evolving Self*

Table II. William James's Theory of Self

Focus	Functions	Attributes
Self as known "Me" (objective)	Physical self	Body properties
	Social self	Relationships, rules, social personality, moral choices
	Psychological self	Consciousness, feelings, moods, all cognition: knowledge, learned skills, motivation, communicative skills, social sensitivity
	Active self[a]	Capacities, typical behavior patterns at age-appropriate levels
Self as knower "I" (subjective)	Continuity	Consistent feelings of individuality
	Distinctness	Unique individuality
	Volition	Personal "willing"[b]
	Self-reflection	Second-order awareness

[a]Added to James's triad by Damon and Hart.[8]
[b]Developed by O. Rank into a psychology of the will.[10]

subject of narcissism and the dialogue about the place for the "self" within the matrix of analytic theory was largely initiated by the provocative writings of Kohut, including *The Analysis of Self*.[2]

While recognizing that any schematic representation of such a highly complex and amorphous psychological construct as the "self" is reductionistic, the hypothetical constructs of Erikson,[11] Loevinger,[12] Selman,[13] and Kegan[5] have been integrated into schematic form in Table III for the purpose of classification and elaboration of the James's "I–me" theoretical model. It should be noted that only a rough correspondence across "stage levels" is implied in this schema. More specific references to these constructs and a brief substantive discussion on self-concept are included in each section of the age-related emotional disorders of childhood and adolescence. The frame of reference for these discussions is an amalgam of the formulations of James,[7] of Kegan,[5] of psychoanalytic

Table III. Theories of Levels and Stages in the Development of Self-concept

Erikson	Loevinger	Kegan	Selman
Trust vs. mistrust	Presocial	Incorporative	Physicalistic self-awareness
Initiative vs. guilt	Impulsive	Impulsive	Awareness of distinction between actions and intentions
Industry vs. inferiority	Self-protective (opportunistic)	Imperial	Emergence of introspective self and second-person perspective
Affiliation vs. abandonment	Conformist	Interpersonal	Completion of introspective self
Identity vs. identity diffusion	Conscientious	Institutional	Concepts of self as observer, taking third-person perspective
	Individualistic		
	Autonomous	Interindividual	Discovery of true self-deception and the unconscious as a natural explanatory concept

theorists, and of the excellent review of the development of self-understanding by Damon and Hart.[8]

SELF-CONCEPT: BIRTH TO 2 YEARS

The early mother–child twosome, or dyad, becomes the critical opening stage of personality growth and development. The mother's attachment with the newborn and the infant's "bonding" response is accomplished, as Piaget noted, during stage 1 of the sensori-motor period of cognitive development by a number of inherited reflexes, including grasping, visual tracking, rooting, and sucking, directed toward searching and seeking interaction and stimulation from the mother.

As early as from birth to 3 months of age, infants appear to have an unlearned attraction to other people, especially to mother and images of young babies.[8] White[14] estimated that at 3½ months a baby has near-mature visual capacity that supports the curiosity of the infant's looking at faces, interest in hand movements, and touching nearby objects. The infant's capacity to respond and enter into rhythmical patterns with important care-taking persons and within himself becomes an important adaptive tool as well as a mainspring in self-concept formation.[15] Beginning as early as 3 months, and usually by 9 months, infants distinguish live TV images of self from other images presented.

In Kegan's model of the "evolving self," this early period is referred to as the "incorporative self," embedded in reflexes, sensing, and moving. It is characterized by close physical presence with "dependence upon and merger with oneself."

Mahler[16] added depth and understanding to the nature of self–object relationships and to the separation–differentiation process in her description of four periods: "hatching" (5–12 months), practicing (12–15 months), rapproachement or moving back to mother (15–24 months), and establishing object constancy or trust in the existence and eventual return of the parents or child-caring person (25–36 months).

EMOTIONAL DISORDERS IN THE FIRST YEAR

The milder developmental disturbances that are transient in nature, as well as reactions to external psychosocial stressors, have been described. More severe emotional reactions in response to separation, deprivation, and the quality of maternal care during the first year of life are the primary focus of the following discussion.

The classic work of Spitz[17] in following 130 children in two settings—61 in a foundling home and 69 in a nursery—documented the importance of maternal care, maternal stimulation, and maternal love during the first year of life. The developmental quotient of children in the foundling home had dropped from 124 to 72 at the end of the first 12 months; there was also a high mortality in that population, with an obvious decrease in their resistance to disease.

The greatest arrest and decline in development occurred between the third and fourth months, about the time of weaning, when much of the human contact and stimulation stopped as nursing stopped. Children in the nursery over that same time frame maintained or showed a small gain in their developmental quotient (101.5–105). Unfortunately, even when placed in more favorable environments after the age of 15 months, the children in the foundling home showed no reversal in their psychological, social, or emotional deficits.

Failure to Thrive

This is classified in DSM III under Reactive Attachment Disorder of Infancy, 313.89. This emotional response in infants is one of the major problems presented to pediatricians. Although the syndrome has been recognizable for many years, it has remained an enigma. The early description by Powell et al.[18] characterized the findings as (1) unstable social history; (2) bizarre polydipsia and polyphagia, e.g., drinking water from toilet bowls and old beer cans and eating whole loaves of bread or jars of mustard at one sitting; (3) developmental delays in walking and talking; (4) short stature (30–66% of chronological age); (5) underweight; (6) social immaturity and withdrawal; (7) onset before second birthday; and (8) radical reversal of all symptoms, including personality and language development, with change of environment, e.g., substitution of a second nurturing caretaker for the mother or primary caretaker.

Egan et al.[19] clarified many of the issues and pointed to clinical interventions that should be considered in case management. The term is currently used to describe infants and children whose weight for height falls below the tenth percentile on standard growth charts. These investigators recognize that some cases may be associated with organic disease, whereas others are nonorganic in origin. Roughly 1–5% of consecutive pediatric admissions may be due to the failure to thrive (FTT) syndrome.

Nonorganic FTT has also been called psychosocial dwarfism, maternal deprivation, deprivation dwarfism, environmental failure to thrive, and growth failure from maternal deprivation secondary to undereating. Egan et al. proposed an effective classification according to etiology, pathogenesis, and treatment (see Table IV).

Economic and Social Deprivation

It has been estimated that in the United States 45% of the young children who function as mentally retarded appear to be the product of low-birth-weight pregnancies due to nutritional deficiencies in the mother. Many of these are teenage mothers or mothers from low-income and disadvantaged communities where adequate food supplies are not available.

Bengoa[20] observed that in 46 Asian, African, and South American communities between 1963 and 1972 more than 80% of the 190,000 children suffered from moderate to severe forms of protein-calorie malnutrition (PCM).

Craviota[21] suggested in his study of a Mexican community of 7000, in which severe malnutrition was highly prevalent, that poverty alone did not explain the occurrence of severe malnutrition. Out of this community, he found some families that continued to produce severely malnourished children over several generations, whereas other families, under similar economic and educational conditions, did not produce severely malnourished children. He recognized that attitudes of parenting, especially mothering, were fed back into their children in patterns similar to their own child-rearing experiences, thus perpetuating the dysfunctional family system in psychosocial as well as nutritional malnourishment.

Table IV Classification of Nonorganic Failure to Thrive

Etiology	Pathogenesis	Intervention
Lack of adequate nutritional information	Inexperienced, poorly prepared mothering skills lead to nutritional and caloric deprivation, resulting starvation leads to FTT	Maternal education and supervision in preparation of nutritional food
Deficiency in maternal care (disturbance in attachment)	Mother may be absent, abusing, indifferent, depressed, overwhelmed, mentally ill, abusing drugs, alcoholic May lack maternal disposition due to childhood deprivation or cultural influences Peak incidence of pathology in first 6 months Prompt intervention imperative or inadequate attachment to mother may lead to severe personality disturbances	Respond to warm, nurturing caretaker Mothers need special instructions on how to care for children, a nurturing figure to assist and support them
Disturbance in separation–individuation	Onset second half of first year "Battle of the spoon" mothers overly involved, meticulous, preoccupied with child's eating Often controlling and mechanical, to which child reacts willfully as a means of achieving degree of autonomy from and control over mother As mother's anxiety increases, so does her coercive effort At first child eats for a third person, may later refuse food in mother's absence Self-imposed starvation results in weight loss and, if chronic, reduced stature	If child is 2–3 years old, individual therapy for child and parent counseling, or family therapy usually necessary If child less than 18 months, counseling with mother, or therapy for mother if indicated

One factor operating in children in every culture would be the mental apathy associated with malnutrition that reduces the child's responsiveness to stimulation. This coupled with the apathy in the adult caring for the child compounds the risks for maldevelopment and learning disabilities.[22]

Child Abuse and Neglect

Each year approximately six million Americans have children, 2.5 million becoming parents for the first time. It has been estimated that 60,000 children will be intentionally injured by their parents, approximately 1500 will die from the "battering," and 15,000 will become permanently brain injured from repeated physical insults.[23]

Cruelty to children is not a new phenomenon. It was not until 1946, however, that pediatric radiology became sufficiently sophisticated to diagnose what Kempe[24] called "the battered child syndrome." Caffey[25] made the association between x-ray markings of a subdural hematoma and x-ray changes in the long bones occurring in physically abused children. It has taken almost a decade to unlock the mysteries of the abusive cycle, but Kempe and co-workers now believe they can describe the sequence of events which take place, from the time of conception of "the" child who becomes the principal focus of abuse, to the actual abusive episode. They have referred to the unusual situations in which these children grow and develop, as a "world of abnormal rearing."[28]

Briefly, the cycle begins when girls choose mates who have been raised in similar abnormal rearing environments. As new parents, they expect the child to resolve one or more of their many problems. If the child conforms, all is well. If the child reacts by crying, not sleeping, not obeying, or not complying with parental expectations, trouble begins. The child tries to be the "good" child and to "take care of the parents," thus missing out on a childhood of his own. The child lacks a normal childhood and adequate role models to engender trust, love, and a sense of worth or value, leading to a lowered sense of self-esteem. The child is also deprived of adequate experiences and familial role models in the handling of angry, hostile-aggressive feelings in outgoing relationships.

This child, now a grown, deprived adult (distrustful, isolated, with a poor self-concept) selects a mate with similar problems, and a generational abusive cycle is potentially carried into another generation. Unfortunately, it is no longer one child in a family who may be abused. It can happen to more than one child. Suggestions for management of child abuse and neglect are outlined in Table V.

SELF-CONCEPT: 2–5 YEARS

Most researchers agree that self-awareness appears around 24 months of age.[5] The self is conceived in physical terms and is believed to be part of the body, usually the head or the whole body. It is described by children of this age in terms of size, shape, or color.[26] Selman[13] refers to this as a "physicalistic conception of self." The child makes no distinction between inner psychological experience and outer world experience.

Young children between ages 3 and 5 think of the "self" more in terms of activities than in terms of body parts or material attributes. This suggests that the notion of the physical self needs to be broadly conceived to include physical action as well as physical body. This observed "active" self predominates during the preschool years.

From a psychoanalytic view, the ego is structured in significant ways through its connection to the body. The genitalia are stimulated early by elimination, cleaning, and diapering; they seem likely to achieve an early mental representation in the ego. The upbringing of parents and their attitude toward genitals, maleness, femaleness, and reproduction influence their handling of their child's body as well as how important body parts are to these children.[27]

Following separation and individuation, the child begins in the second year to recognize physical attributes, functions, and behaviors that distinguish males from females. The formation of gender includes this quality of recognition, plus a recognition of the complementarity of the opposite sex and an identification with the biological reproductive

Table V Suggestions for Management of Child Abuse and Neglect

Assessment of child	Assessment of parents
1 Hospitalize suspected cases (Helfer[21]) (30% may require court action)	1 Avoid making the child the total focus
2 Treat injuries or malnutrition	2 Put violent event in perspective Was it an isolated incident? Is there a pattern of violence? What degree of guilt and remorse is present? How extensive are the parental and child denials?
3 Obtain supportive laboratory tests and radiographs	
4 Examine all siblings within 12 hr	
5 Advise parents of presumptive diagnosis and legal obligation to report findings	3 Place appropriate emphasis on needs of parents
6 Report suspected abuse to local child protective agency within 24 hr	4 Work with total family system and support network in crisis intervention
7 Obtain consultations from social service and other services as necessary within 24 hr	5 Evaluate parental capacities (a) to attend to child's needs, (b) to maintain healthy emotional connections with child, (c) to separate own feelings from child's feelings, and (d) to continue to like the child
8 Submit official written report within 48 hr	
9 When necessary appoint attorney to represent abused child as counsel and guardian	
10 Make home visits to assess safety of child's home	6 Arrange for psychiatric follow-up of parents, including couple group therapy, Parents Anonymous, CALM, day care centers, crisis nurseries, visiting nurses, vocational rehabilitation services, and other local agencies
11 Use multidisciplinary team to consider psychological and legal feasibility of returning child to natural parents	
12 Provide psychiatric follow-up for the child	
13 Plan and expedite court review or informal multidisciplinary team review in 6–12 months	

function.[27] By age 2, gender identity has been established. Meyer concludes his review with the observation that "in the oedipal phase, gender is not reversed once established adequately, although sexual identity and the expression of masculinity and femininity are at issue." The meaning of maleness and femaleness does not reach full maturity until after adolescence.[22]

Kegan[5] sees the preschooler as being in an impulsive balance in his self–object growth. This results in intense attachments, rivalries, and the gradual emerging from the earlier incorporative stage through fantasies, impulsive behavior, and new perceptions. Children of this age are unable either to mediate their impulse life or to hold two perceptions or two competing feelings at the same time. Thus, they lack the capacity for ambivalence. Tantrums at this age serve as a normal vehicle of distress when overwhelmed by internal conflict.

It is now known that from 2 to 4 years of age, toileting experiences will influence critical attitudes in subsequent interpersonal relationships. Such attitudes include feelings about giving and receiving; saving or spending money; degrees of willfulness, obstinacy, and negativism; feelings toward authority figures; and the possible influence of this anal period in the development of obsessive-compulsive patterns of behavior.[28,29]

In elaborating on personality development, Freud observed that around the age of 3 and 4, the boy becomes assertive, seeking to emulate his father as a model. The growing girl may take on a tomboy position, viewing her mother as a love object and her father as a rival. At ages 4 and 5, this negative oedipal stage gradually gives way to a positive oedipal experience for the boy and an Electra stage experience for the girl. At this time the son longs for his mother as a love object and views his father as a rival; he also fears retaliation for these incestual strivings. The daughter shifts from a tomboy to a feminine position (now more broadly defined in our current culture), with the father as the love object; she may become fearful of the loss of her mother's love for these incestual wishes.

EMOTIONAL DISORDERS IN THE PRESCHOOL YEARS

During the toddler and post-toddler years, conflict between parents and child can result in compromises in the assimilation, internalization, and integration of cognitive and affective experiences so essential to shaping personality and daily behaviors. Such conflicts can lead to temper tantrums, poor self-regulatory behavioral control, lack of motor and sensorimotor coordination, varying degrees of negativism, disruption and delay in language development, and disturbed interpersonal behaviors.[15] In their less severe form, these conflicts may be experienced as nightmares, night terrors, and other developmental disturbances. Investigations of infantile autism (DSM III, 299.0X) have pointed to biochemical or organic conditions to explain the lack of responsiveness to other people (autism), the gross impairment in communicative skills, and the bizarre responses to the environment, all developing within the first 30 months, as the cardinal features of this syndrome.

In addition, the affective mood may be labile; there may be an under- or overresponsiveness to light, pain and/or sound; repetitive self-mutilating habits such as hair pulling or biting hands and wrists; and toe walking, rocking, or other rhythmic body movements. It has been suggested that about 40% have an intelligence quotient (IQ) below 50 and 30% an IQ of 70 or more. Because it is so difficult to determine mental functioning in this population, an assessment over time is essential to constructive management. The course of such a pervasive developmental disorder is usually chronic, with social awkwardness and ineptness persisting into adulthood. Development of language for social communication before the age of 6 years and the quality of intact mental functioning appear to be the critical factors affecting outcome. Prevalence studies suggest that this condition is very rare (two to four cases per 10,000), with a frequency in siblings with the disorders 50 times as great as in the general population. Rutter and Schopler[30] wrote one of the most complete reviews of the assessment and management of the disorder, entitled *Autism: A Reappraisal of Concepts and Treatment.*

A second condition, atypical pervasive developmental disorder (299.8X), could be used to describe and designate those cases referred to as a maternal–child symbiotic psychotic reaction. The onset of this condition is also before 30 months. It is characterized by a catastrophic reaction in the infant to separation from the mother, including prolonged crying and screaming, regressive behavior persisting for long periods during separation, and prolonged distortions in the development of social skills and the use of language.

The moderately severe disturbances between parents and child at this age can lead to structural defects in the formation of mental representational data in the child, i.e., the nature of mental picture or image that the child lays down in his mind about his respective parents and the emotional valence, positive or negative, "good" or "bad" attached to that parent.

Table VI. Schematic Representation of Psychoneuroses of Childhood

Inner conflict	Signal anxiety	Mechanisms of defense	Symptom complex[a]
		Undefended anxiety	Anxiety state (300.02)
			Motor activity
			Tic disorder (307.21)
			Hyperactivity (314.01)
			Sleep disturbances (307.46)
External world superego functioning	Incomplete repression →	Denial and displacement on environmental object. Projection, isolation, and condensation	Phobia (300.29)
Internal world	Signal → anxiety	Reversal of affect conversion into somatic system	Conversion disorder (300.11)
Id impulse functioning			Psychological factors affecting physical condition (316.00)
Sexual and aggressive drives expressed in wishes, desires, and fantasies		Reaction formation, isolation of affects and ideas	Obsessive-compulsive disorder (300.30)
		Turning aggression in on self	Adjustment disorder with depressed mood (309.00)

Ages	Critical issues in signal anxiety
0–2	Fear of loss of object
2–4	Fear of loss of love
4–6	Fear of retaliation
6–12	Fear of own conscience
12–18	

[a]DSM III category in parentheses.

Greenspan[15] suggests that such distortions in the mental representational data can lead to fragmentation of the thought processes, to inability of the patient to tolerate internal emotional upheavals, and to symptom complexes, including borderline conditions, psychoses, severe substance abuse, and psychosomatic and impulse disorders.

Childhood phobias, neurotic anxieties, and fears of being hurt or of hurting someone may also be associated with this developmental period. Table VI is a schematic representation of the psychoneuroses of childhood.

Historical Perspective

In 1909 Freud published his analysis of a fear of horses in Little Hans, a 5-year-old boy whose father shared with Freud his observations of his son's fears and verbalizations. Freud did not actually work with the little boy, but he did uncover what he considered an unconscious developmental conflict between the little boy's inner wishes, fantasies, and desires derived from his aggressive and sexual impulse life and the expectations, prohibitions, and admonitions from his parents and the external world. Freud referred to the developmental conflict as the *Oedipus conflict* and to the symptom formation arising from the compromise and the anxiety associated with the compromise as the *infantile neurosis*. These concepts of an infantile neurosis—the Oedipus complex in boys, and the Electra complex in girls—form a cornerstone of psychoanalytical theory and practice.

In 1920 Watson and Rayner reported the conditioning of a small animal (rat) phobia in a 1-year-old infant named Albert. This case added credence to the conditioning theory of behavior that was emerging at that time.

In 1924 Jones published the first systematic application of counterconditioning and social imitation behavioral techniques in treating Peter, a 3-year-old child, who was afraid of rabbits, a fur coat, cotton, wool, a feather, and a white rat. Jones's effort was a forerunner of the behavior-avoidance test (BAT) now used in the assessment of children's fears.

Definition/Classification/Incidence

The Committee of the Group for the Advancement of Psychiatry (GAP) defined the psychoneurosis in childhood as the symptom complex resulting from unconscious conflicts in handling sexual and aggressive impulses that are partially repressed but that continue to remain active and unresolved. The conflicts are present in all children to varying degrees, primarily during the preschool years, and arise in the transactional process that occurs between the child's biopsychosocial development and the significant members of the child's family (adult hierarchy).

In early childhood, conflicts may be expressed in various temporary symptomatic reactions. Depending on their intensity and the absence of a healthy resolution, the unresolved conflicts may become internalized and incorporated as part of the developing personality. If conflicts become syntonic, i.e., experienced without anxiety, they take on the aspect of a character neurosis. If the various symptom complexes are experienced with an associated anxiety, i.e., dystonic, they are considered psychoneurotic in nature.

The various psychoneurotic symptom complexes are classified according to the mechanisms of defense used to cope with the anxiety generated by the incomplete repression. This process operating in the psychoneuroses has been schematically represented in Table VI.

Although common, childhood fears are usually temporary and not serious. Rutter *et al.*[31] on the Isle of Wight, found that only 7 per 1000 of the total population of 10- and 11-year-olds had serious fears, with animals, darkness, school, and disease and illness phobias the most common.

Descriptions

Anxiety States

These repeated panic attacks are not defended against with ego mechanisms of defense, such as denial and more complete repression. They are characterized by motor tension (shakiness, jitteriness, trembling, muscle aches, inability to relax, eyelid twitch, furrowed brow, strained face, and easy startle), autonomic hyperactivity (sweating, palpitations, clammy hands, dry mouth, dizziness, tingling in hands and feet, upset stomach, frequent urination, diarrhea, flushing, pallor, and dilated pupils), apprehensive expectation (worry, fear, rumination, anticipation of misfortune to self or to others, and vigilance and scanning), poor concentration, insomnia, irritability, impatience, and hyperattentiveness.

Phobias

Onset is at 4–5 years of age. Phobias are not rare in childhood. They usually represent attempts to deal with pre-Oedipal conflicts. Usually a partial denial of feelings toward loved and feared objects; detachment of self from conflict; use of projection to transform intolerable inner dangers from sexual and aggressive drives to an outer danger such as a fear of an animal; associated with use of displacement by which fear of parent (e.g., mother) is shifted onto animals; and often utilizing condensation in which all impulses, wishes, and fears of all the objects in the environment can be condensed into a single phobia.

The youngest child on record with a phobia was an 18-month-old who displaced her fear of strict parental toileting and her fear of her own aggressive fantasies into a negative character in a fairy tale (Wulff[32]). Renik et al.[33] described a bamboo phobia in an 18-month-old in which disparity between cognitive functions and self-object mental representations, plus difficulty in taking on separation and individuation issues, seemed to be critical dynamic factors.

In young children the clinician makes a distinction between phobic avoidance, with relatively simple projections and displacements, and the bona fide phobias with greater sophistication and symbolic disguise of the underlying drive-related conflicts.[34,35]

Analysis of the bamboo phobia revealed a fear of castration related to projections onto the father, mother, and sisters. The phobia was seen as a symptom formed to deal with psychosexual conflicts at the time of this child's rapprochement crisis.

School Phobias

This topic has been discussed under school aversion in Chapter 20. Sperling[36] views this symptom complex as one variety of the group of phobias. She recognized that a pathological tie with the parent was a central issue and, unless it could be resolved or partially modified, treatment would not be successful. More recent clinicians have focused on the refusal or avertive symptoms arising out of a hostile–dependent mother–child relationship operating within the family system.

Conversion Disorder

Onset is at around 8 years. Diagnostic criteria include a loss of, or alteration in, physical functioning, suggesting a physical disorder as a predominant disturbance. Psychological factors include one of the following: (1) a temporal relationship exists between an environmental stimulus related to a psychological conflict and the initiation or exacerbation of the symptom, (2) the symptom enables the individual to avoid an activity that is noxious or traumatic, (3) the symptom enables the individual to get support from an environment that otherwise might not be forthcoming (secondary gain), or (4) the internal conflict or psychological need is kept out of conscious awareness (primary gain). In addition, the symptom is not under voluntary control and cannot be explained by any known physical disorder.

A calm mental attitude of *la belle indifférence* indicating a relative lack of concern inconsistent with the severe nature of the impairment is sometimes present. The *DSM III Manual* suggests "this feature has little diagnostic value since it is also found in some seriously ill medical patients who are stoic about their situation." On the pediatric wards, classic cases of conversion hysteria are seen with paralysis of extremities, hysterical blindness, and hysterical (epileptiform) convulsions

Reversal of affect, displacement, identification, and symbolization are the mechanisms of defense in conversion disorders. Sperling[36] suggests that the mother–child relationship is an important dynamic factor in determining the choice of the defense mechanism. The conversion usually arises from regression to pregenital symbiotic phases of development as a defense against the fantasies and wishes of the Oedipal level. All conversions are considered pregenital in origin.

Obsessive-Compulsive Disorder

Onset is between 6 and 7 years. Within a psychoanalytical framework, this disorder is seen as a defense against unconscious conflicts arising from aggressive and sexual impulses, particularly in relationship to the Oedipus complex. The initial defense is by regression to the anal–sadistic level, but the continuing impulsive drives and their derivatives in wishes and fantasies are so intolerable that they are defended against by reaction formation, isolation, and undoing. Reaction formation leads to obsessive thoughts, or compulsive acts, or mixtures of both, which are isolated from the original, unacceptable impulse. Often the resulting behavior, such as excessive hand washing or orderliness, represents the very opposite of the unconscious wish to soil and mess.

Obsessions and compulsions can occur as mild, transient bedtime and feeding rituals by the toddler, without which he cannot function well. Later, obsessional fears can lead to magical thinking and, in the progression of normal development, to obsessional games, such as the avoidance of cracks on the pavement. ("Step on a crack and break your mother's back!")

The diagnostic criteria include a chronic pattern with waxing and waning of obsessional and compulsive symptoms outlined in Table VII.

Prognosis

Continuing studies of the course of the obsessive–compulsive disorders seem to indicate that the prognosis is neither as guarded nor as unfavorable as was once thought. It appears that spontaneous remissions can occur.[37]

Treatment and Management

Adams[38] has written an excellent review of the specific therapies for childhood psychoneuroses, observing that "the conventional wisdom that governs child psychiatry

Table VII. Characteristics of an Obsessive-Compulsive Disorder

Obsessions	Compulsions
Recurrent, persistent ideas, thoughts, images that are ego dystonic, i.e., not voluntary, but experienced as "foreign" thoughts that invade consciousness.	Repetitive and seemingly purposeful behaviors performed according to certain rules, or in a stereotyped fashion. Behavior not an end in itself, but to produce or prevent some future event. May be recognized as senseless, as devoid of pleasure or satisfaction, although it provides release of tension.
Often experienced as senseless or repugnant thoughts.	
Includes thoughts of violence, contamination, and lingering worry and doubt as to whether one has performed some action, such as injuring another person in a traffic accident.	Often experienced as counting, checking, touching, and hand washing.
	Attempts to resist a compulsion increases tension, which is immediately relieved by yielding to the compulsion.

today states that the treatment of choice for neurotic children is psychoanalysis or psychoanalytically oriented psychotherapy." The goal of such therapy is to effect an internal revision of intrapsychic functions so that emotional development may proceed in an optimal way.

Adams touches briefly on behavior therapy, which is covered more completely by Mash and Terdal.[39] These investigators focus on the use of counterconditioning techniques, modeling techniques, operant techniques, and self-control strategies.

Adams concludes his chapter with a brief description of Adlerian, Sullivanian, Rankian, transactional, and Gestalt psychotherapies. He also discusses analytic group therapy, reality therapy, and family therapy.

Family therapy focuses on neutralizing the presenting symptom in the child and reframing the treatment process so as to deal with the child's symptom as representative of distortions and dysfunctions in the larger family system. Unfortunately, family therapists and child psychiatrists have had a tendency to adopt mutually exclusive orientations. Efforts are constantly being made to facilitate an integration of the two orientations[40]. Masten[41] completed a critical review of outcome research on the value of family therapy as a treatment of choice for children and concluded that more and better controlled comparative outcome studies are necessary before such a judgment can be made.

SELF-CONCEPT: 6–12 YEARS

This age or period is called latency, suggesting that the aggressive and sexual drives have been rechanneled from their focus on one's body and one's relationship to mother and father and have been put to use learning more about the world and its symbols and relationships.

At some time during the fifth year, and into the sixth year, there is a resolution of the strong Oedipal and Electra feelings through identification with the parent of the same sex, as well as some internalization of the good and bad aspects of both parents, along with the child's perceptions of the rewarding and punishing, the accepting and rejecting, the loving and not-loving, and the praising and blaming cues from both parents. This process evolves over time and consolidates in the mental construct referred to as the superego or conscience. During the years from 6 to 8, the superego is often strict and harsh, with conflictual guilt feelings over masturbation. From 8 to 10 years of age, it normally becomes less strict and more tolerant. There is also a shift from a phobic stance, or generally fearful organization, to a normal pattern of obsessional thinking characteristic of elementary school-age children.

Most researchers agree that between the ages of 6 and 9 years, there is a shift from a physicalistic to psychological conception of the self. These children begin to understand the mental and volitional aspects of self, apart from links to any body part. They have made a distinction between mind and body, between mental and physical, and between internal and external.[26] Children in this period have an immutable sense of their own humanity (quality of life), sexuality (gender and sex role), individuality (uniqueness), and continuity (connection with one's past and future self).

Seven years seems to be the critical age at which children make comparisons of competence of self in relationship to others. With Kegan's[5] evolving self model, the child aged 5–7 years has moved from the impulsive balance to the imperial one. Kegan notes that before 5 to 7 years the child needs rewards that are fairly immediate, sensual, and communicatory of praise. Going into 5 to 7 years, the child feels more rewarded by learning that he has been correct. He is able to "take command" of his impulses, has developed a conscience, a sense of guilt, and has internalized "the other's voice in the construction of the self." The stage of mutuality is reached in which the self can coordinate and integrate one need system with another: "yours and mine."

Selman[13] also refers to a physicalistic level 0 of self-awareness in very young children that emerges into a level 1 awareness of distinction between actions and intentions. Although Selman does not attach a specific age range to his model of levels of self-awareness, he does state that an attitude at level 2, the emergence of an introspective self and the second person perspective, plays a major role in the social development of the preadolescent child.

EMOTIONAL DISORDERS: 6–12 YEARS

Statistics suggest that the most common difficulty in school-age children who are brought to mental health professionals, pediatricians, and child guidance clinics is some form of school learning difficulty. The various problems uncovered during the early school years are listed in Table VIII.

The contents of this section will focus on three critical issues leading to academic underachievement, namely, primary neurotic learning inhibition, depression in childhood, and the school-age child's reaction to divorce.

Primary Neurotic Learning Inhibition

Sperry et al.[42] describe a pattern of neurotic inhibition of academic learning in boys whose mothers were dominant, often academic achievers or who wished their sons to be, and whose fathers were passive, often underachievers who appeared to devalue educational pursuits.

Table VIII. School Learning Difficulties[a]

Reading difficulties (5, 6, 7)
Developmental dyslexia
Acquired dyslexia
Hyperlexia
Attention deficit disorders (5, 17)
Hyperactivity
Specific developmental disorders
Academic underachievement (20, 21)
Neurotic learning inhibition
Childhood depression
Reaction to divorce
Language and speech problems (10, 13, Appendix B)
Hearing impairment (19, Appendix B)
Receptive and expressive disorders (11)
Articulation and fluency disorders (12)
Visual function disorders (18)
Perceptual disorders (18)
Developmental disorders (1)
Mental retardation (9)

[a]The reader is referred to chapters in this volume in which these specific problems are discussed.

As a defense against identifying with and internalizing the value system and expectations of the mother, these boys often avoided or became passively resistant to academic learning, appeared to take on the underachieving role of the father, and chose vocational–technical pursuits in contrast to academic degree pursuits.

Depression in Childhood

There has been a long delay in the delineation of childhood depression. This has been due partly to its difference from adult depression and partly to the symptomatic manifestations varying with the continuing developmental changes in the child's psychic structure and function.[43]

Diagnosis

A major depressive episode in children is based essentially on the adult criteria in DSM III, with slight modification. Table IX outlines the criteria essential for the diagnosis.

Theories of Etiology of Childhood Depression

There is a burgeoning amount of clinical and technological information about the major affective disorders, generated in clinics and laboratories. Many of the data are derived from adult studies. It is recognized that children are not miniature adults and that the crucial aspect in childhood depression is that the child may be experiencing a loss of such nature that he is incapable of mastering it adaptively.[43] Both children and adults have in common factors related to biogenetics and neurotransmitter activity. This brief review

Table IX. Criteria for Diagnosis of Depression in Childhood

Dysphoric mood (sad, worried, "blue," discouraged, despondent, depressed)
Loss of interest or pleasure (anhedenia) in most activities
At least four of eight symptoms, and in children under age 6, three of the first four
   present nearly every day for a period of at least 2 weeks:

Appetite or weight changes	Loss of energy
Sleep disturbance	Worthless feeling, self-reproach, or
Psychomotor agitation or retardation	guilt
Loss of interest or pleasure in usual	Complaints or evidence of diminished
daily activity (apathy in children	ability to think or concentrate
under age 6)	Recurrent thoughts of death or suicide

of theories of etiology highlights several of the presumed etiological factors that can be subsumed under a broader biopsychological model.

Genetic. Cytryn[44] estimated the lifetime risk of a child of a bipolar responsive parent at about 10% and that of a unipolar parent at 15%. Weitkamp[45] studied 120 families with primary depressive disorders in which 20 met the criteria of containing at least two affected members and 30 sibships. In addition, he found that these families segregate along with the human leukocyte antigen (HLA), suggesting that a locus on the sixth chromosome, but not necessarily part of it, contributes substantially to the risk of depressive disorders. This finding further suggests the possible linkage of depressive disorders to a specific genetic marker as well as the possibility of discovering the gene product through molecular biology.[46]

Biochemical. Mandell[47] has proposed a biochemical theory to explain the persistence of depressive affect after the neurotic conflict has been resolved or been partially worked through. He hypothesizes that infants and young children may be vulnerable in their biochemical responses to psychosocial stressors of child rearing. For example, early and persistent psychological loss or abusive traumata may result in depletion of monoamine transmitter activity. A persistent loss or trauma, over time, could eventuate in the "altered" or "depleted" biochemical state becoming the "normal" biochemical state for that individual throughout his life.

Data that seem to support this hypothesis have been accumulating in children. Puig-Antich *et al.*[48] have demonstrated excessive secretion of cortisol in children with depression. McKnew and Cytryn[49] found a significant reduction in urinary 3-methoxy-4-hydroxyphenylethylene glycol (MHPG), a metabolite of norepinephrine, in a controlled study of nine children aged 6–12 years. More recent MHPG studies have not confirmed this finding in children, however.

Psychological. In his analysis of a depressed child, Cohen[50] traced the development of affect from two simultaneous processes: the origin of the self as the locus of initiative and feelings, and the "good" and "bad" mental representations of the parental images, originating in mutual relationships. These mutual transactions include bonding and attachment of child and parent(s) with the gradual incorporation of personality aspects of the caregivers. Wounds to the self and object representations from distorted and paradoxical child–parent interactions may lead to self-reproach against the internalized love object, to internalization of hostility and ambivalence toward the parents, and to loss of self-esteem and self-worth. Lewis[22] notes that these have been the three classic views of depression from psychoanalytic theory.

Sandler and Joffe[51] emphasized the persistent sense of helplessness and eventual passive resignation in children who have lost or are unable to attain the quality of support and care they feel is essential to their well-being. Belmont[43] focused on the crucial aspect of experiencing at any developmental level a loss of such nature and degree that the child is incapable of mastering that loss adaptively. In fact, the child may become blocked in subsequent personality development.

Social. Two types of family interaction have been reported in depressed children: (1) the scapegoated or the excluded member of the family, and (2) the child "enmeshed" with one parent, usually the sicker one. Deficient rearing, neglect, and physical and/or sexual abuse are the most significant social causes of childhood depression.[52]

Management

Until recently, the treatment of choice has been individual and/or family therapy focused on nurturance, empathy, healthy role modeling, and open verbal expression of socially acceptable hostile–aggressive feelings approved by parents and modeled for the child or children by the parents, and on efforts toward decreasing parental harshness and inconsistency.

In reviewing the use of antidepressants in children prior to 1976, Rappaport found no strong proof of the effectiveness of these drugs on children. The problem arose from the fact that before that time there had been no clear definition of the depressive syndrome in children. More recent investigators have found that imipramine and desmethylimipramine are effective, if a two to three week build-up is allowed, and provided the plasma level reaches 146 μg/ml. Table X highlights the antidepressant drugs considered possibly useful in children and adolescents.

Reaction to Divorce

Perhaps one of the most devastating experiences in a child's life is the divorce of his/her parents. Children survive, but at what cost? Parents feel that their right to marital happiness comes first. As a consequence, from June 1979 to June 1980 there were 1,184,000 divorces in the United States. More than one million children each year are added to the casualty list, and over 12 million children under 18 have experienced divorce in their families since 1972.

It is estimated that 30–45% of all children growing up in the 1980s will experience divorce of their parents or will live with only one parent before they reach 18 years of age. The average length of a marriage is now 6.6 years, hence many of these children are very young and especially vulnerable to the impact of divorce.[53]

Table X. Antidepressant Agents for Children and Adolescents

Drug	Daily use (mg)	Side effects
Imipramine (Tofranil) Tabs 10, 25, 50 mg Capsules 75, 100, 125, 150 mg	2.5 mg/kg per day should not be exceeded in childhood	Cardiotoxic over 75 mg/day Leukopenia Insomnia Dry mouth Jaundice
Widely used for enuresis 25 mg before bedtime to 50 mg	10–50 (max. 100)	
Desipramine (Pertofrane, Norpramin) Tabs 25, 50 mg	25–50	FDA approved for adolescents, not for children
Doxepin (Adapin, Sinequan) Tabs 10, 25, 50, 75, 100 mg	75 (max. 150)	Not recommended for children under 12 years of age
Amoxapine (Asendin) Tabs 50, 100, 150 mg	200–300 (max. 300)	Safety and effectiveness below age 16 not established
Nortriptyline (Aventyl, Pamelor) Liquid 10 mg/5cc Caps 10, 25 mg	30–50	Not recommended for children
Amitriptyline (Elavil, Endep) Tabs 10, 25, 50, 75, 100, 150 mg		Not recommended for children under 12 years of age

Table XI. Central Themes in Child's Divorce Experience[a]

Themes	Child's reactions
Divorce is frightening.	Fear was central response for all children: 30% feared maternal abandonment.
Divorce is time of sadness.	Enormous sense of loss: 50% tearful, pervasively sad; 30% acute depressive: "Widespread yearning for noncustodial father."
Divorce is a time of worry.	50% worried intensely about their mothers; all reacted with increased "sense of vulnerability."
Divorce is a time of feeling rejected.	50% (especially young children); 6–12-year-old boys felt most rejected by fathers.
Divorce is a lonely time.	Loneliness profound, acute, painful, and long remembered.
Divorce is a time of conflicted loyalties.	60% of parents openly compete for children's love and allegiance: "A step toward one parent experienced by child as betrayal of the other."
Divorce is a time of anger.	25% experienced explosive anger at one or both parents; fathers most often object of anger.
Divorce is a time for feeling guilty.	Not all children feel responsible, contrary to popular belief; 30% who felt guilt came from 8-year-old group, or younger.

[a]Data from Wallerstein and Kelly.[54]

Table XII. Specific Reactions to Divorce by Age Groups[a]

Preschool/kindergarten (3–5 years)	Young school-age (6–8 years)	Older school-age (9–12 years)	Adolescence (13–18 years)
Fear	Understood meaning of divorce	Understood complex reality and could withstand stress without regression	Higher quality of "anguish" and "frantic appeals to restore marriage" than researchers anticipated
Regression			
Macabre fantasy	Pervasive sadness and grief; more intense than in any other group		
Bewilderment			
Fantasy as denial		Showed poise, presence, and courage	Profound sense of loss
Play themes	Fear of being left	Attempted mastery through play	Loyalty conflicts
Increased aggression	Yearning for departed parent, especially about father	Fully conscious of their intense anger	Worried about their own marriage in future
Self-blame; guilt			
General emotional neediness; random reaching out to new adults	Inhibition of aggression toward father	Many felt their conscience (superego) weakened by departure of parent who acted as their moral authority	Anger covered over their vulnerability and sense of powerlessness
Efforts at mastery and coping	Anger at custodial mother		Greater maturity and moral growth
	Little feeling of self-blame	Somatic symptoms	A few failed to cope; made a "strategic withdrawal"
	Continued to be loyal to both parents; 25% under heavy pressure from mother to reject father		

[a]Data from Wallerstein and Kelly[54]

From their observations of 131 children from 60 divorcing families in a middle-class Northern California population, Wallerstein and Kelly[54] have written one of the most authoritative books in the field, *Surviving the Breakup*. Table XI summarizes the central themes observed by these workers in the child's experiencing a divorce, for children aged 3–18 at the time of the marital breakup, and in a 5-year follow-up. In addition to these themes, these clinicians recorded the specific reactions by age groupings (see Table XII). Suggestions for helping parents and children through the divorce process are included in Table XIII.

SELF-CONCEPT: 13–20 YEARS

Virtually all researchers agree that adolescent self-understanding shows an increased ability to describe the "me" in psychological and social terms. There is a more consolidated belief in the "I" of the personality as having more power and potential wisdom. There is also a tendency to work toward integrating newly acquired self-attributes into a stable, consistent self-concept during late adolescence. In short, there is a shift from the "Me" to the "I" orientation, with the self as its own evaluator. This transition is also characterized as a shift from action-based conceptions to psychological, belief-system-based self-concepts.

Table XIII Helping Parents and Children through the Process of Separation and Divorce[a]

Phases	Questions and directions

Pre-divorce planning	1 Will divorce lead to better life for each partner?
	2 Can understanding and forgiveness solve the problems?
	3 What is *the basis* for the decision to divorce?
	4 How to prepare children for what is coming
	   a Both parents should tell children about marital difficulties
	   b Make distinction with children between feelings as marital partners, and feelings and ongoing functions as their parents
	   c Be prepared for children to react "as if bolt of lightning struck." Children almost always would prefer to have parents together, even if unhappy, they don't feel emotional impact of marital conflict as parenting is in a different dimension for them
	5 Give children opportunities to ask questions, over a period of time, give them "honest," but sensitive and helpful answers
	6 Don't put children in the middle or make them *pawns*
	7 Explore with respective lawyers information about divorce process, property, issues related to custody, support, and visitation
	8 Explore spiritual–religious issues with priest, rabbi, or minister
	9 Begin to build up a support network for single-parent family to include grandparents, relatives, friends, neighbors, lawyers, clergy, and counselors
	10 Begin to work out practical details

During divorce process	1 Remember it takes a lot of time Allow time for
	   Grieving
	   Wounded self-esteem to parents
	   Family's fear of future
	2 Remember children need help with feelings of sadness, loneliness, rejection, anger, fear of loss of "other" parent, and blame or guilt Parents need help with feelings of failure, betrayal, anger, apprehension of what next, tendency to want to destroy spouse in eyes of children (Put focus on divergence of goals, values, and interests rather than "failure" of marriage)
	3 Remember divorce severs marriage but does *not* have to destroy relationship It is a *different* relationship, but work to support social/emotional growth of children
	4 Remember the need to work out custody, support, visitation, and living arrangements with major changes possible in social and living style Parents that are *now* single, are likely to be excluded from couple activities
	5 Remember experience suggests it will take 2½ years for husband, 3½ years for wife, and up to 5 years for children/adolescents to adjust to impact of divorce

After divorce	1 Changes in social, emotional, and economic realities are felt by each member of family 2 There can be a post-divorce depression in either or both parents 3 "Fall-out" of children's feelings can take on different forms according to age as suggested in Table XII 4 Postdivorce alterations in family system are highly variable Remarriage and move toward a "blended" family, in which new partners bring together children from former marriages, is possible

[a]An outline used by Adamson in teaching at Hahnemann University Philadelphia, PA

The adolescent is now capable of self-reflection, which "establishes a new mode of self-control generated by one's own mental powers of self-reflective self-awareness" (Damon and Hart[8]).

At the top of Selman's developmental sequence, the discovery of true self-deception and of the unconscious as a natural explanatory concept allows the adolescent to become aware of the unconscious mental process at work behind certain behaviors.

In Kegan's theory (see Table III), the adolescent has entered the institutional level associated with an increased sense of self, as in self-dependence and self-ownership. This is a shift from "I am my relationship" to "I have relationships."

The final level of development in this frame of reference is the interindividual level in which the self is separated from its earlier mental construct. At this stage, the self is now able to reflect upon the regulation and purposes of those mental functions which, heretofore, were considered part of the experiencing self.

This level is completed with the process of reciprocity, which allows both (1) the preservation of the other person's distinctness, and (2) the interdependent fashioning of a bigger self-object context in which both individuals can coexist at their highest levels of creativity.

EMOTIONAL DISORDERS: 13–20 YEARS

Although many issues become central to the adolescent's sorting out his own personal identity while reworking earlier phases of his psychosocial and psychosexual development, only four clinical disorders are reviewed in this chapter. They include anorexia nervosa, bulimia, substance abuse, and suicide in childhood and adolescence.

Anorexia Nervosa

It has been estimated that 80,000 Americans, mainly females aged 12–25, have some degree of anorexia nervosa. The figure is 4% for males. There has been a 1000% increase in this malady from 1975 to 1980.

First defined by Gull in 1868 as a "peculiar form of disease, an hysteric apepsia, mostly in young women, and characterized by extreme emaciation," it is now an important syndrome in adolescent psychiatry.

Diagnostic Criteria

DSM III suggests the features essential for the diagnosis (see Table XIV). In recent years much has been written about the condition because of its burgeoning increases in frequency, and the highly visible impact and life threatening nature of the syndrome.

This discussion outlines briefly the central characteristics of the condition (see Table XV) and suggests key resources for therapeutic management.

The successful management of anorexia nervosa depends on the nature of the underlying personality disorder in which the syndrome is embedded and on the clinical competence of the therapist(s) working with the client and his/her family. Risen[57] feels that "psychoanalytic psychotherapy, behavior modification techniques, family therapy, and

Table XIV. Diagnostic Criteria for Anorexia Nervosa

Intense fear of becoming obese, which does not diminish as weight loss progresses
Disturbance of body image, e.g., claiming to "feel fat" even when emaciated
Weight loss of at least 25% of original body weight or, if under 18 years of age, weight loss from original body
    weight plus projected weight gain expected from growth charts may be combined to make the 25%
Refusal to maintain body weight over a minimal normal weight for age and height
No known physical illness that would account for the weight loss

group therapy all have their place . . . provided that one understands . . . what one is trying to accomplish, knows how to proceed, and carefully assesses the individual (and the family system)."

    The resources outlined in Table XVI should be explored in undertaking the treatment of anorexia nervosa.

Table XV. Central Characteristics of Anorexia Nervosa: Clinical Features

Classic picture	Bright, conscientious, often "model" child who shifts from routine dieting to self-destructive obsession over food intake
	Distorted perception of body image, depression, sense of inadequacy, denial of thin appearance, unawareness of fatigue
	Conflict with aggressive and sexual drives which leads to guilt, ambivalence, reaction formation, cessation of menstrual cycle, reduction of breast size, hair loss, waste of muscle tissue, low blood pressure, pulse, hypothermia, and abnormal laboratory findings, including: post-menopausal levels of estrogen and prepubertal luteinizing hormone profile, low BMR, flat glucose tolerance curve, and abnormal liver function studies (e.g., SGOT and SGPT)
Onset	Usually in early to late adolescence
	Rarely in late latency and early 30's
Prevalence	1 in 250 females between 12 and 18 years
	Only 4% of all cases are males
Course	Most commonly single episode with full recovery
	May be episodic
	Occasionally unremitting with death by starvation in 5% to 20% of cases
Complications	Life-threatening situation must be dealt with immediately
	Attention directed toward medical and metabolic status, preferably by a physician other than the active therapist
	Protein supplement three times a day may be sufficient
	Hospitalization may be necessary
Personality patterns	Feighner[55] requires that no other known psychiatric disorder be present
	Rollins,[56] Risen,[57] and others feel the syndrome can be embedded in neurosis, psychotic disorganization, and borderline personalities
	Bruch[58,59] emphasized struggle to control sense of identity, "paralyzing sense of ineffectiveness and powerlessness," deficits in processing internal and external cues, and hostile–dependent relationship to mother
Family system patterns	Minuchin[60] refers to the psychosomatogenic family patterns, including: enmeshment, overprotectiveness, rigidity, and lack of conflict resolution.
	Poor role models for the healthy handling of aggressive and sexual impulses would appear to be another critical arena, especially influencing the preoedipal and oedipal years.

Table XVI. Resources to Explore in Management of Anorexia Nervosa

Treatment modality	Author	Reference
Psychoanalytic orientation	H. Bruch	58
Noninterpretative but "fact finding"	H. Bruch	59
Transference and interpretative	S. Risen	57
"Nurturant authoritative" orientation	S. Levenkron	*Treating and Overcoming Anorexia Nervosa,* Charles Scribner's Sons, New York, 1982.
	P. Zucker	Montefiore Hospital and Medical Center, 111 East 210th Street, Bronx, N.Y. 10467
Family systems orientation	M.S. Palazzoli	*Self-Starvation,* Jason Aronson, New York, 1978.
	S. Minuchin	*Families and Family Therapy,* Harvard University Press, Cambridge, 1974.
	P. Caille *et al.*	A systems theory approach to a case of anorexia nervosa, *Family Process* 16:455–466, 1977.
Group therapy orientation	P. Garfinkel	Clarke Institute of Psychiatry, 250 College Street, Toronto, Canada M5T 1R8
	E. Piazzo *et al.*	Childrens' Hospital Medical Center, 300 Longwood Avenue, Boston, MA 02115
Behavior Therapy orientation[a]	C. Zeller	Treatment of ego deficits in anorexia nervosa, *Amer. J. Orthopsychia.* 52:356–359, 1982.
Centers of information		American Anorexia Nervosa Association, 101 Cedar Lane, Teaneck, N.Y. 07666
		Anorexia Nervosa and Associated disorders (ANAD), Suite 2020, 550 Frontage Road, Northfield, IL 60093

[a]Caution: Systematic desensitization and operant conditioning restore weight gain rapidly, but leave underlying conflicts untouched. This can lead to serious aftereffects. Zeller used behavior therapy in conjunction with a psychodynamic approach.

Bulimia

This condition is characterized by recurrent episodes of rapid consumption of large amounts of food, usually in less than 2 hr, and is commonly referred to as "binge eating." There is an awareness that the eating pattern is abnormal, along with an inordinate preoccupation with food. Often there is a fear of not being able to stop overeating voluntarily. Depressed mood (75%) and self-deprecation often follow such binges, and the eating is often terminated by abdominal pain, sleep, or induced vomiting. The episodes are not due to anorexia nervosa but may interplay with that syndrome. Nor are they related to any known physical disorder. Onset is in adolescence or early adult life, often following an attempt at weight management with self-induced vomiting or laxative use as a "trial technique." It is predominantly seen in females and usually runs a chronic course, up to 6 years or longer. It is seldom incapacitating and is generally not life-threatening, although electrolyte imbalance and dehydration can occur from the repetitious vomiting.

Occasionally parotid gland enlargement, hypokalemia, rectal bleeding, destruction of dental enamel, and alopecia may result from chronic bulimia.[61] Physicians may have a hard time arriving at the diagnosis because patients may be secretive and ashamed of their symptoms.

The high incidence of depressive symptomatology and family history of affective illness suggests that bulimia is a variant of depressive illness.[70]

Substance Abuse and Alcoholism

Teenage drinking of alcohol has led to such a high percentage of traffic fatalities that many states have raised the legal age for drinking. In an urban high school in New Jersey in 1974, 72% of the students in grades 7 through 12 admitted to drinking alcohol; 27% indicated they were problem drinkers. Some children as young as 8–10 years admitted to drinking on a regular basis. An equally distressing observation on the effects of alcohol was made at UCLA, in which 40% of the students in the study showed some brain stem abnormalities.

Statistics from a 1976 study on smoking in the 12–18-year age group showed that more than one million new teenagers begin smoking each year. Eighty-five percent believe it is harmful but persist in smoking.

In that same age group, 12–18 years, a 1979 study of 2100 teenagers in a Central New Jersey School System indicated that 30% used alcohol more than once a month; 22% used marijuana more than once a week; approximately 25% used amphetamines, barbiturates, and hallucinogens; and 9% admitted to using opiates. They began using drugs as young as 13 years and usually obtained them through a friend during school hours.

The approach to the growing problem is not so much to scare as to steer teenagers away from harmful drugs. As professional persons and as parents it is important to let teenagers know the risks, and to help them find alternatives to boredom, to adolescent rebellion, to "acting grown-up," and to "seeking new highs in emotional experiences." Table XVII is an outline of early warning signals for teenagers as to when to go for help. It should be included in all programs on drug-abuse education to alert teenagers to the subtle changes that can take place in their mental functioning and personality development as a result of chronic drug use.

Table XVII. Early Warning Signals: When to Go for Help

Problem in concentrating
Failing memory
Decrease in math ability
Creeping feelings of persecution: that people are talking about you or becoming angry with you
Exaggerated (false) self-confidence or increasing self-doubt
Loss of energy, desire, and drive
Can't say what you want to say: have thoughts, *can't get words out*
Short fuse: "Fly off handle easily"
New "hang-ups" with girlfriends or boyfriends: can't get along!
Sense of hopelessness about life
Total denial that drugs are harmful to you

Suicide in Childhood

Suicidal behavior, threats, thoughts, and ideas are the most common psychiatric emergencies in childhood and adolescence. They should always be taken seriously. Statistics suggest that suicide is more common above the age of 12, and few completed suicides have been reported under the age of 12 years[62,63] It is recognized that parents and others will conceal the true nature of a child's death, and the child's methods, which make it difficult to obtain accurate statistics on incidence of suicide in childhood. It is known that there is a dramatic rise in the frequency and intensity of suicidal ideation in puberty and adolescence. Between 1961 and 1975 the rate of adolescent suicide in America increased 124%. In 1976 there were 4747 suicidal deaths in the 15–24-year age group; in 1978 that number rose to 5115. Also in 1978 there were 153 children between 5 and 14 who killed themselves. It is estimated that the rate continues around 5000 to 6000 per year.

In a Bronx Municipal Hospital study, Pfeffer et al.[64] noted that 13 (33%) of 39 outpatient latency-age children displayed suicidal ideas, threats, or attempts. Eleven were boys and two were girls, with jumping from heights and hanging being the most frequent method. Worries about school performance, disturbed peer relationships, frequency of parental punishment, and parental marital difficulties were most frequently cited as precipitating stresses. Increased psychomotor activity was the most common symptom in the 6 months preceding the attempt; sleep disturbances, firesetting, running away, and depressive symptoms were not seen in significant amounts compared with nonsuicidal children in this same study. No difference in the psychopathology of families in the suicidal and nonsuicidal families was observed. However, the incidence of suicidal behavior of the parents was significantly different for the two groups ($p<0.05$).

In conclusion, the authors noted the specific high-risk factors included the wish to die, an intense preoccupation with death, and significant suicidal behavior in the parents. The literature suggests that the "wish to die" can evolve from feelings of depression, hostility/aggression turned inward, and from the wish to escape from intolerable situations. An increase in motoric behavior appeared to be a specific indicator of potential suicidal behavior. These authors stressed that there appears to be a higher incidence of suicidal behavior in latency-age children than was previously reported and emphasized the need to pay attention to childhood suicidal behavior. Where suicide and attempted suicide do occur in childhood, the methods reflect little premeditation, and primarily impulsive behavior. Successful methods include jumping from high places, hanging, or running into traffic. It must be recognized that Piaget observed that children do not recognize death as finite and irreversible until the age of 9 years.

In most attempts in younger children a disturbed home life was present, including marital conflict, alcoholic parents, incarceration and loss of parents for legal, medical, or psychiatric reasons, family financial problems, and poor peer and sibling relationships. The key factor appeared to be the loss of a significant care-taking person, or loss and deprivation felt within the family system related to a variety of psychosocial and economic stressors.

In a review of 82 consecutive discharges from the Children's Hospital National Medical Center in Washington, Cohen-Sandler[65] found suicidal children ($N = 20$) more depressed and more frequently from a family with a positive history of alcoholism than in the depressed nonsuicidal group ($N = 21$) or in the group with other psychiatric disorders

($N = 35$). These authors also stressed the importance of loss or deprivation in early childhood from parental divorce or death, medical illnesses, and loss of an involved grandparent as underlying factors in suicidal behavior in this age group.

While this notion may hold for children, Tennant et al.[66] have questioned the causal link between early loss and later depression or suicidal behavior among adults, citing evidence that did not support this hypothesis.

In a follow-up study of 73 of the original sample, Cohen-Sandler[67] found that 4 of the 20 suicidal children made further suicide attempts, whereas no children from the other group did so.

Efforts by Tishler and McKenry[68] to compare symptom and self-esteem ratings of parents of suicidal adolescents with a nonpsychiatric control group suggested that mothers of the suicidal children were significantly more likely to have suicidal ideas than mothers in the control group. Recognizing the limitations of the study, it did suggest that factors such as genetic heritability, psychological identification of the suicidal child with a suicidal parent, and the impact of parental suicide intent on the young child all needed to be considered as part of the "language of suicide" communicated within a family system.[69]

Finally, the desire to alter an intolerable living situation beyond their capacity to change and to punish significant persons in their life experience were considered a causative factor in the child's impulsive attempts at suicide.[70]

Suicide in Adolescence

In the United States, suicide is the fourth leading cause of death among young people, exceeded only by accidents, malignancy, and homicide.[71] This phenomenon is a major public health problem, especially because of the increasing rate of completed suicides and attempted suicides among adolescents. Table XVIII highlights several of the critical factors in suicides among adolescents.

Teicher[70] described a three-stage process that leads to social isolation and frequently results in a suicidal attempt: stage 1, a long-standing history of problems from childhood to early adolescence; stage 2, a period of escalation during adolescence; and stage 3, increasing feelings of hopelessness in adolescent characterized by a "chain reaction breakdown of primary (interpersonal) associations" and coping strategies.

Carlson and Cantwell[72] studied 102 psychiatrically referred children, adolescents, and their parents, using the Children's Depression Inventory (CDI) and a semistructured interview. These workers found severe suicidal ideation increased around puberty and correlated with increasingly severe depression. Feelings of "hopelessness" were not described among the suicidal population with the same intensity described by Beck[73] in his adult population. The extent and pervasiveness of family psychopathology in first- and second-degree relatives for all subjects was impressive.

Crumley[74] feels a true adolescent suicidal attempt should be viewed as a cardinal symptom in establishing the identity of a serious psychiatric disorder. It reflects a transient or prolonged break with reality and "at least a partial decrease in reality testing which has serious implications." The seriousness of the attempt is often minimized by the adolescent and his family. Thus, any act of self-damage inflicted with self-destructive intent, however vague and ambiguous, must be taken seriously. Suicidal gestures, or self-

Table XVIII. Factors in Suicide among Adolescents

General	Apparent reasons	Methods[70]
No seasonal variation	Failure in coping efforts; an act of "desperation"[79]	Carbon monoxide gas
40–50% of completed suicides made a previous attempt	Stress of failure in ambition; social and reproductive effectiveness	Hanging
10% of parents of completed suicides also committed suicide	Social isolation	Drug overdose
Antisocial and histrionic personalities with history of drug abuse and secondary depressive symptoms, carry high risk for suicide	Rejection by opposite sex	Firearms
Schizophrenia increases risk 10 times	Anticipation of punishment for "getting into trouble"[70]	Suffocation/plastic bag
Those with bipolar-affective disease, with onset 14–19 years, are at high risk for suicidal behavior	Difficulty achieving biological fitness	Electrocution
	"Hoplessness" is a better predictor than "depression" in adults [80]	Drowning
	This is not totally confirmed in children[81]	Decapitation
	Adolescent incarcerated for criminal activity has increased suicidal risk for first 24 hours	

mutilation in anger, without intended self-destruction, are not considered of the same order of concern. In this category of lesser concern, Crumley would place overdosing to become "high" or intoxicated, and feigned self-injury to dramatize and call attention to oneself.

The partial breakdown in reality testing leading to a suicidal attempt can be seen in borderline personalities, in major affective disorders, or in schizophrenic disorders. The associated depressive syndromes are most commonly reported, along with drug use and alcoholism. Less frequently mentioned are hysterical reactions, compulsive neuroses, and minimal brain dysfunction or ADD. It is important to recognize that underlying all these syndromes one will often find maladaptive personality disorders including impulsive character disorders, antisocial disorders, borderline personality disorders, etc. Mattson *et al.*[75] have deplored the indiscriminate use of the diagnosis of adjustment reaction in the emergency room, which also minimizes the seriousness of the teenager's emotional problems. They also point to the importance of the abnormal Dexamethasone Suppression Tests in 13 of 23 teenagers who attempted suicide, suggesting its relationship to biochemical factors in adolescent depression and in their suicidal behavior.

Treatment of a suicidal attempt is divided into two parts. First, the treatment immediately following the attempt, as outlined in Table XIX. Subsequently, ongoing specific treatment methods must be employed for the different clinical syndromes leading to the self-destructive behavior. The different modalities include individual psychotherapy, group psychotherapy, family therapy, residential treatment, some home placement with treatment, and pharmacotherapy in conjunction with any combination of these approaches. More specific research is needed to determine the most effective therapeutic regimen for the carefully delineated underlying clinical syndrome.

Masterson's follow-up treatment plan[76] indicated the importance of staying with the adolescent over time and of adjusting the clinical intervention to meet the emerging needs of the emotionally developing adolescent.

Table XIX Suggestions for Treatment after Suicidal Attempt

1 Hospitalize, if only briefly, to decompress situation, to explore factors, to organize treatment plan (Suicidal behavior is clinical basis for involuntary admission)

2 Become ''lifeline'' and accessible for child or adolescent whether attempt was motivated as 'attention-getting'' or bona fide attempt to die *Take attempt seriously*

3 Withhold all medications until history of nature of ingested substance is clarified Run drug screens for abused substances

4 Make patient secure from continuing harm from life-threatening objects, or environmental potential for self-destruction

5 Take careful history from parents, patient, peers, and other significant persons in patient's hierarchy to understand facts and dynamic forces behind attempt
    a Identify developmental patterns and premorbid personality characteristics
    b Identify psychostressors and precipitating factors
    c Assess degree of dangerousness in lethality of the attempt, degree of reversibility, and accessibility factors in attempt

6 Request psychological evaluation to determine quality of mental functioning, ego mechanisms of defense, intactness of reality testing, and quality of coping skills

7 Consider neurological assessment, where indicated, to rule out space-taking lesions or residuals from earlier trauma or infection

8 Objectively evaluate degree of depression using Children's Depression Inventory (self-report), K-SADS (Kiddie-Schedule for Affective Disorders and Schizophrenia), Moos Family Environment Scale,[77] and structured and unstructured interviews with adolescent

9 Complete the Dexamethasone Suppression Test [78] [79] [80]

Table XX Prediction and Management of Suicidal Risks

Considerations	Intuitive synthesis of all facts and factors
Prediction is difficult	There is *no* sure way
Nature of circumstances	Degree of personal loss, degree of stress, severe familial or socioeconomic stress
Prior self-destructive behavior	High risk
Suicide note left	High risk
Family history of successful suicide	High risk
''Chain reaction'' with loss of communication, isolation, withdrawal, hopelessness and loss of coping skills	High risk
Degree and nature of depression	Variable risk
Degree of hostility and toward whom	Variable risk
Premorbid personality long-standing history of prior mental illness, personality disorders	At risk
Escalation of problems in adolescence	Variable risk
Reaction of parents from concern to ridicule	Influences risk
Sources of support from family and community	Influences risk
Remove access to lethal weapons (guns, knives) and drugs	
When in doubt lean toward hospitalization	
Management very difficult with strongly determined person	May not be able to prevent suicide
Use careful, consistent, concerned clinical judgment with reasonable cautiousness	

Prediction of suicidal behavior is equally complex and unsettling. Teicher[70] commented that "the belief that suicidal behaviors are predictable is valid as a belief in principle, but not in fact." Table XX is an attempt to state some of the critical factors in predicting suicidal risk. It has also been noted among the persons working with gifted adolescents that some may get caught-up in a personal existential crisis which may lead to self-destructive behavior. To help these brilliant and baffled adolescents, as well as all who struggle with a sense of hopelessness and despair, it is essential to lead them to new bridges and bonds with others who love and understand them, and to bridges of basic faith to cope with the vicissitudes of being and becoming a person in an unfinished (imperfect) world.

REFERENCES

1. Cohen, D.: The pathology of the self in primary childhood autism and Gilles de la Tourette syndrome. *Psychiatr. Clin. North Am.* **3**:383–400, 1980.
2. Kohut, H.: *The Analysis of the Self.* International Universities Press, New York, 1971.
3. Allee, J. G. (ed.). *Webster's Encyclopedia of Dictionaries.* New American edition. Ottenheimer, New York, 1978.
4. Beres, D.: Self, identity, and narcissism. *Psychoanal. Q.* **50**:515–534, 1981.
5. Kegan, R.: *The Evolving Self: Problem and Process in Human Development.* Harvard University Press, Cambridge, Massachusetts, 1982.
6. Ticho, E.: Psychoanalytic theories of the self. *J. Am. Psychoanal. Assoc.* **30**:717–733, 1982.
7. James, W.: *Principles of Psychology.* Holt, New York, 1980.
8. Damon, W., and Hart, D.: The development of self-understanding from infancy through adolescence. *Child Dev.* **53**:841–864, 1982.
9. Mead, G. H.: *Mind, Self, and Society.* University of Chicago Press, Chicago, 1934.
10. Rogers, C.: *The Clinical Treatment of the Problem Child.* Houghton-Mifflin, New York, 1939.
11. Erikson, E.: *Childhood and Society.* Norton, New York, 1950.
12. Loevinger, J.: *Ego Development.* Jossey-Bass, San Francisco, 1976.
13. Selman, R.: *The Growth of Interpersonal Understanding: Developmental and Clinical Analyses.* Academic Press, New York, 1980.
14. White, B.: *The First Three Years of Life.* Prentice-Hall, Englewood Cliffs, New Jersey.
15. Greenspan, S.: *Psychopathology and Adaptation in Infancy and Early Childhood.* International Universities Press, New York, 1981.
16. Mahler, M., Pino, F., and Bergman, A.: *The Psychological Birth of the Human Infant.* Basic Books, New York, 1975.
17. Spitz, R. A.: Hospitalization: An inquiry into the genesis of psychiatric conditions in early childhood. *Psychoanal. Study Child* **1**:53–74, 1945.
18. Powell, G., Brasel, A., and Blizzard, R.: Emotional deprivation and growth retardation simulating idiopathic hypopituitarism. *N. Engl. J. Med.* **276**:1271–1278, 1976.
19. Egan, J., Chartoor, I., Rosen, G.: Non-organic failure to thrive: Pathogenesis and classification. *Clin. Proc. Childrens Hosp. Natl. Med. Ctr.* **36(4)**:173–182, 1980.
20. Bengoa: The problem of malnutrition. *W.H.O. Chron* **28**:3, 1974.
21. Craviota, J.: Mother–child interrelationships and malnourishment, in Baughan, V., and Brazelton, T. (eds.): *The Family—Can It Be Saved?* Year Book, Chicago, 1976.
22. Lewis, M.: *Clinical Aspects of Child Development,* 2nd ed. Lea & Febiger, Philadelphia, 1982.
23. Helfer, R.: *The Diagnostic Process and Treatment Programs.* DHEW Publ. No. (OHO) 75–69, 1975.
24. Kempe, C. H.: *Helping the Battered Child and His Family.* Lippincott, Philadelphia, 1972.
25. Caffey, J.: Multiple fractures in the long bones of infants suffering from chronic subdural hematoma. *Am. J. Roentgenol.* **56**:163–173, 1946.
26. Broughton, J.: Development of concepts of self, mind, reality, and knowledge. *New Directions Child Dev.* **1**:75–100, 1978.

27. Meyer, J.: The theory of gender identity disorders. *J. Am. Psychoanal. Assoc.* **30**:381–418, 1982.
28. Freud, S.: *Character and Anal Eroticism*, Vol. 9. Hogarth Press, London, 1959, pp. 167–175.
29. Abraham, K.: *Selected Papers of Karl Abraham, M.D.* Hogarth Press, London, 1927.
30. Rutter, M., and Schopler, E.: *Autism: A Reappraisal of Concepts and Treatment.* Plenum, New York, 1978.
31. Rutter, M., Tizard, J., and Whitmore, R.: *Education, Health and Behavior.* Longman, London, 1970.
32. Wulff, M.: A phobia in a child of eighteen months. *Int. J. Psychoanal.* **9**:354–359, 1928.
33. Renik, D., Spielman, P., and Afterman, J.: Bamboo phobia in an eighteen month-old boy. *J. Am. Psychoanal. Assoc.* **26**:266–282, 1978.
34. Ritvo, S.: *Current Status of the Concept of the Infantile Neurosis: Implications for Diagnosis and Technique.* Psychoanalytic Study of the Child, No. 29. Yale University Press, New Haven, 1974, pp. 159–182.
35. Nagera, H.: *Early Childhood Disturbances, the Infantile Neurosis and the Adulthood Disturbances.* International Universities Press, New York, 1966.
36. Sperling, M.: *The Major Neuroses and Behavior Disorders in Children.* Jason Aronson, New York, 1974.
37. Anthony, E. J.: Neurotic disorders, in Freedman, A., Kaplan, H., and Sadoch, B. (eds.): *Comprehensive Textbook of Psychiatry*, Vol. 2. Williams & Wilkins, Baltimore, 1975.
38. Adams, P.: Psychoneuroses, in Noshpitz, J. (ed.): *Basic Handbook of Child Psychiatry.* Basic Books, New York, 1979.
39. Mash, E., and Terdal, L.: *Behavioral Assessment of Childhood Disorders.* Guilford Press, New York, 1981.
40. Tseng, W. S., Arensdorf, A., McDermott, J., et al.: Family diagnosis and classification. *J. Am. Acad. Child Psychiatry* **15**(1):15–35, 1976.
41. Masten, A.: Family therapy as a treatment for children: A critical review of outcome research. *Family Process* **18**(3):323–336, 1979.
42. Sperry, B., Gardner, G., Stoner, N., et al.: Renunciation and denial in learning difficulties. *Am. J. Orthopsychiatry* **28**:98–111, 1958.
43. Belmont, H.: Confusing varieties of depression in childhood. *Penn. Med.* **84**(7):41–43, 1981.
44. Cytryn, L.: Biochemical correlates of affective disorders. *Arch. Gen. Psychiatry* **31**:659–661, 1974.
45. Weitkamp, L.: Depressive disorders and HLA: A gene on chromosome 6 that can affect behavior. *N. Engl. J. Med.* **305**:1301–1306, 1981.
46. Matthysee, S., and Kidd, K.: Evidence of HLA linkage in depressive disorders. *N. Engl. J. Med.* **305**:1340–1341, 1981.
47. Mandell, A.: Neurobiological mechanisms of adaptation in relation to models of psychobiological development, in Schopler, E., and Reichler, R. (eds.): *Psychopathology and Child Development.* Plenum, New York, 1976.
48. Puig-Antich, J., Perel, J. M., Lupatkin, W., et al.: Plasma levels of imiprimine and clinical response in prepubertal major depressive disorder. *J. Am. Acad. Child Psychiatry* **18**:617–627, 1979.
49. McKnew, D., and Cytryn, L.: Urinary metabolites in chronically depressed children. *J. Am. Acad. Child Psychiatry* **18**:608–615, 1979.
50. Cohen, D.: Constructive and reconstructive activities in the analysis of a depressed child. *Psychoanal. Study Child* **35**:237–266, 1980.
51. Sander, J., and Joffe, W.: Notes on childhood depression. *Int. J. Psychoanal.* **46**:88–96, 1965.
52. Blumberg, M. L.: Depression in abused and neglected children. *Am. J. Psychother.* **35**(3):330–341, 1981.
53. National Center for Health Statistics: *Advance Report. Final Divorce Statistics. Monthly Vital Stat Report* **29**(suppl. 4), 1980.
54. Wallerstein, J. S., and Kelly, J. B.: *Surviving the Breakup: How Children and Parents Cope with Divorce.* Basic Books, New York, 1980.
55. Feighner, J.: Diagnostic criteria for use in psychiatric research. *Arch. Gen. Psychiatry* **26**:57–63, 1972.
56. Rollins, N., and Piazza, E.: Diagnosis of anorexia nervosa: A critical reappraisal. *J. Am. Acad. Child Psychiatry* **17**:126–137, 1978.
57. Risen, S.: The psychoanalytic treatment of an adolescent with anorexia nervosa. *Psychoanal. Study Child* **37**:433–459, 1982.
58. Bruch, H.: *Eating Disorders.* Basic Books, New York, 1973.
59. Bruch, H.: *The Golden Cage.* Harvard University Press, Cambridge, Massachusetts, 1978.
60. Minuchin, S.: *Families and Family Therapy.* Harvard University Press, Cambridge, Massachusetts, 1974.

61. Herzog, D.: Bulimia: The secretive syndrome. *Psychosomatics* **23**:481–487, 1982.
62. Shaffer, D.: Suicide in childhood and early adolescence. *J. Child Psychol. Psychiatry* **15**:275–291, 1974.
63. Shaffer, D.: Diagnostic considerations in suicidal behavior in children and adolescents. *J. Am. Acad. Child Psychiatry* **21**:414–416, 1982.
64. Pfeffer, R., Conte, H., Plutchik, R., *et al.*: Suicidal behavior in latency-age children. *J. Am. Acad. Child Psychiatry* **19**:703–710, 1980.
65. Cohen-Sandler, R., Berman, A., and King, R.: Life stress and symptomatology: Determinants of suicidal behavior in children. *J. Amer. Aca. Child Psychiatry* **21**:178–186, 1982.
66. Tennant, C., Bebbington, R., and Hurry, J.: Parental death in childhood and risk of adult depressive disorders: A review. *Psychol. Med.* **10**:289–300, 1980.
67. Cohen-Sandler, R., Berman, A., and King, K.: A follow-up study of hospitalized suicidal children. *J. Am. Acad. Child Psychiatry* **21**:398–403, 1982.
68. Tishler, C., and McKenry, P.: Parental negative self and adolescent suicidal attempts. *J. Am. Acad. Child Psychiatry* **21**:404–408, 1982.
69. Kreitman, N., Smith, P., and Tan, E.: Attempted suicide as language: An empirical study. *Brit. J. Psychiatry* **116**:465–473, 1970.
70. Teicher, J.: Suicide and suicide attempts, in Noshpitz, J. (ed.): *Basic Handbook of Child Psychiatry*, Vol. 2. Basic Books, New York, 1979.
71. Healthy People: The Surgeon General's Report on Health Promotion and Disease Prevention, publication 79–55071. US Dept. of Health, Education, and Welfare, 1979, pp. 1–15.
72. Carlson, G., and Cantwell, D.: Suicidal behavior and depression in children and adolescents. *J. Am. Acad. Child Psychiatry* **21**:361–368, 1982.
73. Beck, A. T., Kovacs, M., and Weissman, A.: Hopelessness and suicidal behavior: An overview. *JAMA* **234**:1146–1149, 1975.
74. Crumley, F.: The adolescent suicide attempt: A cardinal symptom of a serious psychiatric disorder. *Am. J. Psychother.* **36**:158–165, 1982.
75. Mattson, A., Seese, J., and Hawkins, J.: Suicidal behavior as a child psychiatric emergency. *Arch. Gen. Psychiatry* **20**:100, 1969.
76. Masterson, J.: *From Borderline Adolescent to Functioning Adult: The Test of Time*. Brunner/Mazel, New York, 1980.
77. Moos, R.: Family Environment Scale, Form R. Consulting Psychologists Press, Palo Alto, California, 1981.
78. Carroll, B., Tarika, J. Albala, A. A., *et al.*: Specific laboratory test for the diagnosis of melancholia. *Arch. Gen. Psychiatry* **38**:15–22, 1981.
79. Brown, W.: The dexamethasone suppression test: Clinical applications. *Psychosomatics* **22**:951–955, 1981.
80. Gwirstman, H., Gerner, R., and Sternbach, H.: The overnight dexamethasone suppression test: Clinical and theoretical reviews. *J. Clin. Psychiatry* **43**:321–327, 1982.

16

Juvenile Delinquency

Peter W. Zinkus and Paul King

INTRODUCTION

Juvenile crime is a problem of epidemic proportions and one that touches every person. The issue has justifiably provoked a national anxiety, both in terms of its staggering economic impact and in the loss of human potential. The necessity for rehabilitation of juvenile offenders, as well as research into the prevention of juvenile crime, has become a priority issue for local and federal governments. Congressional hearings in 1977 reflected a national direction for active intervention into this problem. A literal army of youthful offenders represents a threat to social conscience, economic stability, and personal safety.

Numerous investigators have reported on the alarming increase in juvenile crimes. There has been a marked rise in the incidence since the late 1940s.[1] In relatively recent years, the ratio of juvenile to adults arrests has become disproportionately unbalanced. The apparent dramatic influx in crimes committed by youthful offenders in part reflects improved reporting methods, changes in public attitude, modifications of social values, and the growth in the population of persons under 18 years of age. However, the increase far surpasses the increased numbers of adolescents in the general population. Although these factors appear to be of significance, they do not completely account for the sharp

Peter W. Zinkus • Child Psychology Division, Le Bonheur Children's Medical Center, Memphis, Tennessee 38103. *Paul King* • Child and Adolescent Psychiatry, Adolescent Services, Charter Lakeside Hospital, University of Tennessee Center for the Health Sciences, Memphis, Tennessee 38103.

rise in major offenses committed by delinquent youth. In 1985 it was reported that approximately 3% of American children, 10–17 years of age, appeared in juvenile court each year for offenses other than traffic violations.[2] It has been estimated that one in every nine adolescents will appear in court before the eighteenth birthday. However, the reported incidence in juvenile crime represents only a small sampling of a more pervasive problem. Official juvenile court statistics reflect the illegal acts of those youthful offenders who come to trial in a juvenile court. The statistics do not include those who are arrested but who do not come to trial.

The prognosis for a large percentage of youthful offenders appears pessimistic. The recidivism rate is extremely high. Juvenile delinquency appears to represent a lifelong process of misdemeanancy rather than a transient episode of adolescent misbehavior. Annually in the United States, more than 100,000 children, 7–17 years of age, are confined in jails and similar detention facilities. Institutions for delinquent offenders generally lack the ability to provide a long-term rehabilitation.

Mangel[3] commented as follows on juvenile crime and its long-range sequelae:

> About six of every ten juveniles in jail (and we mean jail with locks and bars and guards) have committed no criminal acts. Eight out of these same ten *do* commit crimes after they leave jail. Some three out of four juveniles who are put in jail as juveniles are convicted of crime as adults. More than one million boys and girls are caught up in America's juvenile justice system each year. On any day more than one thousand juveniles are behind bars.

Mangel further expressed concern about society's priorities in seeking to prevent delinquency by noting that in 1973 approximately $14 million was allocated for delinquency prevention and about $5 billion for highway construction. Juvenile crimes cost approximately $8000 for each delinquent each year and, as an adult criminal, about $27,000 per year.[3] A criminal career is estimated to cost $0.5 million—$250,000 of which can be measured in terms of property loss, higher insurance rates, and costs of maintaining correctional centers. The loss of dignity in a human life and the loss of social potential, however, are factors that cannot be measured in dollars and cents.[4]

Mauser[5] defined a profile of the "typical" juvenile delinquent: (1) average age of 13.5 years, (2) peak years for arrest between ages 13 and 14 years, and (3) an average IQ of 95 (falling within the national norm of average intelligence). Mauser characterized the juvenile delinquent of today as a tougher, meaner, and sicker person than his counterpart of 10–15 years ago, reflecting the influence of the drug culture.

Socioeconomic deprivation and family relationships are recognized as factors influencing delinquent behaviors. Inadequate food, clothing, shelter, and education can adversely influence the physical, intellectual, and attitudinal maturation of children. Deprivation of these essential psychobiological needs as well as insufficient rewards or pleasures of living generally evoke frustration, anxiety, anger, and hostility. The adolescent who by circumstance is deprived of physical and psychological needs may exhibit deviant behaviors by illegally taking what is coveted.

Whether the earlier family experience or the later cultural environment is the more important factor in determining delinquent behavior has not been definitively resolved. It has been suggested, however, that early neglect or abuse is the more essential element influencing subsequent delinquency. The great majority of children growing up within the culture of inner city, with its turmoil, chaos, and violence, may adopt this life style because their early family experiences were associated with significant deprivation, neglect and abuse.

Aichorn[6] was one of the first to focus attention on the relationship between family background and juvenile delinquency, hypothesizing that delinquency was not the end product of poor peer relationships and unsupervised street activities, but, secondary to early disturbed parental emotional interactions. Bender[7] reported on more than 5000 children under the age of 14 years with a variety of psychopathic disorders, including aggressive, delinquent, and antisocial behaviors. Disturbed family relationships, deprivation, abuse, and neglect in early infancy and childhood were defined as etiological factors that distorted the personality development of the child. Parents of juvenile delinquents tend to be more lax, inconsistent, and unkind and more frequently resorted to physical form of punishment than parents of nondelinquent youngsters.[8] It was noted in a review of 5000 abused or neglected children that 12 or more years later, 19% were delinquent. In a county in New York, the incidence of juvenile delinquency among abused children was reported to be 30%.

Juvenile delinquency is apparently a multifactorial disorder, an ill-defined syndrome of behaviors fashioned by a complex amalgamation of cultural, social, psychological, neurological, and educational influences. The remainder of this chapter will focus on psychodynamic factors, as well as the relationship between learning disorders and juvenile delinquency.

A PSYCHODYNAMIC VIEW OF JUVENILE DELINQUENCY

A variety of historical psychodynamic concepts have been proposed to explain types of delinquent behavior. Aichorn[6] demonstrated the use of a therapeutic alliance in achieving a behavioral change, (treatment techniques considered bold by modern standards). He described a type of delinquent who would act out behaviorally through a sense of guilt, which would be expiated when caught. Friedlander[9] dealt with the need to block discharge of impulsive behavior in order to create a level of anxiety high enough for the young person to be psychotherapeutically reached.

The *weakness of conscience* has been regarded as an important factor in developing antisocial behaviors. The parents have been incriminated as the cause of a child's inability to develop a normal conscience.[10] The term *superego lacunae* has been used to describe a young person's weak conscience, as a result of parents' deriving unconscious gratification from the child's behavior. Johnson[11] proposed that neurotic conflicts often accompany the superego lacunae. Redl[12-14] focused on the need to provide attention to specifics of ego function in order to understand and effectively treat delinquent behavior. Rosenthal[15] emphasized the importance of the formation of an ego ideal in the adolescent female, referring to two factors: biological (from mother) and a social culture factor. Conflicts or a poor integration of these factors are expressed in terms of delinquent behavior.

A better understanding of the dynamics of delinquency has been derived from research on hospitalized juvenile delinquents at the Illinois State Psychiatric Institute.[16,17] Delinquent youths treated at this inpatient facility have been categorized into four groups[18]:

1. *Impulsive:* revealing little sensitivity and poor impulse control
2. *Narcissistic:* exhibiting tendency to deny problems; self-centeredness

3. *Depressed:* showing compliance at school and an identification with staff (physical punishment was common during upbringing)
4. *Borderline:* viewed as passive, empty, and less engaging than the other types

Most delinquents presented as a combination of these factors.

CASE HISTORIES

Case History 1   John, a 17-year-old white male, was expelled from school for truancy and being verbally abusive to the principal. John has run away from home about four times in the past year and was jailed in a rural community jail for vagrancy after being found sleeping in the park. He has also been charged with public drunkenness and unlawful possession of a controlled substance. While in detention, he agreed to psychiatric treatment but then would not agree to sign in after the court charges were dropped.

Drug history is significant in that he began smoking marijuana at age 12 and regularly used marijuana since age 13 years. He also admitted to episodic drinking, use of quaaludes, and hallucinogens. John was constantly in conflict with his mother over the lack of responsibility in doing work around the house. One night after an altercation with his mother, John punched holes in the walls, tore a door off its hinges, and took the family car, returning the next morning. Restrictive measures failed to work.

Parents are both high school graduates and the father served in the military. Parents were divorced 5 years ago. John was born without complications and passed through all developmental milestones. He made friends easily and was involved in school sports and wrestling until age 13 years.

John is a good-looking, muscular adolescent male who spoke easily and related well to the examiner. He was casually dressed in jeans and a rock tee shirt and wore his hair long, but neatly combed. He spent much of the interview talking about his girlfriend and how much his girlfriend meant to him. When asked about his problems, he responded with "family problems," giving the examiner the impression that John felt that his parents were the problem. He admitted to the property destruction and stated that he does lose his temper around his parents. He did not consider his drug use a problem, as he primarily used marijuana. John did admit to stealing, but only from his mother or other relatives; he did not consider this criminal behavior. In fact, he showed little empathy toward his parents, feeling that they treated him unjustly.

For about the past 8 months, John would spend much of his time with girlfriend. They were almost always together and she would tell him about her problems. John attempted to get his girlfriend to decrease her drug use, but she overdosed after an argument and John took her to the emergency room. John was also very possessive in his relationship with the girl. He wanted to know all about her whereabouts and would beat her at times, usually after an argument and while he was intoxicated.

John was hospitalized in an adolescent unit for 3 months. Although he spoke in great detail about his girlfriend, he rapidly became provocative toward the girls on the unit and would spend much time in talking with them about their problems. In family therapy, the family can best be described as enmeshed with the mother being overprotective with her son, enabling him to escape from suffering anxiety.[19] It became clear that the mother felt she had a close relationship with her son; she would not date men. She stated that her son would never accept a stepfather. An older brother had moved out 5 years previously. Although the family was not earning a large income, John had the best clothes, a motorcycle, and money to spend. The mother even admitted that she would buy her son a car if he did well in the hospital program.

Individual psychotherapy sessions showed clearly a basic self-centeredness. Problems were denied, minimized, or blamed on someone else. In fact, John had an explanation for every problem incident. He was very demanding of attention and was always angry when limits were set that restricted him in some fashion. He expressed rage at his father and school principals. He constantly needed to be around friends, and especially females, so that he could feel good about himself. Drugs, likewise, would make him comfortable and relieve anxiety.

It is clear that John showed poor impulse control, poor frustration tolerance, self-gratifying relationships, and chemical dependency. As long as adults would give him positive encouragement, he responded favorably, but when frustrated, he was easily hurt and frustrated and would respond with anger. He and his mother maintain an overinvolved relationship that stifles and keeps the boy dependent so the mother can take care of John rather than allowing herself some independence. John's rigid self-centered stance, unconsciously supported by the mother, who has protected him from anxiety, leads to conflicts with authority, poor interpersonal relationships, and little ability to function on an age-appropriate developmental task.

Case History 2 Ann is a 14-year-old white girl admitted after ingesting an unknown quantity of cold pills, Valium, and aspirin, after an abortion. Ann was upset that her 20-year-old boyfriend who had gotten her pregnant and was a strong influence in her heavy drug use was seeing another girl. Ann had a very poor relationship with her stepfather, who was in the home for about 2 years. Ann felt she had lost the "special relationship" she had had with her mother. In addition, she was recently extremely upset by the fact that her stepfather pressed charges against her boyfriend. In addition, he attempted to set firm and consistent limits with Ann, her sister, and her brother. This was poorly tolerated by Ann.

The natural father was described as an individual who had a "drinking problem" and who often resorted to physical attacks on family members. This precipitated several runaway episodes in the past. There is a family history of depressive illness.

There was a history of drug abuse with marijuana and alcohol at age 12, but soon Ann was using Valium, quaaludes, barbiturates, and cocaine. In interview, Ann was openly defiant and hostile. She did not wish to be interviewed and felt forced to see a psychiatrist. She was antagonistic toward her stepfather and showed her mother that she had no respect for her. Ann felt that living with her father would solve all her problems. It was suggested to her that with all her bravado, she was quite dependent on her boyfriend and, in fact, was completely dominated by him. Of course, she rejected this interpretation. Ann did go on to live with her father, but he sent her back to her mother after 3 months. This is not uncommon. The parent without custody, often the father, feels that his daughter's problems are caused by his former wife, especially if the divorce was less than amiable. The child looks at going to the other parent as a way to get out of a limit-setting situation with her stepfather. Once the father began to set limits, Ann began to act up; she was then sent back to her mother.

This time, Ann appeared much less defiant and more depressed. She had no clear conception of herself as a person, without goals, interests, or future plans. She actively considered suicide if her boyfriend were to leave her. She was later able to look at herself as a helpless, depressed, and dependent individual rather than focusing on "family problems." Ann also admitted to being addicted to drugs, that the drugs made her "alive" and gave her personality. "I don't have to care when I'm doing drugs." She was able to see, though, that drugs had completely wrecked her life and had made her miserable in the end. Ann remained rigid in not being willing to deal with her boyfriend. In fact, she was quite protective toward him.

DISCUSSION

Several common features can be identified in both case histories. Dependency on a girlfriend or boyfriend was significantly different from the normal pattern of dating. The presence of the other person serves as an extension of one's self, and when lost, the self becomes lost. *Abandonment depression* is a term used to describe this loss.[20] Poor frustration tolerance and impulse control, and a low depression tolerance were observed in both cases. The adolescents experienced feeling of emptiness, depression, and apathy. The inability to tolerate depression is seen as an ego deficit.[21] Behaviors such as anger, manipulative behavior, poor social skills, and self-centeredness are frequently observed in the borderline adolescent.[22]

Another common feature in the case histories presented is the abuse of drugs. Drug abuse may be a mask for a depressive illness.[23] On the other hand, depression may be induced or released by drug abuse.[24] Drug use has also been viewed as a disease.[25]

Stimulation of the limbic system by "recreational" drugs appears to impart an immediate gratification without exerting an effort.[26] After a period of time, the brain is unable to respond to "normal" stimulation. The seeking of intense thrilling experiences may lead the user to daring robberies, car theft, high-speed chases, and other antisocial or delinquent behaviors. The action is performed in order to achieve a "thrill" or euphoric experience. If the act is committed while the individual is intoxicated with alcohol or other drugs, an added effect is a sense of disinhibition. The combination results in poor impulse control while under the effects of the drug. This phenomenon is readily appreciated with alcohol abuse. Both factors are often in play when a drug abusing young person is engaged in delinquent behavior. Stealing is frequently regarded as a drug-related delinquent behavior. The acts of stealing may first involve parents and other relatives, but soon extends to shoplifting and breaking and entering. These delinquent behaviors are promoted by the need to support an increasing addiction. The delinquent adolescent may be "stoned" much of the time.

If the drug abuse is the primary problem, the psychosocial problems, depression, and family issues are regarded as complications resulting from the abuse of chemicals. Delinquent behavior would similarly be viewed as a result of the drug abuse, rather than in terms of ego or conscience defect. This hypothesis appears to be contrary to most traditional psychodynamic concepts. The conceptual basis for delinquent behavior must be established in order to provide a meaningful treatment program.

Delinquency can be viewed as a character problem or an expression of a family issue. Recent evidence suggests a change in the brain caused by mood altering substances. "Chemical effects" lead to new patterns of thoughts and feelings which are expressed in terms of antisocial behavior. Obviously, treatment techniques must be directed toward the particular problems of the patient and not toward merely modifying behavior. A thorough assessment of the possible origins of delinquent behavior is necessary before a course of treatment can be recommended.

DISORDERS OF LEARNING AND DELINQUENT BEHAVIOR

The juvenile delinquent can be characterized as a nonlearner both in the classroom and in society, seldom profiting from past experience, as attested by high rates of recidivism. Rebellion against society carries over to other social institutions, such as school, and results in deficiencies in academic skills, such as reading. According to this concept, the delinquent reads poorly because he is often truant or inattentive and uncooperative when attending school. A hypothesis, in understanding this complex behavior problem, suggests that a basic learning disorder may in part account for the academic and social maladaptation of the youthful offender.

Reading Disabilities and Juvenile Delinquency

A major academic deficit among delinquent youth is extremely poor reading skill, initially assumed to be a sequel of a wide range of psychosocial deficiencies. The youth offender was traditionally characterized as a psychopathic personality, with reading retardation regarded as a symptom of the psychopathy of the rebellious attitude of delinquent youth. In essence, the hypothesis proposes that the child could learn to read but was not interested in reading! A counterargument proposes that the reading deficits are manifestations of specific learning disabilities among youthful offenders.

McCready[27] suggested a relationship between dyslexia in children and a high-risk potential for delinquency: "the behavior of word-blind children who develop a paranoid reaction toward the teacher and develop a sense of inferiority leading them to respond with behavior disorders in school, truancy and depredation upon school property." Reading problems were described in delinquent youth with average intelligence, who were found to be reading at least 5 years below their chronological age.[28] In a study of children examined at a juvenile detention center, 84% were reading retarded by 2 or more years, and more than 50% were deficient in reading by 5 years or more. The findings suggested that children with learning disabilities must be identified and aided before truancy and subsequent delinquency develop.[29]

More recently, Critchley, in 1968, surveyed a delinquent population and found that 60% were deficient in reading by 2 or more years.[30] Tarnopol[3] confirmed these observations in his sampling of delinquent males, ages 16–23 years. The average reading level of 64% of his subjects was below the sixth-grade level.[31] Mulligan[42] studied delinquents with IQs in the average range and found that they were reading 5.2 grades below their actual grade placement. In addition, many of the children showed classic signs of dyslexia in the form of word and letter reversals and missequencing of letters. Weinschenk[32] supported the concept that many of the children in delinquent populations showed symptoms of congenital dyslexia and dysgraphia.

Whereas many studies confirm that the delinquent reads poorly, there is a paucity of information concerning the nature and etiology of the delinquent's limited reading skills. Investigations of the perceptual capabilities of delinquent adolescents had provided some information on the factors underlying their observed reading disorders.

Perceptual Disorders and Juvenile Delinquency

There appears to be a causal relationship between learning disabilities, reading disorders, and CNS-processing dysfunctions.[33-36] The decoding of transmitted sensory impulses is impaired, presumably at the cortical level, despite intact peripheral sense organs. The child with perceptual lags or dysfunctions may exhibit reversals and rotations of letters and numbers, missequencing of auditory directions, difficulty in integrating auditory and visual symbols, and other modality-associated deficits. Most children with significant perceptual disturbances, despite average or above intelligence, are deficient in academic skills, particularly in reading. In addition evidence of perceptual processing disorders has been found in delinquent populations. Mauser[5] reported that approximately 75% of juvenile delinquents in his study exhibited evidence of specific learning disabilities, corroborating the incidence of 50% in Poremba's study.[4] Neuropsychological studies of delinquent subjects revealed that 55% of the subjects exhibited visuoperceptual or visuomotor disabilities, 31% evidenced impaired nonverbal concept formation, 30% had auditory discrimination or memory disabilities and 28% showed impaired kinesthetic perception.[37] Compton[38] demonstrated similar perceptual abnormalities in a delinquent population, 444 youthful offenders, approximately 46% manifested a significant visual-perceptual deficit and 24% were deficient in language-processing skills. The perceptual disorders were of sufficient severity to compromise academic progress, although overall intellectual abilities were adequate. Petrie *et al.*[39] reported that large numbers of delinquent subjects exhibit atypical visuoperceptual functioning. The etiology of these deficits was defined in terms of subtle organic brain dysfunction, which disrupted normal channels of perceptual learning. The major deficits in juvenile delinquents appeared to be in the areas of visuospatial orientation and visuomotor coordination.[40] Spatial orientation disturbances, as detected on examination such as the Bender–Gestal test, were frequent among youthful offenders.[41] Visual discrimination and visual-perceptual skills were characteristically found among juvenile delinquents.[42] Visual processing disturbances apparently cause considerable stress for the child as he attempts to cope with the standards established by school and society. The sequence of events begins with pressures in school due to academic underachievement caused by perceptual deficits. The resultant anxieties, frustrations, and tensions take the form of behavioral disturbances and finally culminate as antisocial behaviors such as juvenile delinquency.

Auditory processing disturbances and speech/language disorders have similarly been found in groups of delinquents. Disturbances in the ability to process auditory stimuli may be manifested as deficits in auditory association, closure, discrimination, memory and sequential memory and sound blending.[35] Auditory processing deficits as well as speech disturbances often adversely influence educational development and social adaptation.

Critchley[30] reported a higher incidence of articulation deficits among reading-deficient delinquents. The youthful offenders who manifested severe reading disabilities evidenced articulation disorders to a much greater degree than did delinquents with adequate reading skills. Tarnopol[31] studied the verbal skills of a delinquent group and demonstrated a relationship between juvenile delinquency and learning disorders and language function. The poor readers performed poorly on psychological tests measuring functions related to the left cerebral hemisphere, such as speech, language, and auditory processing skills. In addition, delinquents with lower verbal skills had a tendency to commit more crimes and were arrested more often than were subjects with adequate verbal skills. Jacobson[43] noted that many delinquents characteristically learn more efficiently by the visual modality. He suggested that there is a higher incidence of disturbed language and auditory processing disabilities. Faigel[44] noted the relationship between dyslexia and language and reported a high incidence of language-related deficits among delinquent youths. The defective language skills were often expressed as reading disabilities.

A relatively recent study[45] demonstrated the incidence of auditory processing disturbances in delinquent subjects. Institutionalized male delinquents were evaluated with a battery of psychological, educational, and neurological tests. Speech and language as well as auditory processing skills were also assessed. Subjects with significant deficits in auditory processing were also those subjects with the poorest academic skills. Visuoperceptual problems, although present in many of the delinquent subjects, accounted for a much lesser degree of academic deficiency. The results were further extended to hypothesize that the learning-disabled delinquent suffers not only in school but in his ability to profit from past experience as well. The perceptual and learning deficits appear to have a role in reducing his quality of life and adaptation potential.

If a major criticism can be applied to many of the previous studies on the perceptually handicapped delinquent, it is the tendency to look for single-modality perceptual problems. The brain is a dynamic system in which multiple functions operate in a coordinated manner. Multiple modalities of sensory input are integrated by the CNS for the basis of complicated skills such as reading.

Recent surveys of delinquent youth[46,47] support the concept that visual and auditory perceptual disturbances are relatively common causes of academic underachievement. The results further indicate that single-modality perceptual deficits are outnumbered by combinations of both visual and auditory processing disturbances that were present in more than 46% of the youthful offenders. The major areas of weakness included sequential memory, visual memory, and visuomotor coordination. The multiple perceptual disorders, however, were associated with the more severe deficits in reading, spelling, and arithmetic compared with delinquents having only single visual or auditory processing disorders. The combination of deficits appeared to affect more acutely both language and educational development as well as complex multimodal behaviors such as reading.

It is important to emphasize that we do not view learning disorders as confined to classrooms. The child with a learning disability has a pervasive problem that influences his social adaptation and emotional development, as well as his educational progress. Faulty language skills and impaired perceptual skills influence the child's social learning as well as his academic achievements. Parenthetically, the poor classroom learner is potentially the poor social learner. The effects of perceptual disorders on social maturation disturbances is poorly understood, but they may have a profound influence.

Delinquency and Neurological Disorders

The neuroanatomical basis of perceptual processing is poorly understood. Among delinquent youth, neurological investigations have been sporadically reported, but definitive studies relating neurological dysfunction to reading and perceptual skills are lacking. In our initial investigation of youthful offenders,[46,47] the incidence of subtle neurological signs was readily apparent. For example, more than 68% of the subjects in the delinquent population exhibited crossed eye–hand preference. Additional analysis revealed that these subjects were also the poorest readers.

Clements[33] presented data linking neurological dysfunctions with academic and behavioral difficulties in children. Wikler *et al.*[41] analyzed psychometric, neurological, and electroencephalographic (EEG) data in a group of children referred for scholastic and behavioral disorders. Compared with a normal population, the scholastic–behaviorally disturbed group revealed lower scores on psychometric examinations testing perceptual–motor skills. In addition, the disturbed children manifested a greater number of neurological signs and EEG abnormalities. Quitkin and Klein[48] similarly reported a higher frequency of neurological soft, signs, EEG abnormalities, and psychological test deficits among children susceptible to impulsive and destructive behaviors. Many of the children had a history of hyperkinetic behavior during early childhood.

Keldgord[49] found that many of the juvenile offenders committed to correctional centers had evidence of subtle neurological damage. The neurological dysfunctions were not manifested as gross abnormalities but did appear to impair learning and social adaptation. Of particular interest are the behavioral disturbances associated with the minimal brain dysfunction (MBD) syndrome, attentional–deficit disorder characteristics that can also be applied to many delinquent children. Among the more prominent behavioral signs are hyperkinesis, impulsivity, short attention span, aggressive behavior, emotional lability, and learning disorders. Barcai and Rabkin[50] hypothesized that the hyperkinetic child was particularly vulnerable to delinquent behavior, since his behavior and performance "leads to his extrusion from the classroom or his rejection within it." His behavioral difficulties eventually lead to "school aversion, truancy and dropping out. The blocking of normal outlets is finally manifested as deviant behavior or delinquent acts."

Critchley[30] evaluated a group of male juvenile delinquents with a series of neurological examinations, including (1) laterality preference, (2) right–left orientation, (3) finger agnosia, (4) clumsiness, and (5) graphic and spatial tests. Delinquent children had an increased incidence of disturbances in performing these neurological tasks, as compared with a matched control series. Thirty-three percent of the delinquents showed a cross-preference between hand and foot. These mixed dominant subjects were also among the poorest readers. Left–right orientation confusion was also a common problem among the delinquents. Critchley interpreted these findings in terms of a "neurological immaturity" hypothesis. This neurological immaturity was seen as responsible for impaired learning as well as poor social adaptation.

Implications

Educational programs for delinquent children have only recently incorporated special techniques for remediating learning disorders. Rice[51] describes remedial activities useful in improving the perceptual as well as academic abilities of institutionalized youthful offenders. Intensive reading instruction based on behavior-modification techniques has been described. The initial results of many of these innovative approaches suggest that the learning-disabled delinquent can be helped in a significant way that not only improves his ability to cope with the demands of social and vocational adjustment but adds increasingly to his self-confidence and self-esteem. The juvenile justice system traditionally places youthful offenders in institutional settings. This behavior-modification approach has been notoriously unsuccessful with high rates of recidivism common. A well-behaved ex-delinquent who cannot read remains at high risk for a return to his antisocial ways. Regrettably, recent emphasis on deinstitutionalization of youthful offenders has not fully recognized the needs of the learning-disabled juvenile delinquent.

The final common pathway for undiagnosed and untreated learning disabilities is academic underachievement, lack of success experiences, erosion of self-esteem, and, in many children, antisocial behavior. Adequate feelings of self-worth, self-confidence, and self-esteem are important psychosocial elements in maintaining stable character and personality. Deficits in learning abilities threaten behavioral development by endangering the growth of a healthy self-concept.

Kvaraceus[52] was one of the first investigators to suggest a relationship between impaired learning and delinquent behaviors. Delinquency was viewed as a "by-product of the schools" and lack of success in school appeared to foster behavioral difficulties. In addition, Kvaraceus[53] reports on children who fail to react to what they perceive as a hostile school environment. Failure and frustration in school may result in norm-violating behaviors which attempt to mend an individual's loss of self-esteem. Teachers become the hate object for hostile, failing delinquents. Kvaraceus[52] also indicated that more than 60% showed a marked dislike for school and even more hostile feelings toward teachers. As a result, the delinquent child comes to view himself as "a victim of a grand conspiracy by parents, teachers and legal authorities, to keep him a captive in school."

Berman[37] described the sequence of events by which learning disabilities produce behavioral and emotional problems that may culminate in delinquent behavior:

> The cycle begins with early problems at home. The child was showing perceptual and attention problems even prior to school, but the behavior was written off as ornery or uncooperative personality. The child enters the early grades of school already accustomed to the fact that he won't be able to do things as well as expected of him, that he will fail and be humiliated continually. The prophesy is fulfilled in school as teachers, considering the child's behavior problem, punish and ridicule him for failures on behaviors which he cannot control. The child begins to think of himself as a loser, as someone who cannot live up to what people expect of him.

Rather than face continual failure, other forms of attention and recognition must be found. "Clowning around and general disruptiveness become the ways which best insulate this youngster from having to face continual and repeated failure. He becomes much more successful as a clown or troublemaker than he could ever be as a student."

Berman went on to say that the pattern of predelinquent behavior is now set.

> Teachers are now diverted completely away from any learning problems and concentrate solely on how to deal with the child's behavior. He gets further and further behind and becomes more and more a problem. Eventually he's suspended, drops out or is thrown out of school to roam the streets, and the inevitable road to delinquency is well under way. The original problems have never been dealt with; the child is thought of as incorrigible. His problems are seen as psychogenic, not as the result of deflated self-esteem and fears of inadequacy, all of which have been generated by disability. His prophesy of himself as a loser had been fulfilled.

Menkes[54] and Williams[55] reported on the profound effects on self-esteem generated by school failure and the "crippling of the child as an end result of the disease called learning-disabilities." Elliot[56] points out that frustration in school may cause children to attack the system which is causing their discomfort, that is, the school and society. Academic underachievement can evoke pressures from parents and teachers who fail to recognize the child's underlying disorder in learning. Mulligan[42] and Jacobson[43] note that teacher–child relationships are compromised as the child fails to achieve the rewards of success. Often the child is branded erroneously with cruel labels such as "lazy" and/or "retarded." Wagner[57] suggests that hyperactive children may become more aggressive as they attempt to gain recognition, while others[50] see hyperactivity as a "precursor to delinquency."

Not only do problems with self-esteem and confidence arise as a result of disordered learning, but this child may also have increased difficulty with social learning. The learning-disabled child is often impulsive and has a poor ability to learn from past experience. In addition, this child has more than the usual difficulty understanding the consequences of his unacceptable behavior. Poor reception of social cues and a tendency to find himself in conflict with society are difficulties often found in learning-disabled children. The delinquent child's continual conflict with society may reflect a basic deficit in learning the appropriate behaviors that are considered acceptable. This deficit, in combination with the alienation he feels and the effects of poor self-esteem and confidence, renders the delinquent a poor risk to profit from traditional institutional programs.

According to Murray[58]:

> Together, characteristics like these point to a child who is said to be less than ordinarily sensitive to the usual sanctions and rewards. The problem is not initially callousness or street toughness on the part of the child. He might, on the contrary, be extremely receptive to rewards and sanctions. But the messages do not get through in quite the way they were intended, with the result that some of the factors which might restrain the learning-disabled child—the child starts out with a strike against him when exposed to opportunities for committing delinquent acts.

Learning disorders are not the sole cause of juvenile delinquency. However, the suggestion is offered that juvenile delinquency is a complex syndrome and that learning disabilities may be a significant factor contributing to this aberrant behavior. It is further suggested that if learning disabilities can be identified early, and meaningful therapy programs initiated, delinquent behaviors perhaps can be prevented. If child health care professionals have an awareness of the psychosocial complications of impaired learning, they perhaps can be more effective in preserving the self-concept and self-confidence of the victimized child. The socioeconomic and psychosocial liabilities that contribute to delinquent behavior are preventable by early identification and therapy. Ignoring the basic deficits in learning skills may leave a critical area of early intervention unattended.

As early as 1944, Kvaraceus[52] advocated (1) a school curriculum based on a student's needs and interests, (2) closer parent–teacher contact, (3) in-service training for school personnel in recognizing symptoms of early school failure, and (4) special multidisciplinary diagnostic teams and remedial programs designed to identify and intervene in the problem child who will become the potential delinquent. Today, even with our new diagnostic capabilities and special education programs, the appropriate course of action remains unchanged.

REFERENCES

1. Kessler, J.: *The Psychopathology of Childhood.* Prentice-Hall, Englewood Cliffs, New Jersey, 1966.
2. Weiner, I.: Juvenile delinquency. *Pediatr. Clin. North Am.* **22:**673–684, 1975.
3. Mangel, C.: The current state of the art," in Kratoville, B. L. (ed.): *Youth in Trouble.* Academic Therapy Publications, San Rafael, California, 1974, pp. 19–23.
4. Poremba, C.: "As I was saying," in Kratoville, B. (ed.): *Youth in Trouble.* Proceedings of a Symposium, Dallas-Fort Worth Regional Airport, May 1974. Academic Therapy Publications, San Rafael, California, 1974, pp. 74–79.

5. Mauser, A.: Learning disabilities and delinquent youth. *Acad. Ther.* **9**:389–402, 1974.
6. Aichorn, A.: *Wayward Youth*. Viking, New York, 1935.
7. Bender, L.: Psychopathic behavior disorders in children. in Linder, R., and Seliger, R. (eds.): *Handbook of Correctional Psychology*. Philosophical Library, New York, 1947, pp. 378–437.
8. Glueck, S., and Glueck, E.: *Unraveling Juvenile Delinquency*. Commonwealth Fund, New York, 1950.
9. Friedlander, K.: *The Psychoanalytic Approach to Juvenile Delinquency*. International Universities Press, New York, 1960.
10. Johnson, A. M., and Szurek, S. A.: The genesis of antisocial acting-out in children and adults. *Psychoanal. Q.* **21**:313–343, 1952.
11. Johnson, A. M.: Sanctions for superego lacunae of adolescents, in Harrison, S. I., and McDermott, J. F. (eds.): *Childhood Psychopathology*, 5th ed. International Universities Press, New York, 1976, pp. 522–531.
12. Redl, F.: Ego disturbances. *Am. J. Orthopsychiatry* **21**:272–279, 1951.
13. Redl, F.: *Controls from Within*. Free Press of Glenco, New York, 1952.
14. Redl, F.: *When We Deal with Children*. Free Press of Glencoe, New York, 1966.
15. Rosenthal, P. A.: Delinquency in adolescent girls, in Feinstein, S. C., and Giovacchini, P. L. (eds.): *Adolescent Psychiatry*, Vol. VII. University of Chicago Press, Chicago, 1979, pp. 503–515.
16. Offer, D., Marohn, R. C., and Ostrov, E.: Violence among hospitalized delinquents. *Arch. Gen. Psychiatry* **32**:1180–1186, 1975.
17. Offer, D., Marohn, R. C., and Ostrov, E.: *The Psychological World of the Juvenile Delinquent*. Basic Books, New York, 1979.
18. Marohn, R. C., Offer, D., Ostrov, E., *et al.*: Four psychoanalytic types of hospitalized juvenile delinquents, in Feinstein, S. C., and Giovacchini, P. L. (eds.): *Adolescent Psychiatry*, Vol. VII. University of Chicago Press, Chicago, 1979, pp. 466–483.
19. Minnchin, S. M.: *Families and Family Therapy*. Harvard University Press, Cambridge, Massachusetts, 1974.
20. Kernberg, P.: The Psychoanalytic profile of the borderline adolescent in Feinstein, S. C., and Giovacchini, P. L. (eds.): *Adolescent Psychiatry*, Vol. VII. University of Chicago Press, Chicago, 1979, pp. 294–321.
21. Masterson, J. F.: *The Treatment of the Borderline Adolescent: A Developmental Approach*. Wiley, New York, 1972.
22. Grinker, R. R., Sr., Wirble, B., and Drye, R. C.: *The Borderline Syndrome*. Basic Books, New York, 1968.
23. Caper, R. A.: The interaction of drug abuse and depression in an adolescent girl, in Feinstein, S. C., and Giovacchini, P. L. (eds.): *Adolescent Psychiatry*, Vol. IX. University of Chicago Press, Chicago, 1981, pp. 467–476.
24. Easson, W. M.: Symptomatic depression, in Feinstein, S. C., and Giovacchini, P. L. (eds.): *Adolescent Psychiatry*, Vol. V. University of Chicago Press, Chicago, 1977, pp. 257–276.
25. Nahas, G. G.: *Keep Off the Grass*. Pergamon Press, New York, 1979.
26. Newton, M.: *Gone Way Down*. American Studies Press, Tampa, 1981.
27. McCready, E.: Defects in the zone of language. *Am. J. Psychiatry* **6**:267–277, 1926.
28. Fendrick, P., and Bond, G.: Delinquency and reading. *J. Genet. Psychol.* **48**:236–243, 1936.
29. Margolin, J., Roman, M., and Haruri, C.: Reading, disability in the delinquent child. *Am. J. Orthopsychiatry* **25**:25–112.
30. Critchley, E. M. R.: Reading retardation, dyslexia and delinquency. *Br. J. Psychiatry* **114**:1537–1547, 1968.
31. Tarnopol, L.: Delinquency and minimal brain dysfunction. *J. Learning Disabilities* **3**:200–207, 1970.
32. Weinschenk, C.: The significance of diagnosis and treatment of congenital dyslexia and dysgraphia in the prevention of juvenile delinquency. *World Med. J.* **14**:54–60, 1967.
33. Clements, S.: *Minimal Brain Dysfunction in Children*. NINDB Monograph No. 3. U.S. Government Printing Office, Washington, D.C., 1966.
34. Myklebust, H.: *Progress in Learning Disabilities*, Vol. II. Grune & Stratton, New York, 1971.
35. Rampp, L. D., and Plummer, B. A.: Auditory processing dysfunctions and impaired learning. *Learning Disabilities: An Audio Journal for Continuing Education*. Grune & Stratton, New York, **1**(7), 1977. Audiotape.
36. Chalfant, J. C., and Scheffelin, M. A.: *Central Processing Dysfunctions in Children: A Review of Re-*

search. NINDB Monograph No. 9. U.S. Department of Health and Human Services, Bethesda, Maryland, 1968.

37. Berman, A.: Delinquents are disabled, in Kratoville, B. (ed.): *Youth in Trouble*. Proceedings of a Symposium, Dallas–Fort Worth Regional Airport, May 1974. Academic Therapy Publications, San Rafael, California, 1974, pp. 39–43.

38. Compton, R.: Diagnostic evaluation of committed delinquents. in Kratoville, B. (ed.): *Youth in Trouble*. Academic Therapy Publications, San Rafael, California, 1974, pp. 44–56.

39. Petrie, A., McCulloch, R., and Kazdin, P.: The perceptual characteristics of juvenile delinquents. *J. Nerv. Ment. Dis.* **134:**415–421, 1959.

40. Rubin, E., and Braun, J.: Behavioral and learning disabilities associated with cognitive-motor dysfunction. *Percept. Mot. Skills* **26:**171–192, 1968.

41. Wikler, A., Dixon, J., and Parker, J.: Brain function in problem children and controls: Psychometric neurological and electroencephalographic comparisons. *Am. J. Psychiatry* **127:**94, 1970.

42. Mulligan, W.: Dyslexia, specific learning disability, and delinquency. *Juvenile Justice* **23(3):**177–187, 1972.

43. Jacobson, F.: Learning disabilities and juvenile delinquency: A demonstrated relationship, in Weber, R. E. (ed.), *Handbook of Learning Disabilities: A Prognosis for the Child, the Adolescent, the Adult*. Prentice-Hall, Englewood Cliffs, New Jersey, 1974, pp. 189–216.

44. Faigel, C. G.: The adolescent with a learning problem. Experiences and insight with delinquent boys. *Acta Paediatr. Scand. (Suppl.)* **256:**56–59, 1975.

45. Zinkus, P. W., and Gottlieb, M. I.: Disorders of learning and delinquent youth: An overview, in M. Gottlieb and L. Bradford, *Learning Disabilities: An Audio Journal for Continuing Education*. Grune & Stratton, New York, **2**(5), 1978. Audiotape.

46. Zinkus, P. W., and Gottlieb, M. I.: Learning disabilities and juvenile delinquency. *Clin. Pediatr.* **17:**775, 1978.

47. Zinkus, P. W., and Gottlieb, M. I.: Patterns of perceptual deficits in academically deficient juvenile delinquents. *Psychol. Schools* **10:**361, 1979.

48. Quitkin, F., and Klein, D. F.: Two behavioral syndromes in young adults related to possible minimal brain dysfunction. *J. Psychiatr. Res.* **1:**131–142, 1969.

49. Keldgord, R. E.: Brain damage and delinquency: A question and a challenge. *Acad. Ther.* **4(2):**93–99, 1968.

50. Barcai, A., and Rabkin, L.: A precursor to delinquency: The hyperkinetic disorder of childhood. *Psychiatr. Q.* **48:**387–406, 1971.

51. Rice, R.: "Educo-therapy: A new approach to delinquent behavior. *J. Learning Disabilities* **3(1):**16–23, 1970.

52. Kvaraceus, W.: Delinquency: A by-product of the schools? *School Society* **59:**350–351, 1944.

53. Kvaraceus, W. C.: Reading: Failure and delinquency. *NEA J. Todays Ed.* **60(7):**53–54, 1971.

54. Menkes, J. H.: On failing in school. *Pediatrics* **58:**392–393, 1976.

55. Williams, J.: Learning disabilities: A multifaceted health problem. *J. School Health* **46:**515–527, 1976.

56. Elliot, D. S.: Delinquency, school attendance, and dropout. *Social Probl.* **13:**307–314, 1966.

57. Wagner, R.: Secondary emotional reactions in children with learning disabilities. *Mental Hyg.* **54:**577–583, 1970.

58. Murray, C. A.: *The Link Between Learning Disabilities and Juvenile Delinquency: Current Theory and Knowledge*. NIJJDP monograph; U.S. Government Printing Office, Washington, D.C., 1976, p. 27.

17

The Hyperactive Child

Marvin I. Gottlieb

INTRODUCTION

During the past quarter-century, there has been an unprecedented public/professional/legislative advocacy for children with learning disabilities. The generic designation of *learning disabled* generally encompasses a broad spectrum of problems that result in varying degrees of academic underachievement. The heterogeneous population of underachievers includes children with hyperactivity, dyslexia, perceptual motor disorders, attention-deficit disorders, and other nonspecific learning disorders—problems that may occur singly or in combinations. Not infrequently, *hyperactivity* and *learning disabilities* are used as interchangeable terms. Regardless of the etiology of the child's impaired

Marvin I. Gottlieb • Institute for Child Development, Hackensack Medical Center, and Department of Pediatrics, University of Medicine and Dentistry of New Jersey–New Jersey Medical School, Hackensack, New Jersey 07601

learning skills, the bottom-line effects are generally similar: (1) a progressive disparity between intelligence and educational accomplishments (failure to perform at the expected achievement level); (2) a significant risk for developing poor self-concept and lack of self-confidence (often manifested in acting-out behaviors); (3) disruptions in family dynamics, engendered by the associated psychological/social/financial tensions and stresses; and (4) a need for improved communications and coordinated efforts among parents, school professionals, and physicians. The severity of complications frequently associated with learning disabilities has mandated increased professional responsibilities in providing early identification, prompt initiation of remedial strategies, and psychosocial supports for child and family.

Despite intense public and professional concerns during the past 25 years, a myriad of myths, misconceptions, unanswered questions, and controversies still permeate the knowledge base of learning disabilities (and hyperactivity in particular). Markedly divergent descriptions and classifications of the hyperactive child reflect the spectrum of complex and vague psychobiological manifestations associated with hyperkinesis. Discipline-oriented perspectives have variously identified hyperactivity within a range from an ill-defined noncategorizable symptom to a disorder with syndrome status. Difficulties in the quantitative assessment of hyperactivity add further to the dilemma of providing a substantial core of knowledge regarding severity and outcome. Many issues regarding hyperactivity obviously require resolution:[2]

Is hyperactivity a symptom, a syndrome, or a set of syndromes?
Do children outgrow hyperactivity by adolescence?
Is the best management strategy a pharmacological, educational, or behavioral intervention?
Should psychotropic drugs be tried only after all other strategies have failed?

Without question, the early identification of childhood hyperactivity is necessary in initiating and planning effective therapy.[3] However, the multitude of unresolved issues makes the diagnosis and the delineation of a specific therapy program difficult to formulate with a high level of confidence.

As a consequence of persistent areas of uncertainty, the hyperactive child has become a major clinical challenge, particularly when the child is of school age. The child's deviant behavior is disruptive and tension-provoking for peers, teachers, family members, and physicians; it may ultimately be a precursor responsible for molding a negative psychosocial character of the affected child. Anxieties about the child's hyperactivity are further exaggerated by misconceptions of age mates and/or adults. Although hyperactivity may be associated with organic etiologies and a "driven" character, generalizations expressed by the casual observer reflect a psychosocial basis for the deviant behavior:

"The child must be retarded or socially deviant."
"The child is reflecting poor child-rearing practices."
"The child is emotionally disturbed and needs psychotherapy."
"The child could be cured with a pill, a special diet, or a military school."

Needless to say, within the milieu of the child's tension-provoking and embarrassing behaviors, parents and professionals become vulnerable (and at times desperate) to find a "quick cure" to stabilize behaviors. In this atmosphere of vulnerability and haste, confusions in management practices may evolve. As a result, the hyperactive child may be iatrogenically abused by (1) the empirical use of drugs or psychological therapies, without the benefit of a prior diagnostic assessment; (2) injudicious selection of a spectrum of medications to "calm the child down" (e.g., tranquilizers, sedatives); and (3) uncontrolled experimentation with recognized controversial therapies.[1] In view of these divergent and often unsubstantiated approaches (particularly those supported by testimonials in the mass media), the hyperactive child becomes extremely dependent on the expertise and guidance of the professional health care provider. The level of concern and the specific skills of the pediatrician in learning disabilities (i.e., hyperactivity) are critical factors influencing outcome. The role of the physician may significantly influence family dynamics, utilization of educational resources and, design of comprehensive management strategies for the learning-disabled child.

HISTORICAL BACKGROUND

One of the earliest medical descriptions of hyperactivity appeared in a picture book for children, *Der Struwwelpeter* (*Slovenly Peter, or Pretty Stories and Funny Pictures for Little Children*), written and illustrated by a physician, Heinrich Hoffman, in 1844. The book was apparently drawn from Dr. Hoffman's life situations and professional experiences, including the story of "Fidgety Philip," who appears to be the prototype of a classical description of the hyperactive child[4,5]:

> Fidgety Phil
> He won't sit still
> He wiggles
> He giggles. . . .

Scientific interest in behavioral syndromes of brain dysfunction appeared in the medical literature between 1917 and 1926, reporting hyperactivity, short attention span, antisocial behaviors, impulsivity, and emotional instability as common complications of the period-related encephalitis epidemic. The encephalitis-induced "brain-damage behavior syndrome" was later postulated to be a complication of head injury. During the early 1930s, hyperkinesis was regarded as an "organic driveness." In 1937 Bradley reported that hyperactivity in children responded to psychostimulant drugs.[6]

In 1947 Strauss (a neuropsychiatrist) and Lehtinen (a special educator), in their textbook, *Psychopathology and Education of the Brain-Injured Child*, suggested that hyperactivity, disinhibition, and distractibility were the result of brain damage and that brain lesions would elicit these symptoms. In essence, the "Strauss syndrome" implied that perceptual difficulties and behavioral problems were synonymous with brain injury. Hyperkinesis has been postulated by some clinicians to be a complication of underlying perceptual problems; recommending perceptual-motor training for brain-injured children.[6] During the 1950s and 1960s, Pasamanick and Knobloch noted that a spectrum of casualties ("a continuum of reproductive casualty") could result from complications of pregnancy. The "casualties" range from death or cerebral palsy and mental retardation to less life-threatening problems, such as hyperactivity and learning disorders.

Neurological dysfunctions incurred during pre-, peri-, and postnatal periods may not become evident until years later, a phenomenon reported in association with encephalitis, traumatic brain damage, and closed head injuries. The cause-and-effect relationship between perinatal brain injury and long-term psychosocial and educational sequelae is still uncertain. The problem is in part engendered by difficulty in establishing whether or not brain injury has actually occurred. The overall level of behavioral and cognitive deficits following perinatal complications is apparently low, except in children with cerebral palsy or mental retardation.[6]

In 1966, Clements popularized the concept of minimal brain dysfunction (MBD) for children exhibiting a cluster of behavioral and learning problems. The characteristic manifestations of MBD include hyperactivity, short attention span, impulsivity, and disinhibition in association with perceptual, cognitive, and specific learning disabilities. MBD is a misleading term inasmuch as the nature or location of the brain injury cannot be delineated and the syndrome cannot be quantified, as implied by the term "minimal."[4] In part, these vagueries prompted the American Psychiatric Association to redesignate "hyperactivity" and "MBD syndrome" as attention-deficit disorder (ADD), in the 1980 Diagnostic and Statistical Manual of Mental Disorders (DSM III).[7]

TERMINOLOGY/INCIDENCE/ETIOLOGY

An assortment of labels have been used interchangeably in defining the hyperactive child (Table I), reflecting uncertainties in etiology, diagnostic criteria, and management approaches. Among the more common terms are minimal brain damage (implying damage to the nervous system), minimal brain dysfunction or MBD (suggesting a neurophysiological disorder), and developmental hyperactivity (indicative of a maturational lag).[5] Less descriptive diagnostic labels include hyperkinesis, hyperkinetic impulse disorder, hyperkinetic child syndrome, and overactivity disorder. "Hyperactivity" has been

Table I Terms Often Used Interchangeably with or
Suggesting Hyperactivity[a]

Term	Description
Attention disorder	Minimal brain damage
Brain-damaged syndrome	Minimal brain dysfunction
Brain-injured	Minimal cerebral dysfunction
Cerebral dysfunction	Organic behavior disorder
Chronic brain syndrome	Organic brain damage
Developmental hyperactivity	Organic driveness
Distractibility	Overactivity disorder
Hyperactive child syndrome	Perceptual handicaps
Hyperkinetic behavior disorder	Neurological learning disorder
Hyperkinetic impulse disorder	Strauss syndrome
Hyperkinetic reaction of childhood	Specific learning disorder
Learning-disabled	Subtle brain damage
Maturational motor lag	

[a]Adapted from Gottlieb [17]

Table II. Criteria for Classification of Attention-
Deficit Disorder with Hyperactivity[a]

Hyperactivity
    Excess running or climbing
    Difficulty sitting still; excessive fidgeting
    Difficulty staying seated
    Motor restlessness during sleep
    Acts as if "driven by a motor"

Inattention
    Often fails to finish things
    Often does not seem to listen
    Easily distracted
    Difficulty concentrating on task requiring sustained attention

Impulsivity
    Often acts before thinking
    Excessive shifting from one activity to another
    Difficulty organizing work
    Requires a lot of supervision
    Frequently calls out in class
    Difficulty taking turn in games or group activities

Onset before age of 7 years

Duration of illness at least 6 months

Does not meet the criteria for a pervasive developmental
    disorder or manic disorder

---

[a]*Diagnostic and Statistical Manual of Mental Disorders.*[7]

used to define (1) a specific behavior or symptom (i.e., excessive locomotive activity); (2) a complex set of behavioral patterns that tend to covary; or (3) a clinical syndrome or disorder in the medical sense, with a specifiable origin, symptom picture, natural history, and outcome.[2]

Attention-deficit disorder (ADD) with hyperactivity has replaced such labels as "hyperactivity" or "hyperkinesis."[7] The emphasis in the American Psychiatry Association's Diagnostic and Statistical Manual (DSM III) is that attention deficit is the basic disability, rather than other symptoms of the syndrome (Table II). Many children categorized as "hyperactive" do not show major problems in motoric activity levels but manifest difficulties in focusing attention and in modulating behaviors. The new classification in DSM III recognizes two forms of ADD: ADD with and without hyperactivity.[7] Levine[8] subtyped attention deficits into five major categories: primary, secondary to information processing deficits, secondary to psychosocial stresses, situational inattention, and mixed. He meaningfully expanded the profile of children with selective difficulties by noting that they appear to have a variable symptom complex characterized by insatiability, disinhibition, poorly modulated activity, impersistence, inconsistency, social failure, and superficiality.[8] In essence, *hyperactivity* designates children in whom there is a common association between poor selective focus (regardless of subtype) and exaggerated levels of motor output.

The hyperactive child is generally characterized as a child who exhibits a motor behavior that is excessive, poorly organized for age, often clownlike in nature, and disruptive in peer situations. The historical model suggests "a long term childhood pattern characterized by excessive restlessness and inattentiveness."[3] Realistically, an all-inclusive "typical" profile of the hyperactive child cannot be constructed. These children appear to constitute a heterogeneous group, with common but variable behavioral features including: short attention span, impulsivity, excitability, and non-goal-directed motor activity.[9,10] Hyperactivity is probably best perceived as a symptom (a symptom associated with a myriad of problems) rather than as a personality disorder per se.[11]

The hyperkinetic behavioral pattern can also be regarded as a developmental disorder, usually recognized as a consistent manifestation occurring in early or middle childhood and extending into adolescence. Formerly MBD, and more recently ADD, linked hyperactivity with inattentiveness and a learning disorder. Although hyperactivity, MBD, ADD, and learning disability are frequently used synonymously: (1) MBD or ADD is not always associated with learning or perceptual impairment, (2) hyperactivity is not always a learning or perceptual impairment, and (3) hyperactivity is not always associated with ADD. However, the hyperactive child is frequently diagnosed as having ADD.[12]

Teachers, parents, and classmates will attest that hyperactivity is a relatively frequent behavioral problem, particularly among school-age children. Epidemiological surveys suggest a significant but variable prevalence of hyperactivity, ranging from 3 to 15% of school-age children in the general population.[2,11] Higher incidences appear in studies based on teacher assessments and lower incidences from surveys based on physical diagnoses.[2] The reported occurrence of ADD with hyperactivity reveals a wide scatter from 1 in 1000 to 5–6 in 100. A variety of geographical and cultural factors may be responsible for influencing prevalence data, including (1) variations in diagnostic criteria, (2) differences in child-rearing practices, (3) variability in methods of data collection, and (4) real differences in community locations, socioeconomics, and cultural biases.[12] A more universal and consistent finding is that boys are more hyperactive than girls; sex ratios reveal a male preponderance of 5 : 1 to 9 : 1.[2,4,12] The male : female disparity may be even more exaggerated by increasing the stringency of the definition of hyperactivity.

The nonspecific spectrum of terminologies in part reflects confusion regarding the etiological bases of hyperactivity. A variety of possible origins have been postulated: (1) medical (e.g., hyperthyroidism); (2) neurological (e.g., postnatal encephalitis, Sydenham chorea); (3) psychological (e.g., anxiety, situational stress); (4) social–environmental (e.g., boredom, overstimulation); (5) genetic–constitutional (e.g., temperament); and (6) developmental (slow CNS maturation).[13,14] The origin of the child's deviant behavior has been generally associated with organic brain damage and a resultant "driveness" quality to the hyperactivity. Since neurophysiological studies and postmortem examinations do not support a brain lesion postulate, a brain dysfunction hypothesis has received increased attention. A variety of possible genetic and biochemical causes have been suggested, including the role of central catecholamine neurotransmitters (dopamine and norepinephrine), the low central nervous system (CNS) arousal state and inability to inhibit CNS processes, cerebral allergy, CNS toxins (lead), and other environmental factors.[12] Unfortunately, the research on neurological soft signs, neurotransmitters, and other biological variables is incomplete and methodologically subject to criticism and is difficult to replicate.[2]

Many children are recognized as having a psychological basis for their deviant behavior. Perhaps one of the most common nonorganic origins is *situational hyperactivity;* deviant behavior couched in reactions to anxiety, frustration, depression, and poor self-concept. A conservative etiological approach focuses on a search for organic origins with possible primary or secondary psychological overlay.[14] Organic deficits may remain clinically dormant, surfacing only in particular environments (e.g., learning disabilities in classrooms), and therefore the concept of a situational versus a pervasive hyperactivity is important.[6] Children with pervasive hyperactivity appear to be more hyperactive and to have more severe attention deficits, more cognitive deficits, and a worse prognosis.

CLINICAL MANIFESTATIONS/DIAGNOSTIC CRITERIA

The diagnostic assessment of the hyperactive child represents a professional challenge and dilemma. Clinical delineation of hyperactivity depends on identification of a number of associated symptoms that constitute the disorder. Comprehensive evaluation is necessary because hyperactivity may accompany other disorders such as cerebral palsy, mental retardation, and autism. Resolution of the differential diagnosis of hyperactivity requires a systematic search for primary and/or secondary causes of the hyperkinesis. The operational criteria for a diagnosis of ADD with hyperactivity (DSM III) includes (1) excessive general hyperactivity or motor restlessness for the child's age, (2) difficulty in sustaining attention, (3) impulsive behavior, and (4) duration of at least 1 year.[5] The recommended criteria for ADD with hyperactivity are outlined in more detail in Tables II and III.

The clinical manifestations of hyperactivity are in part age dependent (Table IV). Although the classic concept of the "hyperactive child" is usually that of an affected elementary school-age child, tell-tale symptoms in preschoolers and adolescents should not be ignored.[5]

In a study of 100 children referred for interdisciplinary evaluation because of hyperactivity, Kenny et al.[15] assembled a compendium of associated characteristics. Their study sample of 84 boys and 16 girls ranged in age from 2 to 16 years (median 8 years, 4 months). Characteristics of the hyperactive profile included the following: (1) IQs ranged from 50 to 139 (median score 85.3); (2) 52% had normal neurological examinations, and 48% revealed soft neurological signs; (3) 78 had electroencephalograms (EEGs) of which 38 were normal, 25 abnormal, and 15 revealed 14-Hz to 6-Hz positive spike complexes;

Table III Characteristic Features Associated with Hyperactive Behavior in Children[a]

Major features	Minor features
Inattentiveness	Impulsivity
Learning disorder	Peer difficulties
Behavioral problems (misconduct)	Poor self-concept
Immaturity	Emotional deviance

[a]Adapted from Safer and Allen.[3]

Table IV. Clinical Manifestations of Hyperactivity at Various Stages of Childhood

Infants	Toddlers	Preschoolers	Elementary school age	Adolescence
Poor and irregular sleep	Excessive running and jumping	Demanding	Poor attention span	School failure
Feeding problems	Climb out of crib	Do not listen	School difficulties	Antisocial and impulsive behavior
Colic	"Into everything"	Cannot play independently	Better on 1 : 1 situations	Deterioration of innovation
	Flit from one object to another	Poor peer play	Impulsive	Poor peer relations
	Impulsive behavior	Non-goal-directed activity	Low frustration tolerance	Few friends
	No fears	Poor concentration	Poor peer relations	Poor social skills
		Poor response to discipline	Low self-esteem	Poor self-concept
		Rejected by peers and adults		Antecedent of juvenile delinquency

(4) no significant relationship was found among neurological examination, EEG findings, and final diagnosis; (5) 58% were not considered hyperactive by any of the staff (highly significant degree of interjudge agreement); and (6) 64% of families evidenced major environmental pathology. In a relatively recent study, Levine et al.[16] compared youngsters with significant attention deficits with children having other types of learning problems. The children with attention deficits were characterized by (1) increased incidence of behavioral problems during toddler and preschool years, (2) higher prevalence of minor neurological signs, and (3) increased incidence of difficulty on tests of language development. There was significant overlap between the two groups, "suggesting that the clinical characteristic of significant attention deficits is relatively non-specific and is either a primary or secondary finding on a large proportion of a heterogeneous population of children experiencing difficulties in school."

GENERIC ROLE OF THE PHYSICIAN

Specific intervention modalities in the management of childhood hyperactivity are reviewed (pharmacological management, behavioral management, parent counseling, and educational management); however, a more global perspective of the physician's role is warranted. Although the child's physician is often delegated the role of intermittent consultant, there are a variety of reasons why interaction with the physician should be more active and ongoing.[17,18] The physician:

1. Has a long-standing, uninterrupted, unique relationship with the child
2. Is usually the first professional in the life of the child

3. Is often the first to be counseled regarding the child's behavior and/or learning problems
4. Provides an essential contribution in the differential diagnosis of hyperactivity (e.g., recognizing organic disorders such as lead intoxication or thyroid disease)
5. Can prescribe and monitor medications, if necessary, in the management of hyperactivity
6. Provides ongoing comprehensive and longitudinal care, within the context of a family constellation
7. Can serve as the child's advocate while providing necessary family supports

These unique features, in the relationship of physician to child and family, mandate that the physician's role not be limited to that of a medication prescriber. The physician should play a more active role in the life of the hyperactive child, particularly in designing home strategies for the parents. Parental support and reinforcements can be provided by (1) providing a more structured home environment, (2) defining daily routines and avoiding "surprises" for the child, (3) keeping distractions to a minimum, (4) maintaining consistent parental behaviors, and (5) offering suggestions for improving the child's self-concept.

One of the most significant interventions the physician can provide for the hyperactive child is parent counseling.[18] Basically the parents must learn acceptance of their child's strengths and weaknesses, work through their feelings of guilt, become realistic in their expectations, and learn how to address their child's special needs.

Physicians should play a more vigorous role in the child's school life. Although advice on educational programming is inappropriate, the physician should maintain an advocacy role within the educational system. McKinlay and Rosenbloom[19] note "there is no clear cut division between the educational and medical aspects of development or learning disorders." Collaboration between physicians and teachers has increased during the past quarter-century, in part reflecting the mandates of P.L. 94-142. Although P.L. 94-142 neither requires physician participation nor spells out the specifics of the physician's role, it does encourage physician involvement in diagnosis and program planning.[20] The role of the physican in the diagnosis and management of children with educational problems (academics and behavior) is somewhat controversial.[21] Many professionals argue that learning- and school-related behavioral problems are the responsibility of educators and psychologists and that medical intervention serves only to compound the issues.

The arguments against medical involvement in these issues are related to impressions that (1) physicans are not well trained in education, psychology, and child development; (2) physicians do not have sufficient time to make a meaningful commitment for children with these problems; (3) physicians have too narrow a focus in diagnosis and therapy to effectively be involved in learning-behavior problems; and (4) physicians will not be reimbursed adequately for the time to be allocated for assisting these children.[21] The protagonists for medical intervention suggest that well-trained and dedicated physicians can effectively participate in the diagnostic/management process.[1,21,23] In many instances, the physician can become part of the assessment team, providing valuable information regarding the maturation and functional status of the CNS and the neuromotor system. Without question, physicians serve an important function in counseling with school personnel and parents regarding influences of nutrition, chronic illnesses, effects of medications, (both positive and adverse), and controversial therapies. In addition to the more traditional roles expected of physicians, the role of child advocate must be emphasized. The pediatrician is a most significant child advocate, promoting improved community resources, social acceptance, and legislative benefits.

PHARMACOLOGICAL MANAGEMENT

Approximately 50 years ago, Charles Bradley reported on his experiences modifying childhood hyperactivity with stimulant medication.[24] As Bradley noted, "Possibly the most spectacular change in behavior brought about by the use of benzedrine was the remarkably improved school performance of approximately half of the children." Subsequently, numerous reports of clinical trials with dextroamphetamine suggested an improvement in hyperactive behavior. During the 1950s and 1970s, other cerebral stimulants (methylphenidate and pemoline) were reported to have similar beneficial effects. Unfortunately, the overzealous and empirical use of psychostimulant medications created a national concern, prompting the refocusing on the need for accountability when prescribing pharmacological agents.[25]

The psychostimulant drugs (amphetamine, methylphenidate, and pemoline) are the medications most frequently used and are currently the single most effective therapy for hyperactivity in children.[3] Approximately two-thirds to three-fourths of children with hyperactive symptoms appear to respond favorably in one or more behavioral areas to stimulant medications.[2,12] Amphetamines and methylphenidate appear to be effective, as evidenced by improvement noted in parent and teacher behavior ratings, as well as in enhancing performance on tasks of vigilance and attention.[26] The amphetamines and methylphenidate hydrochloride appear to act centrally to enhance catecholaminergic activity. When stimulants fail to modify hyperactivity, after adjusting the dosages, other medications may prove efficacious (Tables V and VI).[27] It has been estimated that approximately 2% of all elementary school-age children receive stimulant drugs for hyperactivity (300,000–400,000 children in the United States).[3]

The administration of behavior-modifying drugs should be an individualized process, requiring close monitoring of behavior and learning, in order to determine their therapeutic effectiveness. Initially in a medication management program, stimulant drugs are prescribed because of their dramatic benefit and relative safety. Ideally, psychopharmacological agents are expected to (1) suppress or decrease hyperactivity, (2) improve impulsivity, (3) prolong attention span, (4) decrease anxiety levels and psychomotor excitation, (5) reduce depression, and (6) improve the child's response to other therapies (e.g., educational interventions).[25] The empirical use of medications, without prior diagnostic assessment, is discouraged. Drugs can temporarily mask meaningful signs and symptoms as well as delay identification of the etiology of the hyperactivity. A meaningful analysis of the causes, relative severity, and associated pathologies of childhood hyperactivity requires the documentation of a comprehensive history, behavioral assessment, physical and neurological examinations, neurodevelopmental evaluation, and laboratory investigation.[25] The judicious selection and administration of behavior-modifying drugs for hyperactivity depends on establishing a more constricted differential diagnosis

Table V. Suggested Guidelines for Pharmacological Management of Hyperactivity[a]

Drugs as an adjunct
  Parent counseling for behavior management at home
  Teacher counseling for behavior management at school
  Supportive counseling for child
Assessment of severity of problem
  Academic impairment
  Social impairment
Choice of drugs
  Ages 6–12 years
    Drug of choice: methylphenidate (Ritalin)
    Second choice: dextroamphetamine (Dexedrine); imipramine (Tofranil)
    Third choice: pemoline (Cylert)
    Fourth choice: thioridazine (Mellaril)
  Under 6 years of age
    Drug of choice: diphenhydramine (Benadryl)
    Other drugs: hydroxyzine (Atarax); promethazine (Phenergan)
  Adolescents
    Drug of choice: imipramine
Drug schedule
  Drugs tried in sequence until maximum allowable dosage is reached or side effects occur
  Dosage adjustments at weekly intervals
  Drugs given only on school days
  Drug "vacation" during summer

[a]Adapted from White.[27a]

of the underlying behavioral problem. Among the more common misuses and abuses of drug therapy are (1) isolated use of drugs, rather than as an adjunct to supportive therapies (e.g., special education programs); (2) prescribing medications without regard for diagnostic interventions and clarifications; (3) using drugs as a therapeutic trial in lieu of evaluation and establishing a diagnosis based on drug response; (4) anticipating that drugs will eliminate all learning impediments; (5) poor monitoring to determine the effectiveness of drug therapy; and (6) failure to recognize drug side effects.[28] Although adverse effects of methylphenidate were not demonstrated on a variety of physiological systems, "The dramatic behavioral improvement following drug treatment should not mislead the physician into believing that he/she has found a simple answer to a complex condition and thus lead him/her to overlook the presence of other handicaps, such as learning disabilities, antisocial behavior and depression. These latter disorders are not usually alleviated by stimulant drugs."[29] Kinsbourne and Swanson[30] recommended guidelines for discussing drug treatment of hyperactivity with parents (anticipatory guidance):

1. The presence of symptoms of hyperactivity does not guarantee a favorable response to stimulant drugs.
2. In a significant minority, an adverse response can occur; therefore, a careful screening phase is necessary.
3. Parents generally perceive drug therapy in a negative connotation, fearing addiction, lack of willpower, or a "drugged" child.

Table VI Pharmacological Agents Used in Management of Childhood Hyperactivity[a]

Drugs	Action	Initial oral dosage	General range of oral dosage	Onset	Duration	Side effects	Comments
Psychostimulants							
Methylphenidate hydrochloride (Ritalin)	Mild nervous system stimulant. Mental effects more prominent than motor effects	5 mg/day (5 mg increments weekly)	5–40 mg/day (split dose age b.i.d.) (0.3–2 mg/kg per day)	30–60 min	4–6 hr	Allergic reactions Anorexia Insomnia Abdominal discomfort Irritability	Not recommended for children under 6 years of age (growth suppression) Not recommended for children over 12 years of age (abuse potential) Lessens distractibility Calms hypermotor activity Monitor with periodic CBC differential and platelet counts Monitor growth May lower seizure threshold
Dextroamphetamine sulfate (Dexedrine)	Marked CNS stimulating action May stimulate reticular activating system and cortex Eventually same therapeutic effects as Ritalin	Children 6–8 years 2.5 mg/day (2.5 mg increments weekly) Children 8–12 years 5 mg/day (2.5 mg increments weekly)	5–35 mg/day (split dose age b.i.d.) (1 mg/kg per day)	30 min	3–6 hr	Anorexia Insomnia Unprovoked crying episodes Abdominal pains Dizziness	Not recommended for children under 6 or over 12 years of age Long term effects not well established May exacerbate symptoms of behavior disturbance in psychotic children May exacerbate motor and phonic tics and Tourette syndrome. Monitor growth
Pemoline (Cylert)	Weak CNS stimulant Pharmacological activity similar to other stimulants but little sympathomimetic effect Precise mechanism and site of action unknown	37.5 mg/day (18.75 mg increments weekly)	37.5–112.5 mg/day	Gradual onset and clinical effect may not be evident for 3–4 weeks	—	Anorexia Insomnia Abnormal liver function tests Abdominal discomfort Increased irritability Hallucinations	Not recommended for children under 6 years of age Monitor growth Liver function tests before and during therapy are indicated

Drug	Action	Dosage	Onset	Duration	Side effects	Remarks
Tricyclics (antidepressants) Imipramine hydrochloride (Tofranil tablets)	Mechanism of action not definitely known	Children 6–8 years 10 mg/day Children over 8 years 25 mg/day		Long acting (24 hr)	Dizziness Constipation Dry mouth Tachycardia Blurred vision Tremor	May exacerbate symptoms of behavior disturbance in psychotic children May precipitate attacks of Tourette's syndrome May be effective in hyperkinetic children who are not responsive to methylphenidate or dextroamphetamine Nonabusable makes it better drug for adolescents Blood counts at 2–3 weeks of therapy and at 6 month intervals for possible agranulocytosis Lowers seizure threshold Not recommended for children under 6 years of age
Neuroleptics (major tranquilizers) Thioridazine (Mellaril)	Inhibitory effect on psychomotor function A weak antagonist of dopamine	10 mg b.i.d or t.i.d (0.5 mg/kg/24 hr)	24 hr	12–24 hr	Hepatotoxicity reported Movement disorders Nasal stuffiness	Drug should be titrated to produce symptomatic improvement
Diphenylmethane derivatives (minor tranquilizers) Diphenhydramine (Benadryl)	Usually cause CNS depression Mechanism of action unknown	5 mg/kg/24 hr Children under 6 years 6.25–12.5 mg/t.i.d or q.i.d Children 5–12 years 50–500 mg/day Children over 12 years 75–100 mg/day	15–30 min	3–6 hr	Dryness of mouth Dizziness Oversedation	Lower seizure threshold in patients with focal lesions of cerebral cortex Should not be used when child has asthma attacks

"Adapted from Jabbour et al.[32] Hershkowitz and Rosman[13] and White.[71]

4. The basis for a ''diagnostic trial'' of medication should be reviewed to determine whether the child is a responder and how the drug affects conduct at home and at school.
5. Careful monitoring by parents, teachers, and physician is necessary to assess response and appearance of undesirable side effects of medication.

BEHAVIORAL MANAGEMENT

Probably the three most important psychotherapeutic interventions that can be offered for the hyperactive child are family counseling, individual psychotherapy, and behavioral therapy. Family counseling is directed toward improving the home environment and enhancing understanding among family members; individual psychotherapy focuses directly on the child's emotional needs, and behavioral therapy addresses the hyperactivity per se and is designed to structure home and school environments.[3]

Behavior therapy (behavior modification) implies the use of behavioral approaches in managing a clinical problem, seeking either to change a specific deviant behavior or to develop a missing desirable behavior. The types of behavior management approaches include ''reducing fears and fantasy in desensitization, increasing self-control by training with biofeedback of physiological states (e.g., heart rate), and manipulating social systems by providing reinforcement for group behavior.''[3] Manipulation of the social system reinforcers is the behavioral approach most applicable to modifying behavior of hyperactive children. ''The essence of this approach consists of: the careful analysis of the relation between behaviors and reinforcers, the definition of desired behaviors, and the introduction of systematic changes in the reinforcement contingencies to establish the desired behaviors.''[3] Safer and Allen[3] recommended a five-step contingency management program for the hyperactive child: (1) define explicitly the behavior to be changed, (2) analyze the consequences reinforcing the behavior, (3) construct new reinforcing contingencies, (4) prime the behavior change to ensure initial success, and (5) evaluate the effectiveness of the change.

Generally it appears that medication is the most successful management approach in rapidly reducing hyperactivity and misconduct, whereas behavior therapy is more effective in improving performance. The best results, however, appear to be a combination of the two treatment modalities in managing deviant behaviors. As Sprague[31] notes, ''From the evidence currently available, it seems likely that no single treatment for hyperkinesis will be successful in the long run, so it is expected that researchers rightly will turn to multimodal approaches. But these raise many major questions, including cost-benefit, possibility of replication, and availability of resources at clinical level.''

PARENT COUNSELING

The physican providing care for the hyperactive child is often mandated a coordinator–counselor role with members of an interdisciplinary assessment team, teachers and school personnel, and parents and child. The counseling role may provide the continuity of care required to assess therapeutic responses of various intervention modalities. The physician is often the most instrumental professional in providing the in-depth counseling to assist parents in adjusting to problems of deviant behavior and learning disorders.[32] Family counseling is an essential component of a comprehensive management strategy for the hyperactive child, particularly if there is an associated learning disability. The success of pharmacological and educational management interventions may depend on parental understanding and compliance. Because of their expertise and rapport with the family, physicians are a significant influence in the counseling process.[25]

Parent counseling may include an orientation into the nature of "hyperactivity," providing realistic expectations about what the child can and cannot control. Discussions may relieve parent(s) of feelings of guilt that their child-rearing practices are responsible for the deviant behavior. Similarly, inappropriate child-rearing practices may require modification. Issues of school and social performance must be refocused in terms of the child's abilities. Parent counseling may also be valuable in interpreting diagnostic data and management strategies recommended by other professionals. Suggestions can be offered to help improve the child's self-concept. Similarly, parent counseling may serve to defuse mounting frustrations and tensions between the parents and other family members.

Parent counseling often necessitates the distribution of reading materials that provide a better understanding of hyperactivity. In some instances, parent group meetings may be of significant value. As a component of parent counseling, review of suggestions regarding the use of various controversial therapies must be addressed.

EDUCATIONAL MANAGEMENT

A variety of educational management approaches have been employed to assist children with hyperactivity and other deviant behaviors. For the child with an associated specific learning disability, the learning-disability specialist generally designs an individualized educational program, as well as a behavioral modification component.

During the 1960s and early 1970s, self-contained classrooms for children with emotional, behavioral, and learning problems were frequently recommended. The hyperactive child was often relocated to a self-contained classroom either for emotionally disturbed children or for children with learning disorders. The most recent emphasis on mainstreaming has initiated intervention by teachers in modifying deviant behavior within the confines of the traditional classroom setting. Mainstreaming has probably also augmented teacher and school personnel interest in pharmacological therapies, as well as the more controversial approaches popularized by the media.

In retrospect, the self-contained classroom served as an "educational valve"; relieving the general educator of the time-consuming responsibility of serving children with deviant and disruptive behaviors.[28] The disruptive influence of the hyperactive child on peers and classroom stability is legend; self-contained classrooms appeared to be the most logical method of dealing with the problem. However, this approach may educationally and socially isolate and stigmatize the child, perhaps engendering a milieu of apathy and hopelessness. By contrast, the hyperactive child in a regular classroom setting creates a challenge and dilemma for teachers and school personnel. Unfortunately, the specific educational program for managing the hyperactive child in a mainstreaming environment is poorly defined and weakly researched.

Without question, the frequent testimonials (usually unsolicited testimonials) underscore the impact that "the hyperkinetic child is extremely difficult to live with at home and at school."[14] Verbal and/or physical restraints, spankings, and other short-term behavioral controls are only marginally effective. The hyperkinetic child generally receives an exaggerated degree of pervasive negative feedback, which impacts heavily on developing self-esteem. In addition to the basic short attention span, impulsivity, and hyperactivity, the child often develops an overlay of manipulative and attention-seeking behaviors. These acquired behaviors generally reflect reactions to social pressures and isolation, frustrations, poor achievement, and family stress, engendered by the hyperkinesis and gradual deterioration of the child's self-concept. As Zinkus[14] notes, "hostility and aggression can become a way of life for the hyperactive child. The child will inevitably be poorly socialized when he enters the classroom situation."

A variety of therapeutic approaches have been used in classroom settings. It is emphasized, however that classroom, home and psychotherapy management approaches must be coordinated in order to provide the child with a consistent and meaningful direction. Approaches that are carefully orchestrated provide the child with consistency in management expectations. By contrast, inconsistencies may serve to exaggerate deviant behaviors. Parents, therapists (e.g., psychiatrist) and teachers should be counseled as to the need for jointly sharing in the most effective management design.

The educational milieu, as a general rule, should be supportive and focused on reinforcing acceptable behaviors, Rewarding desired behaviors tends to increase the likelihood of recurrence of that behavior, whereas nonreward tends to make the behavior decrease in frequency.[14] Teachers may employ star or token reward systems within the context of the classroom. Successful experience in the classroom setting (for peers to view and acknowledge) is most important in bolstering the hyperkinetic child's self-concept; it also serves to encourage behavioral controls. The child's enhanced motivation may serve to improve controls dramatically and to eliminate superimposed attention-seeking-/manipulative behaviors. Teachers should employ "graduated steps" in their expectations; anticipation of overnight cures are unrealistic and serves to increase pressures on the child. Therapeutic approaches to modifying behaviors are generally more effective if applied in a consistent, patient, and understanding manner.

Zinkus[14] described a behavior-modification approach that had been applied to approximately 65 cases, covering a range of children displaying overly aggressive behaviors, hyperactivity, and mild emotional disturbances. The program appears to have effected rapid and dramatic changes in behavior. The basic principles of the program, applicable to teachers and parents, are as follows:

1. Following evaluation of medical and psychological factors, parents (and teachers) are provided a brief orientation to behavior modification techniques and terminology. Aspects of positive and negative reinforcement are reviewed.
2. The concept of long-term behavioral changes occurring through positive reinforcement of appropriate behavior is stressed.
3. New verbal signals are employed, such as "check" rather than "no."
4. A blackboard or large paper sheet is employed to record the checkmark system.
5. No more than three specific behaviors are selected for desired change (e.g., talking out in class, getting out of seat, and not taking turn).
6. Each time a behavior in any of these categories occurs, the teacher says "check" in a firm but modulated voice and places a check on the blackboard or

sheet. If the behavior does not cease, again the teacher says "check," and it is recorded. The child is then given a reasonable time before pronouncing the third checkmark.

7. Following the third checkmark, if accumulated within a half-hour period, the teacher states "time out," and the child is placed in a section of the room, or in another room, for no more than 10 min of quiet. The removal of the child to the time-out area should be accomplished with a matter-of-fact attitude. Verbal contact is not made during efforts to move the child or during the time-out period.

8. In order to leave the time-out area, the child must complete some aspect of schoolwork, such as 10 min of schoolwork (e.g., 10 math problems).

9. If after the first or second checkmark the child ceases in the undesirable behavior, he is allowed to erase the checkmark(s) and to start over again.

10. After a few minutes of good behavior, all checkmarks are removed.

11. The child generally responds to the word "check" and to the matter-of-fact attitude in program administration. In most cases, as the program continues, the number of time-outs decreases dramatically.

This schema represents one behavioral modification approach, capable of administration in a classroom setting (as well as at home). Other techniques such as positive reinforcers (stars) for fulfilling behavioral goals can be used individually or in combination with other approaches. A hyperactive child might be rewarded by a 5-min free time of running in the playground. Regardless of the specific approach adopted, school programs are always complemented with similar programs at home.

CONTROVERSIAL THERAPIES

The hyperactive child and his family are particularly vulnerable and therefore generally anxious to participate in any management program that suggests a "quick cure." This vulnerability is couched in an urgency to control the deviant behavior, which adversely influences peer relations, capacities for learning, social adaptation, and family dynamics. In part, the use and abuse of pharmacological interventions is similarly fashioned by the requests of parents and teachers to "modify the child's behavior, as soon as possible". In addition, as Brown[33] has noted, "paradoxically, traditional medicine is unable to solve some vexing health problems which seem to respond rather well to nontraditional treatments by faith healers, medicine men, or witch doctors." Although the controversial therapies available for hyperactive children were not designed by "faith healers, medicine men or witch doctors," these therapies challenge the effectiveness of less dramatic approaches of "traditional medicine." Brown[33] notes that "traditional medicine is often denounced as being insensitive to the benefits of personal concern and respectful interest in the whole patient." He cites several reasons why patient and physician "remain at uncomforting and untherapeutic distance from one another":

1. There is a hiatus between the patient's concern and expectations from the judgment and decision-making of the physician.

2. Parents expect a specific etiological definition of their child's behavioral problem, a definition that the physician at best can provide infrequently.

3. Parents are familiarized with a variety of therapies, as presented by the media and advocacy groups; physicians may be more critical and less enchanted over the scientific credibility of these management approaches.

The synonymous application of "hyperactive" and "learning disabled" has resulted in interchangeable therapeutic regimens for both. A myriad of controversial therapies have been popularized, including patterning exercises, vestibular sensory-integrative stimulation, visual optometric training, additive and salicylate-free diets, hypoallergenic diets, hypoglycemic diets, orthomolecular and megavitamin therapy, minerals and trace elements, lithium carbonate, coffee, and daylight fluorescent lighting.[28,33]

In a relatively recent survey of primary care physicians, it was reported that almost 50% of the respondents had tried either the Feingold food-additive-elimination diet or a low-sugar diet, or both, as an additional management option, despite mostly negative reports in the pediatric literature. In addition, about 10% of family physicians and general practitioners tried megavitamin therapy.[34] The authors note:

> The findings from this survey raise several important, unanswered questions as to how primary care physicians empirically decide upon specific interventions for clinical conditions and to what extent these decisions are based upon scientific studies and recommendations found in the medical literature. We have found a surprisingly high prevalence of routine utilization of assessment and management approaches which have been repeatedly cautioned, discouraged or negated in published investigations, e.g., assessments such as electroencephalograms, blood chemistry studies, and allergy work-ups and managements such as reliance on long-term medications (stimulant or nonstimulant) and dietary manipulations.

The physician is in a sensitive professional situation in which understanding, patience and guidance is required for families who have elected to try one or more of the controversial therapies. Rather than simply rejecting parental decisions to find the "quick cure," medical supervision, support, and objective analysis are essential. Needless to say, physicians must intervene more aggressively when the child's welfare is at risk because of the empirical trial of a nonscientific treatment approach.

LONG-TERM OUTCOME

The classic reports of Hechtman, Weiss, and their associates during the past decade focused on various aspects of the long-term follow-up of hyperactive children: effects of medication,[35,36] educational and psychosocial status as young adults,[37–39] psychiatric sequelae as adults,[40] and predictors of adult outcome.[41] For purposes of categorizing this discussion, the literature on "follow-up" is reviewed as it relates to four major life periods: (1) the preschool child, (2) the school-age child, (3) the adolescent and young adult, and (4) the adult. Many of the studies performed by Hechtman and Weiss are incorporated into an age-oriented perspective of outcomes of hyperkinesis.

Amado and Lustman[42] recognized that the course (i.e., the outcome) of ADD and hyperactivity past childhood was subject to several variables, suggesting that "each of the various components of the syndrome may vary independently in any given case, receding or acquiring prominence at different rates as the child matures and encounters different environmental challenges." Several generalizations regarding long-term outcome have been formulated: (1) hyperkinetic children tend to become less impulsive, exuberant, and hyperactive by adolescence; (2) hyperkinetic children remain more distractible, restless, emotionally immature, and aggressive; (3) there is an association between hyperactivity and poor school performance; (4) no improvement occurs in tests of intellect or cognitive tasks; (5) motor skills decrease with time; and (6) disabilities in social interactions and academic performances are associated with poor self-concept.[42] These areas are explored in greater detail as they relate to the age-oriented categorizations cited.

Preschool-Age Children

Preschool-age children identified as hyperactive, as anticipated, appear to have continued difficulties when they reach elementary school (school-age). In a study of hyperactive and control children, observed initially in a research nursery in children aged 4 years, and followed until age 6½ years in their elementary school, the results indicated that hyperactive preschool children continue to manifest difficulties during school age.[43] The hyperactive children were reported to exhibit more disruptive behaviors, to receive more negative feedback from teachers, and to manifest lower self-esteem during their elementary school experience. In essence, hyperactive preschool children are reported to have more behavior problems than controls, as elementary school students.[44] Children who were rated as extremely active in the nursery (1) requested more feedback and made more comments in interactions with their mothers, and (2) made more immature moral judgments. However, preschool children who were rated as moderately active apparently did not reveal major differences from the controls.[44]

School-Age Children

Short-term follow-up studies generally confirm Charles Bradley's (1937) observations that stimulant medications improve home and school behavior of hyperactive children, as well as school performance.

In 1975, Weiss et al.[35] studied three groups of hyperactive children matched by age, sex, IQ, and socioeconomic class, by various measures of outcome 5 years after initial evaluation. One group (24 children) were treated with methylphenidate for 3–5 years, a second group (22 children) were treated with chlorpromazine, and the third group (20 children) received no medication during the follow-up period. Weiss et al. noted that "the findings of this study were surprising. All of us had in general been impressed by the efficacy of stimulants for hyperactive children and we probably all expected the study to demonstrate a better outcome in the children who had received methylphenidate than in those who received chlorpromazine or no drugs." The study failed to demonstrate a better 5-year outcome in adolescence in the children who had received methylphenidate for 3–5 years as compared with the children treated with chlorpromazine or no drug therapy. The parameters of measurement included emotional adjustment, delinquency, Wechsler Intelligence Scale for Children (WISC), Bender Gestalt Visuo-motor test, and academic performance.

August et al.[45] defined two subgroups of hyperactive children, excluding brain damaged, mentally retarded, and psychotic children (Table VII). These workers suggested from long-term studies that different treatment modalities are required for each

Table VII. Possible Subtypes of Hyperactive Male Children[a]

	With conduct disorder	Without conduct disorder
Aggressive conduct disorder during childhood	+	−
Parents with serious psychopathology	+	−
Overaggressive/antisocial in young adolescents	+	−
At risk for juvenile delinquency	+	−
Prevalence of cognitive problems	−	+
Respond to training in social skills	+	±
Require special education	+	+
Benefit from stimulant medication	−	+

[a]Adapted from August *et al.*[45]

group; i.e., those with conduct disorder appear to respond well to training in social skills and controlling impulsive behavior, whereas those without conduct disorder need special education and may respond to stimulant medication.[45]

Short- and long-term longitudinal studies of the school-age hyperactive child consistently reveal two major secondary psychoeducational sequelae: (1) difficulties in school characterized by academic underachievement/behavioral problems/disturbed peer relationships; and (2) erosion of self-concept and lack of self-confidence, often manifested in acting-out behaviors.[46] These progressive psychoeducational complications elicit a cyclical phenomenon of superimposed deviant behaviors that further exaggerates the hyperkinetic profile (Fig. 1). A common misperception is that school-age children will outgrow their hyperkinetic behavior problem by the time they are adolescents.

Huessy and Cohen's[47] 7-year follow-up of 500 children confirmed that children identified as having behavioral and learning problems are at risk for subsequent adolescent academic and psychosocial problems. Hyperkinetic children had significantly lower mean grade point averages, depressed achievement scores, and lower IQ scores. The basic premise is that hyperactive children do not necessarily outgrow their symptoms.[46]

Adolescents/Young Adults

Previous discussion has focused on the significant pressures experienced by the hyperactive child from the family, teachers, and peers. The poor psychosocial interactions between the hyperkinetic child and other children and adults in the home and school environments ultimately result in deterioration of self-concept and self-esteem. Hechtman et al.[48] suggested that the persistent negative feedback that the hyperactive child receives from the home and school leaves a definite mark on his self-concept, which extends into young adulthood. In general, review of outcome studies of hyperkinetic children indicates that the significant academic, social, and conduct difficulties encountered during adolescence persist into young adulthood as social, emotional, and impulse problems.[39] Hechtman and Weiss[39] suggested that the clinical outcome of hyperactive young adults can be designated into one of three categories:

Group 1 Hyperactive young adults whose functioning is normal compared with matched controls.

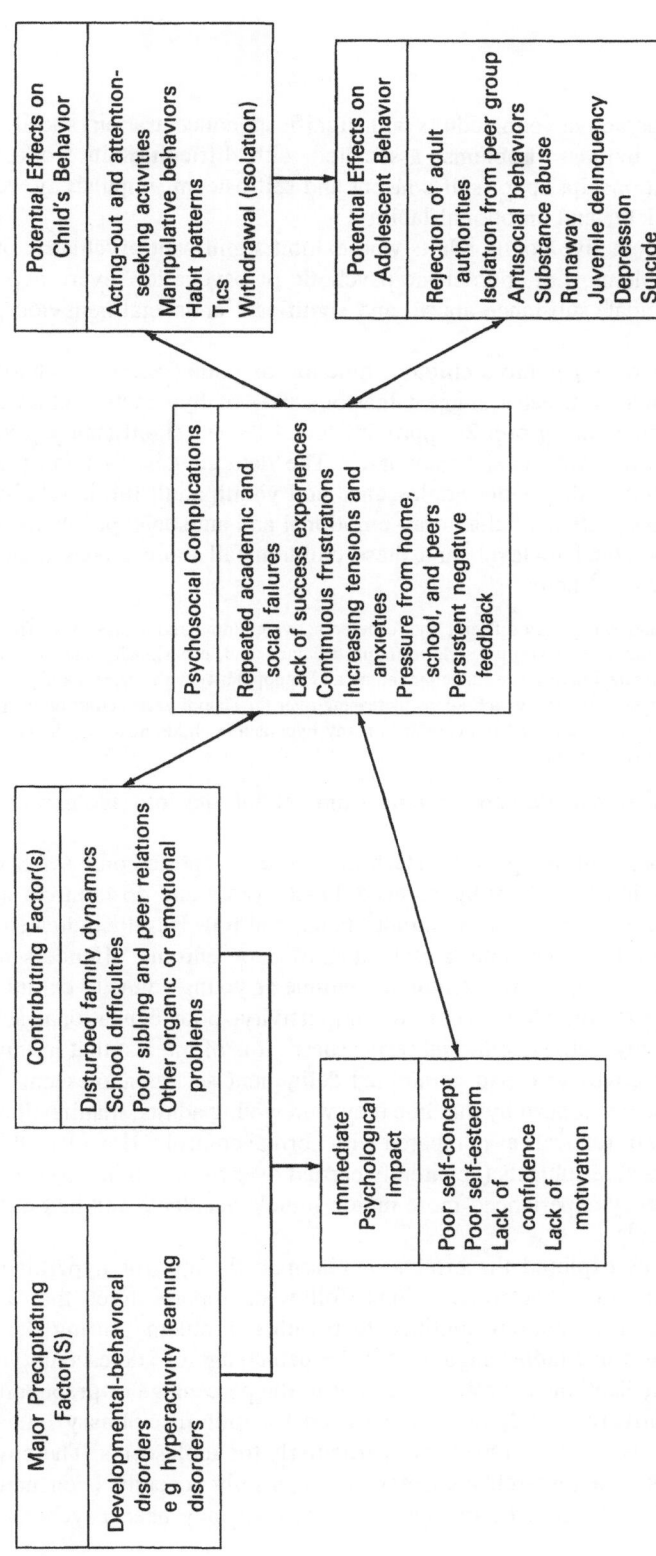

Figure 1 Schema of the possible cyclical, self-perpetuating nature of poor self-concept in hyperactive children and adolescents Adapted from Gottlieb and Zinkus[1]

Group 2 Hyperactive young adults with significant concentration, social, emotional, and impulse problems; associated with difficulties in work, interactive relationships, poor self-concept and self-esteem, impulsivity, restlessness, anxiety, and emotional lability

Group 3 Hyperactive young adults who exhibit significant psychiatric or antisocial problems, i.e., borderline psychotic or psychotic, severe depression and suicidal, substance abuse, and significant antisocial behavior

The vast majority of hyperactive children function as young adults as characterized in group 2. Very rough estimates suggest that 30–40% of hyperactive children fall into group 1 and 40–50% into group 2; approximately 10% are significantly psychiatrically disturbed with serious antisocial behaviors.[49] The data suggest that the prognosis for hyperactive children as they enter adolescence and young adult life is relatively poor.

In addition to significant behavioral–emotional and antisocial problems, school performance is below standard level, and these children fail more grades than do normal controls. Weiss et al.[37] note:

> The school situation is a very difficult one for hyperactive children and adolescents Their poor concentration, impulsive cognitive style, difficult behavior, and, occasionally, specific learning disabilities all interact to produce academic failure and unpopularity with teachers and peers The experience of school failure (which keeps increasing over the school years) contributes towards poor self-esteem and decreased motivation in many hyperactive children, thus enhancing their primary problems of learning

These psychoeducational problems extend from school age into adolescent and young adult years.[37,38]

In a 10–12 year follow-up study, Hechtman et al.[39] reported on a series of outcome variables from 76 hyperactive subjects aged 17–24 years and 45 controls aged 17–24 years (matched for age, sex, socioeconomic status, and IQ). Results indicated that only a few hyperactive children become grossly disturbed or chronic offenders of the law. However, most of the hyperactive children continue as young adults to exhibit symptoms related to the hyperactive child syndrome: impulsivity, poor educational achievement, poor social skills, low self-esteem, and restlessness. It is of interest that in this study, the majority of hyperactives who had committed delinquent acts as adolescents had gained sufficient psychosocial control by the time they were young adults, manifesting no significant increase in court referrals as compared with normal controls. However, the impulsive life-style of hyperactive subjects (apparently carried over from childhood) is suggested by observations that they experienced more motor vehicle accidents and had more frequent residency changes.[38]

Several studies explored the effects of pharmacotherapy for hyperkinesis, with a perspective on long-range outcomes. Some follow-up reports agree that a significant number of hyperactive children continue to manifest problems during the adolescent period. Short-term drug studies suggest that the percentage of adolescents/young adults who respond to medications is probably similar to the percentage of prepubertal children who respond positively.[50,51] However, the need for multidisciplinary interventions in treating hyperactivity must be considered, particularly for adolescents. Therapy for hyperactive adolescents is a research challenge that has only recently been addressed. Of particular interest is the possibility that the adolescent may need psychotherapy as an adjunct to pharmacotherapy.[52] Regardless, long-term studies indicate that our fund of knowledge regarding the efficacy of psychostimulant medications is far from complete. Hechtman et al.[53] reported on a prospective study of young adult outcomes (mean age 21.8 years) of children diagnosed as having ADD with hyperactivity and who had been treated with methylphenidate for at least 3 years. These subjects were compared with matched controls who had not received psychostimulant treatment. The results suggested that as a group the stimulant-treated hyperactives (1) had more residential moves, (2) were significantly more in debt, (3) had fewer car accidents, (4) tended to fail more grades in high school and drop out because of poor grades, and (5) usually got along better with co-workers. In essence, follow-up studies on young adult hyperactives who received no long-term or significant stimulation medication during childhood suggested that the young adult hyperactives were more impulsive and restless, had poorer social skills and self-esteem and lower educational achievement, had more car accidents, had more court referrals, and experienced more nonmedical drug use. There was also a greater incidence of personality disorder (impulsive immature dependent type), but they did not appear to account for a significant percentage of the psychiatric or antisocial population.[53]

Adults

Initial investigations exploring the social functioning of adults previously diagnosed as children presenting with behavioral problems (hyperactivity and learning problems) were generally pessimistic.[54–56] The longitudinal studies revealed a significant incidence of psychiatric disorders, psychiatric hospitalizations, and continued symptoms of restlessness, impulsivity, and mood lability. As a group these adults had not achieved a comparable socioeconomic status to that of their matched controls despite normal intelligence. However, these hyperactive adults were hardworking and performed satisfactorily in their jobs.[56]

Morrison[57] compared 48 adult psychiatric patients who had been hyperactive as children with groups matched for age, sex, and socioeconomic status. The hyperactive subjects exhibited persistent and significant personality disorders of all types, more alcoholism, more sociopathy, and less affective disorders. Hyperkinesis alone is probably not sufficient, however, to produce adult antisocial behaviors. Environmental factors, such as failure of parental control, may act on constitutional hyperactivity, which ultimately results in adult antisocial behavior.[58] In essence, data suggested that social factors may have a significant bearing on the pathogenesis of hyperactive child syndrome.

Hechtman et al.,[59] in a 10-year follow-up study of hyperactive children, focused on the antisocial behaviors occurring in young adults. The hyperactives (1) were not more involved in nonmedical drug use than controls, (2) used alcohol and marijuana only slightly more than did controls, (3) engaged in fewer antisocial behaviors because of fear of adult court systems, and (4) included only a small subset who were involved in drug abuse and antisocial behavior. Although the study was conducted in Canada (representing an environmental variable), the findings suggest a more positive outcome than had generally been expected.

From the studies of Hechtman et al.[53] (Table VIII), several generalities regarding stimulant treatment of hyperactive subjects can be formulated: (1) stimulant treatment in childhood may not eliminate educational, psychosocial, and life difficulties; (2) treatment

Table VIII. Summation of Young Adult Outcome of Hyperactive Children Who Received Long-Term Stimulant Medication Treatment[a]

Characteristics	Hyperactive group		Group matched for sex, IQ, and socioeconomic status
	Stimulant treatment in childhood	No sustained significant stimulant treatment	
Residential moves in past 10 years	+	−	−
Living with girlfriend and/or wife	+	−	−
Expressed satisfaction with present job	+	+	+
No future vocational plans or lower status plans	+	−	−
In debt	+	+	−
Number of car accidents	−	+	−
Physiological variables (e.g., weight, pulse, blood pressure)	−	−	−
Psychological tests (poor performance)			
Matching familiar figures	−	−	−
Embedded figures test	+	+	−
Stroop tests	−	−	−
Tended to fail more grades in high school and drop out because of poor grades	−	−	−
Scored better on doing assigned work, working indepently, completing tasks, and math and language ability	−	−	+
More difficulty getting along with teachers	+	−	−
Difficulty getting along with classmates	−	−	−
Punctuality	−	−	−
Working more independently	−	+	+
Ability to get along with co-workers	+	−	+
Appear to leave school earlier, spend more time doing nothing, start working earlier, have more jobs	+	+	−
Had greater debts (despite similar incomes)	+	+	−
Hospitalizations for psychiatric treatment	+	−	−
Diagnosed as having personality problems	+	−	−
Less positive view of their childhood	−	+	−
Moods, complaints, number of friends, psychosis, perversions, verbal ability	−	−	−
Suicidal attempts or threats	−	−	−
Number of police records or types and degrees of police involvement	−	−	−
Aggression	+	+ +	−
Stealing in elementary school	+	+ +	−
Stealing in high school or as young adults	−	−	−
Number of subjects using alcohol currently	+	+	+
Significant differences currently in use of various drugs	−	−	−
Early age of alcohol usage and more prolonged use of alcohol	+	−	−
Abuse of stimulant medications	+	+	−
Differences in overall scores on three self-esteem tests	−	−	−

[a]Based on study by Hechtman *et al.*[53]

may result in less social isolation and better self-concept; (3) with or without treatment hyperactives have more personality disorders as compared with controls; (4) treatment does not influence the outcome of antisocial behaviors; (5) the incidence of alcohol abuse among hyperactives is not altered by the use of stimulant medication in childhood; and (6) as young adults, stimulant-treated and untreated hyperactives are fairly similar and significantly different from "matched" normal controls.

The hyperactive child syndrome appears to be a pervasive condition in childhood that ultimately affects behaviors, social functioning, learning, and self-esteem.[40] Approximately 50% of hyperactive children seem to outgrow the symptoms before adulthood, but one-half do continue to be chronically disabled by these symptoms. The hyperactive child syndrome appears to be predisposed to various psychiatric disorders, with the exception of alcoholism and schizophrenia. A minority of the subjects exhibit antisocial personality disorders. In general, "all problems found in the adult life of hyperactives are detectable early and are generally already present in the preschool years."[40]

SUMMARY

The hyperactive child represents a clinical management challenge to parents, teachers, and professionals involved in the health care team. The immediate complications of deviant behavior (poor relations, compromised learning abilities, and poor self-concept) may ultimately be measured in poor social adaptation and loss of adult productivity (Fig. 1). Various pharmacological, behavioral, educational, and psychosocial approaches have been employed with varying results. The educational and social vulnerability of the hyperactive child and his family often initiate a trial of controversial therapies touting "quick cures." However, experience suggests that there is no panacea or quick cure for this chronic handicapping disorder of childhood.

The physician is an essential member of the diagnostic and management team. The responsibility for providing medical services for the hyperactive child extends far beyond the administration of medication. The clinical challenge requires skills in coordinating professional team efforts, monitoring effects of therapeutic recommendations, and parent–child–professional counseling. Successful medical intervention can often enhance the quality of life for the hyperactive child by maintaining stability of family dynamics.

REFERENCES

1. Gottlieb, M. I., and Zinkus, P. W.: Education, health and development: The learning-disabled child, in Hughes, J. G., and Griffiths, J. G. (eds.): *Synopsis of Pediatrics.* 6th ed. Mosby, St. Louis, 1984, pp. 33–60.
2. Whalen, C. K.: Hyperactivity, learning problems, and the attention deficit disorders, in Ollendick, T. H., and Hersen, M. (eds.): *Handbook of Child Psychopathology.* Plenum, New York, 1983, pp. 151–199.
3. Safer, D. J., and Allen, R. P. (eds.): *Hyperactive Child, Diagnosis and Management.* University Park Press, Baltimore, 1976.
4. Cantwell, D. P.: The hyperactive child. *Hosp. Pract.* **14:**65–73, 1979.
5. Weiss, G., and Hechtman, L.: The hyperactive child syndrome. *Science* **25:**1348–1353, 1979.
6. Rutter, M. (ed.): Introduction: Concepts of brain dysfunction syndromes and Behavioral studies: Questions and findings on the concept of a distinctive syndrome, in *Developmental Neuropsychiatry.* Guilford Press, New York, 1983, pp. 259–279.

7. DSM III: *Diagnostic and Statistical Manual of Mental Disorders.* American Psychiatric Association, Washington, D.C., 1980.

8. Levine, M. D.: Developmental dysfunctions, in *Levine, M. D., Carey, W. B., Crocker, A. C., and Gross, R. T. (eds.): Developmental-Behavioral Pediatrics.* Saunders, Philadelphia, 1983, pp. 709–755.

9. Varga, J.: The hyperactive child. *Am. J. Dis. Child.* **133:**413–418, 1975.

10. Schuckit, M. A., Petrich, J., and Chiles, J.: Hyperactivity: Diagnostic confusion. *J. Nerv. Ment. Dis.* **166:**79–87, 1978.

11. White, J. H.: The hyperactive child syndrome. *Am. Fam. Physician* **15:**100–104, 1977.

12. Committee on School Health: School Underachievement in *School Health: A Guide for Health Professionals, 1981.* American Academy of Pediatrics, Evanston, Illinois, 1981.

13. Herskowitz, J., and Rosman, N. P. (eds.): Hyperactivity and attentional disorders, in *Pediatrics, Neurology and Psychiatry—Common Ground.* Macmillan, New York, 1982, pp. 403–434.

14. Zinkus, P. W.: Behavioral and emotional sequelae of learning disorders, in Gottlieb, M. I., Zinkus, P. W., and Bradford, L. J. (eds.): *Current Issues in Developmental Pediatrics: The Learning-Disabled Child.* Grune & Stratton, New York, 1979, pp. 183–218.

15. Kenny, T. J., Clemmens, R. L., Hudson, B. W., *et al.:* Characteristics of children referred because of hyperactivity, *J. Pediatr.* **79:**618–622, 1971.

16. Levine, M. D., Busch, D., and Aufseeser, C.: The dimensions of inattention among children with school problems. *Pediatrics* **70:**387–395, 1982.

17. Gottlieb, M. I., Zinkus, P. W., and Bradford, L. G. (eds.): *Current Issues in Developmental Pediatrics: The Learning-Disabled Child.* Grune & Stratton, New York, 1979.

18. Delcau, C. M.: Management of attention deficit disorder. *South. Med. J.* **77:**1273–1276, 1984.

19. McKinlay, N. G., and Rosenbloom, L.: Medical contributions to the management of dyslexia. *Arch. Dis. Child.* **59:**588–590, 1984.

20. Marshall, R. M., and Wojari, D. F.: Medical and educational literature on physician/teacher collaboration. *J. School Health* **55:**62–65, 1985.

21. Levine, M. D.: The child with school problems: Analysis of physician participation. *Except. Child.* **48:**296–304, 1982.

22. Golden, G. S.: Evaluation of the child with school failure: Determining learning disabilities, in Frankenburg, W. K. (ed.): *Children are Different, Behavioral Development.* Monograph 3. Ross Laboratories Publications, Columbus, Ohio, 1982.

23. McDonald, A., Carlson, K., and Palmer, D., *et al.:* Special education and medicine: A survey of physicians. *J. Learn. Disab.* **16:**93–94, 1983.

24. Bradley, C.: The behavior of children receiving benzedrine, *Am. J. Psychiatry* **94:**577–585, 1937.

25. Gottlieb, M. I.: Pills: Pros and cons or medications for school problems. *Acta Symbol.* **6:**35–64, 1975.

26. Solanto, M. V., and Conners, K. C.: A dose-response and time-action analysis of automatic behavioral effects of methylphenidate in attention deficit disorder with hyperactivity. *Psychphysiology* **19:**658–667, 1982.

27. Jabbour, J. T., Duenas, D. A., Gilmartin, R. C., *et al.* (eds.): Disorders of cerebral function, in *Pediatric Neurology Handbook,* 2nd ed. Medical Examination Publishers, New York, 1976, pp. 154–169.

27a. White, J. H. (ed.): *Pediatric Psychopharmacology: A Practical Guide to Clinical Application.* Williams & Wilkins, Baltimore, 1977.

28. Gottlieb, M. I.: The learning-disabled child: Controversial issues revisited, in Gottlieb, M. I., Zinkus, P. W., and Bradford, L. J. (eds.): *Current Issues in Developmental Pediatrics: The Learning-Disabled Child.* Grune & Stratton, New York, 1979, pp. 219–259.

29. Satterfield, J. H., Schell, A. M., and Barb, S. D.: Potential risk of prolonged administration of stimulant medications for hyperactive children. *J. Dev. Behav. Pediatr.* **1:**102–107, 1980.

30. Kinsbourne, M., and Swanson, J. W.: Anticipatory guidance for classroom conduct and learning problems, *J. Dev. Behav. Ped* **1:**112–117, 1980.

31. Sprague, R. L.: Behavior modification and educational techniques, in *Rutter, M. (ed.): Developmental Psychiatry.* Guilford Press, New York, 1983, pp. 404–421.

32. Todd, M., and Gottlieb, M. I.: Interdisciplinary counseling in a medical setting, in *Webster, E. D. (ed.): Professional Approaches with Parents of Handicapped Children.* Thomas, Springfield, Illinois, 1976, pp. 191–216.

33. Brown, G. W.: Learning disabilities: Fads, fallacies and fictions, *Learning Disabilities: An Audio Journal* **3:**1–24, 1979. Audiotape.

34. Burnett, F. C., and Sherman, R.: Management of childhood "hyperactivity" by primary care physicians. *J. Dev. Behav. Pediatr.* 4:88–93, 1983.
35. Weiss, G., Kruger, E., and Danielson, U., *et al.*: Effect of long-term treatment of hyperactive children with methylphendiate. *CMA Journal* 112:159–165, 1975.
36. Hechtman, L., Weiss, G., and Perlman, T.: Young adult outcome of hyperchildren who received long-term stimulant treatment. *J. Am. Acad. Child Psychiatry* 23:261–269, 1984.
37. Weiss, G., Hechtman, L., and Perlman, T.: Hyperactives as young adults: School, employer and self-rating scales obtained during ten-year follow-up evaluation. *Am. J. Orthopsychiatry* 48:438–445, 1978.
38. Weiss, G., Hechtman, L., Perlman, T., *et al.*: Hyperactives as young adults: A controlled prospective ten-year follow-up of 75 children. *Arch. Gen. Psychiatry* 36:675–681, 1979.
39. Hechtman, L., and Weiss, G.: Long-term outcome of hyperactive children. *Am. J. Orthopsychiatry* 53:532–541, 1983.
40. Weiss, G., Hechman, L., Milroy, T., *et al.*: Psychiatric status of hyperactives as adults: A controlled prospective 15-year follow-up of 63 hyperactive children. *J. Am. Acad. Child Psychiatry* 24:211–220, 1985.
41. Hechtman, L., Weiss, G., Perlman, T., *et al.*: Hyperactives as young adults: Initial predictors of adult outcome. *J. Am. Acad. Child Psychiatry* 23:250–260, 1984.
42. Amado, H., and Lustman, P. J.: Attention deficit disorder persisting in adulthood: A review. *Compr. Psychiatry* 23:300–314, 1982.
43. Campbell, S. B., Endman, M. W., and Bernfeld, G.: A three-year follow-up of hyperactive preschoolers into elementary school. *J. Child Psychol. Psychiatry* 18:239–249, 1977.
44. Campbell, S. B., Schleifer, M., Weiss, G., *et al.*: A two-year follow-up of hyperactive preschoolers. *Am. J. Orthopsychiatry* 47:149–162, 1977.
45. August, G. L., Stewart, M. A., and Holmes, C. S.: A four-year follow-up of hyperactive boys with and without conduct disorder. *Br. J. Psychiatry* 143:192–198, 1983.
46. Gottlieb, M. I., and Williams, J. E.: Self-concept in the latency period and adolescence. *Feelings Med. Signif.* 24:23–26, 1982.
47. Huessy, H. R., and Cohen, A. H.: Hyperkinetic behaviors and learning disabilities followed over seven years. *Pediatrics* 57:4–10, 1976.
48. Hechtman, L., Weiss, G., and Perlman, T.: Hyperactives as young adults: Self-esteem and social skills. *Can. J. Psychiatry* 25:478–483, 1980.
49. Hechtman, L., Weiss, G., Perlman, T., *et al.*: Hyperactives as young adults: Various clinical outcomes. *Adolesc. Psychiatry* 9:295–306, 1981.
50. Cantwell, D. P.: Pharmacotherapy of ADD in adolescents: What do we know, where should we go, how should we do it? *Psychopharmacol. Bull.* 21:251–257, 1985.
51. Varley, C. K.: A review of studies of drug treatment efficacy for attention deficit disorder with hyperactivity in adolescents. *Psychopharmacol. Bull.* 21:216–221, 1985.
52. Brown, R. T., Borden, K. A., and Clingerman, S. R.: Pharmacotherapy in ADD adolescents with special attention to multimodality treatments. *Psychopharmacol. Bull.* 21:192–211, 1985.
53. Hechtman, L., Weiss, G., and Perlman, T.: Young adult outcome of hyperactive children who received long-term stimulant-treatment. *J. Am. Acad. Child Psychiatry* 23:261–269, 1984.
54. Menkes, M. M., Ross, J. S., and Menkes, J. H.: A twenty-five year follow-up study on the hyperkinetic child with minimal brain dysfunction. *Pediatrics* 39:393–399, 1967.
55. Morris, H. H., Escoll, P. J., and Wexler, R.: Aggressive behavior disorders of childhood. A follow-up study. *Am. J. Psychiatry* 112:991–997, 1956.
56. Borland, B. L., and Hackman, H. K.: Hyperactive boys and their brothers. A 25-year follow-up study. *Arch. Gen. Psychiatry* 33:669–675, 1976.
57. Morrison, J. R.: Diagnosis of adult psychiatric patients with childhood hyperactivity. *Am. J. Psychiatry* 136:955–958, 1979.
58. Morrison, J. R.: Childhood hyperactivity in an adult psychiatric population: Social factors. *J. Clin. Psychiatry* 41:40–43, 1980.
59. Hechtman, L., Weiss, G., and Perlman, T.: Hyperactives as young adults. Past and current substance abuse and antisocial behavior. *Am. J. Orthopsychiatry* 54:415–425, 1984.

V

Office Management of Developmental Disabilities

18

Visual Problems in Childhood

Roger L. Hiatt

Roger L. Hiatt • Department of Ophthalmology, University of Tennessee Center for the Health Sciences, Memphis, Tennessee 38163.

This chapter briefly reviews visual acuity-associated problems and methods of testing. A classification and discussion is presented including causes of visual loss, such as congenital defects, neurologic disease, inflammation, systemic disease, trauma, and others. The discussion focuses on how visual defects occur and their effect on the development of the child. The special problems encountered in managing the partially sighted or blind child are reviewed.

DETERMINING VISUAL ACUITY

Visual Acuity in Infants

Infants should be able to look at and follow a light source by the age of 3 months. At age 6 months they should reach for objects and be able to hold fixation with either eye, when the opposite eye is covered. An objective normal examination of the eye is very supportive of an assumption that visual acuity is intact. An objective examination generally includes (1) the reaction of the pupils, both directly and consequently; (2) a comparison of the reaction between the eyes; and (3) the presence of the fear reflex, when a movement is made to strike the child in the eye.

Visual Acuity in the Preschool Child

Assessment of visual acuity in a preschool child uses some of the techniques in the infant examination, as well as the kindergarten or picture test chart. Allen cards are good picture test charts because they are individualized. When held singly, they can be held easily at various distances for identification by the child. The E Testing Chart (Illiterate E Chart) is probably one of the more familiar and the best methods for preschool visual acuity screening. The child indicates by finger-pointing the direction of the legs of the table formed by each individual E, which is reduced in size on each line of the chart. To test visual acuity in one eye, the opposite other eye must be properly covered in order to ensure test reliability.

Visual Acuity in the School-Age Child

The Snellen Letter Chart is probably the best method of assessing the vision of a child who is able to read letters. Proper illumination of the chart and correct distances must be maintained before testing can be considered reliable.

COMMON VISUAL DISORDERS AND THEIR CLINICAL CONSIDERATIONS

Amblyopia

Amblyopia refers to subnormal visual acuity in the absence of objectively detectable causes, including ophthalmoscopic or afferent visual pathway disease. The term generally implies a vision defect due to sensory stimulus deprivation, disease, inhibition, or misuse occurring early in life. This topic is reviewed more extensively in a later section of this chapter.

Amaurosis

The term amaurosis means "dim." Amaurosis is generally defined as a total or partial loss of vision but in common usage implies profound loss of vision (blindness or near-blindness). Amaurosis may exist from birth as a result of (1) developmental malformations of the brain and optic nerves; (2) cerebral and optic nerve damage as a complication of gestational and perinatal infections and inflammatory processes, metabolic disturbances, anoxia, or hypoxia; (3) perinatal trauma involving the visual pathways; and (4) early onset of genetically determined optic atrophies and retinal degeneration. Amaurosis developing in an infant or child, who once had good vision has somewhat different implications. A very rapid onset most often indicates an encephalopathy or an acute demyelinating disease affecting the optic nerves, optic chiasm, or cerebrum. Rapid-onset amaurosis may also occur as the result of a rapidly developing hydrocephalus or other conditions that cause increased intercranial pressure and a secondary ischemia of the visual areas. Amaurosis with a more gradual onset and progressive loss is more suggestive of a tumor or a neurodegenerative disease.

Obscurations

Obscurations or transient episodes of visual loss ("blurring") that last only seconds or minutes have special implications. The most important are the visual obscurations of papilledema, which are caused by increased intracranial pressure. These obscurations must be differentiated from the visual symptoms of migraine and cerebrovascular insufficiency.

Photopsias/Visual Hallucinations

Photopsias are abnormal visual phenomena that may take the form of sparks, lightning flashes, luminous rings, fiery globes, and other primitive light sensations. These sensations may be elicited by applying pressure on the eye through the closed lids. Photopsias have no specific localizing value. Visual hallucinations are the apparent perceptions of an external object when no such object is actually present. They may arise from disturbances in the visual pathways, from retina to occipital lobe. Visual hallucinations have no precise localizing value.

Micropsia, Macropsia, and Metamorphopsia

Micropsia is a disturbance of vision characterized by objects appearing smaller than their actual size. By contrast, macropsia is a disturbance in which objects appear larger than their actual size. Metamorphopsia is a visual disturbance characterized by objects and lines appearing distorted and irregular. All these visual disturbances may be of central or peripheral origin and can result from retinal disease, particularly of the macula area.

Nyctalopia/Hemeralopia

Nyctalopia refers to visual deficiency in environments in which there is illumination; the disturbance is generally associated with an impairment in rod function, particularly the dark adaptation time or threshold. Nyctalopia may be further classified into: (1) stationary congenital nightblindness with no associated fundus abnormalities; (2) stationary congenital nightblindness occurring in association with fundus abnormalities; and (3) progressive nightblindness. By contrast, hemeralopia is an unusual condition characterized by deficient vision in good illumination but comparatively better vision in dim illumination. Most commonly it is a congenital disorder of unknown etiology and pathogenesis.

Color Vision Disorders

Colorblindness is usually regarded as being either, red, green, or blue, as either a partial or a complete defect. Achromatopsia is a color vision disorder associated with subnormal vision, nystagmus, and marked photophobia.[1]

Diplopia

Diplopia (double vision) is an abnormal subjective response of seeing one object as two. It is usually a binocular phenomenon, although it may be monocular. The most essential point in assessing a patient complaining of diplopia is to prove that it actually exists. The patient may confuse blurred or distorted vision with double vision.

Oscillopsia

Oscillopsia is an illusory sensation of movement of a stationary object. It is important primarily as a subjective symptom of acquired nystagmus and other eye movement disorders.

Dyslexia

Dyslexia is more comprehensively reviewed in Chapter 6. Dyslexia implies a partial impairment for the patient who may appreciate letters but has difficulty assimilating words; it is manifested as a reading disorder.

Psychogenic Disturbance of Vision

Disturbances in vision due to malingering or hysteria are not uncommon in school-age children. Visual-field constrictions may be a manifestation of psychogenic visual disturbances and may reflect hysteria, anxiety, fatigue, or fabrication.[2-5] (Generally these disturbances follow one of several patterns that can easily be recognized.)

REFRACTIVE ERRORS

A refractive error is the most commonly anomaly of the eye. Children are profoundly affected by refractive difficulties, especially school-age children whose school activities demand good vision. Children, however, may have poor vision in the 20/100 range for relatively long periods, particularly if the vision decrease had a gradual onset. The child may perform poorly in schoolwork and exhibit nervousness and irritability, as a result of visual impairment and excessive focus effort. Fortunately, periodic visual-acuity tests administered in public and private schools uncover most errors of refraction. Conclusive data are unavailable regarding the relationship between headaches and refractive errors. Increased visual effort due to refractive errors can cause headaches at the end of the day or after performing close work; however, its etiological importance is generally overemphasized.

The three types of refractive errors that most commonly affect children are (1) hyperopia, (2) myopia, and (3) astigmatism. The nature of the refractive error is determined by the shape of the eyeball and the relationship of the different refractive surfaces and media to the axial length of the eyeball. The shape of the eyeball is inherited; however, there is evidence that shape may be modified by acquired influences. The eyeball grows as the child grows, until the adult size and shape are reached. While the child grows, refraction may change markedly in some children. Hyperopia increases until about 6 or 7 years and then decreases slowly until adulthood. Acquired myopia may increase gradually from the early or teen years until adulthood.

Hyperopia

In hyperopia (farsightedness) the eyeball is too short, and rays of light passing through the cornea and the lens focus behind the retina. In order to correct this defect, the curvature of the lens must be changed to bring the focus toward the retina. This requires effort by the ciliary muscles which fatigue rapidly; producing symptoms of eye strain. Fortunately children have a relatively great degree of accommodating (focusing) power and despite the strain can overcome the simple hyperopia. Visual acuity is good for distance and near. Hyperopia can be corrected with appropriate eyeglasses or contact lenses, which reduce the excessive muscular effort required for focusing. A child may develop an esotropia as a result of the excessive accommodative effort in the event that focusing is accompanied by a reflex stimuls for the convergent mechanism. These children may have their strabismus completely corrected by medication and/or glasses. Anisometropia, a difference between the two eyes, may either cause a small degree of strabismus or amblyopia, because of the difference in retinal image sizes.

Myopia

In myopia, (nearsightedness) the axis of the eyeball is too long. As a result the focus falls in front of the retina; producing a blurred image for distance. The nearsighted child can often read without excessive muscular effort for focusing. If the myopia is of a high degree, however, the child may hold the print close to the eyes in order to obtain a clear focus. This focusing anomaly can be readily corrected by the use of concave lenses. Acquired myopia has a tendency to increase gradually over a period of years until adulthood. *Congenital myopia* may be of high degree in the range of 10, 15, or even 20 diopters of myopia.[6] Fortunately, visual acuity has a tendency to improve gradually with age and is usually in the 20/40 range by the time the teenage years are reached. Congenital myopia, in contrast to the acquired variety, does not usually increase with advancing age. This may be of some consolation to the parents. Corrective lenses may not be accepted and consistently utilized by these children until near school age, when they become more visually attentive.

Astigmatism

In astigmatism the curvature of the cornea is flatter in one meridian than in the meridian perpendicular to it. As a result, rays of light are focused asymmetrically on the retina and objects viewed appear distorted and blurred. Since the eye constantly attempts to obtain a clear image, the muscular effort expended is nonrewarding and tiring. The deficit is corrected by utilizing a lens (a cylinder) that compensates for the abnormal curvature of the cornea. Testing for glasses (refraction), in young children with significant refraction errors, is performed best when the accommodation or focusing power is completely at rest. The state of rest, or suspension of focusing, permits a more accurate measurement of the refractive error. Cycloplegic drugs, such as atropine, are usually used for the first ophthalmological examination. Atropine is generally used for children up to school age, at which time a shorter-acting agent, such as Mydriacyl or Cyclogyl, is substituted. In refractions in patients beyond the teenage years, cycloplegia may often be omitted.

Modification of the Refractive Error

Various surgical procedures have been tried to reduce myopia or change astigmatism. Currently radial keratotomy, a popular procedure in this country, has been advocated for reducing myopia. The procedure however never increases corrected visual acuity and indeed may decrease it. The risk and the difficulties involved in surgery must be explained to the child and parents. The reduction of myopia in early life with the use of cycloplegics (atropine) is effective and fairly well accepted. However, it requires that the pupils are dilated and accommodation is suspended during the period of treatment. For this reason, many children prefer correcting the myopia with glasses and switching to contact lenses when they reach adolescence.

Additional treatment modalities recommended to reduce the progression of myopia includes use of bifocals, abstinence from near work, and use of contact lenses with a flat-base curve. Simple myopia is not a disease but a refraction error due to the growth of the eyeball. Care must be exercised in trying to modify this condition.

AMBLYOPIA

Amblyopia is commonly caused by three pathological situations: (1) anisometropia, a difference in refraction between the eyes; (2) strabismus, turning of one eye; and (3) visual deprivation, either due to disuse of the eye, or an abnormality which prohibits a clear image during the developmental years.

Anisometropia

In anisometropia there is usually a significant degree of difference in refraction between the eyes. If the difference in refraction is of only minor degree (plus or minus one diopter) the difficulty produced is usually negligible. However, when the disparity is 8, 10, 12, or diopters, the visual acuity in one eye becomes impaired, usually the eye with the higher refractive defect. If detected early, during the first 3 years of life, eyeglasses can produce a clear image; aiding in the development of good vision in the poor eye. Eyeglasses can be augmented by patching the eye with the better vision. A young child, more than older children, can tolerate the unequal correction in the two eyes without must discomfort. If their defractive error is 4 diopters or more between the eyes, the use of a contact lens for the eye with the greater refractive error should be the probability of improved development of vision.

Strabismus

Strabismus in a young child is characterized by possible double vision in one eye or both. If the suppression is alternate, visual acuity usually remains intact and equal in both eyes. There may be short periods of diplopia, but the child (particularly up to school age) learns to suppress one eye or the other rather than seeing double. When suppression occurs, there is interference with binocular vision and visual acuity does not develop properly; indeed, it may deteriorate. Visual acuity may be impaired to a degree that there is a loss of appreciation of hand motion or light perception. Correction of the strabismus, patching of the better eye, and correction of any refraction error is the hallmark of treatment for amblyopia.

Visual-Deprivation Amblyopia

If an infant's eye is patched, for whatever reason, the visual acuity will drop markedly within a matter of days to weeks. There may be an associated deviation of the eyes from the center, particularly if an underlying inequality of muscle pull exists. Visual input is deprived, and a visual deprivation amblyopia results. The same process may occur if the child has a keratic cornea, unilateral cataract, cloudy vitreous, or any pathological condition in which a clear image is not formed on the retina in the early weeks and months of life. Caution must be exercised to avoid producing an iatrogenic visual deprivation amblyopia by patching or similar procedures. Vigorous efforts are necessary as early as possible in the life of a child, particularly in unilateral cases, to remove the obstacles which impair a clear image.[7,8]

VISUAL LOSS SECONDARY TO CONGENITAL DEFECTS

Genetic and Chromosomal Defects

All children with known or suspected genetic and chromosomal anomalies should have an ophthalmological examination. The eye is frequently the target of gene and chromosomal defects. For example, a patient with trisomy 21 (Down syndrome) may present early in life with strabismus and large refractive errors. As the child with trisomy 21 grows, there may be accompanying defects of the cornea (keratoconus) and lens (cataracts). The associated visual anomalies, including nystagmus, may cause subnormal vision in children already cognitively handicapped and who require special education.

Embryological Disorders

Aniridia

In aniridia the iris stump may still be present, producing a huge pupil. The absence of the iris causes photophobia and secondary nystagmus; resulting in visual deprivation and a visual handicap. These patients may be treated with tinted lenses of the conventional or contact form.

Blepharoptosis

In blepharoptosis if one eye is covered by the ptotic eyelid, amblyopia can result due to visual deprivation. In the case of bilateral blepharoptosis, the major clinical sign may be the extension of the head on the neck as the child attempts to look under the ptotic lids. The blepharoptosis should be corrected before the child begins school because the disorder causes difficulties in viewing distance objects, such as the blackboard. Many cases of blepharoptosis can be corrected in the third year of life with satisfactory results.

Corneal Leukoma and Haze in Infants

Haze in infants may be transient due to corneal edema. If haze or leukoma persist, it should be treated promptly, because of the possibility of producing a deprivation amblyopia. The differential diagnosis of corneal leukoma includes metabolic errors, congenital glaucoma, congenital defects (mesodermal dysgenesis), Reiter syndrome, Axenfeld syndrome, and others.

Congenital Cataracts

Congenital cataracts range in severity from mild to severe and may be accompanied by other anomalies. The prognosis is related to the extent that the opacity covers the pupil, rather than the lens involvement per se. If sufficient light can be transmitted, nystagmus will be avoided and some reasonable degree of good vision will ensue; delaying cataract extraction. If the total lens is obscured, immediate bilateral cataract surgery during the early months or weeks of life is indicated. Correction with proper lenses (contact or conventional variety) and occlusion therapy is an adjunct to surgical intervention.

Congenital Glaucoma

Congenital glaucoma may occur in isolation, or it may be associated with other generalized diseases. Treatment is surgical and should be instituted early in the child's life. If surgery re-establishes the proper intraocular pressure, corneal haze or leukoma can be reversed. Children with congenital glaucoma should be examined periodically under anesthesia. Follow-up management is a lifelong process for these patients.

Congenital Retinal Disease

Congenital retinal disease may be manifested clinically in the form of degeneration, such as retinitis pigmentosa. The disorder usually interferes with the child's learning ability and educational progress very early in his school career. Degenerations may involve only the macula as a pigmentary disturbance, ultimately resulting in a progressive visual loss. If the degeneration is accompanied by signs of central nervous system disease, the possibility of Tay-Sachs or Vogt-Spielmeyer disease must be considered.

A retinoblastoma, the most common intraocular malignant tumor in children, may be regarded as a congenital disorder. Retinoblastoma should be considered in the differential diagnosis of any leukokoria, unilateral or bilateral. Early diagnosis and prompt treatment may preserve the globe and permit useful vision.

Albinism

Nystagmus, photophobia, and poor vision form an associated triad in the child with albinism. In generalized albinism, physicians most often associate eye difficulties with lack of tolerance for sunlight. In ocular albinism, however, the ophthalmologist may be the first to detect a lack of sufficient pigment in the retina, iris, and other uveal structures. Associated refractive errors and photophobia usually accompany the deficient pigment.

DISORDERS WITH RADIOLOGICAL IDENTIFICATION

A variety of congenital neurological disorders have profound eye implications. For example, hydrocephalus and cranial stenosis may be associated with visual loss. Craniostenosis is often characterized by eye abnormalities, mental retardation, convulsions, and other neurological defects. In craniofacial dysostosis (i.e., Crouzon disease, hypertelorism, and Treacher-Collins-Franceschetti syndrome) an embarrassment in orbital size may occur, resulting in pressure effects on the optic nerve. Optic atrophy may be associated with achondroplasia, osteogenesis imperfecta, and osteopetrosis. Most of these disorders can be identified on radiological examination.

The single most important neurological disorder that can be detected on a radiological examination is a brain tumor causing optic atrophy (chromophobe adenoma, craniopharyngioma, and other tumors around the circle of Willis, including aneurysms). In cellulitis of the orbit, the radiological diagnosis of sinusitis becomes highly suggestive as a possible site of the infection. In all cases of trauma to the orbit (or around the orbit), the child should be examined radiologically for possible orbital floor fractures.

VISUAL DISORDERS SECONDARY TO NEUROLOGICAL DEFICITS

Cerebral Palsy

More than 75% of all patients with cerebral palsy have associated refractive errors. Hyperopia is the most common visual disorder found with cerebral palsy. At least 50% of these patients have strabismus and esotropia. Treating these problems in a child with cerebral palsy is often difficult because of the multiple handicaps involved. Eye patching, amblyopia, compliance with using glasses, and strabismus surgery are all associated with a lower success rate in patients with cerebral palsy. In some instances, it may be necessary to postpone correcting these defects until the child is older. For example, strabismus surgery may be delayed until the child is of nursery school age.[9]

Nystagmus

Nystagmus may be primary or secondary in a child. Primary nystagmus is present from birth and is a cause of visual loss, abnormal head positioning, strabismus, and other defects. On the other hand, secondary nystagmus may result from visual deprivation, as for example in the amblyopia produced by congenital cataracts. It is critical that the type of nystagmus, primary or secondary, be determined. The causes of secondary nystagmus must be eliminated, if at all possible, very early in the life of the child. Early treatment of primary nystagmus is not recommended, however, other than for correcting accompanying refractive errors. When the child is older (near school age) he/she may be a candidate for the Kestenbaum operation. This procedure consists of finding the eye position that is most quiet for the child, realigning this position into the primary or ''straight ahead'' direction so that he can utilize it for better visual acuity and without abnormal head positions. Alignment in the vertical direction can be performed should the child have an extension of flexion of the head on the neck in order to see. Surgery is best performed when the child is near school age in order to establish confirmation that the visual acuity is definitely better in the abnormal head position than in the opposite field.

Optic Nerve Defects

Hypoplasia

Optic nerve hypoplasia is a common cause of unilateral amaurosis. On ophthalmological examination, the affected nerve head is smaller than its counterpart. The small disc may be accompanied by a sparsity of vessels and by unusual pigmentation around the disc and fundus. When there is a significant degree of hypoplasia, a Marcus Gunn pupil will be present on the side of the hypoplasia. Visual acuity will be compromised, and as the child becomes older further amblyopia ensues. Patching and corrective lenses may be nonproductive therapeutic interventions. Cosmetic corrective surgery may be necessary if esotropia persists into the school-age years.

Optic Atrophy

There are a number of causes of secondary optic atrophy in children, such as tumors of the optic chiasm. Primary optic atrophy may be difficult to define. A pediatric neurologist should be consulted in evaluating a child with optic atrophy.

Optic Neuritis and Papillitis

If visual acuity is significantly decreased, in the absence of evidence of optic nerve congestion, retrobulbar neuritis or neuritis of the portion between the optic nerve head and the chiasm should be suspected. However, if there are signs of swelling, papillitis must be considered. Visual acuity is markedly reduced in association with papillitis usually on the unilateral side. The presence of a demyelinating disease, which could be associated with the neuritis, must be ruled out.

Papilledema

Papilledema in a child is an ominous sign suggesting increased intracranial pressure until proven otherwise. The most common cause of increased intracranial pressure is a brain tumor or other space-occupying lesion.

VISUAL LOSS SECONDARY TO INFLAMMATION

Uveitis

Visceral Larva Migrans

Visceral larva migrans must be included in the differential diagnosis of leukokoria in a child. The ELISA (enzyme-linked immunosorbent assay) test, when positive, is useful in the diagnosis of nematode infestation. The lesions may be isolated or may be confused with a tumor occupying a portion of the vitreous cavity.

Tuberculosis

Tuberculosis of the eye resulting in uveitis may be present as an isolated or disseminated form. It may or may not be accompanied with known signs or symptoms of systemic tuberculosis. In a child with tuberculosis, inflammation of the uveal tract suggests tubercular involvement.

Acute and Chronic Cyclitis (Iridocyclitis)

In a child, acute or chronic uveitis that occurs anteriorly requires diagnostic evaluation to determine the focal or systemic causes of the uveitis. For example, a common cause of uveitis is juvenile rheumatoid arthritis (JRA) or Still disease. In JRA the uveitis may be "quiet" in appearance, i.e., associated with mild flare, few cells, and few symptoms. The pupil, however, may be fused 360° to the lens before it is discovered. The pediatrician and ophthalmologist must work jointly in patient management in the evaluation of a child with iridocyclitis.

Histoplasmosis

Histoplasmosis is endemic in certain areas of the United States, particularly the Southeast. Although more common in adults, it may occur in children, including the hemorrhagic components. A general diagnostic workup for histoplasmosis must be included in any child suspected of having the disease, regardless of the presence of obvious eye involvement.

Toxoplasmosis

Visual acuity may be severely embarrassed in congenital toxoplasmosis. This is due to involvement of the macule with "eat-out" atrophic lesions caused by the *Toxoplasma gondii* organism. Diagnostic evaluation for generalized manifestations of toxoplasmosis includes an investigation of cerebral calcification and cerebral involvement.

Syphilis

Congenital syphilis can manifest itself as luetic keratitis, either early in life or later during the teenage years. General manifestations of syphilis should be investigated if the condition is suspected on the basis of an eye examination.

Rubella

Congenital rubella is often associated with mental retardation, in addition to eye manifestations of retinopathy, iris hypoplasia, and cataracts. The cataracts are most severe and may involve the entire lens. If cataract extraction is performed, a powerful plus lens must be provided in the range of plus 25 in order to correct the huge hyperopia.[9]

Cytomegalic Inclusion Virus

The cytomegalic virus is usually accompanied by signs of an immunosuppressive disease or a condition that has been treated leading to immunosuppression by agents such as cortisone. These lesions are often detected in the chorioretinal layer, manifested as severe inflammation that can mimic other causes of uveitis.

Corneal Ulcers and Inflammation

Bacterial ulcers caused by *Staphylococcus, Gonococcus, Pseudomonas,* and other organisms affect children with poor environmental hygiene. Bacterial ulcers may also occur in children who have generalized systemic disease. Generalized medical treatment of the child is essential in the cure and prevention of such ulcers.

Herpes simplex ulcer may occur in the nutritionally deprived child and particularly in children who have been immunologically suppressed, as an example following kidney transplant procedures. The herpes virus invades the cornea and may undergo subsequent reinvasions depending on the antibody reaction to the insult of the antigen. Herpes on the skin may secondarily invade the eye, although this route is not as common as primary ocular involvement. Herpes simplex ulcers are a leading cause of blindness in the United States and must be suspicioned in any child with a "red eye" that responds poorly to treatment.

VISUAL LOSS SECONDARY TO SYSTEMIC DISEASE

The child with systemic disease and associated visual defects should be jointly evaluated by the primary care physician and an ophthalmologist. For example, a newborn should be examined by an ophthalmologist, particularly if oxygen has been administered. Some premature newborns will exhibit developmental delays, and some will be partially blind as well. Others manifest a high degree of congenital myopia in the absence of retinopathy. Systemic disease requires general treatment as well as specific therapy for the accompanied visual loss.

ACCIDENTS, TRAUMA, AND VISUAL LOSS

Retinal Detachments

Disinsertion of the retina in the periphery, or frank retinal detachments without inflammation, should be suspected in any child presenting with hyphema or with trauma, particularly if there is a vitreous bleed. It is most important to determine the cause of the retinal detachment, and repair should be designed accordingly.

Foreign Body, Lacerations, Burns, and Direct Injuries

Foreign bodies, particularly those that are not inert, must be considered for removal if they penetrate eye structures. Secondary infection is always a significant threat for any foreign body in the eye. Lacerations from sharp instruments or missiles are common particularly during childhood. Lacerations should be repaired under microscopic surgery. Fortunately most are unilateral, but secondary amblyopia is always a threat particularly in the young child. Chemical or thermal burns may cause corneal damage as well as injury to surrounding tissue. Burns must be treated promptly and thoroughly in order to minimize the degree of damage. It has been estimated that approximately 7000 firework injuries occur annually in the United States, 20% involve ocular injuries.[10] BB gun pellet injuries are almost exclusively limited to the eye. These injuries may be accompanied by hyphema. A hyphema requires that the child be at rest and quiet; appropriate bandaging is necessary to prevent secondary bleeds. Penetrating injuries necessitate the removal of the foreign body and appropriate repair instituted. Prevention is the important single factor in management.

MANAGEMENT OF THE PARTIALLY SIGHTED AND BLIND CHILD

In children with subnormal vision (uncorrected by conventional, medical, surgical, and optical means) modification of the educational program is of particular concern. In general the following management principles should be kept in mind: (1) special glasses, or optical aids, should be provided in order to increase the size of the retinal image; (2) reading aids, such as a reading stand and reading markers, are of value; (3) "sight-saving books" are reserved for children who with the best optical correction cannot read the N18 or 18-point type of regular books; (4) the resource room or sight-saving classes are helpful for the visually handicapped, but are unnecessary if the school system provides enough special help in the regular classroom; and (5) the teaching of Braille in schools for the blind is reserved for children who must use a nonvisual method for their primary means of reading. Children should be encouraged to participate in visual learning experiences commensurate with their alertness and interest. The distance utilized in focusing, either for remote fixation or near fixation, has not been proved to produce a physical relationship causing structural changes in the globe. In early life the retina has a very high light sensitivity. Adequate reading is impossible at brightness levels below that which the maturing individual considers adequate.

Subnormal Vision

Children will experience difficulty in recognizing blackboard or remote instruction material when optic and refraction correction, medical treatment, and surgery fail to yield vision within the near-normal range. These children assume fatigue positions for close learning tasks. Visual aids, wherever possible, should be so constructed that the appearance and position required for use approximate normal conditions. Magnifying devices are generally classified into near and far aids. Bifocals are generally not necessary for children, because of their remarkable ability of accommodative focusing. However, they do provide magnification in the near range and represent an unobstrusive visual aid to learning. If bifocal magnification appears to be indicated in excess of 10 diopters, a separate monocular magnification near lens for the better eye should be provided for use at even closer focal distances. Distance magnification is often achieved most inconspicuously with a small pair of ocular glasses, which the student can keep in his desk. The wearing of telescopic lenses, yielding above 2 or 3 magnification, immediately reduces the breadth of visual fields. The child technically becomes "industrially blind" because of the sidewise loss. Large print material is available from the National Aid to Visually Handicapped, the Library of Congress, the American Printing House for the Blind, and some commercial publishers. Large print enables many children with optical visual acuities from 20/100 to 20/200 or even 20/400 to read without magnifying devices and the resultant secondary restriction of visual motility. More than 1000 titles are now available in large-print books and copies can be ordered through various agencies.

Social Implications of Blindness

The social and economic cost of a blind child to society is enormous. In 1972 the total cost for visual disorders in America approximated $5 billion.[11] The expenditures include direct costs (physician's visits) and indirect costs such as supplementary security income payment and loss of federal income taxes. However, this figure does not include state and local government contributions to the support of the blind. To this must be added the cost of at least 5100 cases of legal blindness in the under-20 age group per year. Poor binocular vision is a lifetime disability and usually compromises productive careers. Depth reception is mandatory for surgeons, craftsman, pilots, and other occupations. The cosmetic defects from deviated eyes takes its toll in depriving patients of self assuredness and in reaching certain levels of achievement that demand the highest quality of appearance. Subtle hostile attitudes by the parents toward their strabismic ("crossed eyed") child occasionally are causes of emotional problems.

Education

The psychological aspects of the visual impairment, as well as the direct ocular deficits, significantly influence the success obtained in educating the partially sighted child. The child must feel secure and accepted, in order to respond to therapeutic interventions and to progress in a satisfactory manner.

The best development of the partially sighted child should ideally occur in his own home and community.[12] Parents and teachers should avoid an overemphasis on the educational attainments of partially seeing children, at the expense of all other aspects of psychosocial development. An educational plan adapted for some school systems involves itinerant teachers visiting various classrooms assisting children with special learning needs. A specially trained teacher visits the regular classroom at a stated time, providing special instruction, special reading material, and mechanical aids.

An alternative is the resource room plan in which the child attends a centrally located school that provides special education. The child is enrolled with normal-seeing children in a regular classroom and attends the resource program for special instruction. The resource program includes a specially equipped room, supervised by a teacher trained to instruct the partially sighted.

Consideration of the physical facility and the mechanical aids is necessary in serving partially sighted or blind children in the regular classroom, as well as in the resource room, structure and arrangement of desks, the blackboards and color of the chalk, the type of materials used in papers, among others. Typewriters with very large type can be used as early as the fourth grade. The print is of the 18-point type. Touch type enables students to complete assignments faster. Tape recorders and dictaphones may be useful in taking notes. Television has several advantages for the partially sighted child: (1) the picture is magnified, and (2) the distance from the television set is improved.

Teachers should be aware of some of the behavioral reactions of children with various eye defects. For example, the myopic child will probably wear glasses most of the time, whereas the hyperopic child may prefer on occasion to eliminate the glasses. Children following cataract surgery will probably experience reduced visual acuity, even with the best attempts at correction. The child with nystagmus may be more comfortable holding the head in an "abnormal position" and should be allowed to do so. if this position provides increased visual efficiency. Children with ptosis, congenital glaucoma, and strabismus, because of their "abnormal" appearance, are vulnerable to the development of psychological problems. Children with strabismus may avoid social contacts. Educational programs should be designed to insure consistent and varied associations with normal-sighted children. Schools for the blind are operated for children with extreme visual loss, usually requiring Braille as a means of reading. Admission to the school for the blind is generally based on the child's need for specialized services and the ability to use these resources.[11,14] The National Society for the Prevention of Blindness estimated (1969) that there were approximately 100,000 partially sighted children of school age, defining the "partially seeing child" as one whose best corrected visual acuity is between 20/100 and 20/200. The needs of the child with a temporary handicap (e.g., strabismus) varies considerably from those of a child who is regaining sight (e.g., following cataract surgery) or losing sight (e.g., from a retinitis pigmentosa). When there is a permanent visual handicap, the child and parents must accept the limitations imposed by the disability before successful restructuring therapy can be initiated. Congenital absence of vision, with an associated absence of visual sensory stimulation, may be associated with some delays in overall development. Total blindness from birth with profound sensory deprivation, is generally associated with difficulty in acquiring simple basic orienting skills.[13] Multihandicapped children (e.g., hearing loss and visual loss) will necessitate special resources and specially trained teachers. The recreational and social activities of these children must be individualized. Children with vision loss should be encouraged to participate in various sports that are performed by sighted children (e.g., bowling, swimming). Children and parents may require some ongoing counseling in order to maintain coping skills.

REFERENCES

1 Aristikaitis, M , and Morgan, A   Examination of children, in The Ophthalmologic Staff of The Hospital for Sick Children, Toronto (eds) The Eye in Childhood Year Book, Chicago, 1967, pp 12–18

2 Duke-Elder, S , and Wybar, K C   The anatomy of the visual system, in Duke-Elder, S (ed) System of Ophthalmology, Vol II Mosby, St Louis, 1961, pp 623–636

3 Duke-Elder, S   Congenital deformities, in Duke-Elder, S (ed) System of Ophthalmology, Vol III Mosby, St Louis, 1963, pp 1073–1079

4 Duke-Elder, S , and Scott, G I   Neuro-ophthalmology, in Duke-Elder, S (ed) System of Ophthalmology, Vol XII Mosby, St Louis, 1971, pp 578–581

5 Walsh, F B , and Hoyt, W F   Clinical Neuro-ophthalmology, 3rd ed Williams & Wilkins, Baltimore, 1969

6 Hiatt, R L   Synopsis of Pediatrics, 3rd ed Mosby, St Louis, 1971

7 Duke-Elder, S L , and Wybar, K C   Ocular Motility and Strabismus, Vol VI Mosby, St Louis, 1973

8 Parks, M M   Ocular Motility Lecture Notes Lancaster Course. Colby College of Maine, Waterville, Maine, 1965

9 Hiatt, R L   Synopsis of Pediatrics, 3rd ed Mosby, St Louis, 1971

10 U S Consumer Products Safety Commission. Bureau of Epidemiology Hazard analysis of fireworks injuries, Report No 1313, Nov 1973

11 National Advisory Eye Council Support for vision research, US Department of Health and Human Services, Westat Report. 1976

12 Dennison, A L   Partially seeing children aren't so different Sight Saving Review, 22:208, 1952

13 Lighthouse Nursery School Understanding your blind child The New York Association for the Blind, New York, 1959

14 Committee on Education of Partially Seeing Children Research needs related to partially seeing children Sight Saving Review 24(2): 1954

19

Hearing Problems in Childhood

Marion P. Downs

Primary care physicians responsible for the management of infants and young children should be seriously concerned about hearing during the early years of life. These are optimal (critical) periods for language learning and for full development of the central auditory system. Deprivation of hearing during this time, even as a result of a mild hearing loss, may result in language delay or learning disorders.[1,2] The primary care physician is in the ideal position to identify hearing loss, remediate it, recommend appropriate intervention, and promote preventive measures.

Marion P. Downs • Department of Otolaryngology, University of Colorado Health Sciences Center, Denver, Colorado 80262

THE COMMON HEARING DISORDERS OF INFANCY AND CHILDHOOD

Sensorineural Loss

Most sensorineural losses are congenital and are identified through the use of a high-risk register. However, some sensorineural losses are acquired later in childhood and may be a complication of (1) bacterial meningitis (almost 20% of all cases will have hearing losses as sequelae); (2) high fever; (3) ototoxic drugs (aminoglycosides); (4) encephalitis; or (5) measles, mumps, scarlet fever, or whooping cough (when not immunized). It is these losses, plus a number of hereditary syndromes that appear after birth, that necessitate constant vigilance in the office situation in order to detect their appearance.

Conductive Loss

In infants and children, conductive losses are due mainly to otitis media and to middle ear anomalies. The latter are present at birth and are usually accompanied by some other cranial abnormality such as cleft lip or cleft palate and malformed pinnae. When a child has such a unilateral ear abnormality, the normal-appearing opposite ear should be examined audiologically, as often it too is involved.

The conductive loss from otitis media results in hearing levels of 27–31 dB, whether in the acute stage or in the serous stage that may follow.[3] This degree of loss can be extremely handicapping to an infant learning language for the first time, as many of the softer speech sounds will not be heard with such a loss. It is for this reason that the American Academy of Pediatrics has issued a Position Statement on Middle Ear Disease and Language Development[1] (see Appendix) that states, in part:

> There is growing evidence demonstrating a correlation between middle ear disease with hearing impairment and delays in the development of speech, language and cognitive skills. . . .
> When a child has frequently recurring acute otitis media and/or ear effusion persisting for longer than three months, hearing should be assessed and the development of communicative skills must be monitored.

The identification procedures described in the next section fulfill the stated requirements of monitoring communicative skills and of indicating which children should be referred for audiological evaluations and in-depth language assessments.

IDENTIFICATION OF HEARING LOSS IN AN OFFICE SETTING

Four relatively simple and rapid procedures can be performed in the physician's office; most should be repeated at scheduled visits for immunizations, at 6, 12, and 18 months:

1. Application of the questionnaire of the high-risk register for congenital deafness
2. Screening test for communicative disorders
3. Tympanometry (as a confirmation of pneumatic otoscopy examination)
4. Behavioral testing of hearing

Each of these procedures is rapid and, after experience, should add no more than 3 or 4 min. to the routine office visit. The tests can be performed by nurses, child health associates, nurse practitioners, or other trained office personnel.

The High-Risk Register Questionnaire

A basic tool in the identification of hearing loss is the high-risk register for deafness, which has been recommended by a national Joint Committee on Infant Hearing,[4] composed of representatives from the Academy of Pediatrics, the Academy of Otolaryngology/Head and Neck Surgery, and the American Speech–Language–Hearing Association (see Appendix). It should be applied at the initial health visit to determine whether a condition exists that indicates careful hearing-assessment procedures. The following questions cover the major conditions responsible for congenital deafness, ordered in an ABC mnemonic:

Asphyxia?
    1-min Apgar <3?
    Spontaneous respiration >10 min?
    Hypotonia >2 hr of age?
Bacterial meningitis?
Congenital perinatal infections?
    Rubella or rubella exposure during pregnancy?
    Cytomegalovirus?
    Herpes?
    Toxoplasmosis?
    Syphilis?
Defects of head or neck?
    Craniofacial syndromal abnormality?
    Overt or submucous cleft palate?
    Morphological abnormalities of pinna?
Elevated Bilirubin?
Family history of childhood hearing impairment?
Gram birth weight <1500 g

A positive answer to any of these questions should occasion a referral for a hearing evaluation at an audiology center.

One out of every 75 children who fall into the high-risk register can be expected to have a significant hearing loss. The losses are most always sensorineural, except in the case of defects of head or neck, which are usually associated with middle ear anomalies.

Screening for Communicative Disorders

It is now possible to screen infants and young children (birth to 3 years) for communicative disorders with a fair degree of confidence, and it is this age group that is the principal target. Identification and intervention at this age can forestall later language problems.

The test of choice is the Early Language Milestone (ELM) test.[5] This scale has been validated on a high-risk population, with 97% sensitivity and 93% specificity. Administration time is approximately 1–3 min, and it is scored on a form similar to the Denver Developmental Screening Test (DDST). The optimal time for screening begins at 18 months, around the time the explosive phase of expressive language occurs, and it is at this time that the effects of recurrent middle ear effusion may first be seen.

Early language delays are not outgrown, whether they are caused by recurrent effusions or by environmental deprivation.[6] Early intervention can change the outcome successfully if the problem is identified.[7]

Tympanometry

The most useful aid in identifying a child whose ears should be carefully examined is tympanometry. This test can easily be done by trained office personnel, avoiding the necessity of performing pneumatic otoscopy at every well-child visit. The tympanometer measures the impedance of the eardrum and accurately identifies the presence or absence of fluid in the middle ear. A limitation is that children under 7 months of age who have an effusion may show a normal tympanogram because the infant outer ear canal skin is so pliable it may affect the test results.[8] However, a positive, flat tympanogram (type B) can be relied upon to indicate fluid at this age.

Tympanometry has been shown to have 96% correlation with pneumatic otoscopy under a microscope.[8,9] The latest models require as little as 1–2 sec to take a reading, so that the test is over before the child has time to protest. This fact makes it especially easy for office personnel to handle. Available models are shown in Table I.

Behavioral Testing of Hearing

Hearing can be tested in the physician's office at 6, 12, and 18 months, or when immunizations are given. The tests are designed to identify only losses of 40 dB or greater, (re: audiometric 0) but may detect some of the otitis media problems.

Testing Instruments

Either noisemakers or electronically produced noises can be used for this age group. A kit of noisemakers is available that produce sound levels under 45 dB, with varied frequency representation.* A louder noisemaker is provided that produces sound over 75 dB for the purpose of eliciting a startle response. The best electronic stimuli are those that produce warbled tones or narrow-band noises at difference frequencies and as low as 20–30 dB (re: audiometric 0).

Procedures for Office Behavioral Testing

Behavioral testing of hearing loss can be performed as an office procedure. The stimuli and technique depend on the age of the child.

---

*Hear Kit, BAM World Marketing, 2750 S. Shoshone, Englewood, Colorado 80110.

Table I. Tympanometers: Available Models[a]

Manufacturer	Model	Pressure range (mm H$_2$O)	Features[b]	Comments[c]
American Electromedics	83	−800 to +400	A, B, C, D, E, F, G, J	A, I
	85R	−800 to +400	B, I	B, G, H
	85AR	−400 to +200	B, D, H, I	B, G, H
	86AR	−400 to +200	B, D, E, G, I	B, G, H
Amplaid	70Z	−500 to +500	A, B, C, D, E, F, G, J	A, I
Grason-Stadler	1722	−300 to +200	B, D, E, H, I	B, D, G, H
	1723	−600 to +300	A, C, D, E, F, G, I	A
Madsen Electronics	7073	−600 to +300	A, B, C, D, E, F, H, J	A, I
	7575	−600 to +300	A, C, D, E, F, G, J	B, G, H
	7576B	−600 to +300	A, C, E, G, J	B, G, H
	7577MB	−600 to +300	A, B, C, E, H, J	B, G, H
	Tympanoscope	−300 to +200	B, D, E, H, I	B, E, G, H
Maico Instruments	M15	−300 to +200	B, D, E, H	B, C, D, F, G, H
Teledyne Avionics	TA-20	−500 to +250	A, B, C, D, E, F, G, I	A, J

[a]Adopted by the Committee on Hearing Loss, Section of Otolaryngology and Bronchoesophagology, American Academy of Pediatrics, October, 1981. From Bluestone.[9]

[b]Code: A, manual tympanometry; B, automatic tympanometry; C, contralateral acoustic reflex; D, ipsilateral acoustic reflex; E, pure-tone stimuli; F, noise-band stimuli; G, audiometric intensity range; H, limited intensity range; I, built-in chart recorder; J, separate chart recorder.

[c]Code: A, large desk-top unit; B, small portable unit; C, no chart recorder; D, difficult ear canal seal; E, poor optics for otoscopy; F, digital display of values; G, high sensitivity to patient movement; H, less than 5 sec recording time; I, good with fussy or crying children.

Birth to 5 Months

Technique.   First, select the quietest room available in the office complex; avoiding waiting rooms, bathrooms, air-conditioning vents, or heating blowers, if possible. Place the infant on an examining table or in the mother's arms, fixating attention on a diversion toy. Next, with the free arm, hold the loud stimulus (e.g., a horn) 6 in. from the infant's ear. When the infant is quiet (either watching the toy or asleep), produce the sound, making certain not to direct the end of the horn into the patient's ears (as some air would be felt that way). If any one of the three reflex responses described below is noted, it is classified as a pass. (If the room is sufficiently quiet, the 30–40-dB signals may be used to obtain a reflex or arousal.) If no response is noted, change to the opposite side and present the sound in the same way as before. If any one of the following three responses described is noted, the child receives a passing score.

Responses.   During the early months (birth to 5 months), the only response that can be depended on is a reflex response to a loud sound. The auditory reflexes that can be expected at this age include (1) a startle (a jump, or a Moro-like reflex immediately following the sound); (2) an eyeblink (a sudden constriction of the eyelids immediately following the sound); or (3) arousal from sleep within 2 sec of the sound (an eye movement accompanied by movement of any limb).

Interpretation.   A passing score in one ear indicates that the child does not have a severe hearing loss. It does not ensure, however, that there may not be a mild or moderate hearing loss, under 30 or 40 dB. Mild losses at this age can only be determined by definitive testing in a sound room. A failure or questionable response is a signal that the infant should be further evaluated at an audiology center.

Six Months to 2 Years

Technique.   Select a very quiet room in the office complex. Position the child on the mother's lap, leaning comfortably against her chest or sitting upright. A third person should sit in front of the child and keep attention focused foward (holding up a toy, moving it slowly in a 160° arc, or transferring it quietly from one hand to the other). Observe the baby closely. At this stage, the child should be able to track the toy visually from one side to the other.

The tester is positioned behind the baby with the soft sound signal. Kneeling down, the tester presents the sound at a 135° angle from the child's front vision and at a level near the floor, 1 yard from the baby's ear. It is important to ensure that the baby is unable to see with peripheral vision. Two sounds of different frequency ranges can then be presented to each side.

The observer records responses to the softer sound-signal testing. Then, approaching the child carefully from behind, present the loud sound signal, 6 in. from the right ear. An eyeblink or startle should be elicited. Repeat the maneuver on the opposite side.

This last test provides insurance against false responses in a deaf child. Deaf children are unusually visually alert, constantly scanning their environment. It might thus be easy to assume that a deaf child was turning the head toward the sound when actually the child was really scanning. A deaf child, however, will not give a startle reflex or eyeblink to the loud sound.

Responses.

At 5–10 Months: The head turns toward the side at which sound is being presented. At 5 months it may be a wobbly, beginning head turn that does not completely reach to the side. However, by 6 months of age, the infant should turn the head directly toward the side of the sound source but will not be able to fixate the sound source, when it is on a lower or higher level from his eyes. The child at this age will startle to the loud noise (75 dB+), making a jump like a Moro reflex or an eyeblink.

At 10–14 months: The head turns toward the side of the sound and on a lower level than the eyes. At 10 months of age, the child may first look directly to the side and then downward, but by approximately 11 months he finds the sound directly on the lower level. The child will still startle to the loud sound (75 dB+).

At 14 months to 2 years: The head turns directly toward the sound in all planes. At 14 months of age, the child's eyes may make a sweep to the side and up but soon is fixating directly on the upper as well as lower levels. A startle response to a loud noise (65 dB+) is observed.

MANAGEMENT OF COMMON HEARING LOSSES

Early, zealous interventions are indicated for any hearing loss, whether it be severe sensorineural or mild conductive. The interventions vary with the degree and type of hearing loss.

Sensorineural losses require prompt hearing aid application and subsequent habilitation. The physician will do well to acquaint himself with the facilities available for habilitation and to help guide the parents to those most suitable for the child. Obtaining good advice from educational audiologists is paramount, and the physician should follow the course of the educational treatment to determine that it is satisfactory for the child's needs.

Conductive hearing losses that resist medical treatment should be addressed with the same urgency as sensorineural losses. The language screening test will reveal the child who requires educational intervention. A mild language delay may benefit from a program that can be managed out of the physician's office. Home language-stimulation programs are available for this purpose.

Severe language delays are appropriately handled by speech/language pathologists. Occasionally a persistent mild conductive hearing loss requires amplification, if only for the duration of the hearing-loss period. A low-amplification hearing aid will not harm even a normal hearing ear and will provide help during the time a loss is present. Appropriate therapy with the aid should be given by an educational audiologist.

PREVENTION OF ACQUIRED HEARING LOSS

The keystone of prevention in the physician's office is immunization. Vaccines for childhood viral infections prevent not only acquired hearing losses but, in the case of rubella vaccine, will prevent the severe congenital loss due to rubella from occurring when the child becomes a prospective parent. The new HIB vaccine will greatly reduce the prevalence of hearing losses from bacterial meningitis, and it is hoped that very soon a vaccine for *Pneumococcus* will prevent the escalating numbers of cases of otitis media in the young child.

Other measures include

1. Instructions regarding avoiding exposure to loud noises such as gunfire, firecrackers, cap guns, and amplified music
2. Careful prescriptive doses of aminoglycosides (these ototoxic drugs have not been shown to be harmful during the perinatal period when proper dosages were given, but errors in dosage have produced profound deafness)
3. Proper ear hygiene, with parents given instructions to avoid washing out or medicating ears without a physician's prescription
4. Prophylactic antibiotic regimens for children with persistent middle ear effusion, as well as considerations of surgical interventions for unyielding cases
5. Constant vigilance for child abuse that may produce traumatic hearing loss

Attention to these measures will fulfill the primary physician's responsibility in caring for hearing health.

SUMMARY

The physician can take an active part in identifying all hearing losses, whether profound sensorineural or mild conductive, and has a role in monitoring the language problems that may ensue. The office can be the site of early identification, of evaluation of the hearing as well as the language of children with losses, of active educational interventions as well as medical, and of primary prevention of deafness and hearing impairment.

REFERENCES

1. American Academy of Pediatrics: Policy Statement: Middle ear disease and language development, *News and Comment* Sept. 1984, p. 9.
2. Teele, D. W., Klein, J. O., Rosner, B. A., and the Greater Boston Otitis Media Study Group: Otitis media with effusion during the first three years of life and development of speech and language. *Pediatrics* **74:**282–287, 1984.
3. McDermott, J. C., Giebink, G. S., Le, C. T., *et al.:* Children with persistent otitis media. *Arch. Otolaryngol.* **109:**360–362, 1983.
4. Joint Committee on Infant Hearing: Position Statement, 1982. *Asha* **24(12):**1017–1018, 1982.
5. Coplan, J., Gleason, J. R., Ryan, R., *et al.:* Validation of an early language milestone scale in a high-risk population. *Pediatrics* **70:**5, 677–683, 1982.
6. Silva, P. A.: The prevalence, stability and significance of developmental language delay in preschool children. *Dev. Med. Child Neurol.* **22:**768–777, 1980.
7. Guinagh, B. J., and Jester, R. E.: Long-term effects of infant stimulation programs. *Adv. Behav. Pediatr.* **2:**81–110, 1981.
8. Paradise, J. L., Smith, C., and Bluestone, C. D.: Tympanometric detection of middle ear effusion in infants and young children. *Pediatrics* **58:**198–206, 1976.
9. Bluestone, C. D.: Diagnosis of chronic otitis media with effusion: Description, otoscopy, acoustic impedance measurements, and assessment of hearing. *Pediatric Infectious Diseases* **5**(suppl. 1):S39–S72, 1982.

20

Role of the Physician in the School Life of the Child

Craig B. Liden and Theresa E. Laurie

Craig B. Liden and Theresa E. Laurie • TRANSACT Health Systems, Forbes Regional Health Center, Monroeville, Pennsylvania 15146.

RATIONALE FOR PHYSICIAN INVOLVEMENT

Over the past decade, issues of child development and behavior have moved into a prominent position in the mainstream of general pediatrics.[1] This awareness is characterized by an expanded operational definition of health that includes concern not only for "quantity of life" but "quality of life" for the child as well. As a natural extension of heightened awareness in this regard, physicians are becoming increasingly involved in the major arena of life functioning for children—the school.

The physician is faced daily with the opportunity to facilitate a child's success in school, by consulting to the child's parents or interacting with the appropriate people in the child's school. In 1978 this role for physicians was acknowledged in a report by the Task Force on Pediatric Education.[2] In addition, the Task Force called for revision and expansion of training programs to better prepare the physician to participate fully as a coordinator, manager, and counselor for children with learning and behavior problems. Unfortunately, the changes recommended in this report have not yet been fully realized. As a result, many physicians may totally ignore problems related to the child's educational functioning and may placate parents and teachers by reassuring that the child is "all boy" or "will grow out of it." Others may go to the opposite extreme and expect instant changes in the school environment solely because they demand it.

Physicians have special circumstances that place them in a unique position to effect change in the child's school life. Often physicians are the only professionals who have (and will have) a long-term relationship with both the child and his family. In addition, physicians have the advantage of being respected professionals operating outside the political constraints of the school system. In this position, they can keep the child's needs, not just the system's needs, foremost in mind.

With the appropriate knowledge base and understanding, physicians can translate their heightened awareness and unique circumstances into actions that have a favorable impact on the child's school life. It is the purpose of this chapter to provide the physician with the background and structure to become a responsible facilitator to improve the educational experiences of individual children. Although some may still wish to debate whether physicians should be involved in concerns over a child's school learning and behavior, the previously mentioned factors seem to suggest that physicians have virtually no choice in the matter. There are more cogent questions to be asked: What are the possible roles for physicians in the school life of the child? What are the prerequisite skills to execute these roles? How can physicians function as facilitators within the real-life constraints of their practice? The remainder of this chapter seeks to provide a framework to begin to answer these questions.

POTENTIAL PHYSICIAN ROLES

Many investigators have begun to tackle the difficult question of what the appropriate role is for the physician in the school life of the child.[3,4] There is still no universally accepted answer to this question. Rather, it is possible to describe a spectrum of possibilities. These range from a primary care physician who has limited involvement in the child's school life to a specially trained consultant who becomes intimately involved in school related issues. Given a range of possibilities, the individual physician must responsibly select an appropriate role taking into account his training and expertise, career goals and aims, the needs of the community in which he is practicing, and other practical factors including available time and financial reimbursement possibilities. The first step in preparing to become a responsible facilitator in the school life of the child is to select a realistic role. The following is a brief description of some of these role possibilities. Specific guidelines for actually executing these roles are provided later in this chapter.

General Practitioner

Primary care pediatricians or family practitioners have multiple opportunities to influence the school life of the child without having to have substantial additional training. Within the context of providing continuity of care, physicians can systematically monitor the emergence of various risk factors that have been associated with school dysfunction. These include pregnancy, perinatal, and early health factors, life stress events (including various socioeconomic factors), delayed developmental attainment, temperamental dysfunctions (including behavior management problems), and other life performance failures such as somatic dysfunctions and past school failure. Once identified, such factors can serve as red flags to alert physicians to either monitor the child's development more closely or to make an early referral to the school or other appropriate resource for further assessment and intervention as indicated. The value of such screening and referral, even if done informally, should not be underestimated.

Primary care physicians also play an important role by providing consultation to parents and school personnel. This may mean answering specific questions about the child's health which directly relates to school performance. Alternatively, it may mean maintaining an awareness that some psychosocial and learning problems that children experience may present to the physician as some type of somatic complaint (e.g., headaches or recurrent infections).[5] Therefore, in approaching the assessment and management of such problems, physicians can help uncover an underlying learning or behavioral dysfunction by systematically inquiring about the child's performance at school.

During the course of routine health maintenance visits, general practitioners can review upcoming demands and expectations that the child will face in the school environment with the child and parents. Such anticipatory guidance coupled with a longitudinal awareness of the child's emerging developmental strengths and weaknesses can help identify areas of concern that may require close observation, further assessment, and/or intervention.

Finally, as a consequence of their longitudinal relationship with the child and family, primary care physicians are often viewed as *the* trusted professional advocate, to whom the family can turn when their child experiences school dysfunction. This strong relationship can be mobilized to give physicians access to sensitive family information that may contribute to an understanding of the child's school functioning, to assist in presenting difficult diagnostic information to the family, and to help parents become informed consumers of various resources and programs used to manage school failure.

Nondevelopmental Specialist

The pediatric specialist (e.g., otolaryngologist, cardiologist, allergist), like the general practitioner, has an important role in the school life of the child despite a lack of advanced training in child development. Rare is the medical problem requiring some type of longitudinal tertiary care that does not place the child at risk for some type of minor or major school dysfunction. Therefore, the specialist plays an important role in screening for and identifying school dysfunction in targeted populations such as children with congenital heart disease, cystic fibrosis, leukemia, and other chronic conditions. When dysfunctions occur in these children, specialists play an important role. This includes clearly informing parents and school personnel about the child's limitations with respect to school performance, advocating for a child's school needs, helping secure appropriate consultation and treatment from other professionals, and monitoring the child's school progress.

Specialists also play a direct role in the school life of children when they provide specialty consultation to individual children experiencing school problems. In this role, specialist may answer specific questions or provide treatment that addresses the concerns of parents or school personnel. For example, they may be requested to conduct a neurological or ophthalomologic examination for a child experiencing a reading difficulty. When the findings do not account for the child's problem, specialists can triage the referring person to another more appropriate professional.

General Practitioner-Developmental Specialist

Increasingly, some primary health care providers have obtained additional training in child development or related areas through postgraduate fellowships, participation in specialized inservice training, or simply focused independent study. Consequently, in addition to fulfilling the primary health care roles described previously, these general practitioners have expanded their role in the school life of the child by performing one or two special activities for which they have expertise. Such activities may include serving as the sports team physician; conducting preschool developmental screenings; serving as the physician members of a multidisciplinary team assessing handicapped children (i.e., performing physical assessments); conducting extended assessment of neuromaturation, motor function, attention, or other neurodevelopmental functions; prescribing and monitoring the use of special medical therapies such as stimulant medication; providing short-term behavior management counseling; and conducting parent education groups. These tasks can be performed within the context of a solo or group practice, where other partners have unique areas of expertise. The demands of primary care, including night call and management of hospitalized patients, generally prohibit physicians from expanding beyond a few of the mentioned possibilities. Greater involvement generally requires more time, a structure that allows for regular access to a multidisciplinary team, sufficient indirect time for meetings, phonecalls, and so on and innovative financial reimbursement mechanisms.

Developmental or Behavioral Specialist

With appropriate additional training, the physician can fulfill the role of full-time consultant in the school life of the child. This may take the form of postgraduate fellowship work in developmental pediatrics, behavioral pediatrics, adolescent medicine, pediatric neurology, child psychiatry, or graduate work in such areas as psychology, special education, or speech pathology.

This role generally mandates constant involvement and interaction with a team of professionals with expertise in school problems. Such a team may include social workers, educators, psychologists, or other specially trained professionals. To make such a practice cost effective, the physician and other team members need to develop efficient mechanisms for assessment, management, and interprofessional communication. This may take the form of a traditional multidisciplinary team in which the physician is asked to provide highly specialized assessments and treatment within his disciplinary training that are integrated into a comprehensive management plan. Alternatively, the physician and other team members may subsequently function as transdisciplinarians who provide extended consultation and treatment within and across their traditional disciplinary boundaries. Functioning in this latter role, physician specialists may develop special expertise in integrating and synthesizing information from a variety of sources and thereby be in an ideal position to assume a leadership role within the team.

PREREQUISITE SKILLS NECESSARY FOR EXECUTING ROLES

Once a realistic role has been selected, physicians must acquire certain ''skills'' in order to execute this role efficiently and effectively. By surveying the available literature, it is possible to identify certain core prerequisites that physicians must possess in order to play any of the aforementioned roles. The following section attempts to identify and briefly describe these prerequisite skills.

UNDERSTANDING THE "BASIC SCIENCE" OF DEVELOPMENT AND BEHAVIOR

Before physicians can realistically approach playing a role in the school life of the child, they must have a set of operating philosophical premises that can be uniformly applied to a variety of learning and behavior problems in the school setting. This so-called basic science must include (1) a theory of human behavior that integrates the constitutional and environmental factors that have an impact on a child's school functioning, (2) a practical model of the components of development that contribute to learning and behavior consistent with research in the field, and (3) an understanding of the mechanisms underlying manifest school dysfunction. This set of principles has been synthesized from a review of the contemporary developmental literature.[6,7]

Transactional Scheme of Development

A reductionistic and dualistic medical model is a severe constraint when applied to a child's school functioning. School success or failure cannot be reduced to isolated constitutional or environmental factors that operate in a unidimensional, cause-and-effect fashion. Rather, a child's school status at any point in time is the consequence of a series of reciprocal interactions between the child's intrinsic qualities and life events both within and outside the school environment.[8,9] These reciprocal interactions are constantly evolving and are unique for each child.

Table I Components of TRANSACT

Transactors	Description
Temperament (of child)	Temperament or behavioral style refers to those personality characteristics that modulate the child's interactions with the environment on a day-to-day basis Chess and Thomas[10] have identified nine temperamental characteristics along which an individual's behavior can be rated mood, activity level, rhythmicity, distractibility, approach/withdrawal, adaptability, persistence, threshold or responsiveness, and intensity of reaction
Readiness	Readiness refers to those skills that an individual must use in order to process and act upon information presented to the CNS from the environment These include the perception, integration, and encoding stages of information processing Other terms used to describe these skills include auditory discrimination, auditory processing, receptive and expressive language, auditory and visual sequential memory visual perception, spatial organization, higher-order conceptualization, immediate recall, and short- and long-term memory
Attention	Attention refers to the child's ability to focus and sustain attention during specific tasks from moment to moment The components of attention include arousal level, or state'' cognitive tempo, or the balance between impulsivity and reflectivity, filtering, the ability to purposefully focus and filter out distracting stimuli, vigilance, the ability to sustain a purposeful focus over time, and monitoring, or the ability to appraise information critically attended to (quality control)
Neuromaturation	Neuromaturation refers to the overall organization and maturity of the child's nervous system It is postulated to reflect state of myelinization, degree of integration between discrete CNS systems, and efficiency of neuroregulatory processes Neuromaturation has also been arbitrarily defined to include the integrity of sensory input and motor output systems A child's neuromaturational status is a function of genetic endowment, age, and the intactness of all other body function
Stresses	Life stresses refer to those positive and negative experiences that the child has encountered and had to adapt to in his current or past environment They may come from the child s macroenvironment (e g , society community, family) or microenvironment (e g food, microorganisms medications) They include such things as marriage, divorce, financial difficulty, birth, death, loss of job, failure in school, moving, loss of supports, hospitalizations, acquiring deformities and physical illnesses both acute and chronic
Attitudes	Attitudes include the feelings, values, opinions, and belief systems of the child and the significant others in his environment They are formed in part, by past and present experiences with their family system and its traditions, socioeconomic forces, religion, or other spiritual and moral factors, politics, race, education, and other ethnic and cultural factors A full understanding of attitudes requires a broad awareness of the community in which the child functions

Table I. (Continued)

Transactors	Description
Comparison	Comparisons refer to the standards or expectations that the child and the significant others have set for a given behavior. These norms for behaviors may reflect the child's or significant other's personal goals and motivations, degree of self-centeredness versus concern for others, perceptions of self-competency, self-awareness, and their hopes, fears, and other perceptions about the future.
Temperament (of significant others)	This transactor refers to the temperament or behavioral style of the significant others with whom the child interacts on a day-to-day basis. These significant others include parents, siblings, relatives, peers, teachers, neighbors, clergy, and physicians.

Multiplicity of Factors Contributing to Learning and Behavior

A wide variety of factors participate in the transactions between a child and his environment. Some are more constitutionally determined, whereas others are more environmentally bound. The acronym TRANSACT provides a simple means to remember the major transactors systematically when trying to understand a given child's school-function status. The specific components of TRANSACT are summarized in Table I.

Mechanisms of School Dysfunction

When learning or behavioral dysfunction is demonstrated in the school environment, it is invariably a consequence of a mismatch between the child's constitutional characteristics and the expectations placed upon the child. Two major mechanisms underlie all school dysfunctions. First, it is possible that an emerging and developing characteristic in the child (e.g., rate and dexterity of fine motor output) may not fit with established expectations (e.g., timed written test). Alternatively, an existing characteristic (e.g., high activity level) that may have gone unnoticed or been adapted to in the home environment may not fit with emerging or new expectations in the school environment (e.g., sustained in-seat performance).

Lack of awareness of the mechanisms of dysfunction underlies many of the common but inappropriate responses to school failure. This is particularly true when the child is grossly intact and has experienced no major problems prior to school entry. When such a child first demonstrates school failure, the environment's response may range from accusations of poor motivation ("he's just lazy") to false assurance ("he'll grow out of it") to an overemphasis on other jointly occurring stresses in the child's life ("his parents are having marital problems").

Clearly, school function is not a static phenomenon. A child's intrinsic constitutional characteristics continue to unfold during the school years in progressively more subtle ways. Similarly, performance demands in the school environment continue to increase as the child moves on in grades, while new stress events occur in other aspects of the child's life. Therefore, a child who functions efficiently at one point may experience significant dysfunction at a later point in his school career.

In order to assess and manage school dysfunctions effectively, physicians must be knowledgeable about the structure of the educational system and the specific performance demands that a child faces in his school life. This structure and the emerging demands faced by all children are presented in the section on demands in the regular education program.

Behavioral Commonality of Presentation for Heterogeneous Dysfunction

Dysfunctions resulting from a disparity between constitutional characteristics and demands in the school environment generally manifest themselves as failures in major school performance areas: independent functioning, social interaction, and academic achievement. In order for these problems or failures to be identified, some individual (e.g., the child, parent, teacher, principal) involved in the transaction must feel concern or experience stress and label it as a problem. Because of limitations in our abilities as observers and describers of human behavior, we tend to lump our concerns about children into a relatively limited set of presenting problem sets. During this process, we may use a common label for problems that may have vastly different underlying transactional patterns. For example, children with intrinsic attention-deficit disorders, conductive hearing losses, receptive language disorders, sequential memory difficulties, extreme temperamental traits, and situational anxieties may all look grossly similar in the classroom and be described as ''hyperactive'' by school personnel. In fact, the underlying contributors to dysfunction in these populations differ greatly and warrant radically different management plans. Extreme care must be taken to ensure that all potential contributing factors are systematically considered each time a child presents with school dysfunction.

Too frequently, the assessment process for school problems is of a piecemeal ''ruling out'' nature that focuses solely on one aspect of the child or the environment. If this search results in a positive finding, the diagnostic process may end prematurely before all possible contributors have been uncovered. A narrowly focused treatment plan may be instituted; consequently, the problem may persist, resulting in frustration for the child, family, and involved professionals. Appropriate management of presenting symptoms of school dysfunction always begins with a systematic survey of the operating TRANSACT factors in each individual case.

Systematic Descriptive Analysis as a Key to Establishment of a Diagnostic– Therapeutic Continuum

When a school problem presents, the goals of a systematic survey of the TRANSACT factors should be to develop a descriptive formulation that synthesizes the child's constitutional strengths and weaknesses, the school and home environment's strengths and weaknesses, and their pattern of interaction in relationship to the presenting problem. There are three stages:

Stage I. Identification: Potential components of the problem are systematically categorized by surveying the TRANSACT profile for potential risk factors. This may entail the use of qualitative (e.g., interview and behavioral observations) and quantitative (e.g., rating scales and neurodevelopmental tests) techniques.

Stage II. Refinement: Clinical judgments are made about the relationship of identified risk factors in terms of their contribution to the genesis of the presenting problem.

Stage III. Definition: Specific intervention strategies targeted to each contributor to the presenting problem are generated. Since school problems are always a consequence of a mismatch in expectations, the first step in this stage is always to provide the parents, teacher, significant others, and the child when appropriate with a clarification of the TRANSACT factors operating and their interactions. This is done to facilitate a reordering of expectations. All other intervention strategies fall into one of two categories: providing direct remediation or providing compensatory strategies.

Since TRANSACT is never static, these stages must be reapplied on a longitudinal basis during the child's school career. When dealing with school problems, therapeutic efficacy is measured by the meeting of specific management objectives agreed upon by the child, parents, teachers, physician, and "significant others" when necessary. This process frequently requires contingency planning whereby management objectives and intervention strategies are refined and modified as TRANSACT changes.

EFFECTIVE COMMUNICATION SKILLS

As in all clinical encounters, playing an effective role in the school life of the child begins with effective communication between the physician, child, parents, and involved school personnel. A common complaint that parents of children experiencing school problems have about their physicians is that they do not listen to their concerns or, when they do, their concerns are minimized. Most parents do not expect their child's physician necessarily to have the expertise to assess and manage their child's school problem. However, all parents expect to have their concerns empathetically heard and acted upon in an appropriate fashion through referral, if necessary. In addition, parents and teachers indicate that the information shared by physicians is often too technical and/or is presented in a manner that prohibits the opportunity for them (i.e., parents and teachers) to ask questions.

Physicians must have effective communication skills, including the ability to establish a trusting relationship, refined interviewing techniques, reflective and empathetic listening skills, and the capability of sharing technical or complex information in a clear, concise manner. By employing these skills in dealing with school problems, the physician gains access to observers—the parent and teacher—who may be more reliable and valid than many of our more sophisticated screening or assessment tools. This is a consequence of their longitudinal contact with the child and their built-in access to control populations (i.e., siblings and peers).

Many physicians have not had opportunities to receive formal training or feedback on their communication skills. Consequently, some physicians may be lacking in this area. Professional growth in this area may require consultation with professional colleagues who have special expertise or training in this area (e.g., social workers).

Even when physicians are able to communicate effectively, the lack of sufficient time may prevent them from doing so. There is no escape from the reality that effective communication regarding the child's school life requires time. The amount of time varies according to the role a physician chooses to play. However, this is certainly more than the 90 sec that has been documented to be devoted to "anticipatory guidance" during routine office visits.[11] To mobilize sufficient time, physicians may establish new scheduling routines such as an extended time slot for school entry evaluations or extended times for problem consultation. They can examine the cost effectiveness of their existing office procedures for school aged children (e.g., complete physical examinations) and refine them. They can employ new office procedures (e.g., questionnaires) that save time and/or use other health care professionals creatively.

KNOWLEDGE OF RESOURCES AND POTENTIAL CONTRIBUTION OF OTHER TEAM MEMBERS

The school problems of developing children are multifacted; physicians must therefore cultivate relationships with professionals who possess expertise in a variety of areas: speech and language, psychology, education, social work, and counseling. These individuals must become partners with physicians in helping children with school problems in the community and school. Whenever possible, physicians should develop rapport with school based professionals in these roles as well as similar personnel in the community. It can be useful for physicians to develop a resource file of such individuals for ready access. The physician should develop specific referral criteria and communication patterns in order to work effectively with these professionals.

In addition to developing rapport with a key group of professionals, physicians must become knowledgeable of the vast array of community resources available for families and children. Office staff can be guided to develop a file of resources matched to patient's needs. For example, resources may need to be identified in the following areas: child care or day care; preschools for normal and handicapped; parenting training and education; support groups for parents experiencing problems (e.g., child abuse, alcohol or drugs, problem children, handicapped children, divorce); specific parent organizations for the range of handicaps; legal advice in a variety of areas (e.g., divorce, education); recreational programs for normal and handicapped; and information hot lines.

A file of community resources may take time to develop. Local school systems and parent groups frequently have developed similar files and can be contacted to help reduce duplication of efforts. If physicians have instant access to such information, they can be extremely useful in linking parents to the appropriate resource.

UNDERSTANDING THE EDUCATIONAL SYSTEM

The local school system(s) will be the target of the physician's involvement. To be an effective advocate for children and adolescents, physicians must build rapport with key administrative and educational personnel, have an understanding of the specific demands placed upon children in the school environment, and be knowledgeable about the services available for children with learning and behavior problems.

Building Rapport

Work with a school can be facilitated if the physician knows who to contact for specific problems and has had some contact with these individuals before a problem arises. This task can be accomplished by an information-sharing meeting with the school superintendent if the district is small and/or the administrator in charge of elementary, middle, and secondary schools in larger districts. School personnel may be confused about physician involvement in school matters; physicians must therefore be capable of effectively communicating the role they plan to play in a nonthreatening manner. They must be prepared for facing negative encounters and must understand that such reactions may not be personally directed. Frequently, such reactions are related to the educator's limited contact and unsuccessful experiences with medical professionals. However, through an information-sharing meeting, physicians can learn about the organizational structure of the system and find out who to contact and how to facilitate communication. The names of specific contact people should be obtained in the following areas: (1) medical services; (2) remedial services (reading, math); (3) support services (social worker, psychology, counseling, physical education, speech, and language); and (4) special education services.

School administrators should be asked for information on the range of services available and how to elicit such services. Copies of local and state regulations or guidelines for these special services should be obtained from the district administrators or from appropriate state department personnel. School administrators should also be given an opportunity to obtain information from the physician. This may include call hours, referral mechanisms, scheduling procedures, areas of special expertise, and specifics of any typical assessment or management protocols that are followed. It is hoped that such meetings can help increase the physician's effectiveness in interactions with the schools in the community.

Demands in the Regular Education Program

Schools and classrooms vary from locale to locale and from teacher to teacher. In spite of this variability, some broad similarities in the underlying premises, practices, and procedures used in most schools can be defined.

The chronological age of the child is the most important variable used by the school to determine the child's educational program. In spite of the fact that children grow and develop at varied rates, schools group children according to their chronological age. Thus, children who have lived on earth for equal amounts of time are expected to have attained similar levels of physical, social, and cognitive development. Although teachers may divide the class into several instructional groups, there is an expectation that children should be able to learn at similar rates and respond to similar instructional modes.

In most regular classrooms, only a narrow range of individual differences is tolerated. The large numbers of students in each class greatly affects the degree of individualization which can occur. The programs and procedures used in most classrooms are designed to meet the needs of the group and not the needs of the individual. To meet the goal of educating the masses, teachers are generally required to follow a prescribed curriculum and to use mandated materials and grading procedures. These structures may serve to limit a teacher's ability to modify their instructional procedures. Even when teachers want to alter what or how they are teaching to better meet the needs of individual children, they may not be allowed to deviate from the curriculum or to use supplemental materials.

For many regular classroom teachers, their lack of training in individualizing instruction makes it difficult or even impossible for them to adapt to individual children. Until recently, university training programs did not provide teachers with coursework in strategies for behavior management or modifying instructional materials. Once in the field, practicing teachers rarely have opportunities to learn these skills from other professionals in the school. Little if any time is set aside in most systems for formal staff development activities or for informal opportunities for teachers to exchange ideas.

As a result of these factors, regular educators may express resistance to modifying instructional expectations or methods to match the unique needs of an individual child with variations in physical, cognitive, and affective development. Their reactions may be the result of externally imposed limits or their own frustration at not having the time or know-how to help a child in need. Therefore, in addition to advocating for the child with exceptional needs, physicians may need to advocate on behalf of the classroom teacher and help to obtain for him the necessary support to address a child's problems.

The demands placed on children may vary depending on the community they live in, the school they attend, and the teacher they have. However, there are a set of more general school expectations. Table II summarizes some of the major demands that most children face as they proceed through our educational system. Familiarity with these demands is a key to understanding, anticipating, and managing school dysfunction.

Strategies for Coping with Children with Differences

A prerequisite to interacting effectively with the school system is an understanding of their strategies for coping with children who differ significantly from their peers in either behavior or academic skill development. The following is a brief description of these strategies:

Retention

Occasionally students who show deficiencies in social or academic skills are retained in the same grade level. This solution implies that the student may be immature and will improve if given more time to develop. For a very few students, this additional exposure to the curriculum is beneficial and the results are successful. No federal or state regulations exist to guide schools in making this decision. Therefore, retention may be suggested without a thorough evaluation of the child. Obviously, the problems of children with more extreme learning or behavior needs may not be addressed by exposure to the same content and methods of instruction.

Schools have recognized the fact that retention is not always the best solution. A

Table II Demands Faced by Children in the Educational System

Grade level	Performance demand category			
	General	Independent functioning	Social interaction	Academic achievement
Preschool–kindergarten	Total separation from family and home environment	Complete simple tasks (feeding, dressing) with little or no adult assistance Regulate somatic function (bladder, bowel), conform to school schedule	Follow formal rules for talking, moving, and use of classroom Function in a group, control impulses, and share Understand consequences of his behavior Listen attentively to verbal presentations	Identify likenesses and differences in visual symbols, spoken words, and sounds Understand and use language Identify and reproduce sounds of letters Count, name numerals, and associate numerical value with each numeral
Primary grades (1–3)	Remain in school for whole day Shift emphasis from socialization to instruction in basic academic skills	Eat at school within set time period Transact money Make choices about food, drink Complete mastery of somatic functions Initiate and complete tasks without adult supervision	Decreased reminders of rules Cope with decreased free movement Exert self-control over impulses and attention	Learn to read, extract meaning from longer passage Learn to write, translate spoken to written word Memorize basic math facts in addition, subtraction, multiplication, and division
Intermediate grades (4–6)	Proficiency in basic academic skills Larger quantities of work within specific time frame	Responsible for appearance and possessions Homework, keep track of assignments, organize time, and meet deadlines	Decrease recess and play time Create own social interactions Interact with peers of opposite sex	Silent reading of nonfiction Increased written expression (reports) Apply computation skills to word problems Apply basic skills to content area (social studies and science)
Secondary grades (7–12)	Adjust to larger school Change classes Work with different teachers who are content specialists	Follow strict time schedule Come to class with appropriate materials Meet new problems with minimal teacher support or direction	Peer group pressure to conform Cope with sexuality, dates	Lengthy independent reading assignments Demonstrate knowledge through tests, papers, and reports Meet graduation requirements

variety of services have been developed to help cope with the needs of children for whom this option is not satisfactory. Although the quantity and quality of these services vary tremendously from district to district and from school to school, some level of the programs discussed in the following section should exist in most school settings.

Remedial Programs and Support Services

Remedial programs and supportive services are designed for children with mild academic deficiencies (e.g., reading, speech and language, math and/or mild behavioral problems). These programs and services generally are available at all levels in the educational system, although they make take on several different formats. For example, as a substitute for grade retention, classes may exist for groups of students who are progressing at a slower rate. In the early grades, pre-first grade or *transition* classes may exist. These are generally designed to accommodate somewhat smaller groups of children than are found in the regular program. This allows for more individual attention to the students. The rate of instruction may be reduced and increased opportunities for practice on specific skills may be allowed. In the secondary school, such programs may exist in all subject areas, and a homogeneous group of underachievers may be assigned to a modified version of the standard course offerings.

Some of these programs do not segregate children into a class for the entire day. These programs provide specific instruction to the child in a small group for part of the day. For example, a child may attend a remedial reading or a math program for 40 min each day because of some difficulty in keeping up with the students in the regular class. Similarly, a child may attend weekly group meetings with the school social worker to improve behavior. Like the format described for the transitional class or homogeneous grouping, subject-specific remedial programs enable children to learn at a slower rate and provide more opportunity for individual attention. In most remedial programs, however, the instructional strategies are designed for small group instruction. These programs can be beneficial for children with minor delays in developmental readiness skills. Children with more extreme learning needs require more personalized instruction than most remedial programs can provide.

To qualify for remedial programs or support services, a child must demonstrate mild underachievement in classwork or on standardized testing. The degree of underachievement necessary will vary from district to district. Inappropriate placements can be avoided by a thorough evaluation prior to placement to determine whether such programs would meet a child's needs.

Special Education Service

Historically, special education classes and services have been used to help school systems cope with those students who have extreme learning and behavioral needs. Special education services are flexibly designed to meet the needs of a range of children. The needs of the individual child dictate the amount and type of services needed.

Many differences exist between special and regular education or remedial services. Fewer students are served in special classes than in regular classes. By law, special education services must be matched to the child's individual pattern of functioning. Special education teachers are usually free to select materials, methods, and time lines for teaching specific skills. Therefore, the child's specific needs, not age, the needs of the group, or the mandates of a curriculum, determine what or how he will be taught. For the most part, the training special education teachers receive prepares them for dealing with student's differences and fosters an attitude that is more accepting of variability in student rates and styles of learning.

Until recently, special and regular education have operated as very separate systems. Regular education existed for "normal" children and special education for children who deviated from the norm. Instead of changing the norms and underlying assumptions of basic education to accommodate differences, children were taken out of the mainstream of education. During the 1960s and 1970s, the nature of special education began to change, with increased emphasis being placed on integrating the two programs. As a result of various social, political, and economic forces, federal legislation was enacted during the 1970s that set the foundation for changes in special education. Landmark legislation (P.L. 94-142[12] and Section 504 of P.L. 93-380[13]) provided the following:

1. A free and appropriate public education for all handicapped children
2. A mandate to all local schools to identify all exceptional children
3. The enactment of *due process* procedures (an extension of the Fourteenth Amendment) for parents of handicapped children who disagree with their child's educational program
4. The development of an individualized education program (IEP) for each identified child
5. A guarantee that all handicapped children be educated with their normal peers to the maximum extent possible (least restrictive environment)
6. Equal access to all programs available to children in the district

Any school district receiving federal monies to operate special programs must follow the mandates outlined in these laws. In addition, a district must comply with an elaborate set of identification, classification, placement, and review procedures. Physicians can obtain copies of their state's standards governing special education by contacting the State Director of Special Education.

The type of special education a child receives will depend on the severity of their particular physical, cognitive, or affective needs. A major thrust of the law is to encourage the integration of exceptional children in the mainstream of the educational system. In the law, the terminology used to explain this practice is "least restrictive environment." This term implies that it is preferable to try to maintain a special needs student in close proximity to the nonhandicapped population. Segregation is viewed as less desirable and only appropriate when "the handicap is such that education in regular classes with the use of supplementary aids and services cannot be achieved satisfactorily." This policy is directed at all categories of exceptional children. Therefore, a continuum of services are outlined in the law to be considered as options for children and adolescents with all handicapping conditions.

When the severity of a child's dysfunction necessitates more service than can be provided within the regular classroom or in remedial programs, the child must be formally evaluated to determine eligibility for special educational services. The physician must be aware of special education services and procedures to counsel parents adequately and to play the role of facilitator.

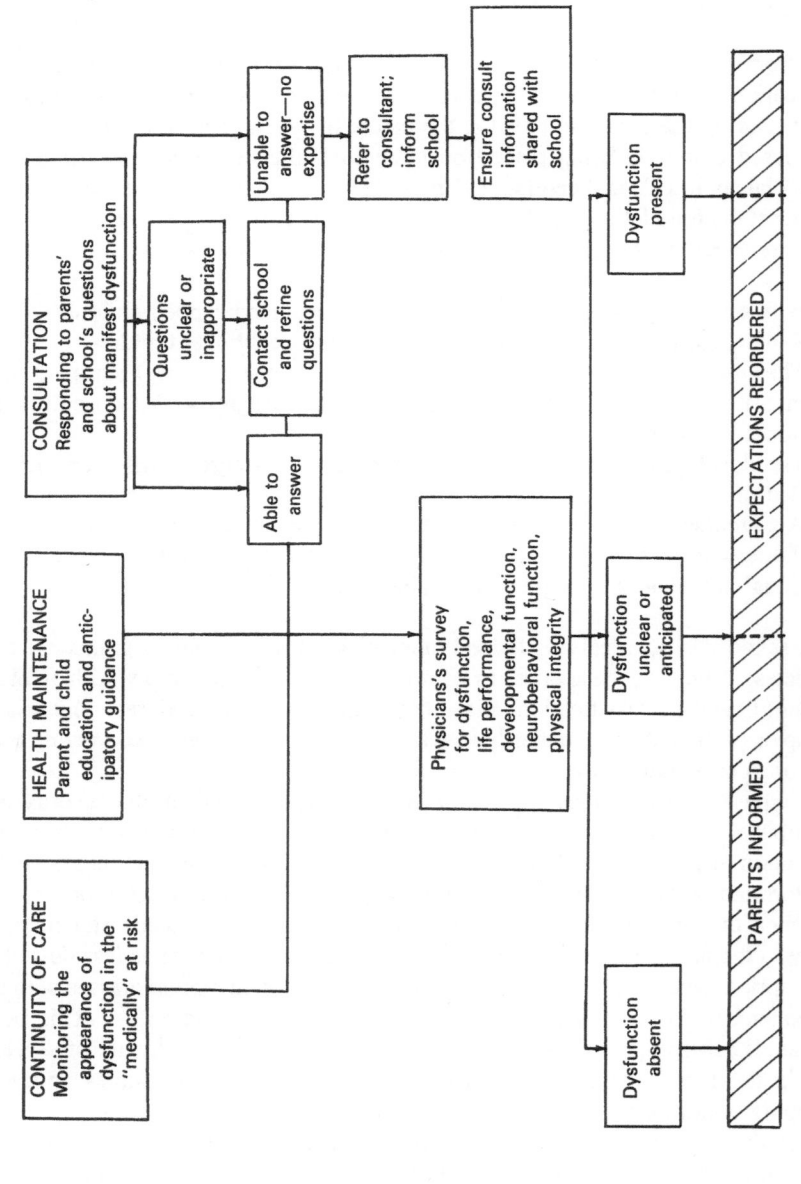

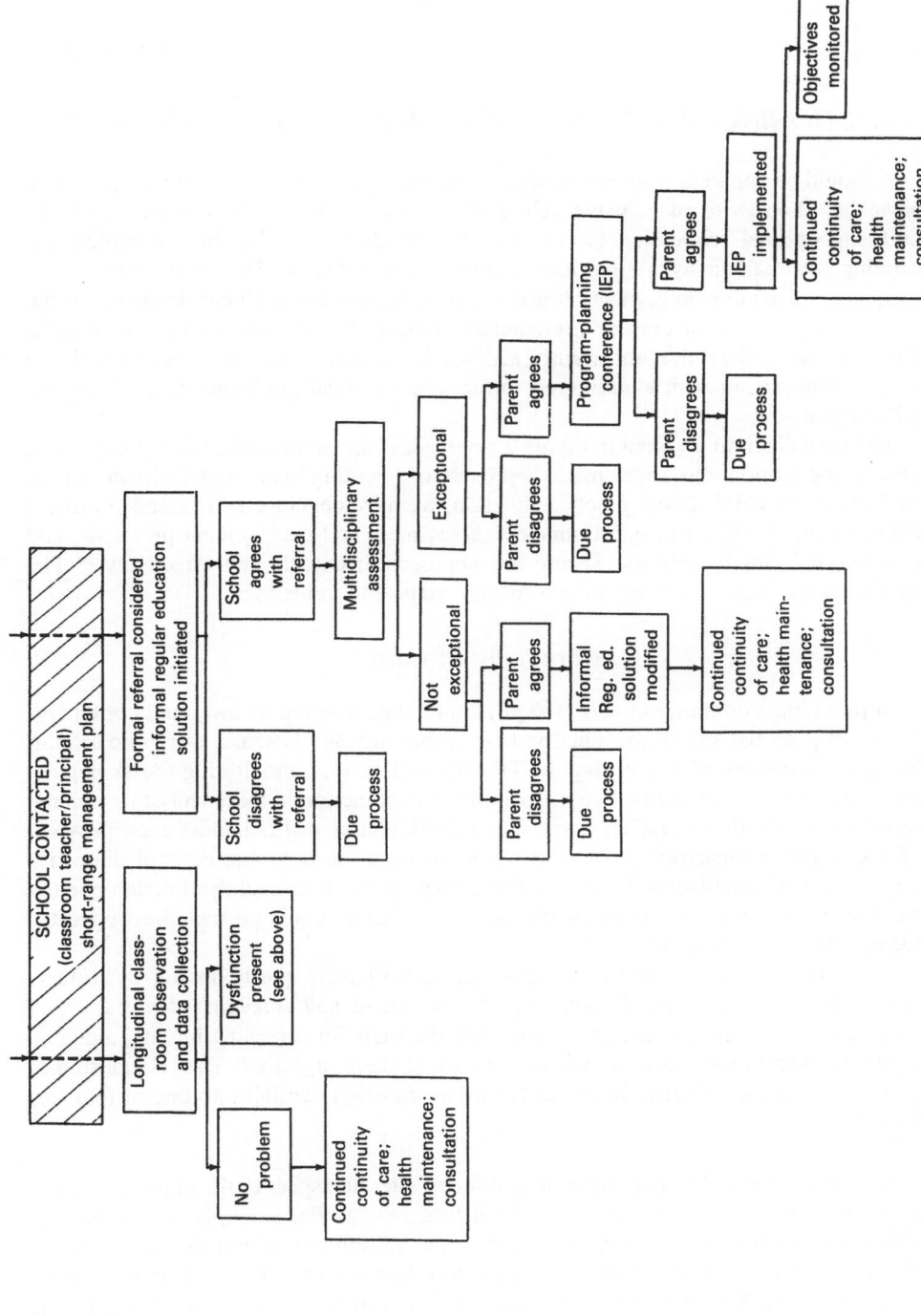

Figure 1. Flow diagram of physician responsibilities as a facilitator of the child's school life.

FUNCTIONING AS A FACILITATOR FOR THE SCHOOL-AGE CHILD

It should be apparent from the foregoing section that regardless of the particular role a physician chooses to play in the school life of the child, this is not an easy task. Facilitating optimal school functioning for an individual child can be a complex and frustrating job marked by a significant degree of uncertainty. This is in large part a consequence of the dynamic, transactional nature of human development. However, if the physician acquires the necessary prerequisite skills and applies them in a systematic fashion, he can reduce this uncertainty and resultant frustration. This section seeks to provide the physician with a structured format and practical guidelines to facilitate the child's school life.

The flow diagram depicted in Figure 1 synthesizes the prerequisite skills presented in the preceding section into a systematic approach to executing the role of facilitator in the school life of the child. In our practice situation, we have developed an extended manual and an accompanying set of questionnaires, assessment and management protocols, and health record forms to help us execute this approach efficiently and effectively.[14] The following is a synopsis of some of the specific steps and guidelines.

Continuity of Care

In providing continuity of care, the physician must develop an awareness of emerging signs of potential school dysfunction long before the child's actual entry into school. This means systematically surveying the TRANSACT factors, monitoring at-risk populations, and identifying the early "signs" of school dysfunction in these and other populations of children in their practice. Some specific risk factors that fall under each TRANSACT factor are summarized in Table III. It is important to note that most of these risk factors have been established through retrospective studies in school dysfunction populations. This is certainly not an exhaustive list of risk factors but is presented as suggested guidelines for the physician.

These risk factors can most efficiently be identified by questionnaire, by history-taking techniques, and through other direct assessment and screening devices. Other chapters in this volume provide physicians with the tools for screening infants, toddlers, and preschoolers in areas that are prerequisite for success in school. The relationship of any one of these specific risk factors to school dysfunction can fall into one of four risk categories:

1. *Direct impact:* The risk factor may directly alter an aspect of the child's constitution that is a prerequisite for efficient school functioning. For example, a hearing loss resulting from treatment with an ototoxic antibiotic will directly inhibit the child's ability to process auditory stimuli. Alternatively, a risk factor may directly alter the child's environment in such a way that it does not fulfill its role of promoting and shaping the child development. Such may be the case when a child's parent may be involved with alcohol or other substance abuse.

2. *Indirect impact:* These risk factors change the child's parents' or school personnel's perception of the child. In this fashion, these risk factors adversely alter patterns of interaction. For example, parents of a previously normal 18-month-old child hospitalized

Table III. At-Risk Factors for School Dysfunction

TRANSACT category	Possible manifestations of at-riskness for school dysfunction
Child's temperament	Difficult and slow-to-warm up temperamental clusters Evidence of extreme temperamental characteristic(s) (hyperactive, colic/irritability, feeding difficulty, sleep disturbance, excessive temper tantrums, obesity)
Child's readiness skills	Global or specific delay in milestone accomplishment (fine motor, sequential memory, receptive language, visuoperceptual motor, higher cognition, expressive language) Requires remedial services in academics Retained in grade
Child's attentional status	Chronic attentional weaknesses during structured tasks in multiple settings (impulsive, short attention span, fatigues easily, distractible, daydreams, poor social perception)
Child's neuromaturational function	Delay in gross motor and articulation milestone accomplishment Gross motor incoordination/clumsiness Persistent primitive reflexes or excessive numbers of soft neurological signs Enuresis, encopresis Permanent brain damage or sensory abnormality Genetic/familial syndrome
Environmental stresses	Pregnancy/perinatal insults (prematurity, low birth weight, small for gestational age, asphyxia, intraventricular hemorrage, hyperbilirubinemia) Intercurrent illnesses (recurrent otitis, meningitis, encephalitis, ingestions, asthma, anemia) Socioeconomic insults (death of parent or pet, divorce, parent loss of job, substance abuse by parent, family move)
Child's/environment's attitudes	Sexual, racial, ethnic or handicapped prejudice in the community Family history of learning– or school-related behavior problems Parental preoccupation with high achievement Insufficient stimulation in environment
Comparisons made by the child and the environment	Parents lack parenting experience and support structures Diminished self-esteem in child Vulnerable child syndrome
Temperament of significant others	Poor attachment/bonding Difficulty in behavioral management Peer-interaction problems Failure to thrive Child abuse

for meningitis may become so fearful for the child's life that they do not resume their usual disciplinary measures, even when the child is discharged without obvious immediate sequelae. As a result, the parents may not set appropriate limits and thereby not provide the child with opportunities to practice the self-control necessary in early school years.

3. *Markers of dysfunction:* These factors may be the earliest manifestations of school dysfunction or associated with specific dysfunctions in high frequency. For example, the

ingestion of a bottle of aspirin by the 2-year-old toddler may be the initial red flag signaling an attention deficit marked by impulsivity and poor monitoring skills.

4. *Chance occurrence:* Some factors bear no relationship to school dysfunction but occur in the life of children experiencing school failure by change. For example, a child having difficulty staying on task and completing assignments in class may be having problems because he is preoccupied with recurrent parental fighting and a possible divorce at home. Thus, divorce can have a direct impact as described above, but not all children whose parents get divorced will experience school dysfunction. Clearly, the simple presence of any given risk factor in a child's past or present history does not necessarily mean it bears any relationship to school dysfunction.

It is important to reinforce the fact that these risk factors do not necessarily have an impact on an individual child in an all-or-none fashion. Rather, the impact on an individual child varies along a continuum raning from not at all to profoundly. Therefore, children can differentially respond to the same risk factor depending upon their age and the status of other TRANSACT variables in that child.

Thus, when identifying a risk factor, the physician must use clinical judgment to determine what relationship, if any, a given factor bears to potential school dysfunction in the child. In turn, the decision regarding which risk category(ies) a given factor falls into determines the appropriate clinical action that must be taken. This decision-making process begins with a clarification of the specific risk factor. This may require a somewhat expanded history-taking session with the parent or other sources regarding their understanding, expectations, concerns, or fears about either the risk factor in question or the child in general. This may also include exploring for the presence of other stresses in the child's life that were previously undetected. Next, the physician must survey the child's life for evidence of life performance, developmental, neurobehavioral, or physical dysfunction (see Table IV). If dysfunction is present in one of these domains, the physician must decide whether the risk factor bears any relationship to this dysfunction. If it is decided that there is a high probability that the risk factor has a direct or indirect impact on the dysfunction, some form of intervention is indirected. This intervention always begins with informing parents and reordering their expectations; it may entail referral for further assessment and management to the school or appropriate community agency. If it is decided that dysfunction is not clearly present in one of these domains, but that early signs of dysfunction may exist, the physician must either make a referral for further clarification or develop a specific plan to longitudinally observe and collect data about the child's developmental and behavioral status. If dysfunction is absent in all these domains, the physician still must continue monitoring the appearance of new risk factors and/or the emergence of dysfunction in the future so that new demands will be placed upon the child. This process of ongoing continuity of care should continue throughout the child's school life.

Health Maintenance

Within the context of health maintenance activities, the physician has a responsibility to review with the child and parent forthcoming demands in the school environment at the

Table IV. Functional Areas

Life performance	Neurobehavioral function
Independent functioning	Neuromaturation
Social interaction	Gross motor
Academic achievement	Temperament
Developmental attainment	Attention
Fine motor	Physical integrity
Visuomotor	General health and nutrition
Spatial organization	Structural
Auditory sequential memory	Physiological
Visual sequential memory	Neurological
Receptive language	Sensory
Expressive language	
Cognitive	

various transition points in the child's school life. (These changing demands have been summarized in the previous section.) Such anticipatory guidance serves two important functions. First, it allows the parent and child to set or reorder their expectations appropriately for the child's performance so that they are in synchrony with the child's intrinsic abilities. In turn, it helps identify areas of concern where the child might not meet upcoming expectations. Such a clinical judgment is generally based on an understanding of the child's past and/or current functional status and matching this against upcoming demands. In such circumstances, the physician may take some preplanning steps with the child, parents, and/or school personnel to minimize the chances for dysfunction. These steps might include providing the parent and child with guidance about how they might begin working or practice to meet a new demand (e.g., separation from parent) that the physician anticipates might be difficult for the child and parent. The physician might also inform school personnel with a letter or phonecall about a problem he anticipates the child might experience and thereby work with school personnel to develop a plan of intervention. Alternatively, the physician may decide to follow the child's school performance closely with a higher index of suspicion.

Consultation

In fulfilling the role of facilitator in the school life of the child, the physician will be asked to respond to specific questions from parents or school personnel about the child's health that influence the child's school life or about manifest school dysfunction. The first step in realizing this role is an honest appraisal of whether the physician can answer the question at hand. This may entail contacting the school and refining the question or referring the parent or school to another consultant who has the necessary expertise.

When the question is appropriate for the physician's expertise, in some instances the physician's interactions with the school will be similar to those with the child's parents. When the child's medical or physical condition warrants, the physician may be acting as an expert communicating the facts or answering questions about the child's health needs and treatment regimens. This can be done in a brief, well-organized letter.[14] School personnel are more likely to understand the information and react favorably if vague terms are replaced by statements in clear behavioral terms.

Survey of the Child's Current Functional Status

When the physician identifies a risk factor(s) that it is felt might contribute to school dysfunction while providing continuity of care or identifies an area(s) of concern during health maintenance activities or is asked a specific question about manifest school dysfunction, a systematic survey of the child's current functional status is indicated. The purpose of this survey is to generate a functional description of the child's strengths and weaknesses in the areas of life performance, developmental attainment, neurobehavioral functions, and physical integrity that can serve as the basis for confirming a suspected school dysfunction, identifying the need for further evaluations/services, and developing a comprehensive management plan. This survey should include an assessment at some level of the functional areas outlined in Table IV. A spectrum of assessment devices and tools can be used to accomplish such a survey. These are identified in other chapters in this textbook; a systematic approach to generating a case formulation is presented elsewhere.[7]

Depending on the level of expertise and training, the physician may play several roles with respect to this functional survey. These roles may include briefly or informally surveying all areas through observation, interview, and review of other testing results or conducting more in-depth assessments of selected areas and relying on other consultants to provide information about the child's functional status in other areas. The physician should seek to make a decision about whether each functional area assessed is efficient. When the physician has identified an inefficient skills area, he must then determine whether this skill area contributes to the school dysfunction that is currently present or to potential dysfunction in the future.

General Management Strategies

Through a systematic and longitudinal review of the child's developmental and behavior history and a survey of the child's current functional status, it is possible for physicians to generate a case formulation that can serve as the basis of deciding whether school dysfunction is present, anticipated, or absent. The next step always entails presenting the generated information to the parents and child, and reordering their expectations as indicated.

If dysfunction is absent, this does not terminate the physician's role. Rather, since the child will continue to develop and school demands will continue to change, the physician must continue longitudinal continuity, health maintenance, and consultation activities.

Facilitating Change in the School When Dysfunction Is Present or Anticipated

Frequently, the physician may recognize that the child's needs may require changes in the expectations or teaching practices used in the current classroom. These types of interactions take more care and require that physicians see themselves as facilitators of change rather than as experts. As facilitators, physicians are acting as peers who are interested in the child. Therefore, they cannot define what should be done. Their role is to stimulate events in the school so that the child's problems are understood and addressed by the appropriate school personnel. Just as a physician may react defensively if a teacher calls and requests or questions a specific treatment for a child, the educators in the school may react if physicians define this role incorrectly.

To experience success in their role as facilitators, physicians should adopt the following approach:

1. *Communicate the boundaries of their role to the school:* For example, a physician may state the following in a phonecall or letter to the principal:

> In my annual screening, I have noted that Tommy J. has been failing in reading. I would like to be helpful in facilitating a plan to improve Tommy's performance. I have encouraged Tommy's parents to ask you for a meeting with Tommy's teacher and the building reading specialist to determine why Tommy is failing and what can be done. If I can be of any help, please let me know. I would also like to be kept abreast of the results of the meeting.

In such an interaction, the physician is defining a role as a person assuring that Tommy's problem is addressed. This also defines the role of a shared problem-solver interested in the child's progress. If the physician wants to be a participant in the analysis of the problem he should clearly indicate a willingness to help and offer to send a report of his records and special findings to the school.

2. *Acknowledge and respect the expertise of individuals in the school:* Trying to help a child by facilitating changes in the attitudes and practices of the adults in the school setting is a difficult job. Physicians are more likely to achieve this goal if they can develop a positive relationship with the educators responsible for the child. An adversarial relationship between the physician and the school can be avoided by communicating a strong respect for the educators' expertise. The physician who explicitly acknowledges that school personnel probably know the child better and probably already have an awareness of the child's problems will be viewed more positively. Asking questions about the educator's views or opinions concerning what can be done will produce more favorable results than will a one-sided communication in which the educator is being told what to do. Once rapport is achieved and the educators feel respected, the physician can move into the role of brainstorming solutions for the problem.

3. *Whenever possible, be an indirect facilitator. Teach the parents what to do:* It is unrealistic to think that physicians can interact directly with the school for every child in need. Physicians may need to define some guidelines for when they will play an active role in the school, for example, if the parents have been unsuccessful in previous interactions with the school or are unable to function in the school on their child's behalf.

Whenever possible, the physician should advise the parents on how to proceed and what to expect. The parents' efforts may need to be supplemented by a brief letter clarifying the physician's concerns.

The child with obvious or subtle dysfunction is likely to produce conflicts in the school throughout his career. The earlier the parents begin learning how to proceed on their child's behalf, the easier it will be to face the constant problems created by the ever-changing demands in school.

If school dysfunction is anticipated but is not clearly present, the physician should involve school personnel if this has not already been done. This means making contact with the classroom teacher and building principal and informing them of his concern. The goals of this contact should be to develop a plan to observe the child longitudinally and collect additional data and/or to implement a short-term management plan if necessary. A specific time line should be agreed on so that the physician, parent, and school personnel can reconvene to review their observations and the impact of any short term intervention. Out of such a meeting it will be determined whether the child is functioning satisfactorily and simply needs regular follow-up or whether school dysfunction is clearly present necessitating a formal referral.

Initiating a Formal Referral

When the physician believes that a child demonstrates significant school dysfunction that cannot be addressed in the current education program, he must assist parents in making a referral to the school for a formal evaluation. To initiate this process, the teacher and building principal need to be contacted both by phone and in writing. It is critical to be as specific as one can be about the reasons for a referral and to share any supporting evidence at this time. The particular procedure for processing referrals may vary from school to school, and these individuals will be knowledgeable about their system's policy. It is also imperative to talk with these important individuals to maintain rapport and cooperation. The physician or parent can build or destroy a relationship by the way he initiates a referral. If a call is made to a district administrator, the teacher and principal are likely to feel slighted and wonder why their involvement or input was not valued. However, if the physician or parent talks with these individuals to obtain their opinions and concerns, a mutual effort can be launched to obtain the necessary services.

At the point of initiating a referral, an informal plan must be implemented to help the child and classroom teacher until the evaluation is completed. The principal's and teacher's cooperation is critical for the implementation of a short-term plan to deal with the child's needs. Therefore, in addition to referring the child, the parent or physician should request a meeting with these individuals. The goal of this meeting is to ask, "What can be done now to deal with the child's problems?" It is useful to request other resource personnel with expertise in the area of the suspected dysfunctions to be present at this meeting. Such knowledgeable individuals can be helpful in generating strategies for coping with the child. Again, any pertinent information that the physician has regarding the child's functioning should be shared with the school in the form of a clear, written statement.

Table V. Assessment of the Individualized Educational Program

Annual goals
  Are the annual goals matched to my child's weaknesses?
  Are these goals clear to me? What expected behaviors will my child learn?
  Is it clear how my child will demonstrate that he has achieved these goals?

Short-term objectives
  Are these objectives matched to the annual goals?
  Are the objectives clear to me? What behaviors will my child learn, and how will my child demonstrate mastery?

Special and related services
  Are special services and materials that I think are critical to my child listed. i.e., large print materials, talking books, adaptive physical education, tape recorder?

Regular education
  Do I understand why my child will be in the specific regular class listed?
  Can I foresee any conflict between my child's needs and the demands in this class?
  Are the teachers from this class present at the meeting?
  If not, how will they be informed about my child's needs?
  How will my child's needs be addressed in the regular class?
  Will the special and regular teacher meet regularly to share information about my child?
  Will anything be done in the special class to help my child in these regular classes?

Monitoring Educational Management

Once a formal referral has been initiated, the physician can play an important role in helping the parents monitor the child's management by the educational system. The following questions need to be systematically reviewed during follow-up:

1. Was a short-term, informal regular education solution initiated?
2. Was a multidisciplinary assessment of the child conducted including psychological, medical, educational, and social input?
3. Was the child determined to be "exceptional"? If so what category (e.g., learning-disabled, mentally retarded, or socially and emotionally disturbed)? If not, what alternative plans were developed to manage and follow the child's difficulties?
4. Was a program-planning conference held and attended by the appropriate individuals?
5. Was an IEP developed for the child? Was it implemented? Were the objectives of the plan reviewed? (Table V provides a list of specific questions that parents can use to review the IEP.)

Should the parents disagree or have difficulty with any steps in this process, the physician can assist them in finding appropriate help and support. The physician can refer the parents to another agency for an independent evaluation and can contact the Department of Special Education in the Office of Education in their state department to inquire about the P.L. 94-142 complaint-management procedures in their state. In addition, the special education administrators in the State Department can provide physicians with names of parent advocacy groups and with copies of printed resources designed for parents of special education students. However, physicians should use caution in advising parents to involve either State Department people or trained advocates. These channels should be used as a last resort if an agreement with the school is impossible or if the parents are not capable of speaking on the behalf of their child.

In addition to monitoring the educational management of the child, physicians must institute and monitor any medical interventions that may be indicated. Once again, it is important to communicate about these treatments on a regular basis to the school personnel so that they can be integrated into the overall management plan.

Follow-up

Once an educational management plan is implemented in the regular education program or with the help of remedial or special education services, the physician can play an important role in monitoring its efficacy. When a child continues to demonstrate significant school dysfunction in the face of an implemented plan, the following questions can help the physician identify reasons for continued difficulty:

1. *Are the child's limitations understood, and have the adult's expectations been altered?* A key to a successful management plan is a clear understanding in the minds of parents and teachers about what a child can and cannot do. The physician is afforded a golden opportunity to help parents translate the findings of an evaluation into a better understanding of their child. The opportunity is extended to the school by helping educators understand that children are not responsible for certain aspects of their performance or behavior, which is primarily constitutional in nature.

2. *Have all the possible factors contributory to the child's problem been considered?* The physician can serve as case manager for dysfunctional children and can obtain copies of all the evaluation data. Once the information is present, the physician can help parents understand what TRANSACT factors within the child and within the home and school environment may be playing a role. Parents frequently feel guilty about their role in the problem. The physician may be able to reframe a parent's understanding by interpreting findings. The same may be true for school personnel.

3. *Has a comprehensive management plan been designed to have an impact on all the factors contributing to the problem?* Frequently, strategies need to be focused on the child, the classroom, and the home in order to improve a child's functioning. Although the physician cannot be the agent influencing all these fronts, he may be the only person capable of a holistic view. For example, to improve a child's inattentive behavior, the following comprehensive plan may be necessary: (1) the child may need to take medication and receive training on how to use language to control his attention; (2) the regular classroom teacher may need to have periodic staffings with appropriate resource people in the building to support him in his efforts to teach the child to complete work; and (3) the family may need the support of a parent course on behavior management. Unless a multifaceted approach to management is taken, little if any improvement in the child's behavior may occur.

SUMMARY

The physician no longer has a choice about whether or not to deal with the school life of children and adolescents in their practice. Instead, the physician must begin to decide how much involvement is realistic.

The physician can begin defining the parameters of his role in the school life of his patients by taking an honest inventory of their strengths and weaknesses in the prerequisite skills outlined in this chapter. The resulting information should point to the level of involvement that is realistic. At the minimum, all physicians can begin by making sure that those children with specific medical conditions have informed teachers who have received clear information on the child's problems and special needs.

For other children and adolescents, the physician can begin asking how children are progressing in school as a means of performing an informal survey of the child's functioning. Those physicians with a desire for greater involvement can develop questionnaires and systematic protocols for surveying the risk of school dysfunction and assessing each child's chances of meeting the forthcoming school demands. In any event, all physicians should begin identifying school dysfunction in their patients and making an effort to see that problems uncovered are systematically addressed.

There is a continuum of roles for dealing with the school problems. Some physicians may prefer to refer identified patients through appropriate channels in the school and/or other agencies and utilize other professionals as consultants. Educators and other team members can be used just as various medical specialists are used: (1) to shed light on a perplexing set of symptoms, (2) to redefine a problem, and (3) to specify a treatment plan. In such instances, the physician is responsible for making a detailed referral and sharing the child's history with the consultants. When the reports return, the physician can review the data to make sure that all factors have been considered and can translate these findings to the families.

Those physicians with more training in the area of developmental issues may select to participate more fully in the assessment and management processes. The physician can conduct more expanded examinations, which include a look at specific neurobehavioral, prerequisite, or life-performance skills. However, this more intensive role in assessment may not be a realistic goal for most physicians currently in practice because of their lack of training and expertise for such tasks.

The range of involvement in the school life of the developing child can be plotted along a spectrum from minimum to maximum involvement. Over time, with more expertise and practice, physicians can become more proficient in their new role in improving the quality of school life for patients in the pediatric age group.

REFERENCES

1. Rogers, D. E., Blendon, R. J., and Hearn, R. P.: Some observations on pediatrics: Its past, present and future. *Pediatrics* **67**:776–784, 1981.
2. The Task Force on Pediatric Education: *The Future of Pediatric Education*. American Academy of Pediatrics, Evanston, Illinois, 1978.
3. Vanderpoole, N., Noble, R. W., and Winters, M.: The physician as school consultant. *Health Values* **4**:20–25, 1980.

4. Levine, M. D.: The child with school problems: An analysis of physician participation. *Exceptional Children* **48**:4–12, 1982.
5. Starfield, B., and Borkowf, S.: Physicians recognition of complaints made by parents about their children's health. *Pediatrics* **43**:168, 1969.
6. Liden, C. B.: Audiologic aspects of learning and behavior. *Pediatr. Clin. North Am.* **28**:981–989, 1981.
7. Liden, C. B., Laurie, T. E., and Murphy, T. F.: Interpreting behaviors of young children. *J. Child Contemp. Soc.* **14**(4): 1982, pp. 59–76.
8. Sameroff, A., and Chandler, M.: Reproductive risk and the continuum of caretaking causalty, in Horowitz, F. (ed.), *Review of Child Development Research*, Vol. 4. Chicago University Press, Chicago, 1975, pp. 187–244.
9. Hetherington, E. M., and Parke, R. D.: *Contemporary Readings in Child Psychology*. 2nd ed. McGraw-Hill, New York, 1981.
10. Chess, S., and Thomas, A.: *Temperament and Development*. Brunner/Mazel, New York, 1977.
11. Reisinger, K. S., and Bires, J. A.: Anticipatory guidance in pediatric practice. *Pediatrics* **66**:889–892, 1980.
12. United States Public Law 94-142: Education for all handicapped children Act of 1975.
13. Section 504 of the Rehabilitation Act of 1973: *Federal Register* **42**:22675, May 4, 1977.
14. McCormick, D., and Levine, M.: Transmission of medical information to school personnel for guidance in management of the individual child. *J. Pediatr.* **89**:333–334, 1976.

Educational Strategies for Children with Developmental Disorders

Bill R. Gearheart

INTRODUCTION

Developmental disabilities is a relatively broad and all-inclusive term. The remediation or amelioration of the associated learning difficulties consequently necessitates the use of a spectrum of educational strategies. Many educators recommend that their "special method" be used exclusively: a like number of educators urge that only a combination of educational methods will be effective for developmentally disabled children. The "only one method" concept has become increasingly unpopular, since it is often inappropriate with many of the wide range of children diagnosed as developmentally disabled. Use of set, established combinations of methods may be equally ineffective. Significant improve-

Bill R. Gearheart • Department of Special Education, University of Northern Colorado, Greeley, Colorado 80639.

ment is often noted, however, when a combination of educational approaches are employed based on valid assessment data and a reasonable rationale. Experienced observers generally concur that no single educational strategy is best, even when attempting to remediate specific subareas of developmental disabilities. Variability and flexibility are mandatory prerequisites for effective teaching of children with handicaps. As a rule these children have highly varied experiential backgrounds, as regards earlier efforts to learn to read, write, or even tie shoelaces, as well as limited control over environmental variables. It is readily recognized that the potential for "curing a disease" is enhanced in a controlled hospital environment. By contrast, most educational programs are implemented within an uncontrolled complex framework of (1) inconsistent home and community conditions, (2) differing degrees of parental support, and (3) widely variable biomedical and psychosocial factors. Prognosticating the potential value of any particular educational intervention must be couched within the context of these cautionary comments. The more successful educational approaches (strategies) frequently used for developmentally disabled children can be classified into several general categories.

THREE LEVELS: PRESCHOOL, ELEMENTARY, AND SECONDARY

A program classification for developmentally disabled children is generally characterized by gross oversimplification and omissions. The recognized categories of preschool, elementary, and secondary-level programs tend to support this generalization. Review of a classification schema enables the presentation of a descriptive analysis of several programs commonly employed for children with chronic handicaps. A program analysis of this type frequently concentrates primarily on resources available at the elementary level, with fewer considerations of the preschool level. Discussions are even more limited regarding resources available at the secondary level. Programming at the secondary level appears to be a distinct consideration from elementary level programming, each requiring a different structure and focus. In order to develop a commonality of concept and terminology, the general characteristics of preschool and elementary programs are reviewed. In addition, an expanded description of some of the educational resources for secondary-age students is presented, highlighting some of the truly unique programs at this level.

Preschool Programs

Preschool programs for developmentally disabled children have a wide range of formats and are usually offered in diverse settings. A national survey and analysis of 103 early-education programs for handicapped children[1] revealed that (1) 95% of the directors regarded their programs as educationally and developmentally based; (2) 97% utilized active parent participation; (3) in programs for children from birth through 3 years, the five most important service components were parent education, infant stimulation, diagnostic–prescriptive teaching, home-based services, and parent support; (4) in programs for children aged 4 and 5 years, the five most important service components were language development, diagnostic–prescriptive teaching, parent education, communication skills, and developmental education; (5) 32% of the early education programs had a formal affiliation with an institution of higher education, and 47% had unofficial or informal ties; and (6) all the programs served children at least 9 months of the year, 44% were operational on a 12-month basis, and 34% served children on either a 10- or 11-month basis.

Considerable variation was noted in the method by which handicapped children were served, depending on such factors as distances between home and facility, population density, and philosophy of the program designers and/or directors. In most early-education programs, efforts were made to obtain background information regarding the child's level of functioning in motor, social, cognitive (or precognitive), self-help, and communication areas. The overall level of performance appeared to be influenced primarily by the type and severity of the disability and the child's functional level of intelligence. The more effective early-education programs established at least a minimum assessment of the child's functional levels of ability that was used in planning goals and activities for the child. The composition of the program is based on the individual needs of the child, as determined by the assessment process. Considerable differences are generally noted in the curriculum content, which is designed for infants and children under the age of 4 years, as compared with programs for children aged 4 and 5 years. There is no automatic cutoff age that dictates program rationale, such as that used in determining placement in kindergarten, first grade, and so forth.

Program directors in the Stramiello study indicated the top five program services for two age groups: birth to 3 years and for the 4–5-year-old children (Table I). It should be noted that many of the projects reviewed in the Stramiello study[1] will be curtailed with reductions in federal assistance. State special-education reimbursements to local school districts may be necessary in order to maintain early-education programs for children aged 3 years and older.

Elementary-Level Programs

Historically, elementary-level programs for developmentally disabled children have been operational for much longer than programs at the preschool or secondary levels. The major focus of most elementary-level programs is the development of basic skills in reading, spelling, writing, arithmetic, and other academic areas. The goal of the curriculum is usually determined by the type and severity of the disability. For example, the goal for a learning disabled student with an IQ in the average range is most often to improve basic reading and/or arithmetic abilities. The ultimate goal is to achieve academic skills commensurate with the child's chronological age. The educational objective is to assist

Table I. Five Most Important Preschool Program Services

Birth to age 3	Ages 4 and 5
Parent education	Language development
Infant stimulation	Diagnostic–prescriptive teaching
Diagnostic–prescriptive teaching	Parent education
Home-based services	Communication skills
Parent support	Developmental education

the child in acquiring the skills necessary to circumvent (or compensate) for the learning disability, thereby functioning as nearly "normal" as is possible. On the other hand, the projected educational expectations for a trainable mentally retarded child would be considerably less. A 10-year-old child with an IQ of 40 is not expected to read as well as a nonhandicapped child of the same age. Realistic objectives for a trainable retarded child would therefore include accomplishing less complex tasks: (1) levels of reading; (2) making correct change; (3) writing name, address, phone number; and (4) academic skills of a more basic nature. Even within the heterogeneous group of mentally retarded children, variation in projected goals will be necessary, even if the IQ levels are similar. (See Appendix for a description of the various levels of mental retardation.) Numerous factors can either improve or impede a child's ability to profit from formal educational programs.

It is essential that the educational system be cognizant of these contingencies; efforts should be directed to the elimination of negative variables. The enhancement of language development is a universal goal and should be pursued within an applied framework, i.e., with application for use in practical situations. For children with lower functional abilities, the focus would be for appropriate social skills. The mentally retarded child may not learn social skills in the "incidental way" in which most children develop this sophistication. It should be noted that the acquisition of social skills is ultimately related with language development.

For children with moderate to severe levels of mental retardation, the "academic" (e.g., reading, spelling) aspects of total programming are of much less significance within the total framework of achievement goals. These subjects receive less emphasis than for a child with higher functional levels. The program design for the more functionally disabled must include an emphasis on enhancing language development and activities that promote skills for maximizing independence. The major educational goals for children with moderate to severe retardation are often similar to the objectives programmed for preschool children. Individualization of the educational program is very important in enhancing the functional abilities of retarded children. Children initially diagnosed as severely mentally retarded may, with consistent, meaningful educational efforts, prove to have significantly higher potentials. There is moral justification and professional obligation in striving for better levels of performance. However, these efforts must always be programmed within the framework of realistic expectations based on the results of an assessment process.

Secondary-Level Programs

The junior and senior high school curriculum for developmentally disturbed students (secondary-level programs), for purposes of this discussion, focuses on children who have the potential for living independently or semiindependently. This goal may be achieved either as a result of effective school programming alone or in conjunction with a sheltered workshop experience. Some school-based programs have made provisions for the very severely mentally retarded; a description of these programs is beyond the scope of this text.

The types of secondary-level programs have been variously categorized. A relatively simple classification system is based on the educational and vocational goals established for the student. Some learning-disabled students are capable of completing a college curriculum; their high school program should prepare them for this experience. Other learning-disabled students attend vocational training programs, and some will terminate their formal academic training at the high school level. Many educable mentally retarded students complete formal schooling with a high school program, at which point they should be prepared for occupational, family, social, and citizenship responsibilities. By contrast, some educable mentally retarded students may participate in an additional 1 or 2 years of vocational training. Students completing programs for the trainable mentally retarded generally enter some type of sheltered employment after high school.

Students of near-average mental ability who have developmental disabilities should seek employment that is both interesting and challenging, but within the restrictive limits of their disability. Programs, designed in high school, should reflect individual planning with the student, parents, and rehabilitation counselors. The major emphasis of elementary-level programs is the development of basic skills. By contrast, secondary-level programs generally focus on possible education following high school and preparation for adult responsibilities. A greater diversification of programs are associated with secondary-level education because of (1) the variability of the adolescent and their problems, (2) the range and severity of the developmental disabilities encountered, and (3) the differing structure of secondary level schools per se.

TYPES OF SCHOOL PROGRAMS

Work–Study Programs

Work–study programs were initially designed for educable mentally retarded students, but recently they have been adapted for learning-disabled students. Usually there is a 1- or 2-year participation in a work–study program. The students are familiarized with the types of jobs available, employer's needs, factors promoting job stability and success, specialized vocabulary associated with particular types of employment, methods of applying for a job, and other related topics. These topics may become the incentive and the vehicle for further learning in reading, arithmetic, and other areas of academic study. Although academic pursuits may occupy as much as one-half of the school day, it is not the dominant emphasis of the program.

During the course of a 1- or 2-year work–study program, the student may be placed "on the job" for at least 50% of the time. Employment may be full time during the last year or semester of the program. Close supervision and monitoring of students in an employment situation make it possible for the instructor to review both positive and negative experiences. Although many issues may have been discussed in a pre-work–study program, such topics as withholding tax, union membership, social security, and related topics take on new meaning and significance when students are actually on the job. Employment attitudes are always a matter of concern and can be discussed realistically if a student experiences difficulty for negative attitudes. In most cases, there is some form of student reimbursement for work–study employment; however, particular programs vary considerably.*

---

*There may be wide variations in the details of how work–study programs are implemented throughout the nation, but the intent is similar in most programs. Our attempt in this description is to provide the reader with a feeling for such programs and not to describe all possible variables.

Work–study programs designed for learning-disabled students usually involve higher skill levels of employment than for the educable mentally retarded students. Initially, both may start at the same level, but more rapid progression is anticipated with the learning-disabled student. Programs for trainable mentally retarded students obviously require much more supervision and involve lower skill levels and responsibilities. Learning-disabled students participate more often in regular academic classes than do educable mentally retarded students. However, trainable mentally retarded students are usually not involved in academic class programs. In many states, the Division of Vocational Rehabilitation may be involved in counseling, job placement, and arranging payments for students in work–study programs.

Individual modifications in work–study programs include (1) the amount of time spent of the job, (2) job location, (3) grade level when the job experience is initiated, (4) courses taught by special-education teachers and regular class teachers, (5) association with outside agencies, (6) grading criteria, and (7) type of diploma or certification of graduation.[2] Although the specific techniques and implementations may vary, the work–study (work–experience) programs have a similar philosophical purpose.

Accommodation and Compensatory Teaching

Accommodation and compensatory teaching are often employed at the secondary level, as substitutes for the more remedial-oriented elementary programs. The emphasis is on modifying the educational environment so that the student learns in spite of learning difficulties. The environmental modifications contrast with efforts directed at remediating the learning problems per se. Work–study programs are based on this philosophical construct. Accommodation and compensatory teaching is believed to be an approach that uses the time of the educational system and the student most efficiently. The concept of adaptive, accommodative, or compensatory teaching, however, is more often applied as an educational strategy for the learning-disabled student. A concerted effort is made to assist students in completing some version of the traditional high school program, with fewer modifications than are required in work–study programs. A more comprehensive discussion of this type of program can be found in *The Learning Disabled Adolescent: Program Alternatives in the Secondary School*.[3] In general, accommodative or compensatory teaching involves (1) adjusting instructional techniques, (2) modifying academic requirements, (3) changing the pace of the regular program (slowing the speed with which students progress through their program), (4) providing advance preparation (with assistance of special teachers) for certain more difficult courses, (5) study skill tutoring, (6) special assignment of particular teachers to learning-disabled students, and (7) special attention to "balance" courses each quarter or semester, and other related efforts. As with most special-education programs, individualized educational planning and specially trained personnel are critical for the success of the program. Remedial/tutorial efforts, although frequently used in the secondary school, are not the major emphasis of special secondary-level programming. In some circumstances, this type of intervention is helpful as a primary resource, but more often it is useful as an adjunct to other programs. Tutorial remediation may be provided either by one-to-one or group contact. The time allocation and content of the tutorial program should be individualized to meet the particular needs of the student. The selection of either a professional remedial expert or a nonprofessional tutor is most important. Interaction between teachers and support personnel is a critical factor in providing a meaningful and maximal remediation effort. Secondary-level programs differ from elementary-level programs because of (1) basic differences in organization and structure of the schools; (2) different goal emphasis; (3) attention focus on certain essential information and concept learning, as opposed to basic skills learning; and (4) the nature and problems of the adolescents in secondary-level programs.

Assessment Results

A well-designed program is based on findings of the educational assessment, an appreciation of the type and severity of the educational deficit, and the nature and/or cause of the underlying disability. Measurement/assessment of these skills is dependent on, and varies with, age and type of disability. There have been persistent difficulties with inappropriate utilization of assessments that do not provide for such variables as secondary disabilities (e.g., sensory deficits) and cumulative effects of environmental deprivation and other influencing factors. In some cases, assessment tools developed for nonhandicapped children may be useful in evaluating developmentally disabled students. Numerous highly specialized examinations have been specifically developed, however, for use with handicapped children. Unfortunately, most evaluations only provide a limited data base that may not provide sufficient information necessary to plan adequately for a child with developmental disabilities. Caution is necessary in order to avoid designing a remedial program based on incomplete information.

In addition to the more traditional academic assessment, a much broader base of information is necessary in order to construct a meaningful program for developmentally disabled students. A variety of developmental factors must be considered, such as the ability to (1) feed one-self with spoon and/or fork, (2) grasp a glass or cup and drink, (3) dress one-self, and (4) express toilet needs—a compendium of motor, language, and social skills. A number of scales, based on normal child-development patterns, have been constructed. These inventories are extremely useful when used by a knowledgeable observer. The use of measurements that are cross-validating or that may suggest the need for additional information is essential. A construct based on too little information about academic, motor, sensory, and social abilities (or combinations of these skills) is a major fault of many program designs. The comprehensive evaluation by a multidisciplinary team, as required by the Education for All Handicapped Act (P.L. 94-142), has helped in reducing this type of restricted diagnostic error. The concept uses an individualized educational program (IEP) designed to meet specific needs of the child, most often necessitating an interdisciplinary approach to therapy design. The law implies that the needs of the child should be extended to include a more liberal interpretation of education, including learning basic skills, such as (1) lacing shoes, (2) understanding and following simple instructions (i.e., "sit down," or "go get the crayons"), and (3) sharing and taking turns. These abilities have traditionally been categorized as "educational" preschool skills. Many of the newly mandated responsibilities for the school in providing for developmental and behavioral needs of the child were formerly grounds for school exclusion. The "educational" frame of reference has been dramatically expanded for many educators (with a remarkable degree of acceptance). Although some backlash has occurred, programs for developmentally disabled students have been successfully incorporated into most public schools. These programs have enjoyed general acceptance by most teachers and administrators.

Approaches Using Behavior Modification

Behavior modification, behavior management, and operant conditioning are similar terminologies referring to a technique commonly employed by teachers of the developmentally disabled. Although some teachers prefer not to be regarded as "behaviorists," nearly all, in some form or another, use many techniques of behaviorists. A review of approximately 100 textbooks for teachers on behavior modification reveals that about one-half of these books were designed for teachers of handicapped students. Many of the texts reviewed were cookbook-type manuals, describing how-to procedures. Acceptance may be inferred from the good sales records.

Behavior modification takes many forms, including modeling, the use of reinforcers such as free time, tokens that represent future rewards, "gold stars," and teacher praise and attention. In many cases, rewards provided for the entire class are effective in encouraging peers to assist in modifying the targeted behavior. In all instances, systematic application of whatever procedure is used is highly essential. This planned systematic intervention is the missing element in many instances when behavior modification is ineffective.

The contracting procedure is a recent trend in program design for developmentally disabled students. The basis for the program involves agreement between teacher and student that if specific tasks are accomplished, a particular reward will be provided. Homme[4] likened this procedure to what he called "Grandma's Law" ("clean up your plate, then you may have dessert"), a description that still seems to apply. Relatively complex contracts can be designed for students with higher IQs and simpler contracts for students with lower levels of functioning. The contract procedure has been very successful in numerous situations. Behavior modification techniques are only a method of attempting to achieve important educational or behavioral goals. Behavior modification is a means to an end, and it is most important that the "end" be carefully defined. The essential role of the teacher is to establish meaningful goals and objectives for change. Occasionally less experienced teachers lose sight of this responsibility.

Perceptual–Motor Approaches

Most developmental psychologists would agree that perceptual–motor development is an important factor in the acquisition of learning. There is continuing controversy, however, as to the extent to which remedial efforts in perceptual–motor exercising will directly improve academic function.[2] The controversy will probably not be settled in the immediate future. Investigations of the casual relationship reveal inferential results regarding the effectiveness (or ineffectiveness) of perceptual–motor training. Some children in perceptual–motor programs (or that incorporate perceptual–motor components) appear to make significant gains. However, most of the children simultaneously receive other types of remedial interventions, making it very difficult to draw accurate conclusions about the value of any one component of the therapy program.

Perceptual–motor training may take many forms, ranging from the relatively simple to the highly complex. For example, a child may be involved with walking a balance beam, pushing an object across the floor with his knee or elbow, working on a trampoline, and lacing (as with a shoe), buttoning, or zipping. Other activities include visual pursuit (visually tracking a ball swinging on a string), placing round and square pegs in a pegboard, and skipping. Climbing, jumping, doing a forward roll, or jumping between the rungs of a ladder placed on the floor may be a part of the motor training program. Perceptual–motor training involves building large muscle capabilities, eye–hand and hand–eye coordination, and internal interpretation of directionality, laterality, and accurate body image. Ocular control, including all its intricacies, is usually accepted as a part of perceptual–motor training, and some perceptual–motor authorities appear to be more interested in visuoperceptual ability than any other specific area of perceptual–motor training.

Regardless of the type of perceptual–motor approach used, one common denominator is hypothesized, that "for the most part, high-level mental processes develop out of and after adequate, integrated development of the motor and perceptual systems, that perceptual abilities provide the base for later conceptual abilities."[2] The hypothesis has its advocates and opponents among experts in the field.

The early pioneers in perceptual–motor research worked with brain-injured students, most of whom were borderline mentally retarded. Subsequently, various modifications of the perceptual–motor approach were used for individuals with lower levels of mental retardation, the learning-disabled, at-risk preschoolers, and children classified as multi-handicapped. The programs reveal varying results, ranging from "near-miracles" in improvement to no discernible benefit. Cratty[5] recommends an examination of verified research findings rather than blind devotion to one of the popular "movement messiahs." In essence, careful application of perceptual–motor training appears to be of value for some children (not all), particularly preschool-age children and those with obvious, diagnosed motor disabilities.

Language Development Approaches

Language is a factor, perhaps the most important factor, that sets humans above other members of the animal kingdom. Children with static impairment of language become increasingly retarded in their general functional development. The development of adequate language is a major goal for all developmentally disabled children. The ability to think symbolically and to produce a variety of sounds makes it possible for children to develop language, but it is the desire to communicate with other human beings that motivates them to learn language. Communication is the basic reason for learning language. Various approaches have been designed to promote language.

It is essential to understand the normal language-learning sequence in order to establish realistic language objectives and goals. Despite disagreement about various facets of language development (e.g., the extent to which language is an innate, as opposed to an acquired, attribute), certain facts are accepted:

1. Infants with normal intelligence have the ability to develop language.
2. In order for language to develop normally, identification with parents (or other significant adults) must be sufficiently binding so that the child feels the desire/need to imitate them.

Table II Acquiring Auditory Receptive Language A Task Analysis

---

Attention
  Attend to vocally produced auditory sound units (noises, speech sounds, words, phrases, sentences)

Discrimination
  Discriminate between auditory vocal sound units

Establishing correspondences
  Establish reciprocal associations between the auditory–vocal sound units and objects or events
  1 Store and identify auditory–vocal units as meaningful auditory language signals Substitute auditory–language signals for actual objects and or events
  2 Establish word order sentences and sentence patterns

Automatic auditory–vocal decoding
  1 Improve interpretation by analyzing increasingly more complex auditory–language signals
  2 Increase the speed and accuracy of the reception of auditory–language signals through variation, practice, and repetition to the point of automatic interpretation

Terminal behavior
  Respond appropriately to verbal commands, instructions, explanations, questions, and statements

---

From Chalfant and Scheffelin [6]

3. Children must hear normal language in order to develop normal language. They must have adequate auditory acuity, intact CNS function, and contact with properly used language.
4. Language learning may be retarded by negative environmental factors.
5. The development of language, and an understanding of it provide the basis for much of the child's evolving ability to think (i.e., we *think* in language, thus we must have language to be able to think effectively).

Tables II and III, developed by Chalfant and Scheffelin,[6] provide a summary, in the form of a task analysis, of the manner in which children acquire auditory receptive language and expressive auditory language. (See Chapters 10, 11, 12, and 13 for a more indepth discussion of language development.)

There are a number of different approaches for enhancing language development and learning. Each attempts to identify where the deficits are in the language-development continuum, with remediation directed specifically at the area of weakness. Most approaches incorporate remedial and developmental components; i.e., there is an effort to correct specific language-acquisition difficulties and to promote accelerated development beyond this point. Individual planning, however, is the key to success! It must be emphasized that understanding of language development is an important prerequisite to meaningful planning because of the complexity of language development.

Multisensory Approaches

A number of approaches have been described as multisensory, but of particular interest to educators working in the field of developmental disabilities are programs utilizing visual, auditory, kinesthetic, and tactile modalities. Most children learn through all these sensory channels. For the general population of children, however, the school

Table III. Acquiring Expressive Auditory Language: A Task Analysis

Intention
  Possess the need to communicate.
  Decide to send message vocally.
Formulate message by retrieving and sequencing the appropriate vocal–language signals.
Organize the vocal–motor sequence
  1. Retrieve the vocal–motor sequence for producing the selected vocal–language signals.
  2. Execute the vocal–motor sequence for producing the vocal–language signal.
Automatic vocal encoding
  1. Combine simple vocal–language signals to form more complex vocal–language signal sequences.
  2. Increase the rate, accuracy, length, total number, and types of vocal–language signal sequences to the point of automatic production.
  3. Shift attention from the mechanics of producing vocal–language signal sequences to the contents of the message to be sent.
Terminal behavior
  Produce appropriate verbal instructions, commands, explanations, descriptions, and questions.

From Chalfant and Scheffelin.[6]

emphasis is usually on the visual and auditory modalities, with little planned utilization of the kinesthetic and tactile. The Fernald method, sometimes called the VAKT method, perfected during the 1920s, with variations and modifications, is still commonly employed.

The Fernald method is described here to exemplify the main thrust of such methods. Specific attention should be given to use the kinesthetic senses (e.g., movement, as interpreted by the proprioceptors in the muscles, joints, tendons) and the tactile senses (sense of touch as interpreted by the fingers).

The Fernald Approach

Although Fernald developed procedures for use in various academic subjects, her major emphasis was in reading; therefore, her methods are illustrated with respect to reading:

1. The first major step is to explain that there is a new way of learning words that really works. The student is told that others have had similar problems and have learned through this new method. The newness of the method is emphasized.
2. The student is asked to select any word he wants to learn, regardless of length.
3. The word is written for the student, usually with a crayon in plain, blackboard-size cursive writing. In most cases, regardless of age, cursive writing is used rather than printing, because it permits the student to see and "feel" the word as a single unit rather than a group of separate letters.
4. The student traces the word with his fingers in contact with the paper, saying the word as he traces it. This is repeated as many times as necessary until he can write the word without looking at the copy.
5. The student writes the word, demonstrating that it is now "his" word. Writing with large letters seems to be more effective than using small letters. Several

words are taught in this manner, and as much time as necessary is taken to master these words completely.

6. When the student has internalized the fact that he can write and recognize words, he is encouraged to start writing stories. These stories are whatever he wishes them to be at first, and the instructor "gives" him any words (in addition to those he has mastered) he needs to complete the story.

7. After the story is written, it is typed, and the student is to read it in typed form while it is still fresh in his mind. It is important that this be done immediately to relate cursive with printed words.

8. After the story is completed and the new word had been used in a meaningful way, the student writes the new word on a card that is filed alphabetically in the student's individual word files. This provides one with a meaningful way to experience the alphabet without undue emphasis on rote memory and often leads to the same end result as rote memory skills.

This procedure has been called the tracing method because tracing is an added feature in contrast to the usual methods of teaching reading or word recognition. However, it should be noted that the child is simultaneously feeling, seeing, saying, and learning the word, a truly multisensory approach.

There are several other points to be observed and followed for greatest success.[7] We will simply list these points, with minimal amplification, to illustrate Fernald's method for maximizing multisensory input:

1. Words should be selected by the student to maximize motivation.
2. Finger contact is essential while tracing.
3. After tracing a word the number of times required to permit writing with success, the student should write the word several times without looking at the copy.
4. In case of errors, the word should be written over from the beginning; erasures should not be permitted, since the total word must be "felt" accurately.
5. Stories must be used at the earliest possible time to reinforce the idea that words carry a message: words should be used in normal context.
6. The student should say the word aloud as it is traced or written. This provides auditory support and additional kinesthetic support through the "feel" of the word (in the lips, tongue, jaws, and throat) as it is said.

Fernald provided for a transition stage in which tracing was seldom or never required and then to a stage at which printed rather than cursive words were used. The final goal is to return to normal reading methods, however, case studies indicate that some students who learn through this approach continue to use tracing intermittently throughout their school career as they have difficulty in remembering specific new words. We might also note that many college students, perhaps the majority, "copy" words, phrases, or ideas they want to remember when studying for tests. They too have apparently found that the kinesthetic and tactile modalities (used in copying) provide excellent support for a sagging or recalcitrant memory.

Other multisensory methods have enjoyed considerable success with developmentally disabled children and adolescents. Most of these programs are sufficiently different from standard teaching approaches to build interest and motivation, which is undoubtedly a great deal of their strength. All involve a more systematic emphasis of the kinesthetic and tactile modalities.

SUMMARY

Educational programs for developmentally disabled children and adolescents are varied and continually evolving. Preschool programs and curricula for adolescents are relatively new, as are the programs for the more severely handicapped.

One educational technique, behavior modification, is used to some extent with all age groups and developmental levels. The technique has no "content" of its own, as far as academic goals are concerned. Accurate determination of academic and/or behavioral goals is critical if objectives are to be achieved in the time available in the school system.

By mandate of federal law (P.L. 94-142) and closely related laws in the 50 states, developmentally disabled children must be provided with an appropriate educational program. An individual program must be planned for each child. The program approaches outlined in this chapter represent those generally used with developmentally disabled students. For the most part, these programs are based on a combination of theoretical considerations and the results of practical "try-it-and-see-if-it-works" efforts. One serious difficulty, if such efforts were to be compared with laboratory research, is that there is usually a mix of children in so-called experimental programs, and it is very difficult to control the effects of outside environment. Progress has been made, and the outlook is relatively bright for many, if not all, developmentally disabled children and adolescents.

REFERENCES

1. Stramiello, A.: *A Descriptive Study of Selected Features of Handicapped Children's Early Education Programs.* University of Northern Colorado, Greeley, Colorado, 1978.
2. Gearheart, B.: *Learning Disabilities: Educational Strategies.* 4th ed. Mosby, St. Louis, 1985.
3. Marsh, G., Gearheart, C., and Gearheart, B.: *The Learning Disabled Disabled Adolescent: Program Alternatives in the Secondary School.* Mosby, St. Louis, 1978.
4. Homme, L.: *How to Use Contingency Contracting in the Classroom.* Research Press, Champaign, Illinois, 1971.
5. Cratty, B.: *Perceptual-Motor Behavior and Educational Processes.* Thomas, Springfield, Illinois, 1969.
6. Chalfant, J., and Scheffelin, M.: *Central Processing Dysfunctions in Children.* NINDS Monograph No. 9. U. S. Department of Health, Education, and Welfare, Washington, D. C., 1969.
7. Gearheart, B.: *Special Education for the 80's.* Mosby, St. Louis, 1980.

22

Guidelines for Physicians

John E. Williams

The office management of developmental disabilities presents several challenges to the pediatrician. Past experience, knowledge, finances, and the desire to serve these children all may be obstacles to caring for handicapped children in an office setting.

Public awareness of the services mandated for children with specific learning disabilities and other chronic handicapping conditions places the pediatrician on the front line for the early identification of these problems. Parents traditionally look to their pediatrician as an authoritative source of information and as an advocate for their children.

Developmental diagnosis can be a formidable challenge for the pediatrician who is not a recent graduate of a residency training program. In the recent past, health maintenance and preventive pediatrics received increasing emphasis in medical school and residency curricula. The American Academy of Pediatrics has recently mandated that developmental assessment be an integral part of well-child care (see Appendix).

John E. Williams • Section of Developmental Pediatrics, Institute for Child Development, Hackensack Medical Center, Department of Pediatrics, University of Medicine and Dentistry of New Jersey–New Jersey Medical School, Hackensack, New Jersey 07601.

In order to help the practitioner bridge this gap in training, the American Academy of Pediatrics has made available their Guidelines for Health Supervision, which includes specific suggestions for developmental assessment. Continuing medical education in pediatrics has also entered the field of child development. Numerous courses on national and local levels are available for pediatricians in practice to increase their fund of knowledge in this area. Many helpful textbooks and timely monographs have become increasingly available. It is important for the practitioner to feel competent in the area of developmental diagnosis. Lack of self-confidence in this area will contribute to the temptation to minimize the parents concerns in the vain hope that the child will "outgrow" the problems. This well-intentioned desire to prevent over-referral tells the parents that they have misconceptions regarding the child and delays accurate diagnosis.

The time and cost involved in handling developmental disabilities in the general pediatric setting have also been obstacles. A thorough developmental examination requires a considerable time commitment as does formulating the findings of the examination, informing the parents, and coordinating consultations. Considerable time must also be spent interpreting findings to parents and assisting them in securing the necessary therapies. When parents are apprised at the initial visit of the time and cost involved, misunderstanding concerning fees is less frequent, and few parents refuse the services. Many third-party payors will reimburse for these examinations and related services if ordered by a physician. The American Academy of Pediatrics is actively pursuing the relationship of the pediatrician to the third-party payors with respect to reimbursement. It is hoped that these efforts will ease the financial burden of parents who have a child with a developmental disability. The pediatrician can also assist the family in registering their child with appropriate governmental agencies that provide support to handicapped children and their families.

Another obstacle has been the pediatrician's personal discomfort in dealing with handicapped individuals. Sometimes this represents a personal decision not to deal with the chronic problems of childhood as opposed to more acute illnesses. Other times, these feelings may represent illogical guilt stemming from having treated the child during a stormy perinatal course. Unfortunately physicians are not immune to prejudice, which can interfere with their dealing with handicapped patients. Attitudes of other parents who are uncomfortable being in waiting rooms with handicapped children can also bring pressure to bear on the pediatrician. Whatever the origin of these feelings, the physician must come to terms with them in order to provide these necessary and valuable services.

The handicapped patient represents a personal and professional challenge. The pediatrician can gain a great deal of satisfaction from knowing that he has participated in helping these children reach their greatest potential. Being a source of support and providing continuity of developmental care for families of children with chronic handicapping conditions is a natural role for the pediatrician even though many times there is no "cure."

EARLY IDENTIFICATION

All "normal" children should be periodically screened for developmental abnormalities. In the past this has taken the form of clinical laboratory testing for disorders that

Table I Prenatal, Intrapartum, and Neonatal Risk Factors[a]

Prenatal factors

Moderate to severe toxemia	Multiparity >5
Chronic hypertension	Uterine malformation
Moderate to severe renal disease	Incompetent cervix
Severe heart disease, class II–IV	Abnormal fetal position
Diabetes, class A II	Polyhydramnios
Previous endocrine ablation	Small pelvis
Thyroid disease	Abnormal cervical cytology
Previous fetal exchange transfusion for Rh	Multiple pregnancy
Previous stillbirth	Age >35 or <15 years
Previous post-term 42 weeks	Positive serology
Previous premature birth	Drug use
Previous neonatal death	Weight <100 or >200 lb
Habitual abortion	History of tuberculosis or hepatitis
Infant >10 lb	Severe anemia

Intrapartum factors

Moderate to severe toxemia	Abruptio placenta
Poly or oligohydramnios	Post-term >42 weeks
Amnionitis	Darkly meconium-stained amniotic fluid
Uterine rupture	Abnormal presentation
Premature rupture of membranes	Multiple pregnancy
Demerol >300 mg	Aberrations of fetal heart rate
$MgSO_4$ >25 g	Prolapsed cord
Labor >20 hr	Fetal weight <1500 g
Labor <30 hr	Breech delivery
Placenta previa	Shoulder dystocia

Neonatal factors

Prematurity <2000 grams	Hypocalcemia
Apgar at 5 min <5	Hyper or hypomagnesemia
Apgar at 1 min <5	Hypothyroidism
Resuscitation at birth	Failure to gain weight (SGA)
Fetal anomalies (renal, GI) musculoskeletal, etc	Major cardiac anomalies
	Congestive heart failure
Low birth weight (SGA)	Hyperbilirubinemia
Feeding problems	Hemorrhagic diathesis
RDS type I	Chromosomal anomalies
Meconium aspiration syndrome	Sepsis
Cogenital pneumonia	CNS depression
Anomalies of the respiratory system	Meningitis
Apnea	Seizures
Hypoglycemia	

From Hobel et al Prenatal and intrapartum high risk screening Am J Obstet Gynecol 117·1–9 1973

have developmental consequences, such as congenital syphilis More recently, screening for inborn errors of metabolism has been instituted The American Academy of Pediatrics has published guidelines for a timetable of developmental screening during well-child visits These practices will identify most children who are at no particular risk for developmental abnormalities Effort should be made, however, to identify a subpopulation of

Table II Pre- and Perinatal Infections as Developmental Risk Factors[a]

Infection	Effect
Rubella virus	Intrauterine growth retardation, cataracts, chorioretinitis, glaucoma, cardiac defects, deafness, thrombocytopenic purpura, microcephaly, retardation, hepatitis, hepatosplenomegaly
Cytomegalovirus	Prematurity, low birth weight, thrombocytopenia, meningoencephalitis, chorioretinitis, intracranial calcifications, microcephaly, hydrocephalus, congenital heart disease, sensorineural hearing loss, mental retardation
Toxoplasma gondii	Prematurity, stillbirth, hydrocephalus, microcephaly, microphthalmia, chorioretinitis, convulsions, mental retardation
Treponema pallidum	Rhinitis (''snuffles''), skin lesions, osseous lesions causing pseudoparalysis, osteomyelitis, periostitis, hydrocephalus, convulsions (late form shows mental retardation)
Herpes virus	Coma, convulsions, hepatosplenomegaly, jaundice, skin lesions, mental retardation

[a]Manifestations and sequelae of these infections are variable, depending on such factors as when during gestation they are acquired as well as treatment

children in whom the incidence of developmental abnormalities is higher than that of the general population.

Many factors that occur alone or in combination have been associated with developmental abnormalities. A multitude of pre- and perinatal risk factors have been identified that place infants at developmental risk (Tables I and II). Although no absolute cause-and-

Table III Maternally Administered Drugs as Developmental Risk Factors

Drug	Developmental effects
Aminopterin and amethopterin	Intrauterine growth retardation, multiple anomalies
Amphetamines	Congenital heart disease
Chlorambucil	Renal agensis
Chloroquine	Retinal damage, mental retardation (?)
Cigarette smoking	Low birth weight
Corticosteroids	Cleft palate (?)
Dicumarol	Fetal hemorrhage, death
Diethylstilbestrol	Vaginal cancer
Diphenylhydantoin	Fetal hydantoin syndrome
Estrogen	Masculinization, advanced bone age
Ethanol	Multiple congenital anomalies, mental retardation
LSD	Chromosome damage
Mepivacaine	Bradycardia, convulsions, death
Methimazole	Goiter
Morphine, heroin	Withdrawal syndromes
Progesterone	Masculinization of female fetus
Propylthiouracil	Goiter
Quinine	Abortion, thrombocytopenia
Streptomycin	Deafness
Tetracycline	Tooth stain, retarded skeletal growth
Thalidomide	Phocomelia, anomalies

effect relationships have been established for many of these factors, conditions that are easily diagnosed at birth, such as Down syndrome, are obvious predictors of developmental difficulties. Prenatal factors such as maternally administered drugs (Table III), family history of genetic disorders affecting development, and adverse socioeconomic factors may also place infants in an at-risk category.

Untoward postnatal events must also be considered risk factors. Children who have suffered central nervous system (CNS) infection or trauma require close developmental follow-up. Children who have been victims of child abuse or who have been found to have organic or nonorganic failure to thrive also require close developmental scrutiny. Children who because of postnatal events have compromised vision or hearing also require special medical follow-up. Appliances such as hearing aids and glasses may be necessary in order to maximize residual hearing and vision. These children also require additional developmental supervision to ensure that language development and learning are optimized.

When children are identified as being at increased risk for developmental difficulties, special care must be taken so that they receive systematic developmental followup in addition to general health supervision. This special timetable of developmental examinations can be incorporated into a busy office practice with the aid of a card file (Fig. 1). This file may be updated at each neurodevelopmental follow-up visit to summarize immediately the results of assessments and consultations. Unkept appointments become immediately apparent, and one is less likely to lose track of at-risk infants.

Name	Date	Age	Vision	Hearing	Developmental assessment	Referral to:	Follow-up dates
Address							
Telephone							
Birth date							
High risk							
Date and age of incurred high risk							

Figure 1. Neurodevelopmental follow-up record sheet.

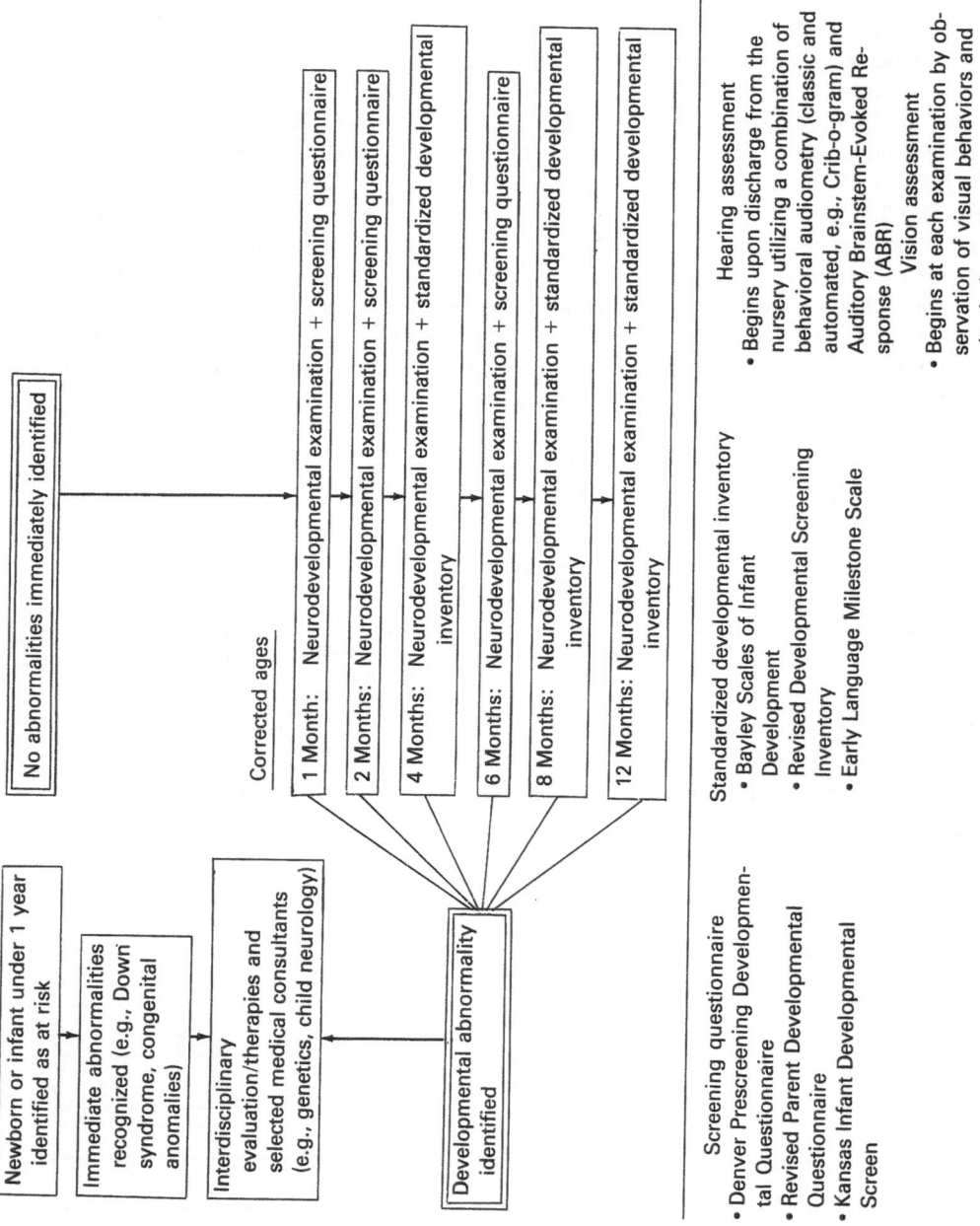

Figure 2. Neurodevelopmental examination schedule for at-risk infants, birth through 1 year.

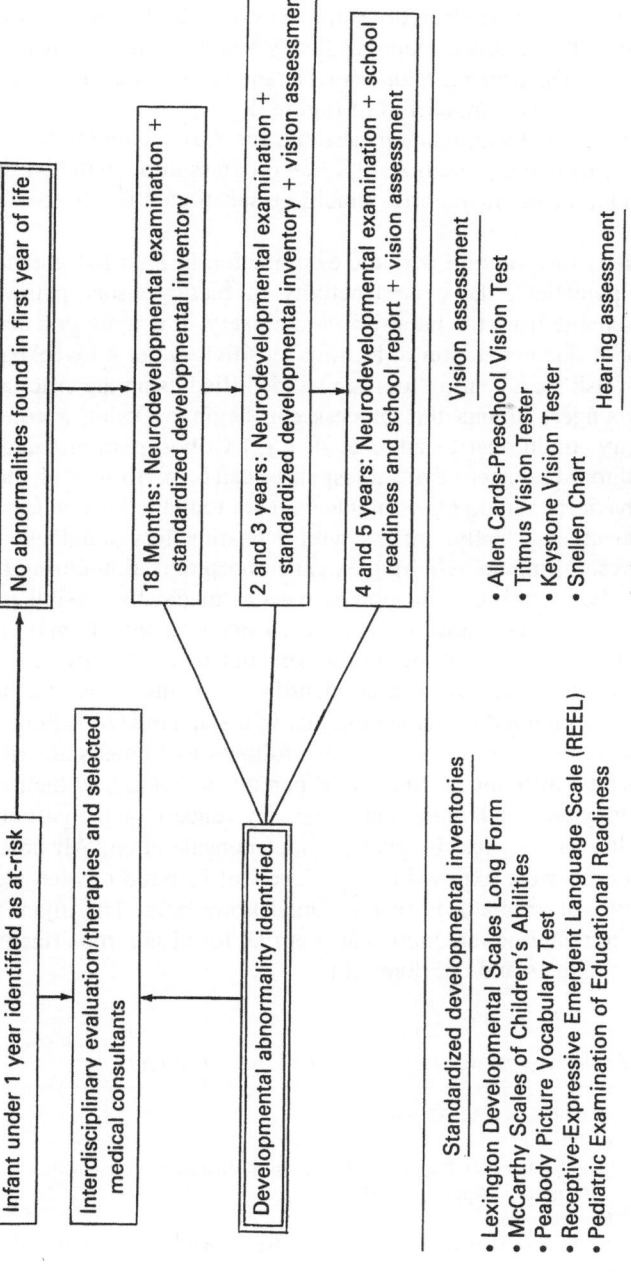

Figure 3. Neurodevelopmental examination schedule for at-risk children, 18 months through 5 years.

Screening tests that were designed for use on normal populations have been used to evaluate children identified as at risk for developmental difficulties. It is the opinion of the author that children previously identified as being at risk for having developmental disabilities should skip the screening stage of testing. These children deserve closer scrutiny and should be periodically examined, both physically and neurodevelopmentally, using a more in-depth approach. The neurodevelopmental examination schedule for at-risk infants from birth to 1 year of age is summarized in Figure 2.

The neurodevelopmental examination schedule for at-risk children from 18 months to 5 years of age is outlined in Figure 3. As children progress through the preschool years, age appropriate developmental inventories should be substituted for those used at earlier ages.

The special senses also require periodic examination in high-risk infants. Through the use of evoked potentials, the central activity of these sensory pathways can be examined before discharge from the intensive-care nursery. It is more practical however, to begin the process of documentation of hearing sensitivity after 40 weeks postconceptional age. Infants at risk for a hearing loss can be identified using the criteria outlined in Table IV. In the youngest infants this process can begin by using a combination of behavioral audiometry, traditional or automated, e.g., Crib-o-gram and auditory brainstem responses. Auditory brainstem-evoked responses can be performed on those children who do not pass behavioral audiometry. Infants who are found to have a hearing loss can benefit from amplification. Ideally, infants with a hearing loss should be aided by 4 months of age. Therefore, infants requiring extended hospitalization during the newborn period should begin their hearing evaluation as soon as medically feasible.

Traditionally, hearing screening has been performed on infants and children in a somewhat haphazard fashion. The use of noisemakers in a non-sound treated environment is not appropriate for infants who have been identified as being at risk for hearing loss. These infants must be examined by an audiologist in a standardized fashion.

Vision should also be assessed as a part of the follow-up of infants identified as being at risk for developmental difficulties. Many new parents do not expect their infants to be able to "see" until they are much older. However, any concern on the part of the parents for their child's ability to see must be given, serious consideration. All infants who are born prematurely or who were exposed to high levels of inspired oxygen are at risk for developing retinopathy of prematurity or retrolental fibroplasia. The infant who is suspected of having an intrauterine infection is also at risk for visual impairment because of the development of cataracts and chorioretinitis.

Table IV Risk Factors for Hearing Loss in Infancy

Family history of hearing loss in childhood
Low birth weight (<1.5 kg)
Unconjugated bilirubin greater than the accepted level for exchange transfusion
Severe perinatal asphyxia (i.e., Apgar score 0–3)
Congenital TORCH infection
Malformations of the head or neck (e.g., cleft palate, atypical pinnae, otic stenosis/atresia)
Any CNS infection
Pre- or postnatal exposure to drugs known to be ototoxic

As pediatricians become more systematic in their follow-up of infants and young children who have been identified as being at risk for developmental disabilities, greater numbers of children will be diagnosed at earlier ages. These children can benefit from the many special services available to them before their entry into the school system. The early diagnosis of a remedial handicap has obvious positive consequences. When a more chronic condition is identified, long-range planning for specific therapies and special education can begin early. Parent education/support can also begin at this time and can be of benefit in avoiding the anxiety that often accompanies a late diagnosis.

HISTORICAL DATA BASE

In the evaluation of the child with a developmental disability, the historical and background information of the patient and his family form the groundwork upon which diagnostic and therapeutic decisions are made. This information can come from a variety of sources, and every effort should be made to obtain as complete a historical data base as possible.

Physicians are taught as medical students to ask parents for the ages at which various developmental milestones were attained. The importance of the milestones will vary according to the age of the patient and his current problems. Although the parents' recollection of the milestones are not as reliable as well documented periodic developmental testing, they can be used to point out developmental areas of concern. For example, if the parents are only concerned with language development, a history of late milestones in motor areas may identify a child who has problems that were unidentified by the parents. Developmental milestones can also be used to help document the time of onset of a condition that is affecting the neurodevelopmental sequence. A range of the ages at which developmental milestones should be attained can be found in most developmental assessment tools (see Appendix).

The developmental milestones can also be of use in developing a historical profile of a particular child's development. The traditional areas of development can be compared with one another in order to point out specific areas that are lagging behind. If all areas are lagging behind to the same degree, suspicion of an overall developmental abnormality should be aroused. In this situation, the late acquisition of milestones, but with steady progress, should be emphasized. This pattern is characteristic of a developmental problem of a static nature. If the history of the developmental milestones reveals the loss of previously acquired skills, suspicion should be aroused for the existence of an underlying disorder that may be progressive in nature. Children with inborn errors of metabolism may present in this manner during infancy. For example, children with Canavan disease, a lipodistrophy, may at first appear normal and may attain several early developmental milestones. In the following months they may lose the ability to follow objects with their eyes or roll over, milestones they previously attained.

In older children, the onset of progressive neurological disorders may be heralded by a change in personality. Later, deficiencies in school performance or motor control become evident. Thus, although early developmental milestones can be reported as normal, efforts must be made to contemporize the developmental history in order to track development into the school-age years.

Several methods are available for obtaining background information prior to the parent interview. One efficient method of obtaining information from parents is the use of a questionnaire (see Appendix). Because the questionnaire is completed at home, uneducated or bilingual parents can spend as much time as necessary to answer questions. They may also enlist the aid of friends or relatives, if necessary. They may also telephone office personnel in order to clarify questions. If a questionnaire is used, it should be exhaustive and include medical, developmental, family, environmental, socioeconomic, and behavioral areas. This produces a source that can be referred to at a later date for information that is not dependent on the immediate recall of the parents. It also provides a means of identifying problem areas that can be fully discussed during the parent interview. Although questionnaires can be lengthy and time consuming for parents, most favorably accept the task as evidence of concern on the part of the physician. They are frequently pleased that such a thorough history is being taken.

Before the parent interview, effort should be made to obtain records from previous hospitalizations and agency contacts. Frequently the parents' recollection of perinatal events are unclear. Details of medical importance such as fetal bradycardia during labor, Apgar scores, neonatal anthropometric measurements, medications, bilirubin levels, and other risk factors are documented in the birth records. Obtaining records from previous agency contacts will not only provide past diagnostic impressions but will also help prevent the inappropriate repetition of recent medical and psychological testing.

The parent interview is an important part of the evaluation process. Within the context of general office practice, parents will often voice developmental concerns during a well-child visit or during a visit for a minor medical complaint. At that time the physician should acknowledge the parents' concern and explain that it may be necessary to obtain further background information before scheduling an appointment to address their specific developmental concern. If the patient and his past history is already known, a separate appointment can be scheduled so that both parents may be interviewed. Adequate time must be allotted for the parents to voice their concerns. An atmosphere of frequent telephone interruptions is not conducive to conducting an interview during which very sensitive issues may be discussed. By simultaneously interviewing both parents, their individual perspectives of the problem can be obtained.

During the parent interview, a chronological history of the chief complaint can be obtained. Particular points of interest to the physician found on the parent questionnaire can be amplified. Special emphasis can be placed on current developmental, social, or academic performance, and the parents' appraisal of the child's strengths and weaknesses can be obtained. The parent questionnaire and the records of hospitalizations and previous agency contacts should be reviewed before the parent interview. This will help the physician direct the interview toward problem areas identified from these sources. It will also help prevent covering redundant or irrelevant information and thereby decrease the time needed for the interview.

The parent interview also presents an opportunity for the assessment of cultural, environmental, and socioeconomic factors. The influence of siblings and extended family members can be assessed. Ethnic and cultural background may influence diagnostic and therapeutic recommendations. The geographical availability of educational and therapeutic facilities may also be explored. At this time, an estimate can be made of the parents motivation to invest their time and resources necessary to complete the evaluation and follow through on the recommendations. A single-parent family or a very chaotic family may require contact with a social agency to provide support. A family in which both parents are employed full time may require a great deal of adjustment in order to ensure that a handicapped child is taken to various consultants or therapists. All these factors must be considered before recommendations are made.

Through the parent interview, the parents become members of the evaluation team. One must not lose sight that the parents have the most detailed, and usually the most accurate, knowledge of the child's past development and behavior. Their input into the diagnostic and therapeutic process must not be underestimated.

PHYSICAL EXAMINATION

When a child is suspected of having a developmental disability, a thorough physical examination is indicated. In a general pediatric setting, the pediatrician may feel that the patient has been physically examined in the past and that no findings have been overlooked. This attitude should be abandoned because when examining a child from a developmental perspective, more subtle findings may be apparent that could have been overlooked or judged insignificant in previous examinations. In addition, findings may be present that were not evident in earlier examinations, e.g., neurofibromas or subtle seizures.

The general pediatric examination is well described in standard textbooks of pediatrics. Emphasis should be placed, however, on the assessment growth and physical maturation and the search for major and minor physical variations.

The cornerstone of the assessment of physical growth is accurate measurement. Infantometers and stadiometers are commercially available (see Appendix). The measurement devices attached to most scales provide only an estimate of stature. By custom, recumbent length is measured in children under the age of 18 months rather than height. For older children, standing height is measured. Present and past determinations of stature, weight, and head circumference should be plotted on standard growth charts. Velocity graphs may be used when growth rate is in question. Tables for the influence of parental stature are also available. Analysis of the patterns of growth can be a significant aid in identifying children in whom further laboratory investigations are indicated. Sexual maturation should be assessed according to the Tanner scale and compared with age-appropriate norms.

As part of the physical examination, effort should be made to identify major and minor variations in morphology. Whenever a single major or minor congenital anomaly is identified, one should search for the presence of other anomalies. Clusters of certain anomalies may lead the examiner to suspect the presence of a malformation syndrome (Table V).

Major anomalies, such as cleft lip and/or cleft palate, congenital heart disease, and skeletal anomalies, have obvious medical consequences. Other anomalies, such as variation in head shape, may signify underlying anomalies, i.e., malformations of the CNS. In addition to the medical consequences of major anomalies, the physician must consider the emotional impact on the family and their developmental consequences.

The pediatrician is frequently called upon to inform the parents of the presence of a

Table V Minor Congenital Anomalies

Head
 Atypical head shape
 Double or frontal hair whorls
 Wry hair
 Head circumference >1 5 SD or <1 5 SD
 Hemangioma over nose or philthrum
 Low hairline

Eyes
 Hypertelorism
 Epicanthal folds
 Atypcial size or shaped palpebral fissures

Ears
 Atypical placement of the pinna
 Preauricular pits or tags
 Asymmetrical pinnae
 Cartilage hypoplasia
 Abnormal ear length

Mouth
 Small mandible
 Enamel hypoplasia
 Fused teeth
 High-arched palate
 Geographical tongue
 Furrowed tongue
 Philtrum length

Hands
 Short fourth or fifth metacarpals
 Hypoplastic or hyperconvex nails
 Camptodactly or hyperextensibility
 Clinodactly
 Transverse palmer creases
 Arachnodactly
 Supranumerary digits
 Lymphedema

Feet
 Hypoplastic or hyperconvex nails
 Lymphedema
 Short metatarsal (low-set first or third and fourth toes)
 Partial syndactly of second and third toes
 Long third toe
 Large gap between first and second toes

Limbs and trunk
 Hypo- or hyperextensibility of joints
 Increased carrying angle of the elbows
 Assymmetrical axillary folds (absent pectoralis)
 Webbing or excess skin folds
 Congenital dislocation of the hip
 Nipple placement and number

major anomaly or genetic syndrome in their newborn infant. Many parents later express the extreme dissatisfaction with the method whereby this information was conveyed. Care must be taken to ensure that up-to-date and accurate information is given to parents regarding the nature and prognosis of their child's particular condition. Equal emphasis should be placed on the parent–infant attachment process. Parents should be allowed the opportunity to accept the infant as "their child." Obviously these events cannot be adequately conducted in a hallway, over a telephone, or during busy hospital rounds. Although parents must be informed very soon after birth, the session must be well planned and conducted in an unhurried fashion, preferably with the infant present. Several sessions may be necessary in order to answer questions and assess the adequacy of the parental coping style.

Minor congenital anomalies often fail to be identified at birth. If they are found in the comprehensive physical examination, a more thorough search for other congenital anomalies, including hidden major anomalies or genetic syndromes, should be carried out. The relationship of minor congenital anomalies to developmental disabilities, such as specific learning disabilities, is controversial. The hypothesis that minor physical anomalies are somehow related to minor anomalies of neuronal organization has not been confirmed by scientific investigation.

The presence of the clinical features of specific chromosomal disorders is an obvious indication for chromosomal analysis. The recently described syndrome of X-linked mental retardation associated with a fragile site on the X chromosome has been shown to be a major cause of mental retardation. Chromosomal analysis for fragility of the X chromosome is therefore indicated for all retarded boys who have the clinical features of this syndrome. It has also been reported to be found in higher incidence among populations of boys with autism. Multiple major and minor congenital anomalies, especially when associated with mental retardation, are also indications for chromosomal analysis. Typical historical and physical findings can be indications for testing for the presence of genetically determined inborn errors of metabolism. Prenatal diagnosis and genetic counselling regarding these conditions have become major tools in the prevention of developmental disabilities.

In summary, the comprehensive physical examination of children with suspected developmental disabilities should not be underemphasized. Many times this search for more subtle abnormalities that might have been previously overlooked can provide clues for accurate diagnosis. Negative findings on the physical examination can reassure both the physician and the parents that a condition that could be interfering with normal growth and development has not been overlooked.

NEURODEVELOPMENTAL EXAMINATION

The neurodevelopmental examination of children consists of several components that must be individually tailored to each child's developmental level. A major component is the neurological examination (including testing of vision and hearing), which must be performed on all children suspected of having a developmental disability. The neurodevelopmental examination must also include assessment of emerging developmental milestones and in older children a thorough search for signs of more subtle neurological dysfunctions. The discussion that follows is divided for convience into infants, preschoolers, and school-age children.

INFANTS

The general neurological examination of infants is well described in standard pediatric and child neurology textbooks. A primary aim of the neurological examination is to identify abnormalities that may be amenable to correction, e.g., hydrocephalus. It is equally important to diagnose progressive/degenerative diseases of the nervous system in this age group.

The assessment of vision in infancy is carried out primarily by physical examination and observation for visual behaviors. The physical examination of the eye can reveal cataracts, strabismus, colobomas, retinal disease, abnormalities of the optic disc, intraocular tumors, pupillary abnormalities, and other abnormalities that can impair vision. Visual function is primarily assessed by observing ocular reflexes and behaviors that are dependent on vision. For example, facial regard, following, and opticokinetic nystagmus may be observed early in infancy. Reaching for large objects and, later on, regarding smaller objects are also evidence of visual function. The presence of wandering/searching eye movements or nystagmus should always arouse the suspicion of visual impairment. Visual evoked responses can be used to document visual deficits or evaluate the presence of white matter disease.

Color vision and visual acuity are developmental phenomena. The cone cells of the retina are developed by 2 months of age, and the macula is mature by 6 months. Newborns are hyperopic. By age 2 visual acuity is approximately 20/70. By age 5, it has improved to 20/30. The 7-year-old child should have 20/20 vision.

Progress in the neurophysiological assessment of hearing has made the diagnosis of hearing loss possible during the neonatal period. In the past it was customary to wait until infants were 6 months of age or older for behavioral audiometry to be carried out. Even lengthier delays in diagnosis were common when motor or cognitive disabilities interfered with behavioral audiometry. All infants at risk for a developmental disability should have audiometric testing in order to document the presence of hearing necessary for the development of speech and language.

The developmental examination of infants begins with observation of the mother and child together. How the infant cuddles and its ease of consolability may provide clues to its particular temperament. The mother's ease of handling, manner of holding, and "reading" the infant's signals can help in describing the maternal–infant relationship. Observation of the child's sociability, interest in the environment (i.e., following objects and reaching), and interaction with unfamiliar adults also provide clues to the infant's personality and individual behavioral style.

The office assessment of cognitive/linguistic development of infants has traditionally been carried out by the use of the pediatrician's built-in-Gesell scales; a "guesstimate" of normalcy made by observing the presence or absence of one or more milestones. This obviously fallacious approach to developmental diagnosis has been replaced by the administration of standardized assessment instruments. The pediatrician working outside an interdisciplinary setting should become familiar with instruments such as the Early Language Milestone Scale and the Baley Scales of Infant Development (see Appendix). Knowledge of the prelinguistic milestones can also be a valuable aid to the early diagnosis of cognitive/linguistic delays (Table VI).

The motor development of infants is best carried out on a mat rather than on an

Table VI. Linguistic Precursors in Infancy[a]

Birth to 4 months	5–9 months	9–12 months	13–16 months
		Expressive	
Crying	Imitations/exchange	Imitations/exchange	Jargon more elaborate
Nondistress vowel and consonant sounds	Nondistress vowel and consonant sounds	Jargonlike strings of sounds.	Imitations/exchange
		Gesture/sharing objects	Single words with meaning
		Prewords	
		Receptive	
		Looks for absent familiar persons when asked	Points to one body part
		Gestural imitations (e.g., wave, patting)	Follows simple directions with example
		Responds consistently to "no"	Retrieves familiar object on request
		Object permanence	
Follows in a complete arc	Returns glance to origin of object	Retrieves covered object	Retrieves object from under screen after displacement out of view of child
	Retrieves paritally covered object		
		Means–ends/operational causality	
Hand watching	Drops one of two held cubes to hold a third cube	Pulls string to obtain toy	Moves mechanical toy in imitation
		Moves to retrieve toy	
Movement to activate object	Pulls support to gain a distant object		Gives toy to adult for activation
Procedure to reinstate spectacle	Plays peek-a-boo		
Grasping			
		Feeding	
Sucking	Cup drinking	Self-finger feeding (soft chewable)	Self cup feeding (untidy)
Spoonfeeding nonchewable	Biting/chewing single pieces (soft)	Neat assisted cup drinking	
		Uses spoon (untidy)	Representational play: pretends to drink from cup; feeds doll with toy bottle

[a]From Uzgiris and Hunt (1975).

examining table. On the mat, movement and position can be assessed free of the limitations of working on an examining table. The mother can be allowed close proximity to the infant to provide consolation if the infant becomes upset. The infant's desire to be close to mother can also be used as a motivation for rolling, crawling, and taking steps.

In the assessment of motor development in infancy, the observation of posture and movement provides valuable information. A sequence of postural development can be observed in all positions. Deviations from this sequence signal the presence of abnormal or atypical motor development.

In the prone position during the early days of life, the face can be momentarily lifted and the head rotated from side to side. As neuromaturation continues, the face comes to a 90° angle with the mat, and more weight begins to be borne by the chest and elbows. By 4 months of age, weight is borne by the radial surfaces of the forearms and hands. Next weight shifting for reaching takes place. By 6 months of age, weight bearing on the palms of the hands and pelvis occurs.

It is also important to observe posture in the supine position. The flexion seen in the early weeks of life gives way to a more relaxed extensor posture. The position of the hands is also important. In weak or hypotonic infants, the hands are characteristically braced in supination on the mat beside the head. In the normal infant 3–4 months of age, midline play and hand regard should be present. The "frog leg" posture in the supine position is also characteristic of weak or hypotonic infants. Symmetry of movement while the infant is supine should also be observed. After 6 months of age, kicking should be more reciprocal than tandem. In the supine position, consistent asymmetry in the quantity of movement of the extremities could represent the presence of a paresis.

All infants should also be observed in the sitting position. During the first few weeks of life, the infant should be able to pick his head up momentarily when held in sitting and prevent it from falling consistently forward or backward. Over the next 3 months, head control should become more well developed and can be estimated by gently rocking the infant in the lateral and anterior–posterior planes. Spinal curvature should also be observed in supported sitting. Dorsal curvature should decrease as the infant approaches independent sitting. Independent sitting is usually preceded by sitting while using the hands for anterior propping. As the sitting posture becomes more frequent, the lateral propping reflexes become more active. Trunk rotation in sitting should also be noted. This can be observed by having the child reach for objects on the mat to the side or slightly behind.

Fixing is the stabilization of joints in order to provide a stable proximal platform for movement to occur elsewhere. Abnormal fixing occurs when muscle tone interferes with the normal sequence of proximal-distal and cephalo-caudal development. Effort should be made to observe abnormal fixing in all of the postures described above. For example, in the sitting position hyptonic infants frequently exhibit fixing of the shoulder girdle by using shoulder retraction in order to maintain stability for the arms and head.

The infant's movement should be observed not only for the age at which movement milestones are reached, but also for patterns of movement. For example, an infant may be able to roll from supine to prone by 6 months of age. When this activity is observed by the examiner, however, one may see that an atypical sequence of movement is used to achieve this milestone. For example, excessive arching onto the vertex and heels may allow the infant to "flip" into the prone position rather than using the normal sequence of scissoring the lower extremities, rolling the pelvis and following through with the shoulders. Similarly, the age and method that an infant uses to move in and out of sitting independently should be observed. The pediatrician should also make note of the infant's preferred means of locomotion. An infant with atypical motor development may prefer rolling from one place to another, "bunny hopping" on hands and knees (knees and hips flexed, legs moving together), or buttock scooting. In observing an infant creeping or crawling, strength, reciprocal use of the extremities, and whether the movement is fluid or ataxic should be noted.

The neurodevelopmental examination of infants should also include an evaluation of muscle tone. The neurological evaluation of gestational age in newborns has been applied to the normal evolution of muscle tone through the first year of life (Fig. 4). Abnormalities in muscle tone are reflected by the limitation or exaggeration of these maneuvers. Because of the dependence of muscle tone on the state of arousal of the infant and type and quality of proprioceptive and extroceptive influences, the pediatrician should also make an effort to observe the effects of abnormal muscle tone on the infant's natural postures and spontaneous motor behavior. For example, when handling a hypertonic infant, the examiner typically feels undue resistance toward antigravity movements and exaggerated resistance when moving with gravity. The hypertonicity will also be evidenced in spontaneous movement, such as extension of the legs, while commando crawling with the arms. The hypotonic infant also lacks proper antigravity postural control. However, in this case there is decreased resistance to the forces of gravity. In the prone position, this may be evidenced by shoulder elevation and neck hyperextension. Hypermobility of the joints is also usually present.

The primitive and postural reflexes may also provide clues to abnormalities in the normal pattern of motor development. Although there is presently no profile of primitive reflexes that allows the diagnosis of cerebral palsy to be made with infallibility, the ages at which these reflexes are expected to be present or absent are well established, and effort should therefore be made to elicit primitive reflexes as a part of the neurodevelopmental examination of infants. Their degree, presence, or absence can be considered with other motor findings as a part of the overall diagnostic picture. Clinical experience has shown the palmar grasp, rooting, moro, sucking, and asymmetrical neck reflexes to be of particular value.

During the integration of the primitive reflexes into the infant's movement patterns, the postural reflexes begin to appear (Table VII). As anterior and lateral propping reactions begin to develop, the infant becomes more able to sit independently. Later posterior propping becomes evident. By 4 months of age, neck righting begins. Between 6 and 9 months, the parachute reflex becomes evident. After 1 year of age, the Landau reflex is present. Reflexes should be evaluated with regard to timing, strength, and symmetry.

When motor abnormalities are found in infancy, the physician must consider labeling the child as having cerebral palsy. Unfortunately there is no pathognomonic sign for making this diagnosis, and routine laboratory investigations are of little value. Therefore, infants who are suspected of having a nonprogressive injury to the developing CNS that affects their movement and posture could be included in this group of disorders. The diagnosis of cerebral palsy is therefore primarily descriptive of many pathological conditions that affect the motor system. The label of cerebral palsy conveys little clinical information and should be qualified by a description of the type of motor disturbance, its distribution, and severity, as outlined in Table VIII. When considering diagnosing an infant as having cerebral palsy, the physician must consider its impact on the family. Unfortunately, cerebral palsy is poorly understood by the lay public. Most parents' conception of the disorder is limited and may not accurately reflect their child's particular problems. The physician must therefore anticipate the parental reaction to this diagnosis

Popliteal angle

The infant is supine, buttocks kept on the table. The thighs flexed onto the abdomen, then the legs are extended until there is resistance.

Adductor angle

The infant is supine. The legs are opened as far as possible.

Heel to ear

The infant is supine, buttock kept on the table. With the leg straight, the foot is moved to the ear. The angle found by the leg and table surface is measured.

Foot dorsiflexion

The foot is flexed onto the leg and the acute angle is measured.

Scarf sign

The infant is supine. One hand is pulled across the chest until resistance is felt. The position of the elbow is noted.

1 to 3 months

80° to 100°

40° to 80°

80° to 100°

60° to 70°

Elbow does not reach midline

4 to 6 months

90° to 120°

70° to 110°

90° to 130°

60° to 70°

Elbow slightly passes midline

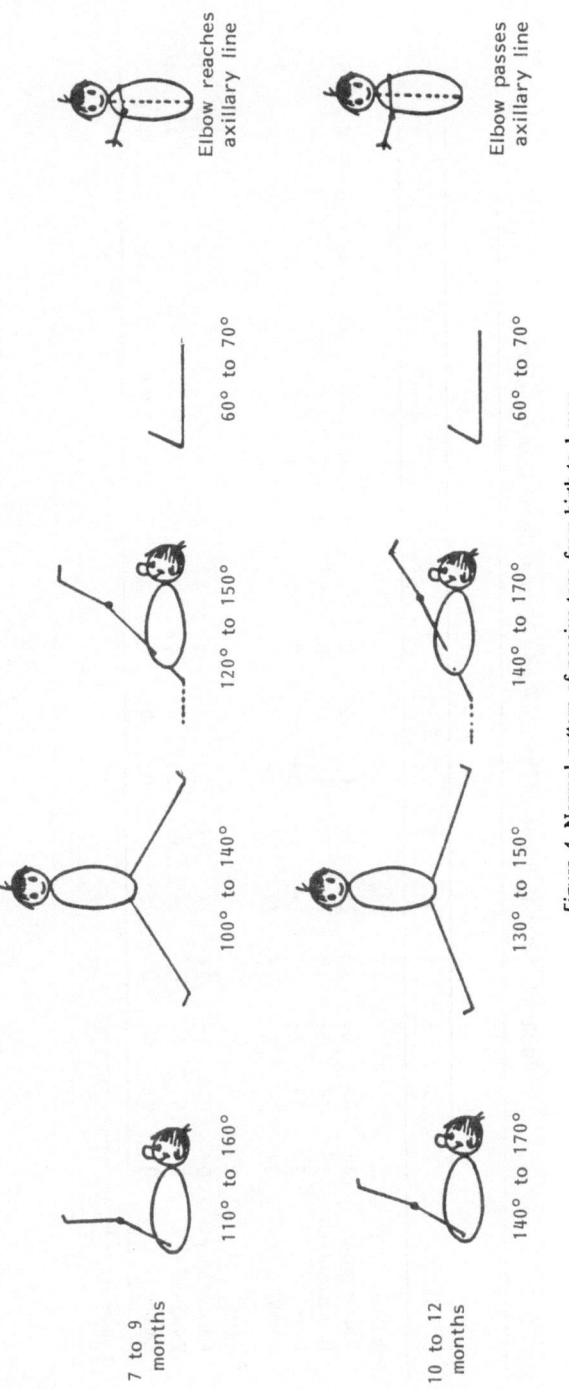

7 to 9 months   110° to 160°   100° to 140°   120° to 150°   60° to 70°   Elbow reaches axillary line

10 to 12 months   140° to 170°   130° to 150°   140° to 170°   60° to 70°   Elbow passes axillary line

Figure 4. Normal pattern of passive tone from birth to 1 year.

Table VII Normal Pattern of Primitive and Postural Reflex Development[a]

| | Months | | | | | | | | | | | | | | | | | |
Reflexes	1	2	3	4	5	6	7	8	9	10	11	12	14	16	18	20	22	24
Primitive																		
Palmar grasp	3+	3+	2+	1+	1+	1+	0	0	0	0	0	0	0	0	0	0	0	0
Rooting/sucking	3+	3+	2+	1+	1+	1+	0	0	0	0	0	0	0	0	0	0	0	0
Moro	3+	3+	2+	2+	1+	1+	1+	0	0	0	0	0	0	0	0	0	0	0
ATNR	2+	3+	2+	1+	1+	1+	1+	1+	0	0	0	0	0	0	0	0	0	0
Postural																		
Neck righting	0	0	1+	2+	2+	3+	3+	4+	4+	4+	4+	4+	4+	4+	4+	4+	4+	4+
Parachute	0	0	0	0	1+	3+	3+	4+	4+	4+	4+	4+	4+	4+	4+	4+	4+	4+
Landau	0	0	0	0	0	0	0	0	0	1+	3+	4+	4+	4+	4+	3+	3+	2+

[a]0, absent expression; 4+, strongest expression

Table VIII. Classification of Cerebral Palsy

Type of motor disturbance	Distribution		Severity
	Location	Description	
Spasticity	Quadraplegia	All extremities with equal involvement	Mild
Athetosis (tension, montension, dystonia, tremor)	Diplegia	Tetraparesis with mild upper extremity involvement	
Rigidity			Moderate
Ataxia			
Tremor	Hemiplegia	Upper and lower extremity on one side	
Hypotonia (atonia, rare)			Severe
Mixed	Paraplegia	Both lower extremities, upper extremities normal	
	Monoplegia	One extremity	

and the need for ongoing educational and supportive counseling regarding the ramifications of this diagnosis.

PRESCHOOL CHILDREN

As in infancy, the assessment of preschool children must consist of physical, neurological, and developmental examinations. The pediatric physical and neurological examinations are not described in detail here, as they are well described elsewhere. The focus of the physical examination is to assess growth and to search carefully for subtle medical and genetic disorders that may have been previously overlooked. The neurological examination will reveal any focal neurological signs or findings that may indicate the presence of an underlying progressive neurological disorder.

Vision and hearing must be assessed in all children suspected of having a developmental disorder. Vision in this age group is assessed by physical examination and by the testing of acuity. The cover–uncover test and symmetry of the corneal light reflex can be used to detect the presence of strabismus. The method of testing the child's visual acuity, however, is dependent on attentional, behavioral, and cognitive factors. Children at lower developmental ages can be tested with Allen Picture Cards. Distant visual acuity can be assessed in higher functioning children with the Snellen Illiterate E Chart or the Snellen Chart. Visual testing instruments are also available (see Appendix). Hearing should be assessed in a sound-treated environment. Routine screening can miss a significant hearing loss. Testing under earphones for auditory acuity and tympanometry should be performed in this age group.

The developmental examination of preschool children should begin with an assessment of their behavioral style. Effort should be made to describe any atypical behaviors that are present and the child's degree of relatedness to his parents and unfamiliar adults. Observation in both a free-play environment and in more structured situations can provide an informal assessment of physical activity and the child's ability to focus attention. One must always be aware of the influence of the environment on attention span. One should

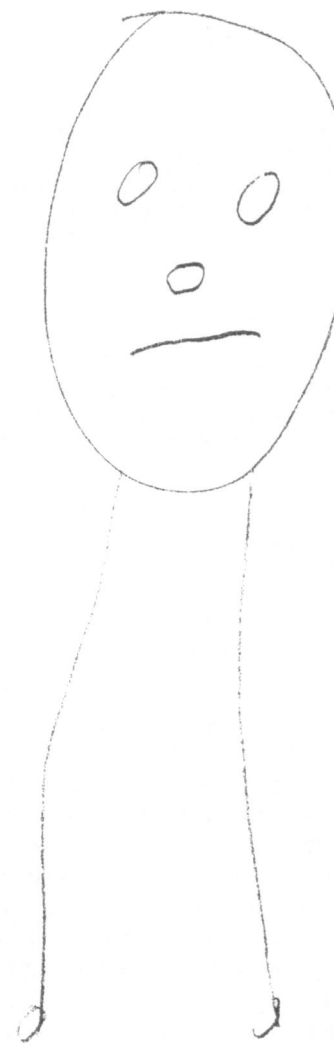

Figure 5. Typical tadpole drawing of a person by a 3-year-old girl.

therefore not discount the parents' history of the child's ability to focus attention and level of motor activity on the basis of a brief period of observation. A discrepancy between the two may identify a child who can modify these behaviors with changes in his environment, i.e., a child who might respond well to behavior modification techniques.

In the preschool child, fine motor skills are superimposed on the basic patterns of movement that were laid down in infancy. The observation of progressive facility with stacking blocks, stringing beads, using scissors, handling buttons, snaps, and zippers, can provide an estimate of individual child's fine motor skills. As walking becomes more refined, skills that require additional motor planning become a part of the child's motor repertoire. Activities such as walking up steps, kicking a ball, jumping in place, and pedaling emerge in the early preschool years. By age 4, skills such as walking up and down stairs without support, balancing on each foot, and smooth running at different speeds have evolved.

The developmental assessment of preschool children should also include an examination of speech and language skills. In order to obtain a language sample, one can observe the child in spontaneous play with children or adults or interact directly with the child using story books, pictures, and other items of interest to stimulate conversation. It is also useful to engage the older preschool child in conversation about recent events. This allows the examiner to observe how the child uses language to communicate ideas from long-term memory that are not rote.

In addition to the developmental milestones of language, one should make note of fluency, prosody, and intelligibility in connected speech. While naming objects or imitating words, sound omissions and substitutions can be compared with age-related norms (see Appendix). The physician should also make note of the presence of any atypical use of language. The presence of jargon, an atypical use of pronouns, or echololia may be evidence of a profound communication disorder.

Older preschool children should be observed while drawing with a crayon or primary pencil. The Gesell drawings; circle at 3 years, cross at $3\frac{1}{2}$ years, and a square at 4 years can be presented. In addition, the physician should also ask the child to draw a person. During the early preschool years, there should be little differentiation of parts, although some children may be able to name parts while drawing. Older preschool children may draw a figure that resembles a tadpole with increasing detail on the head and little detail for the rest of the body (Fig. 5).

Developmental disabilities identified during the preschool period obviously require interventions according to their nature and severity. Nevertheless, controversy continues to surround the identification of children with learning disabilities during the preschool years. The possibility of subtle findings representing a difference in the individual's neuromaturational timetable versus a true disorder makes labeling a child as learning-disabled prior to kindergarten difficult. In older preschoolers, however, the assessment of attention, speech and language function, visuoperceptual/graphomotor skills, and fine and gross motor coordination may identify a child at risk for failure to achieve in a traditional educational setting. Many standardized inventories of a language, social, motor, adaptive, and perceptual development in the preschool child are available (see Appendix). With training and experience in administration, the physician can use these developmental inventories in combination with the history and neurodevelopmental examination as an aid to deciding which children should be referred for a more complete interdisciplinary developmental/educational assessment.

SCHOOL-AGE CHILDREN

As in younger patients, a complete physical examination should be carried out as outlined previously. Emphasis should be placed on the identification of signs of minor biological variation. Effort should also be made to identify those children in whom

*Table IX. Neurological Disorders That May Present as Slowly
Progressive Learning Problems*

Seizures
Wilson disease
Neuronal ceroid-lipofuscinosis
Juvenile-onset metachromatic leukodystrophy
Juvenile Huntington chorea
Subacute sclerosing panencephalitis
Adrenoleukodystrophy
Friedreich ataxia
Hallervorden-Spatz disease
Neimann-Pick disease variants
Other organic brain syndromes (e.g., substance abuse, lead encephalopathy)

underlying metabolic disorders could have been overlooked at earlier ages. Progressive
CNS disorders can present as slowly progressive learning or personality problems in this
age group (Table IX). The traditional neurological examination and history may uncover
more specific signs or symptoms of these disorders.

Vision and hearing should be tested in all school-age children suspected of having a
learning disability or other developmental disorder. By age 7, 20/20 vision should be
present in each eye. Vision testing should include near and far visual acuity, color vision,
and muscle balance. The Snellen Letter Chart or mechanical vision testers can be employed (see Appendix). Hearing testing should be conducted in a sound-treated environment. A mild conductive hearing loss may be missed in routine office screening. Although classified as mild, this degree of hearing loss can become quite significant in a
regular classroom setting. Even if the hearing loss is transient, communication with the
classroom teacher regarding special seating and instruction is indicated (see Appendix).
Audiological consultation may also help delineate the nature of a learning disability by
administering a central auditory battery. This usually consists of various listening tasks
that require selective auditory attention, discrimination, and memory. Although the
clinical interpretation of such a battery remains controversial, strengths and weaknesses
may be identified that can be of help in the classroom.

As an extension of the neurological examination, the neurodevelopmental assessment should include a search for neurological soft signs (Table X). These soft signs
appear in the areas of motor function, directionality, cortical sensation, body image, and
spatial perception. These findings are prevalent in normal preschool children and less so
in older children. This implies that soft signs are maturational in nature and should not be
present in average older school-aged children. The significance of the presence of soft
signs remains controversial. It is generally agreed that they do not imply brain damage and
that they are not pathognomonic for learning disabilities. It is also believed that they are
not helpful for recommending changes in curriculum, nor is special training to improve a
particular soft sign helpful. They are helpful, however, in making decisions concerning
the relative contribution of intrinsic versus environmental influences on the learning
disabled child's performance. Soft signs may also be helpful in demonstrating to parents
the intrinsic nature of learning disabilities and that their child is not just poorly motivated
or oppositional.

Table X. Soft Neurological Signs[a]

Choreiform movements of outstretched hands
Motor impersistence
Hyperactive or slightly assymetrical deep tendon reflexes
Awkward gait
Mild tremors, nystagmus, or ataxia
Mild hyper- or hypotonia
Dysdiadochokinesis
Poor identification of stimulated fingers
Inability to discriminate simultaneously stimulated fingers
Awkward repeated finger-to-thumb apposition (+/−synkinesis)
Extinction of distal stimulus when face and hand are simultaneously stimulated
Incorrect identification of left and right

[a]In general, these signs are prevalent in preschool children and decrease in incidence over the next 4–5 years.

The physician must also take into account how the presence of such minor neurological dysfunctions affect the child's function in his peer group. A child who is viewed as clumsy and poorly coordinated may have difficulty in peer-related activities, such as sports, which may affect self-esteem.

Unfortunately, by training or experience, pediatricians find themselves talking to parents and looking at children. As part of the neurodevelopmental examination, however, it is important to set aside time to speak with the child without the parents being present. This time can be used to establish rapport and find out the child's perspective of the problems. It is often useful to ask the child why he believes he is undergoing examination. In addition to performing a standard mental status examination, looking at memory, concentration, contact with reality, and affect, the physician can ask the child how he views himself in relationship to his family, peers, and school. Many school-age children with developmental disabilities may feel victimized and scapegoated by their teachers and peers and view their home environment as a place of constant punishment and disapproval. During the interview, the physician should be alert for signs of depression, bizarre ideation, and other indications of emotional disorders.

During the interview, an appraisal of the child's communicative abilities can be made. As children reach school age, the demands and expectations of their language abilities change. During the primary years, children are expected to decode symbolic language in the process of learning to read. As they progress through the primary years, more demands on encoding take place. This is a change from the analysis of language to the formulation of ideas, putting them into sentences, and writing them down on paper. This occurs at a time when demands on memory are also changing. In the early school years, children depend on recognition and associational memory. Later they are required to retrieve greater volumes of more specific information. As these demands increase, the child must fight fatigue and ignore the social and environmental distractions of the classroom.

As children progress through the school years, language expectations become more complex. Up to the fourth grade, the language level of school reading materials approximates the child's social language. In the fifth grade, the language level of reading materials surpasses the child's social language. In the sixth grade, the complexity of the

Table XI. Characteristics of the Conversation of
Children with Language Disorders[a]

Frequent self-revision
Inordinate response latency
Overuse of nonspecific words (e.g., things, stuff, play)
Seemingly inappropriate responses
Frequent pauses, hesistancy, and repetitions
Poor topic maintenance
Numerous requests for repetitions and clarifications

[a]Damico and Oller. Pragmatic versus Morphological/Syntactic criteria for language referrals. *Lang. and Hear. Ser. in Schools*
11:85–94, 1980.

reading language greatly exceeds their social language and children with subtle language disorders may begin to have academic difficulties. Children with more overt language disorders may present at earlier grades.

While interviewing the school-age child, the physician should be aware of the manner in which the child communicates verbally. In addition to taking note of errors in articulation and dysfluency, one should notice phonation and prosody. The physician should also be listening for the conversational symptoms of an underlying language disorder (Table XI). Children with language disorders tend to overuse nonspecific words and often answer questions after an inordinate pause. Their conversation may be characterized by frequent pauses, self-revision, and poor topic maintenance. These children also make numerous requests for the repetition and clarification of directions. Children with severe language disorders may make remarks in conversation that superficially appear inappropriate or tangential but are instead attributable to their language disability. This difficulty in communication will many times interfere with peer relationships, making them appear odd or "weird."

Expressive language abilities may also be examined by observing the child's ability to describe a recent experience. Joke telling and retelling stories will also provide opportunities to observe how the school-age child communicates verbally. Children with very good expressive skills can hide a mild receptive language problem for many years. Their language problems may not appear until demands become so great that they can no longer use coping strategies in order to achieve academically.

Older children with receptive language disorders frequently have difficulty following directions. They may also confuse words that sound alike, e.g., lap for lack, chair for bear. They may also have difficulty focusing their attention during tasks that require verbal processing, such as listening in class. These children are easily distracted by extraneous verbal information and have difficulty picking out the important information in verbally presented material. The physician may demonstrate this problem by having the child read a paragraph and then orally summarize it for the examiner.

Audiological assessment is mandatory for all children suspected of having a language disorder or other specific learning disabilities. This is especially true for bilingual children in whom language difficulties may be explained away by having English as a second language. A mild hearing loss will interfere greatly with the reception and interpretation of verbally presented information; it will also contribute to the attention difficulties in the classroom.

School-age children with academic problems will many times have weakness in the area of memory as a part of their specific learning disability. Memory is directly related to one's ability to focus attention on a task so that the event may be retained. When a child with attentional problems is superficially involved in a task, learning is obviously impaired. The episode may be recalled, but many times the child's memory will be cluttered with irrelevant events.

When children reach the later school years they must be able to hold an entire task in memory while working on only a part of the project. Children with weakness in this memory modality may have difficulty completing projects or complex classwork without close supervision.

As children begin to read and write, they must begin simultaneously to combine academic modalities involving memory. For example, while writing a child must remember how to form letters and at the same time must remember how to spell. If a child has a discrepancy in the memory for these two areas, his performance will deteriorate. One may also see children who have difficulty with specific memory modalities. For example, some children may have good verbal memory and can remember what they have heard yet have very weak visual memory and have difficulty remembering what was presented through the visual modality.

During the examination, the physician must remain alert for this unevenness in the way a particular child handles different memory tasks. Specific sequencing difficulties may be assessed by having the child recite a sequence of digits given at 1-second intervals. Other modalities can be assessed in conjunction with specific sequencing skills by asking the child to remember a sequence of geometric figures or to imitate a sequence of gestures. Sentence repetition may also be used in children who do not have language problems. By increasing the length and complexity of these tasks, one may decide whether this is a particular area of weakness.

As academic demands increase, school-age children must develop more sophisticated mnemonic strategies. A child who has difficulty making mental associations or who lacks the ability to divide memorization tasks into small pieces will have difficulty when required to perform tasks such as remembering a sequence of events in history or recalling the attributes of a foreign country.

Memory problems should also be suspected in children who have trouble in specific academic areas. Different school subjects tap different memory skills. For example, children may have problems with specific memory involving spelling. Children with memory problems may also demonstrate a gap between their comprehension/conceptualization skills and their daily classroom performance. Their test scores are frequently inferior to their ability to participate in classroom discussions. These children are able to recall the generalities but not the specific details of a subject.

Successful academic performance in the school-age child also depends on visuoperceptual processing and graphomotor abilities. Gross motor coordination may be thought of as a base on which fine motor activities are superimposed. Poor gross motor function can interfere with fine motor performance. Gross motor abilities in the school-age child are assessed by looking primarily at higher-level motor-planning activities, such as throwing and catching a ball, skipping, balancing with eyes closed, and gesture imitation. School-age children with gross motor coordination difficulties are frequently ridiculed by their peers. They have difficulty competing in sports and other motor-related activities.

Poor peer acceptance and being ridiculed or labeled clumsy serve to create a poor self-image.

School-age children who have fine motor dysfunction frequently have a history of failure in writing output. Children with this difficulty frequently produce a low volume of written work and can develop a "writing phobia" that fosters a lack of practice. Caution must be used in judging fine motor dysfunction by artistic or mechanical ability. In artistic or mechanical activities, the eyes drive the hand. Difficulty with writing involves a dissynchronization of ideational, verbal, and graphomotor fluencies, not just poor eye–hand coordination. Therefore, difficulty in any of these areas can produce nonfluent writing.

Fine motor abilities that affect graphomotor performance and writing involve several neuromotor functions. Eye–hand motor coordination must be well developed in order for a child to have legible handwriting that follows the lines and maintains margins. Fine motor function is also influenced by nonvisual feedback arising from the kinesthetic perception of the movement of finger joints and the feel of the movement of the pencil on the page. These all influence the motor plan. Thus writing is not a purely visuomotor task. Visual feedback is much too slow for writing.

Handwriting problems may be demonstrated by having a child copy a line drawing on graph paper or by having him write his name with eyes closed. If there is a fluctuation in motor memory or motor plan, true writing dyspraxia results. The examiner must keep in mind that by the middle school years, writing should not require effort.

During the examination, the physician can observe how the child uses a pencil in letter and number formation and spatial orientation. The child may also be asked to draw familiar objects and a human figure. The presence of laborious or illegible handwriting should always raise the possibility of fine motor dysfunction.

School-age children with fine motor dysfunction also suffer ridicule and derision. If children cannot "get it down on paper," they cannot complete their assignments or prove they know their lessons. The imperfect transcription of ideas to written language can significantly impair motivation because a faulty product is produced. These children's work is labeled sloppy or careless, both of which have the connotation of purposeful misconduct or a lack of motivation on the part of the child.

Visual-perceptual processing can be assessed during the examination by standardized instruments (see Appendix). The physician may assess such areas as visual memory by asking the child to copy designs after a few seconds of study. Matching designs can reveal visual processing weaknesses unrelated to fine motor/graphomotor dysfunction that may contaminate copying tasks.

The physician must also consider behavioral and attentional factors when assessing the neurodevelopmental status of the school-age child. Problems in these areas can greatly affect academic performance. The attention-deficit disorder with and without hyperactivity is well described in Chapter 17. However, symptoms in older school-age children may vary from those in the classic description of younger children.

Subtle problems in selective attention may greatly affect school performance. The ability to facilitate attention selectively for the activity at hand while simultaneously inhibiting extraneous stimuli allows children to persist successfully in an activity. The examiner must carefully consider whether the present activity is actually different from what the child's attention is truly focused on. With deficits in selective attention, the child's degree of arousal and cognitive stamina may be decreased. These children appear to be fatigued in the classroom or at the homework desk. Many children fight this feeling with increased motor activity. Poor selective attention also affects performance consistency and produces a varying motivational state. These children also have difficulty simplifying their work because they are unable to identify the recurring patterns of many tasks (as in arithmetic). These children also lack the ability to modify their approach to a task while working because they have difficulty paying attention to the feedback and reinforcement of their performance.

Although children with the attention-deficit disorder show a decline in hyperactivity in middle childhood, they continue to have difficulty focusing attention. Many of these children are greatly distracted from academic endeavors by sports, dating, and other extracurricular activities. Their distractability may also present as an aggravation of their fatigability. Most of these children have a preference for "big picture" subjects and do not pay attention to detail. This selective underarousal creates extreme performance inconsistency. Test scores typically vary from A's to F's within a subject. These children also retain a degree of impulsivity that interferes with their ability to formulate sound problem-solving strategies.

Older children with the attention-deficit order tend to be future oriented and often appear restless in their present life situation. The social and academic effects of this disorder create feelings of frustration and anxiety. If academic and social dysfunction are considerable, the physician must be alert for signs of depression and poor self-esteem.

During the neurodevelopmental examination of the school-age child, the pediatrician should make an effort to describe the child's behavioral style in addition to the child's selective attention and ability to focus on various visual and auditory tasks. The child's level of physical activity should be noted. The presence of physical activity during various tasks that challenge areas of strength and weakness may provide a clue as to whether increased motor activity is a pervasive problem or one that may be related to situational anxiety. The presence of vocal or motor tics and habits such as nail biting should also be noted.

Limit testing and oppositional behaviors during the examination should also be described. The response of these behaviors to limit setting, structuring, or praise and reward during the examination may also help the physician assess how firmly rooted these problems are in the child's behavioral style.

There are several approaches to obtaining the information described earlier during the neurodevelopmental examination of the school-age child (see Appendix). These range from eclectic to formal standarized examinations. Whichever method, or combination of methods, the physician chooses, one should strive to make the examination a positive experience for the child. The scrutiny of evaluation automatically implies deviance, and the examiner should be aware of the possibility of negative feelings and anxiety regarding the testing situation.

CASE FORMULATION AND THE INFORMING INTERVIEW

The synthesis of the findings of a neurodevelopmental examination should place emphasis on a profile of the child's strengths and weaknesses. Too much emphasis should not be placed on any one finding. This is important because in a single examination a "red herring" may overshadow other equally important findings. The physician must exercise great care in amalgamating the history and neurodevelopmental findings. One must carefully weigh functional versus environmental influences on the child's performance. The history is important in comparing problems reported by the parents with those observed during the examination. For example, a child may be reported to have behavioral problems or a poor attention span in the classroom. If these problems are not observed during the examination, one should consider the effects of the environment on behavioral and cognitive style.

The synthesis of the findings of the neurodevelopmental examination should also identify those areas that require more detailed or expert evaluation. The physician will need to choose medical and other professional (e.g., speech pathologist, special educator, psychologist, physical therapist) consultations. Thus, the physician will find that the neurodevelopmental examination will rarely be done in isolation. This approach will provide a profile of the child's neurodevelopmental status from several professional perspectives. After the child has been evaluated by this team of consultants, the physician will have a more precise delineation of the problem areas discovered during the neurodevelopmental examination. These evaluations will also serve as a base for therapeutic interventions by these specialists. This team approach also provides a set of diagnostic checks and balances that has been shown to be a most effective approach to the management of children with developmental disabilities.

The informing interview must always be conducted with both parents present. A parent should never be placed in the vulnerable position of having to explain findings to the other parent. This approach will also help foster the involvement of a parent who has become detached from the problem. His importance will be confirmed by the physician's insistence on his presence.

The informing interview should take place in an unhurried atmosphere and in an environment with few distractions. Young children should not be present. Diagnostic findings should be explained to parents in terms appropriate to their level of understanding. Although parents generally ask about prognosis, the physician should resist the temptation to make specific long-range predictions regarding any child's future functional capacities. At early ages it is difficult to predict the adult capacities of even retarded children. Speaking to parents in broad generalizations, such as how adults are functioning today who have similar IQ's, may foster misconceptions and does not take into account the effects of modern-day or future educational and therapeutic techniques. Handicapped children of 20 years ago did not enjoy the interventions available to children today; therefore, such analogies may be fallacious.

It should be stressed to parents that periodic developmental testing will be necessary in order to assess the effectiveness of therapy and to build a developmental growth chart from which a rate of developmental progress can be extrapolated. For example, a parent might be told that if a child who is 1 year behind in development today is 2 years behind 3 years from now, he is obviously making very slow progress. Thus, one could prognosticate that over the short term the child's developmental status will be commensurate with this rate of development lag. Helping parents to become more focused on progress over the short term can help them deal with their anxieties regarding issues in the distant future.

During the informing interview, the physician should also demystify developmental disabilities, particularly those of their child. The neurodevelopmental aspects of such problems as attentional deficits and specific learning disabilities can be explained to parents and, at their request, to their child's teachers and therapists. It should be emphasized to the parents that children with these problems are not inherently lazy, poorly motivated, or bad.

The physician should stress the ongoing nature of his involvement with the family. Children with developmental disabilities face new crises each time they must change teachers, therapists, or neighborhoods, upon entering puberty, and when they begin dating or plan to live independent of their families. The pediatrician must understand that every time they face one of these crises, parents of children with developmental disabilities will again experience the feelings of anger and denial that occurred when they first suspected or were told that their child was developmentally disabled. The pediatrician must therefore anticipate these problems and serve as an ongoing resource to the family. Support, advocacy, and guidance from the physician can facilitate these transitions as the developmentally disabled child grows to adulthood.

SELECTED READING

Accardo, P. J.: *A Neurodevelopmental Perspective on Specific Learning Disabilities*. University Park Press, Baltimore, 1980.

Accardo, P. J., and Capute, A. J.: *The Pediatrician and the Developmentally Delayed Child:A Clinical Textbook on Mental Retardation*. University Park Press, Baltimore, 1979.

Boyce, N. L., and Larson, V L.: *Adolescent's Communication: Development and Disorders*.Thinking Publ., Eau Claire, 1983.

Dworkin, P. H.:Learning and behavior problems of schoolchildren. *Maj. Problems Clin. Pediatr.* **27**:1–244, 1985.

Field, T. M. (ed.): *Infants Born at Risk: Behavior and Development*.S.P. Medical and Scientific Books, New York, 1979.

Frankenburg, W. K., Emde, R. N., and Sullivan, J. W. (eds.): *Early Identification of Children at Risk: an International Perspective*. Plenum, New York, 1985.

Frankenburg, W. K., Thornton, S. M., and Cohrs, M. E. (eds.).: *Pediatric Developmental Diagnosis*. Thieme-Stratton, New York, 1981.

Gottlieb, M. I., Zinkus, P. W., and Bradford, L. J. (eds.): *Current Issues in Developmental Pediatrics: The Learning Disabled Child*. Grune & Stratton, New York, 1979.

Hallam,H. (ed.): *Symposium on continuing care of the high-risk infant. Clin. Perinatol.* **11**:1–127, 1984.

Harel, S., and Anastaslow, N. J. (eds.): *The at-Risk Infant*. Paul H. Brookes, Baltimore, 1985.

Illingworth, R. S.: *The Development of the Infant and the Young Child, Normal and Abnormal*. Churchill Livingstone, Edinburgh, 1975.

Knobloch, H.: *Manual of Developmental Diagnosis*. Harper & Rowe, Hagerstown, Maryland, 1980.

Levine, L D., Carey, W.B., Crocker, A. C., *et al.* (eds.):*A Pediatric Approach to Learning Disorders*. Wiley, New York, 1980.

Scheiner, A. P., and Abrams, I. F.: *The Practical Management of the Developmentally Disabled Child*. Mosby, St. Louis, 1980.

Scherzer, A. L., and Tscharmuter, I.: Early diagnosis and therapy in cerebral palsy: A primer on infant developmental problems, *Pediatr. Habil.* **3**:1–289, 1982.

Shaywitz, S. E., Grossman, H. J., and Shaywitz, B. A. (eds.): Symposium on learning disorders. *Pediatr. Clin. North Am.* **21**:279–518, 1984.

Uzgiris, I. C., and Hunt, J. McV.: *Assessment in Infancy-Ordinal Scales of Psychological Development*. University of Illinois Press, Urbana, 1975.

Controversial Therapy

George W. Brown

INTRODUCTION

Deeply rooted in modern experience with developmental disabilities are a number of interventions that survive in defiance of criticism, scorn, and exposure as "therapeutically senseless." Before examining specific treatments, it is informative to explore the interac-

George W. Brown • Los Lunas Hospital and Training School, Los Lunas, New Mexico 87031.

tions of those served with those providing the services. Specifically to be considered is the role that the professional may play in turning away patients–clients, families, advocates, and friends from established therapies—pushing them toward unproved, nonstandard, controversial treatment programs.

VULNERABILITY OF FAMILIES

Sooner or later, most families encounter distress of some kind; these occasions seem to be inherent to the human condition. Families in which there is a person with a developmental handicap experience these occasions in magnified form, added to the burdens of the disability in the loved one. There is an abundant literature on the impact of disability on family members' aspirations, interpersonal dynamics, and life patterns.[1] These discussions vary in emphasis, sometimes stressing chronic sorrow and grief in loss of the "expected" child. Others discuss anger, resentment, hostility, and other external reactions. Still others focus on guilt, self-blame, and feelings of unworthiness as prominent reactions among the families of handicapped children.

Reaction patterns are variable within a family, from one family to another, and in a given family from one time to another. A parent or other caregiver may vacillate from overprotecting the impaired person, to feeling a sense of martyrdom and depletion, to rejection and blaming the victim. But one element appears to remain constant: The family wants a treatment program that will help the loved one.

This universal, persisting, powerful yearning for helpful intervention is felicitous, but it is associated with a vulnerability, a danger of indiscriminate adoption of insubstantial therapy, that is, the yearning to "do something." This is often the sad pathway to fad treatment, therapeutic recklessness, and perhaps to outright quackery.

MESSAGES TO FAMILIES

Families are sometimes given the covert message from trusted sources that standard interventions are not likely to be beneficial and that they are invariably expensive, demanding, and drawn out. Standard interventions include physical and occupational therapy, language training, orthopedic procedures, and other chronic treatment efforts.

In contrast to the guarded ambiance surrounding traditional modes of therapy, the family is often provided optimistic and "sunny excitement" from the activists providing nonstandard therapy. The nonstandard interventions are generally presented with clichés suggesting that they are highly successful, prompt results are promised ("the cure will be dramatic"), and the costs in time and money will be eminently worthwhile. The promoters of the bright and new treatment methods will answer questions usually without hesitation. By contrast, cautious spokespersons for traditional therapy may turn families away by failure to answer questions fully. Families report that they feel they are misled and that uncertainties are ignored, questions evaded, and fears are exacerbated. They feel patronized and excluded by the detached "efficiency" of the professionals or by the elitism of the technical jargon. When they feel pushed aside, families may turn to other nontraditional sources of help.

Some of the shame, guilt, or feelings of stigmatization may result from the unanswerable questions that haunt parents and other family members.[1] These questions may hide self-blame for imagined transgressions in diet, physical activity, medication use, or simply bad thoughts. The unanswerable questions (''Why did this happen to us?'' ''Why are we being punished?'' ''Who is really to blame?'') cause families to feel adrift when professionals cannot answer these questions. Questions that do not have long answers may seem just as crucial as questions that do (''If you know what causes Down syndrome, why don't you prevent it?'' ''My friend's daughter has a seizure disorder that is controlled by medication—why can't our child's seizures be stopped?'')

Professionals bring only finite knowledge to their interactions with families. The professional, striving to be objective yet empathetic, explains what is known about a particular impairment. He thinks, ''I will outline what little is known and what might be done. We will share our disappointment that more is not available.'' The family, however, may perceive a subtly distorted message, interpreting it as, ''We professionals will tell you what you need to know; don't press for knowledge beyond your depth.'' Or perhaps, ''You relatives are too emotionally involved to grasp the mysteries that we experts are bringing you—leave these complex matters to us.''

Families may be endowed with a general feeling of ominous futility. The professional's inability to provide a therapeutic solution may be perceived as confusion as to what is wrong. Parents are heard to say, ''The pediatrician didn't know what was wrong, even after all those tests.'' Perhaps the pediatrician knew what was wrong but did not know what to do about it. With many developmental disabilities, the diagnosis is certain but the problem lies in recommending an effective program of care. Sometimes families are not told enough because professionals simply cannot know all about the many genetic, chromosomal, and other birth impairments and the hundreds of degenerative, metabolic, infectious, and traumatic disorders that can lead to a handicap. Fredrickson[2] discussed the rising volume of information and the new devices and techniques used to study complex and unusual illnesses, urging that every health professional be exposed to the new diagnostic and therapeutic methods, at least to some small degree. It may be tempting for families to turn to naturalistic ''cures,'' if they sense that their health care professional may not have kept abreast of the new ideas and machines whirring away in the ivory towers of biomedicine.

The health care professional is often in a curious no-win situation. The services provided may strike the family as being disappointingly limited but still quite burdensome and expensive. The prospects for marked improvement or cure are dim. However, when the family raises the issue of a nonstandard, alternate therapy, the expert reacts with self-serving objections: ''Don't try that quackery; it won't do anything.'' The family may well react: ''Well, if may not do much, but its advocates are a lot more enthusiastic and optimistic than you experts are.'' The less to be expected from a standard treatment, the more attractive an exciting, highly touted, alternative program appears to be. As fads become more appealing, the more unsympathetic and ''theoretical'' the health care skeptic appears. When the standard disciplines have little to offer, skeptics are not persuasive when ''scientifically'' denouncing fads and snake oil remedies. Even when the professional team has considerable information about a specific condition, that does not necessarily provide dependable insights on the prospects for every newly diagnosed person. Developmental disabilities do not always run true to form; the variation from one child (e.g., with Down syndrome) to another may be as great as the differences between a handicapped child and an unimpaired one.

PROFESSIONAL STYLES

Professionals have a tendency to devise routine systems for handling recurring issues, although frequently these routines fail to meet the special needs of the family.[3] The professional, in the interest of his own sanity, confronts each client and family in a somewhat detached "scientific" mode. The professional may experience each contact as being "business as usual," but the few minutes of contact between client and professional may be highly charged emotionally for the family and the identified patient.

Medical professionals are often engrossed in causation. This process of "looking backward" may confuse family members who are concerned with the present and a plan for the future. One group of professionals may talk about the patient's past and then try to communicate with others who are centering on the program for the future. This is fertile ground for controversy, with each group wondering what makes the other act and talk in such strange ways. Another disturbance of focus is the tendency for some professionals to center on how much the client lacks, i.e., how defective he is. The family, however, takes a hopeful look at what is present, i.e., how successful the person is. Communications can be difficult when one group of helpers is looking at what is missing and others at what is present. This divergence of viewpoints is seen when test results are discussed with families, especially tests of mental function. The tests are performed by a stranger, in a strange place, in a brief and uncharacteristic slice of time. The parents are anxious and hopeful and the client may sense the tension. When the results are discussed, families often react with suspicion: "But he does those things at home all the time," or "Your results seem to be about a different person than the one we know."

One theme suggests that handicapped people are too often treated much like ethnic and other minorities, rather than like complete, fully accredited persons.[3] Part of the difficulty might be the widespread application of the "medical model" by professionals, even nonmedical ones. The potential for alienation, even humiliation, is high when the worst features of the biomedical-deviance model are invoked. The tendency to conduct procedures and tests "behind the backs" of the involved patient may leave them and others feeling more like specimens, rather than participants in a conjoint venture. There is some risk, under the best of circumstances, that clients will view professionals as engaging in a subtle conspiracy. Quiet procedures that have a "behind special doors" flavor may push families toward more open and "personalized" providers.

Families may be overwhelmed by the diverse kinds of professionals who contribute to the interdisciplinary team effort. It is not unusual for team members themselves to be puzzled by technical jargon and specialty turf. If professionals are confused, clients are confused even more by the babel of language and the diffusion of responsibility that they experience with the habilitation team.

Clients and families may object to their assigned role of "patient" rather than full participant. The contacts seem to be at the convenience of the professionals and at their place of activity. Professionals may imply that they expect unchallenged acceptance of their judgments as well as unquestioning compliance, often in matters that are distressingly complex, such as medications, special devices, documents, consultations, and so on.

Considering the stories of professional disregard and imposition, it is hardly surprising that families drift toward therapists who are more flexible and considerate. Many of the promoters of the unproven seem as interested in making the client comfortable as they are in pushing their therapeutic acrobatics.

Burnham[4] discussed the passing of American medicine's "golden age." He reviewed the erosion of the image of the physician, including the often repeated charges of greed, imposition, pretension, and the growing suspicion that many physicians may be deficient in technical knowledge and skill. There is concern that physicians are also profligate in their use of drugs, surgery, and other chancy therapies. The public's increasing awareness of medical details and the widespread recognition that people should challenge professionals on technical matters have tarnished the image of the physician. Despite medicine's remarkable leaps in technical competence, the sometimes distant, austere style of the health professional contributes to making people unhappy with their own health care and suspicious of professionals in general.

The vulnerability of families grows as standard interventions seem to offer limited benefits, and as alternative programs are put forward by enthusiastic and persuasive proponents. Our best hope for avoiding controversial therapies is some combination of valid advance in habilitation and health care methods, along with improvements, among professionals, in presenting, explaining, justifying, and advocating well-founded therapies, even those with limited compass and tentative prospects.

UTILITY OF THERAPY

Moving away from treatment modalities, consider the pitfalls of assignment of therapy. There are complex ethical and legal controversies surrounding the imposition of arbitrary training programs on people who, by any reasonable standards, cannot possibly achieve meaningful habilitative progress.

The ideal confluence of therapy and client is the application of a good treatment program to a receptive client who has enough responsiveness to benefit from the program. A less satisfactory, but common, situation is one in which the client has large reserves of response potential, but is provided with a poor treatment plan, which is given credit for providing benefits that would have occurred naturally without therapy.

A sensitive issue, frequently overlooked, is intervention with a good program with a client who has a fixed or deteriorating condition and who cannot benefit from any program. The best of interventions may degenerate into invasions when ritualistically applied to clients who deserve a more considerable, less intense program. The professional staff, in these cases, may become discouraged; they lose faith in their methods, and scarce resources are used up in activities that benefit no one.

The worst situation is the application of a poor or harmful program with clients who are unable to benefit from any therapy, even the best. The concerned observer may believe that someone must be to blame when therapy does not succeed; the observer may be quick to blame the professionals who are managing the therapy. Saddest of all, the professionals may be blaming the client for not responding as expected.

If data were systematically collected, appropriate value judgments could be made by the interested parties, and outcome utilities could be assigned to the four results possible in every treatment decision: (1) client treated—client benefits (true-positive), (2) client not treated—would not have benefited (true-negative), (3) client not treated—would have benefited (false-negative); and (4) client treated—no benefit (false-positive). If enough experience and data are gathered, and some values are agreed upon by the interested parties, it is theoretically possible to quantitate the moral, economic, and technical costs of each of the four outcomes.[5]

INSTITUTION OR COMMUNITY

Another controversy in treatment involves implementation of institutional versus community care. The uncritical, kneejerk allegiance to the idea of closing down all residential facilities for the developmentally disabled has been questioned. Zigler[6] comments, "Public policy is now committed to such concepts as deinstitutionalization and normalization. I join many workers in the field who view these concepts as little more than slogans that are badly in need of an empirical data base." Ellis[7] stated succinctly, "No one has demonstrated that learning is facilitated in clients by their movement to smaller facilities in the community."

A complex challenge in habilitation for the profoundly handicapped must be faced. A misconception about habilitation among legal advocates and others is the confusion of the "right to a program," the opportunity; with the "right to be benefitted," the outcome.[8] We can always provide a program, but not always benefit! There are no good methods available to predict those clients who will profit from training programs. Many serious scholars[7-9] have suggested that arbitrary, singleminded, ritualistic training programs should be replaced by "enrichment" programs that provide physical exercise, pleasant job activities, guidance in leisure time management, and other day-to-day experiences that have meaning and provide dignity to the recipient. There are uncertainties about the efficacy of the technology (behavioral programs) in training the profoundly neurologically impaired.[8] The efficacy of behavioral change has to be judged on several levels: the performance goal desired, the emotional and other costs of the training, the stability of the induced behavior, the staff resources available, and the likelihood that the acquired behavior will generalize to other areas of performance.

The quality of training programs depends on availability of trained staff, staff morale and enthusiasm, access to appropriate technology, and financial support.[7] The misuse of training resources on the nonresponding client may be degrading to the subject and defeating to the therapist. The training staff is at risk of burning out in unfruitful programs, when they might better be using their skills with clients who respond in meaningful ways.[9]

Many of the clients remaining in residential facilities, after the higher-level residents have been moved into the community, have formidable impairments. They are mainly adults, i.e., beyond the "developmental years." They often have serious health problems, multiple impairments, and difficult, self-abusive, aberrant conduct, and most have already failed to benefit from past training programs.[7] Only a small number of the profoundly impaired could be expected to manage, much less thrive, in a community setting. Training programs have not been shown to reduce the dangerous and defeating maladaptive behaviors. Many of the habilitation goals set by legal advocates are so inappropriate and artificial that professional judgment is often preempted and neutralized.

There are no clear answers to these problems, primarily because of the ethical concerns of the professionals and the value systems of the families and advocates. The issue is raised here only to indicate that it is alive and pulsating; there are humane and sensitive people, professionals and lay persons, ethicists and scientists, who are searching for persuasive guidelines for decisions in these controversial areas.

ATTITUDES TOWARD SCIENCE

It is not appropriate to attempt a detailed account of controlled therapeutic trials in this chapter, although the subject of unproven therapies requires a brief look at the concepts and methods of experimental design.

One requisite for meaningful research is a belief in science rather than intuition or hunch. The effort to establish medical therapeutics as a respected branch of experimental science has not been uniformly successful. Day[10] relates some experiences in pediatric research and the difficulties of carrying out clinical research and interpreting it to non-scientists, especially to legal and ethicist observers. He suggests that clinical research often allows too many variables to act simultaneously: "The lesson, it seems to me, is to make only one change at a time, and to test it . . . for both side effects and benefits." Day urges that medical students be exposed to courses that emphasize the logic and critical thinking of biostatistics, rather than the computation.

Werry[11] commented on the impact of social trends on the attitude of the general public toward science, especially therapeutics:

> The discovery in the sixties by a whole generation of Americans of injustice, poverty, racism, sexism, imperialism, exploitation, and ecological irresponsibility has led to many positive attitudes and developments but it has also resulted in a new form of totalitarianism based on anti-intellectualism and a contempt for patiently established truth, especially by the scientific method. . . . Much of the anti-medication movement not only views doctors as mere tools of the System, but regards the scientific method with suspicion. . . . [The scientific method] is unsurpassed in preventing the accumulation of knowledge based solely on superstition and self deception.

Elegant science is not as easy to accomplish as it is to endorse. A recent study of coronary heart disease[12] required follow-up of more than 12,000 men for several years, to evaluate the (controversial?) treatment of hypertension, reduction of smoking, and diet advice to lower cholesterol. The results of this laborious and expensive project were mixed: both the experimental and the control groups did better than expected. However, special health care interventions did not appear to produce greater benefits than the routine health care provided the control men. When we see unimpressive results from such elaborate and costly studies, using treatments that most health care professionals believe are effective, it is not surprising that promoters do not take eagerly to trying such prolonged and chancy ventures.

Der Simonian et al.[13] reviewed the methods required to ensure reliability and validity in therapeutic trials. Simeonsson et al.[14] discussed design features that are often neglected in evaluations of therapeutic programs, with special emphasis on child development: (1) careful definition of inclusion criteria, (2) random assignment of therapy, (3) control/contrast groups, (4) objective data collection, and (5) interrater reliability reports. Other safeguards are reviewed which prevent the capricious intrusion of wishful thinking, finagling, or self-deception.

The problem of inclusion criteria is particularly prominent in research in developmental disabilities, because of the variety of impairments and the idiosyncratic classification systems used by some researchers. Two recent reports on the benefits of megavitamins,[15,16] for example, leave the reader uninformed as to the specific disorders that the subjects had. Palframan et al.[17] discussed the multiple causes of hyperactivity in childhood. They list several diagnostic classes that are easily confused with attention-deficit disorder with hyperactivity: anxiety, conduct disorders, psychoses, mental retardation, cerebral palsy, seizure variants, and others. The investigator must carefully define the subjects studied, or the results are not interpretable and applicable to other people.

In a previous essay on controversial therapy,[18] careful attention was urged to the trial protocol: (1) definition of the subjects, (2) nonbiased selection criteria, (3) controls, (4) blinding techniques, (5) objective reproducible measurements, (6) standard analysis methods, (7) publication in peer-reviewed journals, and (8) acceptance of the impermanence of science. As Golden[19] and others[18,20,21] have indicated, the burden of proof of the efficacy of a new therapy is on the proponent, not on the audience or on the potential user. Golden notes that, "Critics of the technique need not prove noneffectiveness, but should insist on positive data from the proponents."

HALLMARKS OF QUACKERY

Health care sects of peculiar bent are not recent inventions. King[22] recounts the colorful ideas and methods of various schools of herbal medicine in this country and describes the bizarre flowering of the theories of homeopathy. Interwoven in this account is the clear evidence that the controlled clinical trial has been slow to gain acceptance and a place of respect among the aggressive and impatient leaders of therapeutic "causes."

Carlova[23] described the "healers" waiting to move into health care whenever standard medicine seems to fail. These pushers are at times denounced as mobs trying to break into the mainstream of health care by brute force, rather than by earning credibility through study and hard work. Carlova makes another compelling warning: If traditional medicine is to be persuasive in opposing unproven therapies and health fads, the opposition must be voiced on the basis of danger to patient care and not on the basis of financial loss.

The promoters, whether charlatans or self-deceiving humanists, show an antic array of tipoffs that a strange game is afoot. Golden[19] mentions that the theories are often eccentric; benefits are claimed for a wide range of diseases; the treatments are touted as completely harmless; testimonials and anecdotes abound; and the therapies often have a gripping emotional appeal, i.e., they are "natural," "organic," and unsullied by modern technology.

A brochure published by the American Council on Science and Health[24] cites ploys used by the pusher of the panacea (Table I). The Galileo ploy is the device of identifying with some authentic genius who once was derided and scorned, but who eventually was vindicated. The conspiracy theory implies that the government, big industry, and the medical establishment are conspiring to suppress life-saving therapies because of greed.

Table I. Ploys Used in Promoting
Nonscientific Therapeutic Approaches[a]

Exploitation of the natural fear of disease
Uncertainy about traditional medical care
Promises of painless treatment
Promises of good results
Claims of miraculous scientific breakthroughs
Simpleton science
The Galileo ploy
The conspiracy theory
The moving target
Reliance on testimonials
Appeals to freedom of choice

[a]Adapted from American Council on Science and Health.[24]

The moving target is the ploy of shifting claims so rapidly that the critic is always several steps behind the latest assertion. Cassileth[25] presented an excellent discussion of the conspiracy theory, body purification, and related "naturopathic" schemes. Brown[18] provided several tipoffs to weakly supported therapy. Two techniques have a rather engaging, ingenious quality. One is the reflected glory ploy of claiming intimacy with an eminent person, then using this familiarity as evidence of validation. "As I said to Denton (or Jonas . . . or Linus), this is a boon for mankind. And he didn't disagree!" The second ploy with panache is one in which a promoter broadcasts his contempt for an obvious fraud (e.g., bee pollen to stop aging), then urges that "we reasonable people" stick together to support truth. If we stand united against "that quackery," we therefore must share a bond with our righteous comrade's therapeutic theories. A comment by Ferry[21] applies to all these controversial therapies: "Surely it is time for us to plan *rational* therapeutic endeavors for the handicapped children and families we serve. . . ."

UNPROVEN

Historians of the future may call the epoch of the middle years of this century the age of the randomized clinical trial in therapeutic research. Spodick[26] noted that we are in an era that devotes considerable effort to avoid major research pitfalls. The careful investigator strives to avoid conclusions based on tradition, zeal, questionable data, and the perenniel siren song, "It can't hurt," or the contrapuntal refrain, "Prove me wrong." Spodick discussed the rather "schizoid behavior" of the therapeutic community in setting high standards for assessing new medications, but few for new surgical procedures. "There is no FDA for the surgeon." Similarly, there are no standards for evaluating nutritional interventions and other management protocols, such as stroke rehabilitation, language therapy, and special education.

The controlled therapeutic trial continues to meet opposition from some professionals and many nonscientists. Some of the pressures against such trials include (1) uncritical respect for authority ("My professor taught . . . "); (2) reverence for hearsay and tradition ("Preoperative enemas are necessary"); (3) the urge to do something, no matter how antic; (4) the fear that patients will be harmed in clinical trials; and (5) the conviction that uncontrolled, pilot trials will lead to knowledge. In spite of regular warnings against uncontrolled pilot trials, they continue to be done; their chief contribution is to lead us into accepting the unproven or rejecting the potentially provable.[13] The word "unproven" in a legal context assumes a glacial, slightly scornful, aspect—"your case is weak, your evidence is unconvincing." In a scientific context, *unproven* has a devasting impact. The work of a lifetime can be swept away by a distributed verdict among the experts: "The thesis is unproven!" In Scottish law the decision of "not proven" can be reached, in contrast to our "not guilty." The accused is not given a clear bill of moral health; instead, the prosecution simply has not established its accusations. The distinction is similar to accepting the null hypothesis in an experiment; the researcher concludes that, if an effect is present, it is not apparent. The word "unproven" denotes many layers of inference for the scientists: (1) claims are being promoted that lack supporting evidence; (2) there is a suspicion of unseemly haste to get the attention of an uncritical audience; and (3) there is a hint of exploitation or pecuniary expediency. The scientist who castigates Drug X as "unproven" may sound to the nonscientist as if he is still willing to be convinced. If the individual were open to persuasion, comments such as "the early data are suggestive . . . or encouraging . . . or tentatively persuasive," would be employed. When the label "unproven" is used by a scientist the implication is that judgment is close to firm: the claims are not valid.

REVIEWS OF CONTROVERSIAL THERAPY

During the past decade, there have been several carefully reasoned reviews of controversial therapy in developmental pediatrics.[13,18,27,28,29] In each review, similar arrays of nonstandard therapy are discussed. Apparently some unfounded therapies seem to have amazing staying power. Golden[19] warned that we must be wary of not just controversial therapies; reminding us that many standard therapies have become "entrenched in clinical practice by many years of use" without critical controlled trials. Golden emphasizes that there has been a surprising general acceptance of many therapies founded on weak research. He reviewed the flimsy "science" behind megavitamins, mineral supplements (based on hair analysis), special diets, hypoglycemia therapy, motor patterning rituals, and optometric training; he cautioned that, "Each person must decide whether to practice science or magic."

Educators are becoming increasingly cognizant of the presence of pseudoscience in educational interventions. In the inaugural chapter of a new publication, *Learning Disabilities*, McCarthy[30] deplores the "plethora of panaceas" that parents are bombarded with, including eye training, megavitamins, elimination diets, special lights, yoga, biofeedback, and multisensory cutaneous stimulation. With some asperity McCarthy commented, as "one bud of our hydra breaks off and fades into oblivion . . (the promoters) come up with two or three more. . . ." McCarthy commented on the teaching of reading: "In spite of the monumental amounts of research in the teaching of reading, *there are no important facts* about methods of teaching reading which are incontestably known."

Brown[18] suggested that there might be a shared element between the lapses that lead to fraud (and finagling) in big science and the credulous acceptance of pseudoscience by the general public. A link between the peccant scientist and the gullible nonscientist may be a "loss of nerve." The scientist under pressure may cave in, he may cut corners; the nonscientist under pressure for a successful treatment may turn to the charlatan, the mountebank, the snake oil salesman.

Culbertson and Ferry[31] reviewed optometric exercises, perceptual–motor training, sensory integrative therapy, and special diets. They sum up: "To date all of the treatment modalities (for learning disabilities) remain unproven in their efficacy."

Hyperactivity in children has been the target of a multitude of interventions. Levine and Melmed[32] cite orthomolecular diets, megavitamins, motor patterning, antihistamines, optometry, and allergy desensitization. These workers are sanguine about the influence that pediatricians might have on treatment decisions: "Pediatricians have an important role to play as scientific consumer advocates." Does anyone listen?

Brief mention of mental illness is appropriate at this point. Wender and Klein's[33] monograph on the "new biopsychiatry" suggests that

> Mental illness, which brings not only suffering but also disrupted lives to both the patient and the patient's family, is distressingly common. Unfortunately, disagreement about how to approach it is equally common: sects abound, each claiming that it has discovered the basic truth and the perfect cure, and that all others worship false gods.

They comment on the interest in the general public in matters of the mind:

> Literary critics, philosophers, popular psychologists, and hordes of analysands consider themselves qualified to expound upon matters of mental health. This self-confidence is no substitute for convincing evidence. The prevailing belief in the overall effectiveness of many of the popular panaceas is unfounded.

Controversial therapies fall into three groups: (1) the currently accepted (stimulants for hyperactivity), (2) the still tentative but encouraging (biofeedback), and (3) the thoroughly discredited (patterning). These lists make dull reading, and they may make even the fairest critic look like a cynic or a therapeutic nihilist. In the sections that follow, a few specific controversial therapies are reviewed. The real issue however is how and why unfruitful interventions get established so quickly, firmly, and capriciously. Overattention to the fad itself may obscure the generic problem: Why do so many people eagerly repudiate or drift away from traditional therapy?

PATTERNING

The neurological constructs and the therapeutic acrobatics of the advocates of the motor patterning therapy, and related "neuromuscular" relearning programs, have not been shown to be valid. Chapanis[34] reviewed the theory of the Doman-Delacato intervention program; the critique is lucid and fair, and clearly demonstrates the lack of scientific credibility in the treatment. The American Academy of Pediatrics[35] issued a policy statement that should (but unfortunately will probably not) finally close the book on this kind of therapy. It is clear that the theories of neurological function are unsupported, the diagnostic techniques are bizarre, and the therapy is exhausting, demanding, and futile.

A tangent from patterning is a new manipulation applied directly to the skull. Gilmore[36] in a newsletter for parents, talks about "craniosacral therapy"—a kind of phrenology, molding personality by cranial massage. The therapy involves fine tuning the cerebral functions, e.g., language, thinking, attending, by inducing subtle movement in the plates of the cranium. The sad thing is not that such therapies are taken seriously by otherwise sensible people, but that they get respectful attention in a newsletter that is supposed to be helping families, not misguiding them.

SENSORY INTEGRATIVE THERAPY

A pioneer in the treatment of cerebral palsy makes a neurological assertion that may explain why developmentalists are wary of some muscle movement therapies: "It is therefore the body musculature which guides and directs the central nervous system."[37] This sounds like the neurologic theories articulated by the practitioners of sensory integrative therapy.

An investigator strongly identified with integrative and vestibular stimulation therapy is A. Jean Ayres. She describes her theories in a number of publications.[38,39] Her writing is replete with words like "possibly," "conceivably," and other qualifiers. A typical assertion sounds like this: If language requires complex motor integration, and people with poor integration have language problems, then enhancing general motor integration may help language. It is equally compelling to believe that spending a lot of time on "integration" may be time spent away from language. Cratty[40] is more precise and circumspect on his recommendations, warning that there are no adequate supporting data for many of Ayres's theories and therapeutic claims. He suggests that the program is probably an educational fad, but that there is some danger that the intrusion of the therapy could take the child away from more appropriate academic activities. Sensory integrative therapy may be a trendy therapy, as pointed out by Lerer, a pediatrician, in an Open Letter to An Occupational Therapist.[41] He aroused a number of people who stated that the therapy was firmly grounded in neurologic and educational data, and that Lerer was either short-sighted or malicious in challenging the program. This form of therapy appears to receive its most ardent support from occupational therapists employed by school systems. Unfortunately, these advocates do not seem to have interest in, or time for, controlled therapeutic trials to evaluate the various movement and sensory treatments that they advocate.

MEGAVITAMINS/ORTHOMOLECULAR THERAPY

The American Academy of Pediatrics[42] issued a policy statement in 1976 on the lack of scientific support for megavitamin therapy in childhood psychosis or learning disabilities. However, an article by Harrell et al.[15] reawakened the dormant interest in megadose vitamins as a treatment for mentally retarded children. The study is weakened by (1) vague criteria for selection of subjects, (2) loss of several subjects to follow-up, and (3) the peculiar use of thyroid in 13 of the 16 subjects reported. The American Academy of Pediatrics[43] was highly critical of the report by Harrell et al. Brenner[16] reported on a mixed group of children treated with a variety of high dose vitamins. The report illustrated many of the methodological problems often seen in studies of this type. The subjects are not described, random selection is not reported, the controls/contrasts are unclear, the methods of judging improvement are not stated, and there is great difficulty in telling what was done to whom.

Therapy with large doses of vitamins has been suggested for many years and for many disorders, especially chronic neurologic disease. There has been no convincing data on the efficacy of vitamin therapy for these disorders. It is therefore slightly unsettling to see in an Association for Retarded Citzens newsletter[44] that megavitamin therapy is still being viewed as an exciting prospect for treatment of the mentally retarded. A carefully designed study of vitamin and mineral supplements in Down syndrome has been reported by Bennett et al.[45] Observer bias was strictly controlled, and the assessment procedures were objective and thorough. These investigators found no benefits from the vitamin–mineral supplements in the patients' physical appearance, general health, intelligence, behavior, or adaptability as a result of the therapy.

The report mentions that many of the parents expressed gratitude that the controversial and overblown propaganda about megavitamin therapy had been at last clarified for them. They were relieved that they could go ahead with sensible programs for the children, without the fear that they were missing a breakthrough or were neglecting their loved ones.

VITAMINS IN GENERAL

In 1981 the sales of vitamins in the United States amounted to more than $980 million—almost $1 billion. One wonders whether some of that money might be better spent in other ways, perhaps in research in metabolic disease. *Prevention,* a monthly magazine devoted to promoting health, shows how editorial material can be tied in with advertising. About 20–30% of the magazine contains full-page ads for vitamins and other nutritional products. The articles, written for popular consumption, contain the expected mix of stories of short-term dramatic cures and testimonials. The articles reflect lack of controls and other defects of method that seem to invest the popular accounts by proponents of "natural" intervention.

There is a relationship between certain restricted diets, usually for food allergies, and vitamin deficiencies or excesses.[46,47] Silverman and Lecks[48] reported on an allergic child who had received a number of bizarre treatments, including severe restriction of protein and calories in the diet. However, the child was given vitamin supplements and gradually developed signs of vitamin A toxicity: fever, headache, stiff neck, dry skin, and fissured lips. The authors comment forcefully on the explosion in the mass media of "dietary fallacies, pseudoscientific nutrition, and food faddism." They also suggest that certain kinds of patients seem more susceptible to strange and nonstandard treatments, especially children with complex allergic diseases, hereditofamilial disorders, neurological impairments, and those with rare and obscure conditions for which there are no known treatments.

ALLERGY

Grieco[49] reviewed several controversial diagnostic and treatment programs in allergic disease. He discussed some rather antic methods, indicating the lack of supporting data for some of the more outlandish procedures, e.g., sublingual testing and treatment of food allergy. Grieco also discussed the lack of evidence in support of treatment with autogeneous urine immunization.

The matter of elimination or "defined" diets is a confused one. The confusion is not just in how to select patients and the diet they are to get. There is also the physiological question of whether the patient has a true allergy or some other anomaly of metabolism requiring avoidance of certain substances and foods.

Crook[50] frequently comments in journal letter sections, asserting that a variety of behavior problems can be managed by diet. He reported on a set of symptoms he terms the allergy-tension-fatigue syndrome. In lieu of a verified data base, the skeptic is invited to the clinic to see cures firsthand. Rapp,[51] an allergist, has also published letters in journals about the benefits of diet for a variety of childhood behaviors.

DIET AND HYPERACTIVITY

The literature on defined diets and hyperactive children is growing in size and complexity, but with heat rather than light. Wender[52] concluded that the evidence suggests that only a few children, if any, are likely to benefit from the "defined" diets that are included under the umbrella, Feingold diet.

Rapoport et al.[20] discuss diet and behavior in childhood:

> The Feingold hypothesis . . . seems to have assumed the status of dogma despite the fact that it remains only a hypothesis, not a proven fact. . . . The time has come when the promulgation of a treatment to an anxious and credulous public before it has been properly tested . . . should be regarded as a possible breech of medical ethics.

The NIH Consensus Development Conference[53] has been reported in several journals. The *Journal of the American Medical Association* published a news item on the conference[54] and later published the report of the panel, with an editorial by Gilbert B. Forbes,[55] a respected expert in metabolic disease. Forbes is reserved in his judgments on the correct state of knowledge about nutrition in relation to behavior, noting the possibility that diets act mainly through a placebo effect. He suggested that physicians face an interesting ethical problem when a family asks about a nutritional program that the physician firmly believes acts only as a placebo. In general, the Consensus panel comes to no firm recommendations about the benefits of defined diets in the treatment of childhood hyperactivity. The report stresses the need for more well-designed and well-conducted clinical trials, especially on the matter of uniform and consistent diagnostic groupings for children enrolled in the research. There do not appear to be sound theories behind the claimed benefits of dietary therapy of behavior problems in childhood. In the absence of sound theory, progress in research will be difficult.

STIMULANT MEDICATION

There is probably more controversy surrounding the issues of stimulant medication than the issue merits. Cowart[56] indicated that the consensus of experienced therapists is that these medications work very well in the short run; there are no major growth side effects, and many children seem to benefit from even the prolonged use of stimulant medications. Cantwell and Carlson[57] endorsed the use of stimulants in children who have been properly evaluated: "this form of therapeutic intervention for children with Attention Deficit Disorder with Hyperactivity has more empirical evidence to support it than any other therapeutic intervention in child psychiatry for any other condition.'' Other than a general aversion by the public to the use of medication in children, there may be a practical reason why families find stimulants unacceptable. That is, the patient himself violently or steadfastly opposes the medication. Sleator et al.[58] studied the opposition of children to taking stimulant medications. The children give a number of reasons for resisting, regardless of the benefits. This aversion may lead families to look for an alternative therapy that will be more acceptable to the patient, perhaps something like a change in diet that will involve the entire household. In any case, therapy with stimulant medication (in carefully diagnosed children with ADD with hyperactivity) should no longer be considered a controversial therapy.

DIETS IN GENERAL

Special diets and other colorful nutritional practices have been with us for a long time, and there are no indications (despite professional desires) that general interest will abate. White and Selvey[59] presented an overview of current activities in nutrition, including the Cambridge diet, starch blockers, megavitamins, hair analysis, and the new ''superoxide dismutase'' theory. This last theory hypothesizes that cellular scavengers ''clean out'' the cells, delaying aging while making the user beautiful. Also included in their review (with admirable restraint) are metabolic fads like laetrile, elmination diets, enzymes, cell injections, gland extract, colonic irrigations, and coffee enemas.

Several relatively recent articles have reviewed vegetarian diets, which are used in a variety of forms.[60–64] The main concerns of nutritionists are the dangers of interference with growth, the occurence of vitamin deficiencies, and the risk of mineral shortages. Finberg[61] suggested that we may have been lax in not forcefully voicing the risks of nonstandard diets: ''one of the major failings of present-day pediatricians lies in our not having effectively communicated to the public the things we know well, while frequently publicizing speculative and untested hypotheses.'' The public however is not always interested in or convinced by scolding from the nay-sayers in the ivory towers of biomedicine. The Beverly Hills diet is supported by a book that Nirkin[65] analyzed for nutritional inaccuracy. Innumerable errors of theory and fact seemed to undermine the credibility of the promoters of the diet. The Cambridge diet is discussed in *The Medical Letter*.[66] This diet is very low in calories (330 per day), and previous diets with very low calorie content, especially those with poor quality protein, have been associated with serious health problems, even death. The Cambridge diet is probably too restricted in calories to be safe for some people over a significant period of time, making medical supervision essential.

POTPOURRI

A miscellany of offbeat nutritional projects merit brief mention. Adler,[67] a language expert, reported on the beneficial effects of nutritional interventions on children with learning disabilities. He made this peculiar assertion: ''These conclusions cannot be documented by formalized and objective research (why not?), but only through subjective perceptions.'' Prinz et al.[68] reported that hyperactive children consume more sugar than do normal children. The possibility that the hyperactivity leads to more sugar intake is not mentioned, only that greater sugar intake leads to hyperactivity. They also looked for evidence in support of the Feingold hypothesis, but found none. Pueschel *et al.*[69] studied 5-hydroxytryptophan (5-HT) and pyridoxine therapy in young children with Down syndrome and found no significant changes in muscle tone or cognitive ability in the treated children.

The Medical Letter[70] reported on fish oil capsules as a new supplement to prevent atherosclerosis. The capsules are sold in health food stores, but there is no evidence that the material helps the cardiovascular system or that it is safe for long-term use. Page[71] reported on herbal medicine obtainable by mail from Hong Kong. The pills contain prednisone and indomethacin, as well as high levels of lead.

Morgan[72] reviewed a fascinating chapter on self-treatment in this country in an account of the partial paralysis of about 50,000 Americans during the 1930s due to poisoning with Jamaica ginger. The condition was also called "jake leg." Jamaica ginger, an extract of ginger root, was added to water as a treatment for respiratory symptoms, digestive disorders, and menstrual irregularities. The specific poison found in Jamaica ginger is triorthocresyl phosphate (TOCP), which caused poisoning of about 10,000 Moroccans when airplane hydraulic fluid was used in cooking oil.

Some non-nutritional controversies are of passing interest. Burkitt,[73] with ill-disguised asperity commented on the fatuity of routine preoperative enemas, which have been abandoned in many European countries, Australia, New Zealand, and South Africa. The place of optometric exercises for treatment of learning disorders continues to be controversial. The December 1981 issue of *The Journal of Learning Disabilities* was devoted to optometry.[74] To the skeptical reader, the case for optometric exercises for learning disabilities remains unproved.

A controversy recently flared about a research report suggesting that alcoholics can be taught to drink moderately rather than being urged to refrain completely.[75] Adequate follow-up indicates that alcoholics allowed moderate drinking may do very poorly. And a final controversy: Does aspirin contribute to the risk of developing Reye syndrome?[76,77] This is a rather pathetic parade of examples of our gullibility.

TWO PERSONALITIES

Two eminent men show how success in nonscientific areas may be weak preparation for dealing with complex technical matters in therapeutics. Mr. Jack Dreyfus became a multimillionaire at an early age; he founded the Dreyfus Fund and was a renowned investment prodigy. He became interested in the anticonvulsant, phenytoin (Dilantin); he is convinced that phenytoin is an effective treatment for a remarkably long list of diseases, including depression, alcohol withdrawal, muscle disorders, heart disease, fear reactions, anxiety, various allergic conditions, and pain syndromes. Mr. Dreyfus's views are presented in his book, *A Remarkable Medicine Has Been Neglected*. Sun[78] described the obsessive focus of Mr. Dreyfus on phenytoin and his persisting attempts to get more widespread attention for the drug.

Norman Cousins, a distinguished editor and author, illustrates how uncertain the trip may be from the literary to the scientific world. The strange saga of Norman Cousins's illness and self-cure are recounted in his book.[79] It is reported that he has received thousands of letters from physicians expressing moral support and complimenting him on his eloquent appeal to physicians to listen to their patients.[80,81] While in his forties, Cousins came down with an obscure, still undiagnosed, illness with a bizarre mix of manifestations that suggest some kind of arthritis or other connective tissue disease. He diagnosed the disease as "adrenal exhaustion" and decided on his own therapy. Cousins began the treatments in a hospital. After moving into a hotel, Cousins set up his own therapeutic domain, including facilities to provide laughter, positive emotions, and equipment and staff for intravenous vitamin C. Cousins's reasons for selecting vitamin C and the dosages utilized are unclear. He assiduously watched his sedimentation rate decrease as his symptoms subsided. As time passed, Cousins made remarkable improvement (the natural tendency for some sick people to get better was ignored). He favored the theory that his physicians could not diagnose his illness; therefore, he had to take matters into his own hands, leading to self-cure by humor, positive emotions, and intravenous vitamin C. Some standard (but unspecified) medications may have also been used. Although Cousins received a large outpouring of support from physicians, there has been surprisingly mild reaction to the lack of scientific support for his assertions. There are two critical reviews of Cousins's account of his self-cure.[82,83] There seem to have been no formal comments from physicians about the passivity of Cousins's physician during this self-treatment.

Cousins and Dreyfus illustrate the dangers of assuming that a person who is outstanding in a literary or commercial enterprise is also equipped to handle the logic and detached objectivity required of the scientist. Neither appears to have a rudimentary grasp of experimental design, controls, measurement criteria, the dangers of testimonials, or other technical requirements for therapeutic research.

CONCLUSIONS

Keeping up with fad health and controversial therapies is a never-ending festival of wondrous claims, clever ploys, antic endorsements, and charismatic personalities. If many people were not being bilked of their money and time, or actually physically harmed, it would be a carnival of delight. The harsh reality, however, is that the rigors and ponderousness of the scientific method are easily circumvented, and the parade goes on. One aim of this chapter is to suggest that health care professionals re-examine their interactional styles in the hope that families will not be driven by us into the hands of promoters. Another aim is to invite attention to the rigorous and demanding protocols that must be followed in clinical therapeutic trials. The health professional can judge for himself, in the light of his own scientific standards, whether to believe assertions about dramatic new therapies. And a final aim: Perhaps the discouraging prevalence of unproven therapies can be softened by making a game of classifying the "hallmarks of quackery" that tip off the strident and self-serving antics of the promoters.

REFERENCES

1. Schild, S.: The family of the retarded child, in Koch, R., and Dobson, J. C. (eds.): *The Mentally Retarded Child and His Family.* Brunner/Mazel, New York, 1976, pp. 454–465.

2. Fredrickson, D. S.: "Venice" is not sinking (the water is rising). Some views on biomedical research. *J.A.M.A.* **247:**3072–3075, 1982.
3. Gliedman, J., and Roth, W.: *The Unexpected Minority.* Harcourt, Brace, Jovanovich, New York, 1980.
4. Burnham, J. C.: American medicine's golden age: What happened to it? *Science* **215:**1474–1479, 1982.
5. Miller, M. C. III, Westphal, M. C., Jr., and Reigart, J. R., II: *Mathematical Models in Medical Diagnosis.* Praeger, New York, 1981.
6. Zigler, E.: National crisis in mental retardation research. *Am. J. Ment. Defic.* **83:**1–8, 1978.
7. Ellis, N. R.: On training the mentally retarded. *Anal. Intervent. Dev. Disab.* **1:**99–108, 1981.
8. Baumeister, A. A.: The right to habilitation: What does it mean? *Anal. Intervent. Dev. Disab.* **1:**61–74, 1981.
9. Bailey, J. S.: Wanted: A rational search for the limiting conditions of habilitation in the retarded. *Anal. Intervent. Dev. Disab.* **1:**45–52, 1981.
10. Day, R. L.: Faith, doubt, and statistics. *Pediatrics* **67:**101–106, 1981.
11. Werry, J. S. (ed.): *Pediatric Psychopharmacology: The Use of Behavior Modifying Drugs in Children.* Brunner/Mazel, New York, 1978.
12. Multiple Risk Factor Intervention Trial Research Group: Multiple risk factor intervention trial. *J.A.M.A.* **248:**1465–1477, 1982.
13. DerSimonian, R., Charette, L. J., McPeek, T. S., *et al.*: Reporting on methods in clinical trials. *N. Engl. J. Med.* **306:**1332–1337, 1982.
14. Simeonsson, R. J., Cooper, D. H., and Scheiner, A. P.: A review and analysis of the effectiveness of early intervention programs. *Pediatrics* **69:**635–641, 1982.
15. Harrell, R. F., Capp, R. H., Davis, D. R., *et al.*: Can nutritional supplements help mentally retarded children? An exploratory study. *Proc. Natl. Acad. Sci. U.S.A.* **78:**574–578, 1981.
16. Brenner, A.: The effects of megadoses of selected B complex vitamins on children with hyperkinesis: Controlled studies with long term follow-up. *J. Learn. Disab.* **15:**258–264, 1982.
17. Palframan, D. S., Balmaceda, R., and Dimock, J.: The multifactorial etiology of hyperkinetic syndrome. Psychiatr. J. Univ. Ottawa **6:**161–169, 1981.
18. Brown, G. W.: A loss of nerve. *J. Dev. Behav. Pediatr.* **3:**88–95, 1982.
19. Golden, G. S.: Nonstandard therapies in the developmental disabilities. *Am. J. Dis. Child.* **134:**487–491, 1980.
20. Rapoport, J. L., Mikkelson, E. J., Werry, J. S.: Antimanic, antianxiety, hallucinogenic and miscellaneous drugs, in Werry, J. S. (ed.): *Pediatric Psychopharmacology.* Brunner/Mazel, New York, 1978, pp. 316–355.
21. Ferry, P. C.: On growing new neurons: Are early intervention programs effective? *Pediatrics* **67:**38–41, 1981.
22. King, L. S. III: Medical sects and their influence. *J.A.M.A.* **248:**1221–1224, 1982.
23. Carlova, J.: Will low-cost "healers" replace M.D.s? *Med. Econ.*, Aug. 9, 84–90, 1982.
24. American Council on Science and Health: "Vitamin B-15": Anatomy of a health fraud. Summit, New Jersey, 1981.
25. Cassileth, B. R.: After laetrile, what? *N. Engl. J. Med.* **306:**1482–1484, 1982.
26. Spodick, D. H.: Randomized controlled clinical trials—The behavioral case. *J.A.M.A.* **247:**2258–2260, 1982.
27. Silver, L.: Acceptable and controversial approaches to treating the child with learning disabilities. *Pediatrics* **55:**406–415, 1975.
28. Arnold, L. E.: Parents of hyperactive and aggressive children, in Arnold, L. E. (ed.): *Helping Parents Help Their Children.* Brunner/Mazel, New York, 1978, pp. 192–207.
29. Gottlieb, M. I.: The learning-disabled child: Controversial issues revisited, in Gottlieb, M. I., Zinkus, P. W., and Bradford, L. J. (eds.): *Current Issues in Developmental Pediatrics: The Learning-Disabled Child.* Grune & Stratton, New York, 1979, pp. 219–259.
30. McCarthy, J. M.: Cross currents and prevailing winds: 1982. *Learn. Disab.* **1:**3–10, 1982.
31. Culbertson, J. L., and Ferry, P. C.: Learning disabilities. *Pediatr. Clin. North Am.* **29:**121–136, 1982.
32. Levine, M. D., and Melmed, R. D.: The unhappy wanderers: Children with attention deficits. *Pediatr. Clin. North Am.* **29:**105–120, 1982.
33. Wender, P. H., and Klein, D. F.: *Mind, Mood, and Medicine.* Farrar-Straus-Giroux, New York, 1981.
34. Chapanis, N. P.: The patterning method of therapy: A critique, in Black, P. (ed.): *Brain Dysfunction in Children: Etiology, Diagnosis, and Management.* Raven, New York, 1981, pp. 265–280.

35. American Academy of Pediatrics: The Doman-Delacato treatment of neurologically handicapped children. *Pediatrics* **70**:810–812, 1982.
36. Gilmore, N. J.: Right-brain, left-brain asymmetry. *ACLD Newsbriefs* 19, 1982.
37. Bobath, K.: A neurophysiological basis for the treatment of cerebral palsy. *Clin. Devel. Med.*, no. 75. Lippincott, Philadelphia, 1980.
38. Ayres, A. J.: *Sensory Integration and Learning Disorders.* Western Psychologic Services, Los Angeles, 1973.
39. Ayres, A. J.: Learning disabilities and the vestibular system. *J. Learn. Disab.* **11**:18–29, 1978.
40. Cratty, B. J.: *Remedial Motor Activity for Children.* Lea & Febiger, Philadelphia, 1975.
41. Lerer, R. J.: An open letter to an occupational therapist. *J. Learn. Disab.* **14**:3–4, 1981.
42. American Academy of Pediatrics, Committee on Nutrition: Megavitamin therapy for childhood psychosis and learning disabilities. *Pediatrics* **58**:910–911, 1976.
43. American Academy of Pediatrics, Committee on Nutrition: Megavitamins and mental retardation. *AAP News Comments* p. 11, Sept. 1981.
44. The ARC, Association for Retarded Citizens: *Newsletter* July/Aug., p. 6, 1982.
45. Bennett, F. C., McClelland, S., Kriegsmann, E. A., *et al.*: Vitamin and mineral supplementation in Down's syndrome. *Pediatrics* **72**:707–713, 1983.
46. Herbert, V.: *Nutrition Cultism: Facts and Fictions.* GF Stickley, Philadelphia, 1980.
47. Farris, W. A., and Erdman, J. W., Jr.: Protracted hypervitaminosis A following long-term low-level intake. *J.A.M.A.* **247**:1317–1318, 1982.
48. Silverman, S. H., and Lecks, H. I.: Protein-calorie deficiency and vitamin indiscretion in an atopic child who developed hypervitaminosis A. *Clin. Pediatr.* **21**:172–174, 1982.
49. Grieco, M. H.: Controversial practices in allergy. *J.A.M.A.* **247**:3106–3111, 1982.
50. Crook, W. G.: Adolescent behavior. (Letter.) *Clin. Pediatr.* **21**:501, 1982.
51. Rapp, D. J.: Diet and hyperactivity. (Letter.) *Pediatrics* **67**:937, 1981.
52. Wender, E. H.: New evidence on food additives and hyperkinesis. *Am. J. Dis. Child.* **134**:1122–1128, 1980.
53. NIH Consensus Development Conference: Defined diets and childhood hyperactivity. *Clin. Pediatr.* **21**:627–630, 1982; *J.A.M.A.* **248**:290–292, 1982; *Science* **215**:958, 1982.
54. Bolsen, B.: No agreement on diets for "hyperactive" kids. *Med. News J.A.M.A.* **247**:948; 953; 956, 1982.
55. Forbes, G. B.: Nutrition and hyperactivity. *J.A.M.A.* **248**:355–356, 1982.
56. Cowart, V. S.: Stimulant therapy for attention disorders. *Med. News J.A.M.A.* **248**:279; 283–287, 1982.
57. Cantwell, D. P., and Carlson, G. A.: Stimulants, in Werry, J. S. (ed.): *Pediatric Psychopharmacology.* Brunner/Mazel, New York, 1978, pp. 171–207.
58. Sleator, E. K., Ullmann, R. K., and vonNeumann, A.: How do hyperactive children feel about taking stimulants and will they tell the doctor? *Clin. Pediatr.* **21**:474–479, 1982.
59. White, P. L., and Selvey, N.: Nutrition and the new health awareness. *J.A.M.A.* **247**:2914–2916, 1982.
60. Dwyer, J. T., Dietz, W. H., Jr., Hass, G., *et al.*: Risk of nutritional rickets among vegetarian children. *Am. J. Dis. Child.* **133**:134–140, 1979.
61. Finberg, L.: Human choice, vegetable deficiencies, and vegetarian beliefs. *Am. J. Dis. Child.* **133**:129, 1979.
62. Zmora, E., Gorodischer, R., and Bar-Ziv, J.: Multiple nutritional deficiencies in infants from a strict vegetarian community. *Am. J. Dis. Child.* **133**:141–144, 1979.
63. MacLean, W. C., Jr., and Graham, G. G.: Vegetarianism in children. *Am. J. Dis. Child.* **134**:513–519, 1980.
64. American Academy of Pediatrics, Committee on Nutrition: Nutritional aspects of vegetarianism, health foods, and fad diets. *Pediatrics* **59**:460–464, 1980.
65. Mirkin, G. C., and Shore, R. N.: The Beverly Hills diet, dangers of the newest weight loss fad. *J.A.M.A.* **246**:2235–2237, 1981.
66. The Cambridge diet. *Med. Lett.* **24**:91, 1982.
67. Adler, S.: Nutrition and language-learning development in pre-school programs for children with learning disabilities. *J. Learn. Disabl.* **15**:323–325, 1982.
68. Prinz, R. J., Roberts, W. A., and Hantman, E.: Dietary correlates of hyperactive behavior in children. *J. Consult. Clin. Psychol.* **40**:760–769, 1980.
69. Pueschel, S. M., Reed, R. B., Cronk, C. E., *et al.*: 5-Hydroxytryptophan and pyridoxine: Their effects in young children with Down's syndrome. *Am. J. Dis. Child.* **134**:838–844, 1980.

70. Fish oil for prevention of atherosclerosis. *Med. Lett.* **24:**99–100, 1982.

71. Page, H.: Mail-order medication contains some surprises. *Med. News J.A.M.A.* **248:**623, 1982.

72. Morgan, J. P.: The Jamaica ginger paralysis. *J.A.M.A.* **248:**1864–1867, 1982.

73. Burkitt, D. P.: Procedures of unproved value. *J.A.M.A.* **247:**1278–1279, 1982.

74. Focus on optometry. *J. Learn. Disab.* **14:**546–590, 1981.

75. Norman, C.: No fraud found in alcoholism study. *Science* **218:**771, 1982.

76. American Academy of Pediatrics: Aspirin and Reye syndrome. *Pediatrics* **69:**810–812, 1982.

77. FDA Drug Bulletin: Salicylate labeling may change because of Reye syndrome. **12:**9–10, 1982.

78. Sun, M.: Book touts Dilantin for depression. *Science* **215:**951–952, 1982.

79. Cousins, N.: *Anatomy of an Illness, as Perceived by the Patient.* Norton, New York, 1979.

80. Holden, C.: Cousins' account of self-cure rapped. *Science* **214:**892, 1981.

81. Ingelfinger, F.: Listen to the patient—once again. *N. Engl. J. Med.* **295:**1478–1479, 1976.

82. Kahn, S.: The anatomy of Norman Cousins' illness. *Mt. Sinai J. Med.* **48:**305–314, 1982.

83. Ruderman, F. A.: A placebo for the doctor. *Commentary* 54–60, May 1980.

Appendixes

Psychoeducational Testing

PSYCHOEDUCATIONAL TEST BATTERY USED IN THE DIAGNOSIS OF DEVELOPMENTAL DISABILITIES[a]

Name of test	Age range of test (years-months)[b]	Comments
	I. Intelligence and Readiness Tests	
Stanford-Binet Intelligence Scale for Children—Revised (Houghton-Mifflin, 1960)	2-0 to 18-0	Test of general intellectual development. Series of subtests grouped into age levels measuring comprehension, abstract reasoning, concept formation, and visuoperceptual skills. Predominantly tests verbal intelligence.
Wechsler Intelligence Scale for Children (WISC) (Psychological Corporation, 1944)	5-0 to 15-0	Excellent test of general intellectual ability. Full-scale IQ reflects overall intellectual level. Verbal IQ indicates intellectual ability related to verbal skills such as comprehension, abstract reasoning, vocabulary, memory, and arithmetic. Subtests are sensitive to auditory perceptual and language deficits. Performance IQ indicates intellectual ability related to nonverbal skills such as visual sequencing, visuospatial relationships, and visuomotor coordination. Subtests are sensitive to deficits in visuoperceptual skills. Difficulty with certain subtests may reflect the presence of a learning disability.
Wechsler Intelligence Scale for Children—Revised (WISC-R) (Psychological Corporation, 1974)	6-0 to 16-11	1974 revision of the WISC. Reduces cultural bias of the WISC.
Wechsler Preschool and Primary Scale of Intelligence (WPPSI) (Psychological Corporation, 1967)	4-0 to 6-6	Provides a general IQ score; verbal and performance IQs. Separate subtest scores useful in comparing skills.

(continued)

PSYCHOEDUCATIONAL TEST BATTERY USED IN THE DIAGNOSIS OF DEVELOPMENTAL DISABILITIES[a] (Continued)

Name of test	Age range of test (years-months)[b]	Comments
Peabody Picture Vocabulary Tests (PPVT) (American Guidance Service, 1959)	2-3 to 18-5	Essentially measures receptive language and ability to recognize pictures. Raw scores converted into mental ages and standard score IQ. May reflect a cultural bias. Can be used with language-impaired children.
Lorge-Thorndike (Group Intelligence Test) (Houghton-Mifflin, 1964)	Grade: kindergarten to 12th	Less reliable than individual intelligence tests. Usually administered by teachers and/or school personnel.
Otis-Lenon (Group Intelligence Test) (Harcourt, Brace, Jovanovich, 1968)	Grade: kindergarten to 12th	Less reliable than individual intelligence tests. Usually administered by teachers and/or school personnel.

II. Special Intelligence Tests for Handicapped Children

Peabody Picture Vocabulary Tests (PPVT) (American Guidance Service, 1959)	2-3 to 18-5	Useful for language-impaired children.
Leiter International Performance Scale (C. H. Stoelting, 1948)	2-0 to 12-0	Useful for deaf or speech-handicapped children.
Hiskey-Nebraska Test of Learning Aptitude (Marshall S. Hiskey, 1966)	3-0 to 16-0	Useful for language- and/or hearing-impaired children.
Hayes Adaption of the Stanford-Binet (Houghton-Mifflin, 1960)	2-0 to 18-0	Useful for the visually handicapped.

III. Developmental Scales and Screening Tests

Bayley Scales of Infant Development (Psychological Corporation, 1969)	0-2 to 2-6	Provides a score of mental and psychomotor development.
Catell Infant Intelligence Scale (Psychological Corporation, 1969)	0-2 to 2-6	Basically an extension of the Stanford-Binet.
Columbia Mental Maturity Scale	3-0 to 12-11	Nonverbal test measured as mental age and IQ. Developed for use with cerebral palsy patients.
Denver Developmental Screening Test (DDST) (LADOCA Project and Publishing, 1969)	Birth to 6-0	Screening test for early development (gross motor, fine motor, language, and personal-social skills).
First Grade Screening Test (American Guidance Service)	Grade: late kindergarten or early first	Readiness screening test for first grade.
Gesell Developmental Schedules (Psychological Corporation, 1969)	4 (weeks) to 6-0	Test of early development.
Raven's Colored Progressive Matrices	4-6 to 11-6	Nonverbal test of general intelligence. Useful in assessing perceptual accuracy, reasoning ability, and visual discrimination.

PSYCHOEDUCATIONAL TEST BATTERY USED IN THE DIAGNOSIS OF DEVELOPMENTAL DISABILITIES[a] (Continued)

Name of test	Age range of test (years-months)[b]	Comments
Slosson Intelligence Test for Children and Adults (Slosson Educational Publications)	2-0 to adulthood	Verbally oriented screening test based on Gesell Scales and Stanford-Binet.
Vineland Social Maturity Scale (Psychological Corporation, 1953)	Infancy to 25	Assesses competence for daily living; social age and social quotient determined. Administered to child or guardian.
IV. Achievement Tests		
Wide Range Achievement Test (WRAT) (Psychological Corporation, 1965)	Kindergarten to college	Test of oral word reading, arithmetic, and spelling.
Peabody Individual Achievement Test (PIAT) (American Guidance Service)	5-3 to 18-3	Test of general information skills, mathematics, reading, and spelling.
California Achievement Test (Group) (California Test Bureau, 1963)	Grade: First to 12th	Screening of academic skills.
Metropolitan Achievement Test (Group) (Harcourt, Brace, Jovanovich, 1964)	Grade: First to 12th	Screening of academic skills.
V. Perceptual Development		
Illinois Test of Psycholinguistic Abilities (ITPA) (University of Illinois Press, 1968)	2-4 to 10-3	Evaluates auditory and visuoperceptual skills expressed in age. Assesses receptive, associative, and expressive processes.
Southern California Sensory Integration Tests (Ayers) (Western Psychological Services, 1972)	4-0 to 10-0	Useful in assessing visual, tactile and kinesthetic functioning.
VI. Auditory Perceptual Development		
Carrow Test for Auditory Comprehension of Language (Learning Concepts, 1973)	3-0 to 6-11	Useful in assessing auditory comprehension.
Goldman-Fristoe-Woodcock Test (American Guidance Service, 1970)	4-0 to adulthood	Test of speech sound discrimination skills.
Wepman Auditory Discrimination Test	5-0 to 8-0	Test requires that subject understands concept of "same" and "different."
VII. Visuoperceptual Development		
Bender Visual Motor Gestalt Test for Children (Western Psychological Services, 1962)	5-0 to adulthood	Test for visuomotor coordination and visuospatial orientation. Reflects brain damage and emotional disturbances. Test of figure copying; checking for distortions, angulations, rotations, fragmentations, and general disorganization.

(*continued*)

PSYCHOEDUCATIONAL TEST BATTERY USED IN THE DIAGNOSIS OF DEVELOPMENTAL DISABILITIES[a] (Continued)

Name of test	Age range of test (years-months)[b]	Comments
Frostig Developmental Test of Visual Perception (Consulting Psychologist Press, 1961)	3-0 to 9-0	Test of various visual-processing skills.
Slosson Drawing Coordination Test (Slosson Educational Publications, 1973)	1-0 to 12-0	Test of visuomotor coordination and visuospatial perception.
Visual Retention Test (Benton)	8-0 to adulthood	Test of visuomotor skills, visual memory, and spatial perception.
VIII. Neuropsychological Test		
Reitan Indiana Neuropsychological Test Battery (Neuropsychology Laboratory, 1955)	5-0 to adulthood	Assesses presence of brain dysfunction, perceptual and cognitive abilities.
IX. Emotional Development		
California Test of Personality (California Test Bureau, 1953)	Kindergarten age to adulthood	Inventory is self-reporting of areas such as sense of personal worth, family, and school relationships.
Child's Apperception Test (CAT) (C.P.S., 1961)	3-0 to 10-0	Series of animal picture cards focusing on problems of early childhood. Child projects experiences and problems from card interpretations.
Children's Personality Questionnaire (Institute for Personality and Ability Testing, 1963)	8-0 to 12-0	A self-report measurement.
Draw-A-Person Test (DAP) (Western Psychological Services, 1963)	3-0 to 13-0	Measures IQ on drawing of a human figure. Provides insight into child's self-concept.
Early School Personlity Questionnaire (Institute for Personality and Ability Testing, 1974)	6-0 to 8-0	A self-report measurement.
House–Tree–Person Projective Technique (Western Psychological Services, 1964)	3-0 to adulthood	Provides insight into child's self-concept and perception of the environment.
Rorschach Inkblot Test (Grune & Stratton, 1960)	3-0 to adulthood	Projective test involving 10 inkblot designs. Patient projects needs, anxieties, and conflicts.
Symond's Picture Story Test	Adolescent	Personality inventory for adolescents.
Thematic Apperception Test (Psychological Corporation, 1943)	4-0 to adulthood	Projective test in which child responds to pictures and constructs a story. Subject projects self into scenes he interprets, which may suggest emotional conflicts.

[a]Adapted in part from Sanders, M.J.: Psychological tests, in Gottlieb, M.I., Zinkus, P. W. and Bradford, L. I. (eds.): *Current Issues in Developmental Pediatrics: The Learning Disabled Child.* Grune & Stratton, New York, 1979.
[b]All age ranges are in years and months, except when noted otherwise.

TESTS COMMONLY EMPLOYED IN ASSESSING SPEECH AND LANGUAGE BEHAVIORS

Name of test	Age range of test[a] (years–months)
I. Language	
A. Receptive/Expressive	
Detroit Test of Learning Aptitude (The Bobbs-Merrill Co., Inc.)	3–0 to 19–0
Illinois Test of Psycholinguistic Abilities (ITPA) (University of Illinois Press)	2–4 to 10–3
Northwestern Syntax Screening Test (Northwestern University)	Up to age 8–0
Porch Index of Communicative Abilities in Children (Consulting Psychological Press)	Preschool to 12–0
Preschool Language Scale (Bell & Howell Co.)	1–0 to 7–0
Receptive-Expressive Emergent Language Scales (REEL) (Computer Management Corp.)	Birth to 3–0
B. Receptive	
Assessment of Children's Language Comprehension (Consulting Psychologist Press)	Grade: prekindergarten to school age
Boehm Test of Basic Concepts (Psychological Corporation)	Grade: kindergarten to 2nd
Peabody Picture Vocabulary Test (PPVT) (American Guidance Service)	2–3 to 18–5
Test for Auditory Comprehension of Language-Revised (Carrow) (DLM Teaching Resources)	3–0 to 10–0
Test of Receptive Language (G-B Services, Canada)	7–0 to 12–0
Test of Syntactic Abilities (Quigley) (Dormac, Inc.)	10–0 to 18–0
B. Expressive	
Test of Expressive Language (written) (G-B Services, Canada)	7–0 to 12–0
II. Articulation	
Fisher-Logemann Test of Articulation Competence (Houghton-Mifflin, Co.)	Grade: prekindergarten (to adulthood)
Goldman-Fristoe Test of Articulation (American Guidance Service)	Grade: prekindergarten (to school age)
McDonald's Deep Test of Articulation (Stanwix House, Pittsburgh)	School age
Preschool Language Scale (Bell & Howell Co.)	2–0 to 7–0
The Templin-Darley Tests of Articulation (University of Iowa Bureau of Educational Research and Service)	School age
III. Auditory Processing: Discrimination	
Wepman Auditory Discrimination Test Language Research Associates (Chicago)	5–0 to 8–0
IV. Memory/Sequencing	
Detroit Test of Learning Aptitude (The Bobbs-Merrill)	3–0 to 19–0
Clinical Evaluation of Language Functions (Charles E. Merrill)	6–3 to 9–2; grade: kindergarten to 12th

[a]All age ranges in years and months, except when noted otherwise.

DIRECTORY OF DEVELOPMENTAL TESTING INSTRUMENTS

Developmental Inventories

Bayley Scales of Infant Development
  Psychological Corporation
  7500 Old Oak Road
  Cleveland, Ohio 44130

Cattell Infant Intelligence Scales
  Psychological Corporation
  7500 Old Oak Road
  Cleveland, Ohio 44130

Revised Gesell Devlopmental Schedules
Revised Parent Developmental Questionnaire
  In: manual of Developmental Diagnosis,
  Knoblock et al. 1980
  Harper & Row, Hagerstown, Maryland

Goodenough-Harris Drawing Test
  Harcourt, Brace, Jovanovich, Inc.
  Test Department
  757 Third Avenue
  New York, New York 10017

Lexington Developmental Scales
  UCPB Child Development Center
  P.O. Box 8002
  465 Springhill Drive
  Lexington, Kentucky 40503

McCarthy Scales of Childrens Abilities
  Psychological Corporation
  7500 Old Oak Road
  Cleveland, Ohio 44130

Developmental Screening Inventories

Denver Developmental Screening Test (DDST)
Denver Developmental Screening Test-Revised
  (DDST-R)
Denver Developmental Questionnaire (PDQ)
LADOCA Project and Publishing Foundation, Inc.
  51st Avenue and Lincoln Street
  Denver, Colorado 80216

Kansas Infant Developmental Screen (KIDS)
  University of Kansas Medical Center
  Department of Community Health
  225 Family Practice Building
  39th and Rainbow Blvd.
  Kansas City, Kansas 66103

Lexington Developmental Scales (Short Form)
  UCPB Child Development Center
  P.O. Box 8003
  465 Springhill Drive
  Lexington, Kentucky 40503

Minnesota Child Development Inventory (MCDI)
Minnesota Preschool Inventory
  Behavior Science Systems, Inc.
  Harold R. Ireton, Ph.D.
  Box 1108
  Minneapolis, Minnesota 55440

Revised Developmental Questionnaire
  Revised Developmental Screening Inventory
  Benjamin Pasamanic
  Albany Medical College
  Albany, New York 12208

Language Assessment

Peabody Picture Vocabulary Test (PPVT)
  American Guidance Service
  Publishing Building
  Circle Pines, Minnesota 55014

Receptive-Expressive Emergent Language Scale
  (REEL)
  Computer Management Corp.
  Language Education Division
  Gainesville, Florida

Test For Auditory Comprehension of Language
  DLM Teaching Resources
  P.O. Box 4000
  One DLM Park
  Allen, Texas 75002

Early Language Milestone Scale (ELMS)
  Modern Education Corporation
  P.O. Box 721
  Tulsa, Oklahoma 74101

Readiness/Education Screening

Aggregate Neurobehaviorial Student Health and Educational Review (ANSER)
  Educators Publishing Service, Inc.
  75 Moulton Street
  Cambridge, Massachusetts 02138

Slosson Drawing Coordination Test
Slosson Oral Reading Test
  Slosson Educational Publications, Inc.
  P.O. Box 280
  East Aurora, New York, 14052

(continued)

DIRECTORY OF DEVELOPMENTAL TESTING
INSTRUMENTS (Continued)

Detroit Tests of Learning Aptitude
  Bobbs-Merrill Co., Inc.
  4300 West 62 Street
  Indianapolis, Indiana 46206

Gray Oral Reading Paragraphs Test
  Bobbs-Merrill Co., Inc.
  4300 West 62nd Street
  Indianapolis, Indiana 46206

Preschool Development Inventory (PDI)
  Behavior Science Systems, Inc.
  Harold Ireton, Ph.D.
  Box 1108
  Minneapolis, Minnesota, 55440

Pediatric Examination of Educational Readiness
  (PEER)
  Educators Publishing Service, Inc.
  75 Moulton Street
  Cambridge, Massachusetts 02138

Wide Range Achievement Test
  Guidance Association
  1526 Gilpin Avenue
  Wilmington, Delaware

Vision Testing

Allen Cards—Preschool Vision Test
  Mead Johnson
  Evansville, Indiana 47721

Keystone Vision Tester
  Mast Development Co.
  2212 East 12th Street
  Davenport, Iowa 52803

Snellen Chart
  American Optical Company

Titmus Vision Tester
  Titmus Optical Co., Inc.
  Pettersburg, Virginia 23803

Speech/Language and Hearing

DEVELOPMENTAL NORMS: EXPRESSIVE AND RECEPTIVE LANGUAGE[a]

Age	Expressive language	Receptive language
1 month	Sighs, grunts, and small throaty noises Meager vocalizations Undifferentiated crying	Activity may cease with sound stimulus Attends to human voice
2–3 months	Differentiated crying, cooing, or babbling sounds Vocalizes as a result of need fulfillment Repetitive vocalizing ("dadada")	Attends to human voice with smiles and cooing May anticipate sounds associated with feeding Soothed by adult voice
4–5 months	Babbling Socialized vocalization (oo's, chuckles, laughs) Uses sound to get attention Uses some consonants	Turns to voice on hearing name May turn head to familiar sound
6–9 months	Lalling Coos to music Crows and squeals Some intonations Syllables, consonants, and front vowels	Turns to bell Smiles in response to speech Listens to familiar words Begins response to words with gestures ("bye-bye")
9–12 months	Beginning of speech ("dada") First words distinct Echolalia Imitates inflections Imitates syllables and words	Adjusts to words Imitates vocalizations of others Understands "no," "dada" Responds to name and simple commands Enjoys listening to words Responds by gesture to "patty cake" and "bye-bye"
12–18 months	Attention seeking by making noises Repeats familiar words Uses expressive jargon At 18 months has 15–20-word vocabulary Indicates wants	Responds to simple commands (hands you a block) Understands a demand
18–24 months	Meaningful speech Abandoning baby speech Beginning to combine words Hums and sings Approximately 300-word vocabulary Two words in sentence Specifies need for food, drink, etc. Uses two concepts ("Daddy gone")	Identifies some pictures from name Responds to simple commands ("Put doll on chair") Listens to rhymes and songs Attempts to follow more complex directions Points to body parts Increased comprehension
2–3 years	Speech intelligible and differentiated 450 words in vocabulary by 30 months Sentence length of 3–4-words Repeats syllables Occasional nonfluencies	Understands two prepositions Identifies pictures Responds to suggestions Memory span improves

(continued)

DEVELOPMENTAL NORMS: EXPRESSIVE AND RECEPTIVE LANGUAGE[a]   (Continued)

Age	Expressive language	Receptive language
3–4 years	Vocabulary of approximately 1000 words by 36 months Begins to use compound and complex sentences Sings phrases of songs Sentence lengths of 5 words Knows name, sex, address Expresses feelings and problems	Comprehends complex and compound sentences Listens to stories Answers simple questions Generalizations common in comprehension
4–5 years	Speech intelligibility approximately 98% Speech is forthright Can tell stories mixing fact and fiction Questions at a peak Sentence length 5+ words Talks about everything Conjunctions used	Sophistication of comprehension Tries to use new words Can define simple words Understands some abstract words Likes to be read to
5–8 years	Uses basic structures of sentences Language becomes more symbolic Learning to read and write	Begins abstracting and categorizing Defines and explains words

[a]Adapted in part from Gottlieb, M. I., Zinkus, P. W., and Thompson, A.: Chronic middle ear disease and auditory perceptual deficits. *Clin. Pediatr.* **18**:725–732, 1979.

HEARING IMPAIRMENT AND ASSOCIATED DIFFICULTY WITH SPEECH DISCRIMINATION

ANSI (dB)	Degree of hearing loss	Associated difficulty with speech discrimination
25	Slight	Faint speech causes difficulty
40	Mild	Difficulty with normal speech at 1 m
55	Marked	Difficulty discriminating loud speech
70	Severe	Difficulty with amplified or shouted speech
90	Extreme	Generally no understanding of speech even when it is amplified

PARENT/PHYSICIAN HEARING CHECKLIST

Age	Hearing behaviors
Birth to 3 months	Startled by loud sounds Soothed by mother's voice
3–6 months	Head and eyes turn to locate sound Responds to mother's voice "Oohs, ba-ba's" Enjoy's sound-producing toys
6–10 months	Responds to name Responds to telephone ring Responds to conversational level voice Understands "no" and "bye-bye"
10–15 months	Can point to familiar object on command Imitates simple sounds Imitates simple words
15–18 months	Follows simple directions Vocalizes first words Many words by 18 months

COMMON NEURODEVELOPMENTAL COMPLICATIONS OF HEARING LOSS

Severity of hearing loss	Possible etiological origins	Complications		Types of therapy
		Speech/language	Educational	
Slight (15–25 dB)	Serous otitis media Perforation of tympanic membrane Sensorineural loss	Distant or faint speech may present a difficulty.	Possible auditory learning dysfunction; may reveal a slight verbal deficit.	Preferential class seating.
Mild (25–40 dB) (ASA)	Serous otitis media Perforation tympanic membrane Sensorineural loss Tympansclerosis	Difficulty with conversational speech over 3–5 feet; limited vocabulary and speech disorders may be observed.	May miss 50% of class discussions; auditory learning dysfunction.	Special education resource help; hearing aid; favorable class setting; lip-reading instruction; speech therapy.
Moderate (40–65 dB) (ASA)	Chronic otitis media Middle ear anomaly Sensorineural loss	Speech must be loud to understand; defective speech; deficient language use and comprehension.	Learning disability; difficulty with group learning or discussion; auditory processing dysfunction; limited vocabulary.	Special education resource or special class. Special help in speech/language development; hearing aid and lip-reading; speech therapy.
Severe (65–95 dB) (ASA)	Sensorineural loss Middle ear disease	Loud voices may be heard from ear: +/– identification of environmental sounds; defective speech and language. If before 1 year: no spontaneous development.	Marked educational retardation; marked learning disability; limited vocabulary.	Full-time education for deaf children; hearing-aid, lip-reading, speech therapy; auditory training; counseling.
Profound (≥95 dB) (ASA)	Sensorineural or mixed loss	Relies on vision rather than hearing; defective speech and language; speech and language will not develop spontaneously if loss present <1.	Marked learning disability due to no understanding of speech.	As above; oral and manual communication; counseling.

AMERICAN ACADEMY OF PEDIATRICS: JOINT COMMITTEE ON INFANT HEARING*

Early detection of hearing impairment in the affected infants is important for medical treatment and subsequent educational intervention to assure development of communication skills.

In 1973, the Joint Committee on Infant Hearing Screening recommended identifying infants at risk for hearing impairment by means of five criteria and suggested follow-up audiological evaluation of these infants until accurate assessments of hearing could be made (*AAP Newsletter Supplement*, October 1973). Since the incidence of moderate to profound hearing loss in the at-risk infant group is 2.5–5.0%, audiological testing of this group is warranted. Acoustical testing of all newborn infants has a high incidence of false-positive and false-negative results and is not universally recommended.

Recent research suggests the need for expansion and clarification of the 1973 criteria. This 1982 statement expands the risk criteria and makes recommendations for the evaluation and treatment of the hearing-impaired infant.

I. Identification

A. Risk criteria

Factors that identify those infants who are at risk for having hearing impairment include the following:

1. Family history of childhood hearing impairment
2. Congenital perinatal infection (e.g., cytomegalovirus, rubella, herpes, toxoplasmosis, syphilis)
3. Anatomic malformations involving the head or neck (e.g., dysmorphic appearance, including syndromal and nonsyndromal abnormalities, overt or submucous cleft palate, morphological abnormalities of the pinna)
4. Birth weight <1500 g
5. Hyperbilirubinemia at level exceeding indications for exchange transfusion
6. Bacterial meningitis, especially *Haemophilus influenzae*
7. Severe asphyxia that may include infants with Apgar scores of 0–3 or who fail to institute spontaneous respiration by 10 min and those with hypotonia persisting to 2 hr of age

B. Screening procedure

The hearing of infants who manifest any item on the list of risk criteria should be screened, preferably under the supervision of an audiologist, optimally by 3 months of age but not later than 6 months of age. The initial screening should include the observation of behavioral or electrophysiological response to sound. (The Committee has no recommendations at this time regarding any specific device.) If consistent electrophysiological or behavioral responses are detected at appropriate sound levels, the screening process will be considered complete except in those cases in which there is a probability of a progressive hearing loss; e.g., family history or delayed onset or degenerative disease, or history of intrauterine infection. If results of an initial screening of an infant manifesting any risk criteria are equivocal, the infant should be referred for diagnostic testing.

---

*Modified from AAP. Joint Committee on Infant Hearing: Position statement 1982. *Pediatrics* **70**:496, 1982. Copyright American Academy of Pediatrics, 1984.

II. Diagnosis for Infants Failing Screening

A. Diagnostic evaluation of an infant 6 months of age should include the following:
    1. General physical examination and history including:
        a. Examination of the head and neck
        b. Otoscopy and otomicroscopy
        c. Identification of relevant physical abnormalities
        d. Laboratory tests such as urinalysis and diagnostic tests for perinatal infections
    2. Comprehensive audiological evaluation:
        a. Behavioral history
        b. Behavioral observation audiometry
        c. Testing of auditory evoked potentials, if indicated
B. After the age of 6 months, the following are also recommended:
    1. Communication skills evaluation
    2. Acoustical immitance (impedance) measurements
    3. Selected tests of development

III. Management of the Hearing-Impaired Infant

Habilitation of the hearing-impaired infant may begin while the diagnostic evaluation is in process. The Committee recommends, however, that whenever possible, the diagnostic process should be completed and habilitation begun by the age of 6 months. Services to the hearing-impaired infant <6 months of age include the following:

A. Medical management
    1. Re-evaluation
    2. Treatment
    3. Genetic evaluation and counseling when indicated
B. Audiological management
    1. Ongoing audiological assessment
    2. Selection of hearing aid(s)
    3. Family counseling
C. Psychoeducational management
    1. Formulation of individualized educational plan
    2. Information about implications of hearing impairment

After the age of 6 months, the hearing-impaired infant becomes easier to manage in a habilitation plan but he will require the services listed above.

Selected Readings

Early Intervention

Ling, D.: Early speech development, in Mencher, G., Gerber, S. E. (eds.): *Early Management of Hearing Loss*. Grune & Stratton, New York, 1981, pp. 319–335.

McFarland, W. H., Simmons, F. B.: The importance of early intervention with severe childhood deafness. *Pediatr. Annu.* **9**:13, 1980.

Skinner, M.: The hearing of speech during language acquisition. *Otolaryngol. Clin. North Am.* **11**:631, 1978.

Identification of Hearing Impairment in Infants

Bess, F. H.: *Childhood Deafness: Causation, Assessment and Management*. Grune & Stratton, New York, 1977.

Greenstein, J. M., Greenstein, B. B., McConville, K., *et al. Mother–Infant Communication and Language Acquisition in Deaf Infants.* Lexington School for Deaf, New York, 1976.
Northern, J., and Downs, M.: *Hearing in Children.* Williams & Wilkins, Baltimore, 1978.

Diagnosis and Management

Gerber, S. E., and Mencher, G. T.: *Proceedings of Saskatchewan Conference on Early Diagnosis of Hearing Loss, Saskatoon, Saskatchewan, May 7–9, 1978.* Grune & Stratton, New York, 1978.
Mencher, G. T., and Gerber, S. E.: *Early Management of Hearing Loss.* Grune & Stratton, New York, 1981.
Simmons, B. F.: Diagnosis and rehabilitation of deaf newborns: Part II. *ASHA* **22:**475, 1980.

Evoked Potential Audiometry

Despland, P. A., and Galambos, R.: The auditory brainstem response (ABR) is a useful diagnostic tool in the intensive care nursery. *Pediatr. Res.* **14:**154, 1980.
Galambos, C., and Galambos, R.: Brainstem evoked response audiometry in newborn hearing screening. *Arch. Otolaryngol.* **105:**86, 1979.
Starr, A., Amlie, R. N., and Martin, W. H., *et al.*: Development of auditory function in newborn infants revealed by auditory brainstem potentials. *Pediatrics* **60:**831, 1977.

GUIDELINES FOR ASSISTING THE SCHOOL-AGE CHILD WITH AUDITORY DIFFICULTIES

Present materials slowly
Present materials as concretely as possible
Minimize background noise
Minimize distractions
Repeat materials as needed (question whether the child understands what is required)
Preferential classroom seating
Ensure teacher's awareness of problem
Resource assistance as needed

AMERICAN ACADEMY OF PEDIATRICS: MIDDLE EAR DISEASE AND LANGUAGE DEVELOPMENT*

There is growing evidence demonstrating a correlation between middle ear disease with hearing impairment and delays in the development of speech, language and cognitive skills. A parent or other caretaker may be the first person to detect such early symptoms as irritability, decreased responsiveness, and disturbed sleep. Middle ear disease may be so subtle that a full evaluation for this condition should combine pneumatic otoscopy, and possibly tympanometry, with a direct view of the tympanic membrane. This statement is not meant to be a recommendation for specific treatment methods. When a child has frequently recurring acute otitis media and/or middle ear effusion persisting for longer than 3 months, hearing should be assessed and the development of communicative skills must be monitored.

The Committee believes it is important that the physician inform the parent that a child with middle ear disease may not hear normally. Although the child may withdraw socially and diminish experimentation with verbal communication, the parent should be encouraged to continue commu-

*Modified from AAP: Policy statement: Middle ear disease and language development. *News Comment* **35**(9):9, 1984. Copyright American Academy of Pediatrics, 1984.

nicating by touching and seeking eye contact with the child when loudly and clearly speaking. Such measures, along with prompt restoration of hearing whenever possible, may help diminish the likelihood that a child with middle ear disease will develop a communicative disorder. Middle ear disease can occur in the presence of sensorineural hearing loss. Any child whose parent expresses concern about whether the child hears should be considered for referral for behavioral audiometry without delay.

Committee on Early Childhood, Adoption and Dependent Care

Selma Deitch, M.D., Chairman
David L. Chadwick, M.D.
Thomas Coleman, M.D.
Donna O'Hare, M.D.

Burton Sokoloff, M.D.
George G. Sterne, M.D.
Virginia Wagner, M.D.

Liaison Representatives
Elaine Schwartz, Children's Bureau, OHD, DHHS
Jeanne Hunzeker, DSW, Child Welfare League of America

Kenneth Grundfast, M.D., Section of Otolaryngology
Carol Gerson, M.D., Section of Otolaryngology

Selected Readings

Hanson, D. G., and Ulvestad, R. F. (eds.): Otitis media and child development: Speech, language and education. *Ann. Otol. Reninol. Laryngol.* Suppl. 60. **88**(5):part 2.

Bluestone, C. D., Klein, J. O., Paradise, J. L., *et al.*: Workshop on effects of otitis media on the child. *Pediatrics* **71**:639–652, 1983.

Date of approval by Executive Board: July 1984. Date of publication: September 1984

The Physician and the School

AMERICAN ACADEMY OF PEDIATRICS: SPORTS AND THE CHILD WITH EPILEPSY*

The 1968 statement of the Committee on Children with Handicaps, "The Epileptic Child and Competitive School Athletics," is restated with considerable modification.

The responsibility for weighing the risks involved in athletic participation should be shared by the parents, the physician, and the child. Such risks should be weighed against the psychological trauma resulting from unnecessary restriction of physical activities. Parents should participate in all decisions. To the degree appropriate to the age and judgment of the child, his wishes should be considered. The young athlete must be.taught that there is a risk of injury and that he should be prepared to impose voluntary restrictions on physical activity depending on the nature and frequency of seizures.

Proper medical management, good seizure control, and proper supervision are essential if children with epilepsy are to participate fully in physical education programs and interscholastic athletics. Common sense dictates that situations in which a seizure could cause a *dangerous* fall should be avoided. These situations include rope climbing, activity on parallel bars, and high diving. Swimming should be supervised; no competitive underwater swimming is acceptable. Participation in contact or collision sports should be given individual consideration according to the specific problem of the athlete. Epilepsy per se should not exclude a child from hockey, baseball, football, basketball, and wrestling.

Physicians who take care of children who are involved in athletics should realize that in today's culture, sports and athletic activity are extremely important to young people and that unnecessarily strict interpretation of medical conditions may in fact do more harm than good.

Committee on Children with Handicaps, 1982–1983

Albert C. Fremont, MD, Chairman   J. Albert Browder, MD, ARC–U.S.
Herbert J. Cohen, MD   Jane C. S. Perrin, MD, AAPM
James W. Coker, Jr., MD   Barry Russman, MD
Alfred Healy, MD   Section on Neurology
David W. MacFarlane, MD   Herman Saettler, EdD
Bernard Weisskopf, MD

Committee on Sports Medicine, 1982–1983
Thomas E. Shaffer, MD, Chairman   Henry Levison, MD
Paul G. Dyment, MD   Section on Diseases of the Chest
Eugene F. Luckstead, MD   James H. Moller, MD
John J. Murray, MD   Section on Cardiology
Nathan J. Smith, MD   Arthur M. Pappas, MD
Frederick W. Baker, MD   Section on Orthopaedics
  Canadian Paediatric Society   Richard Malacrea, NATA

*Modified from AAP. Committee on Children with Handicaps and Committee on Sports Medicine: Sports and the child with epilepsy. *Pediatrics* **72**:884, 1983. Copyright American Academy of Pediatrics, 1983.

Selected Readings

Bennett, P B , and Elliott, D H *The Physiology and Medicine of Diving and Compressed Air Work* 2nd ed
  Williams & Wilkins, Baltimore, 1975
Committee on Children with Handicaps, American Academy of Pediatrics The epileptic child and competitive
  school athletics *Pediatrics* **42:**700, 1968
Committee on the Medical Aspects of Sports, American Medical Association Epileptics and contact sports
  J A M A **229:**820, 1974
Committee on School Health, American Academy of Pediatrics *School Health A Guide for Health Profes
  sionals* American Academy of Pediatrics, Evanston, Illinois, 1981
Korezyn, A D Participation of epileptic patients in sports *J Sports Med* **19:**195, 1979
Livingston, and Berman, W Participation of the epileptic child in contact sports *J Sports Med* **2:**170 1974
Pearn, J , Bart, R , and Yamaoka, R Drowning risks to epileptic children A study from Hawaii *Br Med J*
  2:1284, 1978

AMERICAN ACADEMY OF PEDIATRICS ADMINISTRATION OF MEDICATION IN SCHOOL*

Many children with chronic disabilities or illnesses are able to attend school because of the effectiveness of their prescribed medication Any student who is required to take prescribed medication
during regular school hours should do so in compliance with school regulations These regulations
should include the following

1. A physician should provide written orders with the name of the drug, dose, time interval
   when the medication is to be taken, and diagnosis or reason the medicine is needed
2. The parent or guardian should provide a written request that the school district comply with
   the physician's order
3. Medication should be brought to school in a container appropriately labeled by the phar-
   macist or the physician
4. When the student does not regularly take his own medication, or if the parent or physician
   requests that school personnel administer the medication, provision should be made for the
   medication to be kept in a locked cabinet Designated personnel must be available to
   administer the medication at agreed-upon times, and arrangements should be made for
   alternate personnel to perform the task in case of absence The person administering the
   medication must keep a written record
5. When the child is usually responsible for taking his own medication, he may do so in school
   without supervision by school personnel, provided the physician and parent have provided
   the required authorizations The school administration should cooperate with the physician,
   parent, and child In such instances, it is understood that the school bears no responsibility
   for safeguarding the medication or assuring that it is taken, and the parent should provide a
   written statement relieving the school of such responsibility
6. Individual school districts should seek the advice of counsel as they assume the responsibility for giving medication during school hours Liability coverage should be provided for the
   staff including nurses, teachers, athletic staff, principals, superintendents, and members of
   the school board

Committee on School Health, 1983–1984
Joseph Zanga, MD, Chairman   Maxine M Sehring, MD
Michael A Donlan, MD   Martin W Sklaire, MD
Jerry Newton, MD   John Trieschmann, MD

*Modified from AAP Committee on School Health Administration of medication in school *Pediatrics* **74** 433 1984
Copyright American Academy of Pediatrics 1984

Liaison Representatives
Thomas Coleman, MD
  Section on Child Development
Janice Hutchinson, MD, AMA
Betty McGinnis, CPNP, NAPNAP
Marjorie Hughes, MD
  American School Health Association

Jerry Jacobs, MD
  Section on Rheumatology
Charles Zimont, MD
  American Academy of Family Physicians

AMERICAN ACADEMY OF PEDIATRICS: CORPORAL PUNISHMENT IN SCHOOLS*

Since 1978, various committees of the American Academy of Pediatrics have intermittently addressed the question of corporal punishment and discipline.

A review of recent psychiatric, psychological, and educational literature continues to accumulate evidence in opposition to corporal punishment in schools, although 47 states still have legislation permitting this management.

The American Academy of Pediatrics is opposed to the use of corporal punishment in schools, and urges all parents, educators, school board members, legislators, and other adults to seek the abandonment of corporal punishment and its legal prohibition in all states.

Employment of alternative methods[1,2] for implementation of self-control and responsible behavior is recommended.

Committee on School Health, 1982–1983
J. Ward Stackpole, MD, Chairman
Conrad L. Andringa, MD
Michael A. Donlan, MD
Leonard L. Kishner, MD

Kenneth D. Rogers, MD
Maxine M. Sehring, MD
Joseph R. Zanga, MD

Liaison Representatives
Janice Hutchinson, MD, AMA
Betty McGinnis, NAPNA/P
Marjorie Hughes, MD, ASHA

Charles Zimont, MD, AAFP
Michael A. Hogan, MD
  Section on Child Development

References

1. American Academy of Pediatrics: Committee on Psychosocial Aspects of Child and Family Health: The pediatrician's role in discipline. *Pediatrics* **72:**373, 1983.
2. Christophersen, E. R.: The pediatrician and parental discipline. *Pediatrics* **66:**641, 1980.

Selected Readings

Hiner, N. R.: Children's rights, corporal punishment and child abuse. *Bull. Menninger Clin.* **43:**233, 1979.
Hyman, L. A., and Lally, D.: Discipline in the 1980s: Some alternatives to corporal punishment. *Children Today* Jan.–Feb.:10–12, 1982.
Hyman, L. A., and Wise, J. H.: *Corporal Punishment in American Education: Readings in History, Practice, and Alternatives.* Temple University Press, Philadelphia, 1979.

*Modified from AAP. Committee on School Health: Corporal punishment in schools. *Pediatrics* **73:**258, 1984. Copyright American Academy of Pediatrics, 1984.

Smith, J. D., Polloway, E. A., and West, G. K.: Corporal punishment and its implications for exceptional
    children. *Except. Child* **45**:264–268, 1979.
Wessel, M. A.: The pediatrician and corporal punishment. *Pediatrics* **66**:639, 1980.
Wise, J. H. (ed.): *Proceedings: Conference on Corporal Punishment in Schools: A National Debate.* U.S. Dept
    of Health, Education and Welfare document No. 729–222/565. National Institute of Education, Wash-
    ington, D.C., 1977.

AMERICAN ACADEMY OF PEDIATRICS: GUIDELINES FOR URGENT CARE IN SCHOOL*

Minor injuries and illnesses can occur in children during the course of the school day. They are usually well handled by the nurse in consultation with the school medical advisor; true medical emergencies are quite rare. Many school systems, however, have part-time school medical advisors and nurses who cover more than one school building and who may not be readily available. Therefore, the burden of emergency recognition and management may fall on teachers, principals, or other personnel in the local school. Inappropriate and delayed care may result in increased morbidity or possible death. Finally, consideration must be given to the question of malpractice or assault charges being filed by the families of inappropriately treated children.

In order to solve this problem, it is important for school administrators in consultation with the school medical advisor and nursing service to formulate a guide for emergency care. The Committee of School Health of the American Academy of Pediatrics suggests the following:

1. Every school district should have an identified, qualified administrator with decision-making status.

2. An emergency care manual and standing orders for first aid should be written and made available to nurses, athletic staff, and faculty volunteers. A sample manual[1] is available from the Connecticut State Department of Health, 540 Nortontown Rd., Guilford, Connecticut 96437 ($8.50).

3. The school nurse in each building should be the key person to carry out the program as she or he is most familiar with the student's health problems. All nurses should be trained in a program of emergency care developed by physicians, emergency medical technicians, and/or other nurses with special training in emergency care.

4. As school nurses or physicians cannot always be available, two or more regular members of the school staff, depending on school size, should be designated and trained to handle emergencies according to established protocols until the nurse, physician, or other emergency personnel can be reached. Programs should include training in first aid and cardiopulmonary resuscitation and recognition and treatment of anaphylaxis. These programs can be directed by school nurses trained in emergency care with the physician's supervision as described in the preceding paragraph. If this training is not available, the standard Red Cross or Emergency Medical Technician training may be used. Training should be on a voluntary basis with certificates provided jointly by the school medical advisor, Director of Health, and Board of Education; or state certification could be offered, if available. Periodic recertification should be required to assure competence.

5. Legislation should be encouraged in each state, under the "Good Samaritan Act," to provide legal protection for emergency care givers.

6. An emergency medical kit and anaphylaxis kit (e.g., Anakit, Epinen) should be kept with the medications in each school, and the kits should be made available to trained staff volunteers.

7. Emergencies related to participation in athletics may be handled by a trainer or athletic staff member who has received training in sports medicine and emergency care.

8. Description and disposition of illnesses or injuries of a serious nature (those injuries or illnesses in which a student, staff member, or visitor is released from school to see a physician or be

*Modified from AAP. Committee on School Health: Guidelines for urgent care in school. *Pediatrics* **74**:148, 1984. Copyright American Academy of Pediatrics, 1984.

seen at a hospital) should be recorded on an illness and accident form. A copy should be filed in the student's cumulative health record, a copy should be sent to the principal, and a copy should be forwarded to the regular health care provider and to the hospital or physician treating the child's acute problem.

Further description and classification of school medical emergencies and sports injuries and their treatment may be obtained from *School Health: A Guide for Health Professionals.*[2].

Committee on School Health, 1983–1984
Joseph Zanga, MD, Chairman   Maxine M. Sehring, MD
Michael A. Donlan, MD   Martin W. Sklaire, MD
Jerry Newton, MD   John Trieschmann, MD

Liaison Representatives
Marjorie Hughes, MD   Jerry Jacobs, MD
  American School Health Association   Section on Rheumatology
Janice Hutchinson, MD, AMA   Charles Zimont, MD
Betty McGinnis, CPNP, NAPNAP   American Academy of Family Physicians

References

1. Connecticut Chapter, American Academy of Pediatrics: *Providing Emergency Care to Students in Connecticut Public Schools.*
2. Committee on School Health, American Academy of Pediatrics: *School Health: A Guide for Health Professionals.* American Academy of Pediatrics, Evanston, Illinois, 1981.

AMERICAN ACADEMY OF PEDIATRICS: THE PEDIATRICIAN'S ROLE IN PROMOTING THE HEALTH OF A PATIENT IN DAY CARE*

American families have changed. More mothers are working, and more young children are being cared for outside the home. The stresses inherent in this sociological change are great.

Pediatric practice has also changed. Increasingly, pediatricians are involved not only in the medical care of the child but in the ecological system in which the child exists. The pediatrician has traditionally worked with parents and children to promote healthy functioning, which encompasses the physical, emotional, cognitive, and social health of the growing and developing child. The pediatrician must now expand this role to include working with significant other adults who interact closely with the child who spends much of the day away from home. In this way, the pediatrician will contribute to the promotion of the child's general wellbeing, and some maladaptive behaviors will be prevented.

Parents and adults whom parents delegate to provide child care on a regular basis have the greatest responsibility for children. With increasing numbers of single-parent families and families in which both parents work, there is a greater use of the variety of alternative care-giving arrangements involving adults who are neither parents nor relatives of the child. Effective communication among the child's pediatrician and regular care givers is more difficult to achieve than in the past when parents provided most of the child's care. When developmental irregularities or a chronic illness are a concern, it is particularly important for pediatricians to communicate to the person(s) providing child care the unique features of the child and family. Thus the care giver will be better able to prepare an individualized program that enhances the child's development, increases self-esteem and supports the parents' child-caring capacity.

Current methods of communication between pediatricians and child care providers are often

*Modified from AAP. Committee on Early Childhood, Adoption, and Dependent Care: The pediatrician's role in promoting the health of a patient in day care. *Pediatrics* **74:**157, 1984. Copyright American Academy of Pediatrics, 1984.

woefully inadequate. Much useful and important data are not shared. Often, the child care provider receives only certification of immunization status and documentation of a visit to the pediatrician's office. In providing continuing health care for the child, the pediatrician acquires a great deal of information about the child's medical status, adaptability, and temperament, as well as family strengths. This information could be used to enhance the family's successful use of a day care resource. Pediatricians underestimate the value of this wealth of information they have gathered, and it is often only loosely documented in the child's health profile required for entry into a day care setting. Conversely, pediatricians could increase their understanding of the child and contribute more effectively to the child's growth and development with access to the behavioral observations made by the significant adults involved in the child's day care program.

In order to advise the family about whether day care is timely, or to counsel the family regarding preparation for the separation, or to answer such questions as, "Is this a good setting for my child?" and "Is the child able to participate in all aspects of the day care program?" the pediatrician must not only know the child and the family but must have some understanding of the specific programs. Will the day care program be supportive to the family's parenting style? Will the parent be able to participate in decisions regarding the child's daily activities? Can the staff adapt to the parents' needs? Can the staff members show spontaneous affection? Is there a schedule of activities? Is nutritious food provided? What accident precautions are enforced on special trips? What are the sanitary precautions for the care of the young child? What are the policies regarding the ill child? Is there an identified staff person responsible for issues related to health? Is the program licensed? Most of these questions may be answered by a parent; others may be answered by the program director or the local licensing agency. Most, but not all, needs can be met.

In the child's best interest, there should be system for exchanging information about the child between the physician and the day care provider. This exchange is generally infrequent and used primarily to understand a child for whom there is concern, e.g., the child with asthma, the clumsy child, or the child who is less or more mature than expected for his chronological age. The parent will usually be transmitting his or her own concerns and the concerns raised by the two systems, but with prior approval from the parent, telephone calls and/or notes between physician and day care provider may be more efficient and effective.

Common topics for communication between a physician and a day care provider may include: (1) current state of health and nutrition, including management of colds, diarrhea, bruises, chronic illness, handicapping conditions, and poor or exuberant appetite; (2) growth pattern observed over time and its significance to physical adaptation in the day care environment, such as size of chairs, height of steps, fatigue; (3) hearing and vision function, e.g., the child with recurrent middle ear effusion who may be irritable and unresponsive to auditory stimuli or the child who requires glasses but does not wear them; (4) sequential development and its expression in body management, fine motor skills, communications, self-care, social interaction with adults and children, and the characteristics of play; (5) integration of family members into the program at some level to contribute to the maintenance of a positive parent–child relationship; and (6) the child's initial and ongoing adjustment to the program.

Pediatricians should have an increasing role in addressing the needs of their own patients who are in day care programs, particularly those children who may be at risk for adapting poorly or who may need special considerations. They should be knowledgeable about the variety of child care settings available in their communities. Pediatricians who are aware of the resources in their communities and who have the skills to recommend a good program, to provide a useful health profile of the child and family, and to be receptive to the concerns of members of the day care program staff will contribute immeasurably to their patients' well-being and successful participation in the day care program.

Committee on Early Childhood, Adoption and Dependent Care, 1982–1984
Selma R. Deitch, MD, Chairman   Jean Pakter, MD
David L. Chadwick, MD   Burton Sokoloff, MD
Thomas Coleman, MD   George G. Sterne, MD
Donna O'Hare, MD   Virginia Wagner, MD

Liaison Representatives
Elaine Schwartz
   Children's Bureau, OHD, DHHS
Helen Felitto
   Child Welfare League of America
Jeanne Hunzeker, DSW
   Child Welfare League of America

Kenneth Grundfast, MD
   Section on Otolaryngology
Consultant
Susan Aronson, MD

D

Learning Disabilities

Problem	Parents	Teacher
Specific learning disability	Usually report no problems until school age. Good peer relations initially.	May perform well in some areas. Depressed performance spreads. May develop behavior problems.
Mental retardation	May be regarded as "slow." Plays with younger children.	Cannot compete at age and grade level. Depressed in all areas.
Organic disorder (e.g., hearing loss)	Concern over problem. Functions well in uninvolved areas.	Functions well in uninvolved areas. Generally good behavior and peer relations.
Somatic illness	May detect recent changes in behavior and performance.	Performance poor during period of illness, otherwise no problem noted.
Psychosis	Disturbed family relationships. Poor social interaction.	Bizarre responses. Poor school performance.
Behavioral disorder	At home may not be a major concern. Often does well on a 1:1 basis.	Attention-seeking behaviors. Can do well in structured environment.
Socioeconomic deprivation	Usually no problems reported. Functions well in home environment.	May be labeled as having "poor motivation" or as "not prepared."

[a]In part adapted from Schulman, J. L.: *Management of Emotional Disorders in Pediatrics.* Year Book, Chicago, 1969.

ACADEMIC UNDERACHIEVEMENT[a]

Observations and findings

Physician	Psychologist	Speech pathologist
May detect "soft" neurological signs.	Identifies areas of depression on battery of examinations.	May identify specific deficit (e.g., auditory processing disturbance).
Varies with extent of brain damage. Identifies specific syndrome.	Depression in all areas tested.	Depressed in language and all areas tested.
Identification of organic handicap (e.g., hearing loss).	Depressions in area of affected modality.	May identify specific handicap (e.g., hearing loss).
Identification of cause of illness (e.g., kidney disease).	Depression in test results may be temporary due to illness.	Results may be depressed temporarily due to illness.
Identification of psychotic behavior and disturbed emotionality.	Reports bizarre responses and wide scatter on battery of examinations.	Reports bizarre responses.
Usually normal findings on physical examination and neurodevelopmental testing.	Good results if child cooperates. May identify cause of behavioral difficulty.	May identify attention seeking behaviors or good performance.
Usually normal findings on physical examination.	Reflection of cultural bias on examination. Test scores may be depressed.	May identify influence of deprivation (e.g., language).

AMERICAN ACADEMY OF PEDIATRICS: CHILDREN WITH LEARNING DISABILITIES*

The learning-disabled child is being recognized more frequently in the schools. Children with learning disabilities display a range of characteristics that vary in kind and severity. Typically, the child is of "normal" intelligence but fails to learn at a "normal" rate even though he is given the same educational opportunities as children with equal intelligence.

The magnitude of the problems posed by learning disabilities is becoming more widely known, and the public and professional concern are increasing. Physicians are frequently asked to provide medical diagnoses and treatment to augment educational evaluation and management. Some of the medical considerations are as follows:

Is there a sensory abnormality (i.e., vision, hearing)?
Is there a central nervous system dysfunction caused by a genetic defect or perinatal injury, infection or trauma, convulsive disorder, or other dysfunction of unknown etiology? Are there "soft" neurological signs?
Are there significant, environmental health factors, particularly severe undernutrition?
Are there relevant psychological or sociocultural factors with the child and family? Familial incidence?
What are the physician's diagnostic tools and techniques?
How early can diagnosis be made?
What medical management will help? Are drugs, "perceptuomotor training," or orthoptics useful?
What should the physician know about educational techniques? Which techniques help?

The American Academy of Pediatrics, through the Council on Child Health, is presenting a series of statements on learning disabilities. The first, "The Eye and Learning Disabilities" (published in a *Newsletter supplement,* January 1, 1972, and in *Pediatrics* **49:**454, 1972), was prepared jointly with the American Academy of Ophthalmology and Otolaryngology and the American Association of Ophthalmology. Other statements will include early identification, techniques in office diagnosis—special diagnostic methods, drug therapy, and special education methods.

The role of the physician will be delineated, and emphasis will be placed on the important interdisciplinary function with educators, school administrators, psychologists, child guidance personnel, school health staff, community resources, and, most importantly, the child and family.

Council on Child Health
M. Harry Jennison, MD, Chairman
Howard C. Mofenson, MD, Committee on
    Accident Prevention
Richard B. Feiertag, MD, Committee on
    Adoption and Dependent Care
Robert B. Kugel, MD, Committee on Children
    with Handicaps

William B. Forsyth, MD, Committee on
    Infant and Preschool Child
Andrew Rinker, MD, Committee on School
    Health
Sprague W. Hazard, MD, Committee on
    Youth

Liaison Representatives
Effie O. Ellis, MD, American Medical Association

Sarah H. Knutti, MD, National Institute of
    Child Health and Human Development, NIH

*Modified from Statement, American Academy of Pediatrics, November 1973. Copyright American Academy of Pediatrics, 1973.

AMERICAN ACADEMY OF PEDIATRICS: EARLY IDENTIFICATION OF CHILDREN WITH LEARNING DISABILITIES: THE PRESCHOOL CHILD*

The term "learning disabilities" too often has been applied indiscriminately to all children who, for one or a combination of reasons, may experience difficulty in performing within normal expectancy levels on certain learning or behavioral tasks. Care must be taken to determine whether a child's inability to function according to established norms results from the absence of skills stemming from specific disabilities, limited exposure to certain learning opportunities, culturally different experiences and behavior, or a combination of these or other factors. Labeling should be used only insofar as it contributes to recognition of the basic problem, so appropriate remedial measures can be instituted. Mislabeling is a disservice not only to the child but also to his parents and others who are attempting to assist them.

Definition

Children with true, *specific* disabilities in learning generally evidence near average to above average intelligence. They manifest specific learning or behavioral abnormalities characterized by mild to severe deficits in auditory or visual perception, association, conceptualization, language competence, motor function, or control of attention and impulse. Historically, children with generalized depressions in intellectual functions (mentally retarded); peripheral (sensory), visual, auditory, or motor handicaps; and emotional disturbance have been excluded by definition from the classification of learning disabilities. Children with these primary handicapping conditions may have concomitant specific disabilities resulting in multiple handicaps affecting their psychosocial and/or educational adjustment. Care must be taken not to confuse *cultural differences* with *deficits*.

Screening, Assessment, and Reassessment

Early identification programs should be established in each community to follow children considered at risk because of history or unusual behavior that might interfere with normal learning at home or in the school environment.

The spectrum of biological and psychological processes involved in human learning encompasses multiple disciplines and requires multiteam screening and assessment procedures. Certain principles must be stressed:

1. At the present, there is no simple screening technique of scientific validity and reliability to detect learning disabiity.
2. A high percentage of children at risk for learning can be identified early through formalized multidisciplinary screening and assessment procedures which are extremely reliable when done on an individualized basis.
3. Standardized intelligence, readiness, achievement, and specialized tests (i.e., language or visuomotor) can be valuable if they sample a group of skills and information known to be prerequisites to learning academic skills. The deficiencies and culturally biased aspects of each test must be carefully weighed by the examining team before selection and, especially, before interpreting test results.
4. Children evidencing symptoms of disability in the screening procedure should be provided with in-depth assessment prior to any diagnosis of learning disability or special program placement, other than one with a diagnostic–teaching provision.
5. Assessment is ongoing; formal reassessments should be provided at regular intervals, especially when the child demonstrates appreciable changes in behavior or learning that suggest a need for comprehensive reassessment.

*Modified from AAP. Council on Child Health: Statement, American Academy of Pediatrics, November 1973. Copyright American Academy of Pediatrics, 1973.

Techniques

Screening Procedures

Information should be obtained about the child's present physical, mental, social, and emotional development in addition to formal sampling of the following:

1. Visual acuity and perception
2. Auditory acuity and perception
3. Tactile acuity and perception
4. Language comprehension and expression (including the primary language of the home)
5. Cognitive—associative and conceptual skills
6. Motor integration (gross and fine) and development

In-depth Assessment

Children judged to be at risk on screening should have formal evaluations in the following areas:

1. Medical, neurological, and emotional health and needs of the child, including a complete history of the pregnancy, birth, and development prior to assessment
2. Visual and auditory development, including acuity, discrimination, memory, sequencing, and integration
3. Language and speech development, including comprehension, grammatical construction, articulatory ability, rhythm, and voice
4. Ability to integrate visual, auditory, and motor systems
5. General information level or intellectual development (care should be taken to assess his intellectual functioning on verbal and nonverbal tasks)
6. Environment for learning, including an understanding of the family's attitudes, priorities, and learning proficiencies

Special attention should be given to children whose behavioral patterns are frequently inappropriate, withdrawn, or disruptive. Observation or reports of such behavior in the home or a preschool setting should be evaluated thoroughly to determine its nature and frequency. Certain children display behavior patterns derived from temperamental characteristics that are often stabilized enough to appear innate. A substantial number of children display involuntary irregularities and deviations that apparently result from actual neurological dysfunction. Others demonstrate learning patterns of volitional aberrant behavior or emotional disturbance. Many children enter the learning situation preoccupied by fears or personal conflicts with parents, peers, or teachers, and, they do not learn well in the classroom. No single assessment tool will help the child specialist distinguish among the aforementioned behavior patterns. Much time and effort by a team of specialists, parents, and teachers is generally required to determine the causes of aberrant behavior and the most appropriate plan for positive modification.

There are programs that offer intelligent and well-designed plans of remediation for children with specific learning disabilities. The condition is neither imaginary nor trivial. Early identification is of the upmost importance to the child and his family, if for no other reason than to provide the parents with an understanding of the child's difficulty and the knowledge that he is neither retarded nor unduly stubborn.

Council on Child Health
Robert B. Kugel, MD, Chairman
William B. Forsyth, MD
Sprague W. Hazard, MD
Jean L. McMahon, MD
Rowland L. Mindlin, MD

Howard C. Mofenson, MD
Andrew Rinker, MD
Henry M. Seidel, MD
Robert G. Scherz, MD
David W. Van Gelder, MD

Subcommittee on Early Identification
Jean L. McMahon, MD, Chairman
Joseph Brinkley, MD

Norman B. Schell, MD
Earl Siegel, MD

Liaison Representatives
Effie O. Ellis, MD, American Medical Association
Sarah H. Knutti, MD, National Institute of Child Health and Human Development
William C. Healey, PhD, American Speech & Hearing Association

Dallas Beyer, Association for Childhood Education International
Milton Akers, EdD, National Association for Education of Young Children

Selected Readings

Ahr, E.: The development of a group of preschool screening test of early school entrance potential. *Psychol. Schools,* **4:**59, 1967.

Bateman, B.: Learning disorders. *Rev. Ed. Res.* **36:**93, 1966.

Bateman, B., and Frankel, H.: Special education and the pediatrician. *J. Learning Disab.* **5:**178, 1972.

Central Processing Dysfunctions in Children: A Review of Research. NINDS Monograph No. 9. Washington, D.C.: Government Printing Office, 1969.

Crichton, J., Catterson, J., Kendall, D., and Dunn, H.: Learning Disabilities. A Practical Office Manual. Sherbrooke, Quebec: Canadian Paediatric Society, 1972.

Denhoff, E.: Detecting potential learning problems at preschool medical examinations. *Tex. Med.* **65:**56, 1969.

Denhoff, E., Hainsworth, P. K., and Hainsworth, M. L.: The child at risk for learning disorder—Can he be identified during the first year of life? *Clin. Pediatr.* **11:**164, 1972.

Evans, J. S., and Bangs, T.: Effects of preschool language training on later academic achievement of children with language and learning disabilities: A descriptive analysis. *J. Learning Disab.* **5:**585, 1972.

Fitzhardinge, P. M., and Steven, E. M.: The small-for-date infant. II. Neurological and intellectual sequelae. *Pediatrics* **50:**50, 1972.

Gallagher, J. J., and Bradley, R. H.: Early identification of developmental difficulties. *71st Yearbook of the National Society for the Study of Education,* Part II. Chicago, Illinois: p. 87, 1972.

Gofman, H. F., and Allmond, B. W., Jr.: Learning and language disorders in children. Part I: The preschool child. *Curr. Prob. Pediatr.* August, 1971.

Gregory, W. C., and Hylton, P. H.: The physician's responsibility in predicting learning disabilities in preschool children: The evaluation of children with school failures. *Va. Med. Mon.* **98:**89, 108, 1971.

Haring, N. G., and Ridgway, R. W.: Early identification of children with learning disabilities. *Excep. Child.* **33:**387, 1967.

Kenny, T. J., Clemmens, R. L., Cicci, R., *et al.*: The medical evaluation of children with reading problems (dyslexia). *Pediatrics* **49:**438, 1972.

Lerner, J. W.: *Children with Learning Disabilities: Theories, Diagnosis and Teaching Strategies.* Houghton-Mifflin, Boston, 1971.

McGrady, H. J.: Learning disabilities: Implications for medicine and education. *J. School Health* **61:**227, 1971.

McMahon, J. L.: Organic brain syndrome—Early detection in the child. *Rocky Mt. Med. J.* **64:**76, 1967.

Minimal Brain Dysfunction in Children: Terminology and Identification. Phase One of a Three-Phase Project. NINDB Monograph No. 3. Washington, D.C.: Government Printing Office, Public Health Service Publication No. 1415, 1966.

Minimal Brain Dysfunction in Children. Educational, Medical and Health Related Services. Phase Two of a Three-Phase Project. N and SDCP Monograph. Washington, D.C.: Government Printing Office, Public Health Service Publication No. 2015, 1969.

Snyder, R. D., and Mortimer, J.: Diagnosis and treatment: Dyslexia. *Pediatrics* **44:**601, 1969.

Taichert, L. C.: *Childhood Learning, Behavior and the Family.* Behavioral Publications, New York, 1973.

Tarnopol, L. (ed.): *Learning Disorders in Children: Diagnosis, Medication, Education.* Little Brown, Boston, 1971.

Thompson, L. J.: Learning disabilities: An overview. *Am. J. Psychiatry.* **130:**393, 1973.

AMERICAN ACADEMY OF PEDIATRICS: READING DISABILITY: DO THE EYES HAVE IT?*

Poor school performance is an increasingly common presenting complaint in pediatric clinics and offices.[1] The underachieving student can be an exasperating challenge to parents, teachers, and pediatricians. Delays in learning to read are among the most common manifestations of the so-called low severity-high prevalence disabilities of schoolchildren. Various subtle developmental lags interact with environmental conditions, educational experiences, and the child's intrinsic temperamental repertoire, with resultant delays in the acquisition of academic skill. It is difficult to stand by and observe passively a precipitous decline in self-esteem, as a schoolchild becomes aware that peers are learning to read and he is not. The temptation is great to succumb to an urgent longing to uncover, thence to heal, the causative lesion. Reading at first glance appears to be a visual process, so it is not surprising that investigators, teachers, and clinicians have first sought answers in the realms of ocular and visuoperceptual function. Consequently, many children with reading delays have found themselves in intervention programs based on the assumptions that they have functional visual deficits, that these are etiologically linked to their reading problems, and, therefore, that visual therapies will correct the academic impairment. The critical review by Metzger and Werner[2] seriously challenges these widely accepted premises.

Metzger and Werner[2] cite gaping flaws in experimental design among studies that support various visually based hypotheses. Furthermore, as they point out, recent literature suggests that apparent deficiencies of pure visual perception or visuomotor function are as common a finding in youngsters with normal reading skills as in those with problems.

Disabilities of reading and other forms of disordered learning derive from a wide range of possible intrinsic and exogenous deficiencies. In some instances, discrete impairments of verbal labeling interfere with the matching of sounds with symbols.[3] Weaknesses of recognition or of retrieval memory, problems with selective attention, or trouble interpreting and retaining sequences of data (e.g., letter order, syntax, or narrative flow) are among a multitude of dysfunction that have been described within the heterogeneous population of youngsters with reading delays.[4]

In all cases, there exists a serious need to differentiate between normal variation, association, causality, and secondary effect. Thus, the coexistence of erratic eye movements and reading delays in a child need not comprise an etiologic interaction. One recent study suggests, in fact, that uneven visual pursuit may be a compensatory strategy some youngsters employ because they have trouble appreciating or remembering all the letters in a word at once.[5] Their eyes quickly scan back and forth to overcome a weakness of memory. To train such students to track symbols more evenly thus might thwart this laudable spontaneous compensation.

A substantial body of research has sought to isolate the cause of reading disability, a quest akin to seeking a unitary explanation for all chronic coughs. Future investigations would be enriched by uncovering contributing factors predisposing to reading difficulties. Instead of asking whether an ocular or visual processing deficit, for example, is the cause of reading disability, there is a need to determine whether some youngsters with impaired reading indeed have such handicaps and, if so, whether the association is in any way relevant (i.e., causal, secondary, or aggravating).

Several heuristic tendencies have undermined the scientific basis of research into the causes and treatments of learning disorders. These have included (1) overreliance on anecdotal evidence; (2) a lack of carefully matched comparison groups (both normal and dysfunctional) and, consequently, a poor appreciation of what constitutes normal variation and factors common to multiple forms of deviation; (3) an initial preconception that a factor in isolation causes a reading disability in contrast to a condition being the end result of multiple convergent influences; (4) an exclusive stress on mean differences between groups of good and poor readers rather than on cluster analyses that consider multiple interactive factors and subgroups of affected students; (5) an assumption that there exists only one method by which normal children read; (6) a tendency to interpret findings narrowly, so that inattention to visual detail, for example, might be regarded as a visual defect rather than a broader manifestation of attentional weakness in all modalities; (7) a failure to control for non-

*Modified from Levine, M D Reading disability Do the eyes have it? *Pediatrics* **73**:869, 1984 Copyright American Academy of Pediatrics, 1984, and the author

specific gains accrued simply by bestowing more attention upon a child (such as through tutoring, visual training, a rigid diet, or even oboe lessons); and (8) a peculiar tendency for research on therapy to be undertaken by individuals with a vested interest (often pecuniary) in a positive outcome.

Many pediatricians find themselves isolated amid the crossfire between hard science and ardent testimony, as optometric and visuomotor training programs expand in number and influence throughout North America. Aggressive marketing, dramatic presentations at national meetings, loosely reviewed journal articles, and fervent anecdotal reports of cure may convince school personnel and parents that visual training is the answer. In such cases, the pediatrician may be bypassed and considerable family and community resource diverted toward as yet unsubstantiated interventions, which may delay or abort the implementation of more appropriate educational measures and counseling strategies.

For pediatricians, the challenge extends beyond visual diagnosis and training. In their hunt for simple explanations of complex phenomena, susceptible parents, teachers, and professionals have sought to medicalize prematurely a varied assortment of learning and behavioral problems. Currently, there is burgeoning consumer demand for diagnoses of hypoglycemia, oversensitivity to sugar, vestibular dysfunction, idiosyncratic reaction to foods, allergy, and vitamin deficiency. Thus, implied treatments include elimination diets, megavitamin therapies, labor-intensive physical exercises, questionably effective drugs, and allergic hyposensitization. Ironically, over time development develops; consequently, when such allegedly therapeutic measures are undertaken, subsequent gains are conveniently attributed to the intervention with some appearance of plausibility.

It is easy to construct attractive hypotheses with sufficient allure to attract a cultlike following. For example, one could argue for the appealing and timely notion that impurities in modern industrial air are causing most reading difficulties. Therefore, it would follow that children with reading problems require special facial masks to filter out such contaminants. Pediatricians might then prescribe the requisite respiratory protective gear. Students indeed would gain in reading in association with the wearing of their masks. After all, youngsters with these problems are likely to make some progress anyway. Wearing masks would probably cause them to talk less and listen more in class, and some parents and teachers would want and perhaps need to perceive the appliance as working. In addition, the nonspecific positive impact of monitoring compliance to see that a child wears his mask might superimpose new structure and discipline. Word could spread throughout North America that we had discovered the cause and treatment of reading disability. Moreover, replacement cartridges for masks might provide an ongoing source of revenue for those who promoted and prescribed them. Although this example is bizarre, it may not be all that divergent from the identification and promotion of other highly appealing "pseudoscientific" explanations and treatments.

Pediatricians must serve as scientific consumer advocates, helping parents, teachers, and the community at large to evaluate claims and insist on hard evidence regarding diagnostic and therapeutic modalities. Literature reviews, such as that of Metzger and Werner, serve to inform advocacy and should be read and quoted by physicians whose patients receive or are considering seductive therapies. Within academic developmental pediatrics and other disciplines, there needs to be effectively designed research undertaken without bias or self-interest in the outcome, either to prove or disclaim the efficacy of proposed measures. While being skeptical, especially with regard to prematurely disseminated therapies, it is important that we remain open minded, entirely willing to be convinced that for some problem students, dietary, visual, metabolic, and other appealing explanations actually may emerge as relevant factors. On the other hand, the wholesale endorsement of single explanations and treatments for large numbers of children with clinical disorders as complex as reading disability deserves our outspoken mistrust.

References

1. Dworkin, P. H., Shonkoff, J. P., Leviton, A., et al.: Training in developmental pediatrics: How pediatricians perceive the gaps. Am. J. Dis. Child. 133:709, 1979.
2. Metzger, R. L., and Werner, D. B.: Use of visual training for reading disabilities: A review. Pediatrics 73:824, 1984.
3. Vellutino, F.: Dyslexia: Theory and Research. Cambridge.

TYPES OF EDUCATIONAL MANAGEMENT STRATEGIES FOR GIFTED CHILDREN

Type	Program design	Advantages	Disadvantages
Ability grouping	Special schools or classes "Pullout" programs Summer workshops "Afterschool" programs	Opportunity to work at level of ability Program designed to meet needs of individual child Learning experience continuous	Requires specially trained teachers Program often not individualized Student may not be gifted in all subjects Exaggerates feelings of being different Expensive program design
Acceleration	Early school entrance Grade "skipping" Move through the material at an accelerated rate Less time to complete school	Can be used in any school Enter careers earlier, more productivity Educational costs lowered Less boredom with academics Social/emotional adjustments high	Bias of teachers, administrators, and parents Possible social disruptions Law does not permit early entrance Teacher not specially trained
Enrichment	Addition of areas of learning not normally in curriculum Resource programs	Children not separated Less expensive than ability grouping	Used in a traditional classroom Teachers may not be specially trained Poor program coordination

*In part adapted from Clark, B.: *Growing up Gifted*. Charles E. Merrill, Columbus, Ohio, 1979.

E

Behavioral Issues

DIAGNOSTIC CRITERIA FOR ATTENTION-DEFICIT DISORDER WITH HYPERACTIVITY: DSM III[a]

Hyperactivity (at least two of the following)
  Excessive running or climbing
  Difficulty sitting still or excessive fidgeting
  Difficulty staying seated
  Motor restlessness during sleep
  Always on the go or acts as if "driven by a motor"

Inattention (at least three of the following)
  Often fails to finish things he or she starts
  Often seems not to listen
  Easily distracted
  Difficulty concentrating on schoolwork or other tasks requiring sustained attention

Impulsivity (at least three of the following)
  Often acts before thinking
  Excessive shifting from one activity to another
  Has difficulty organizing work (not due to cognitive impairment)
  Needs a lot of supervision
  Frequently calling out in class
  Difficulty waiting for turn in games or group situations

Onset before age 7 years

Duration of illness at least 6 months

Does not meet the criteria for a pervasive developmental disorder or manic disorder

[a]From the *Diagnostic and Statistical Manual of Mental Disorders* American Psychological Association, Washington, D C , 1980

DIFFERENTIAL DIAGNOSIS OF HYPERACTIVITY AS A SYMPTOM

Type of hyperactivity	Descriptive labels	Possible value of EEG	History of prior neurological injury	Significant findings on neurological examination	Associated learning problems	Behavioral problems	Response to drug therapy	Diagnosis possible during preschool period
Neurological hyperactivity								
Attention-deficit disorder	Minimal brain dysfunction	−	+/−	+/− (soft signs)	+	+/−	+/−	+/−
Acute and progressive cerebral deterioration	Depends on specific etiology	+	−	+	+	+/−	−	+
Mental retardation	"Slow", "Retarded"	+/−	+/−	+/−	+	+/−	+/−	+
Developmental hyperactivity	"Immature" "Disinhibited"	−	−	−	+/−	+/−	−	+/−
Psychogenic hyperactivity								
Mild (situational anxiety type)	"Acting out" "Active because of being under pressure"	−	−	−	+/−	+/−	−	+
Severe (psychosis or severe neurosis)	"Emotionally disturbed"	−	−	−	+	+	+/−	+

[a] Adapted from Schmitt, B.D., et al.: 1973.

APPROACHES TO MANAGEMENT OF HYPERACTIVITY[a]

Type of hyperactivity	Parent's home management program (with professional guidance)	Special educational assistance	Pharmacological management
Neurological hyperactivity			
Attention-deficit disorder	+	+	+/−
Acute and progressive cerebral deterioration	+	+	−
Mental retardation	+	+	+/−
Developmental hyperactivity	+	+/− (usually not required)	
Psychogenic hyperactivity			
Mild (situational anxiety type)	+	+ (if school is source of anxiety or contributes to it)	−
Severe (psychosis or severe neurosis)	+	+	+ (under psychiatric program)

[a]Adapted from Schmitt, B. D.: et al.: 1973.

CATEGORIES OF PSYCHOTROPIC DRUGS

Category	Generic name	Tradename
Cerebral stimulants	Dextroamphetamine	Dexedrine
	Methylphenidate	Ritalin
	Pemoline	Cylert
Sedatives and tranquilizers	Barbiturates	Phenobarbital
	Phenothiazines	
	Chlorpromazine	Thorazine
	Thioridazine	Mellaril
	Others	
	Diazepam	Valium
	Diphenhydramine	Benadryl
	Chlordiazepoxide	Librium
	Meprobamate	Equinil, Miltown
Antidepressants	Imipramine	Tofranil
	Amitryptyline	Elavil
Anticonvulsants	Barbiturates	Phenobarbital
	Diphenylhydantoin	Dilantin

FAMILY DYNAMICS[a]

Type of relationship	Parental interactions	Effects on child
Confused	Concerned but unsure of how to cope with child's difficulty. Usually has tried unsuccessfully to work with child; frustrated. Sense of failure, guilt. Ambivalence may interfere with seeking professional intervention.	Child appears anxious; always testing limits. Child's self-concept reflects parents' confusion, frustration, and anxieties.
Inconsistent	Parent uses varying methods to control child, no pattern. Parents transmit two opposite messages at the same time.	Child confused and frustrated. Child may withdraw or become anxious and rebel.
Denial	Minimizes or does not admit to child's difficulty. Parents' goals, expectancies, dreams for child have been thwarted. Parent usually first reacts by feeling child will outgrow problem.	Child confused and frustrated because of dichotomy between reality and parents' denial. This confusion may bring withdrawal or acting out. Feeling of insecurity may occur. Self-confidence is shaky.
Vicarious	Parent lives through the child. Child is to realize aspirations parents could not achieve. Child's handicap destroys the parents' dreams for the child.	Child may be pressured to achieve despite handicap. Child may be pushed to overcome handicap. Child may have poor self-concept.
Symbiotic	Abnormally close tie between one parent and child. Parent begins to devote his/her life to this child. May reflect deep-seated emotional problems in the parent.	Child does not develop an independent personality. Lack of independence, infantile reactions, fear of separation.
Overprotective	Parents try to shield child from ordinary hazards of life, exaggerated with a child with a handicap. Parents' concerns are limitless. Parents may reflect guilt feelings.	Child may become fearful; self-confidence and esteem are low. Handicap becomes exaggerated and out of proportion to reality.
Overpermissive	Parents permit a wider range of behavior than normal and cannot set limits. Parents may be ineffectual. Parents may be responding to guilt feelings.	Child with handicap may be given free rein because of misconceptions, pity, etc. Child may not conform socially. Child may become overly dependent.
Rigid	Parents set very high and unrealistic standards. Parents may be perfectionists, organizers, and compulsive at times. Applies these standards and rules for child; expectations higher than child's capability.	May be disappointment to parents because of handicap. Child may also strive for perfection. Child may rebel actively or passively. Child may withdraw and regress.
Disinterested	Often seen in multiproblem or disorganized households. Child's problems secondary to more pressing problems/conflicts family faces each day.	Child is usually withdrawn or passive; "loner." Later, child is likely to act out; run away, delinquent. More likely not to conform socially.

FAMILY DYNAMICS[a] (Continued)

Type of relationship	Parental interactions	Effects on child
Neglectful	Parent exhibits lack of responsibility for child. Child's handicap may create negative feelings in parent. Parent has ambivalent feelings toward child.	Rnage of neglect, including physical and emotional needs of child. Child feels unwanted and unloved and may focus on handicap as cause.
Fragmented	Parental discord to pathological degree. Parental separation usual result.	Child may see handicap as cause of parental problems. Feelings of insecurity and rejection.
Rejecting	Parents may actually reject child; may be precipitated by handicap. Something about child may cause negative feeling.	Child feels unwanted or unloved. May blame handicap for feeling of rejection. Results in poor self-concept; apprehensive about all peers and adults.

[a]Adapted in part from Schulman, J. L.: *Management of emotional disorders in pediatric practice.* Year Book, Chicago, 1969; and Webster, E.: *Professional Approaches with Parents of Handicapped Children.* Charles C Thomas, Springfield, Illinois, 1976.

AMERICAN ACADEMY OF PEDIATRICS: THE PEDIATRICIAN'S ROLE IN DISCIPLINE*

With declining availability of extended family to support and advise young parents and with the growing numbers of single-parent families, the pediatrician is increasingly consulted about the behavioral management of children and especially about appropriate discipline. Discipline means "to impart knowledge and skill to" rather than corporal punishment.

The emotionally mature adult is a disciplined person, able to postpone pleasure appropriately, tolerate discomfort when necessary, and be assertive without being hostile. Such abilities are learned over time and the process begins in earliest childhood.

As the human newborn matures physiologically and neurologically and as his care givers gradually impose limits in relationship to feeding, toileting, or sleeping, the child's biological rhythms become more regular and adapt to family routines. Signals of discomfort, such as crying and aimless thrashing of limbs, are modified and abandoned as the infant acquires memories of past relief of distress provided by the environment (parents).

As the infant becomes more mobile, he will initiate contacts with the environment; some of the potentially dangerous contacts include electric cords and plugs, peanuts, or valuable bric-a-brac. Actions must be taken to protect the infant or toddler: the use of safety plugs or removal of the danger, signals of "No," or physical removal of the child to a "safer" area. Some persistent, active children pose a real discipline challenge to their parents; other children are quite adaptable and "easy." And just as children vary in their behaviors, some parents find it difficult to say "No"; some parents are neglectful; and still others are overly restrictive, controlling, and harsh. It is the responsibility of the care giver to set limits for the child, but as the child grows and incorporates the attitudes and practices of his or her care givers (modeling), the child develops an inner self-responsibility, a conscience. Concurrently, responsibility for behavior is gradually transferred from the care-giving adult to the child as he or she slowly becomes more autonomous and independent.

If children are to attain self-discipline and a healthy conscience, it is incumbent on responsible care givers, parents, teachers, physicians, and others to: (1) know and accept age-appropriate

*Modified from AAP. Committee on Psychosocial Aspects of Child and Family Health: The pediatrician's role in discipline. *Pediatrics* **72**:373, 1983. Copyright American Academy of Pediatrics, 1983.

behavior, (2) set reasonable, consistent limits, (3) reinforce desirable behavior (accentuate the positive), and (4) recognize the individuality of each child and range of response to restriction. Punishment or restriction, when necessary, must be immediate and not physically harmful to the child.

Alternatives to corporal punishment and ways of avoiding parent-child conflict include: (1) structuring the physical environment, e.g., placing breakable objects out of reach, providing play areas, and making proper toys available; (2) structuring the emotional environment, for instance, "Five more minutes to play before your nap," or "We have to pick up before eating"; (3) admitting and exploring feelings about restrictions and limits: "I know you want to play more, but it is time for your nap," or "I know you don't like to sit on the potty now, but you have to try a little"; (4) reinforcing desirable behavior: "What a big girl you are to tell me and not wet your pants!" "You are a good picker-upper!" Sometimes one can distract or interrupt undesirable behavior. "If you are going to hit, you have to sit over there until you can play nicely again"; and (5) modeling. Children unconsciously adopt the behaviors of their care givers. Ideally, parents must be sensitive to the child's feelings and to their own behavior.

Because they are human beings, parents will seldom behave perfectly; likewise, they cannot expect their children always to behave perfectly. Punishment should seldom be necessary in an environment in which mutual respect has been established. When punishment does become necessary, measures such as brief isolation or restriction of privileges are recommended. One must consider the potential modeling effect of punishment on how children respond to their environment. Adults who were harshly treated or abused in their childhood are at high risk for similar treatment of their own children.

Committee on Psychosocial Aspects of Child and Family Health
Morris Green, MD, Chairman   John B. Reinhart, MD
T. Berry Brazelton, MD   Irwin L. Schwartz, MD
David B. Friedman, MD

Liaison Representatives
Peter Wallace, MD   Katerina Haka-Ikse, MD
   AAP District VI   Canadian Paediatric Society

YOUTH SUICIDE: WARNING SIGNS

Becoming withdrawn and uncommunicative	Running away from home and/or truancy
Deep depression and feeling of worthlessness	Broken home and family crises
Sudden disruptive, violent, and/or explosive outbursts	Evidences of poor self-concept
School failure or drop in achievement levels	Insomnia or excessive sleep
Previous suicide attempt or talking about suicide	Hyperactive or hypoactive behaviors
Significant loss of a family member	"Getting life in order"
Friend or relative a recent suicide victim	Giving away prized possessions
Loss of concern for previous interests	Sudden interest in religion and afterlife
Becoming socially isolated	

ABNORMAL MOVEMENTS:
INVENTORY OF TICS

Head and face
- Twisting hair
- Grimacing
- Raising eyebrows
- Eyelid blinking
- Winking
- Wrinkling nose
- Twitching mouth
- Biting lips
- Protracting lower jaw
- Head banging and rolling
- Extruding tongue
- Fingering ear
- Nodding, jerking of head
- Twisting neck
- Looking sideways
- Sucking fingers
- Picking nose
- Displaying teeth

Arms and hands
- Jerking hands
- Swinging arms
- Writhing fingers
- Striking head or body
- Scratching
- Manipulating genitalia

Body and lower extremity
- Shaking foot
- Shaking knee
- Shrugging shoulder
- Writhing body
- Jumping

Respiratory
- Hiccoughing
- Coughing
- Hysterical laughing
- Grunting
- Barking
- Clearing throat
- Yawning
- Sighing
- Blowing through nostrils
- Blowing through lips
- Increased respiratory effort

Alimentary
- Belching
- Sucking movements
- Vomiting
- Swallowing
- Spitting

[a]Adapted from Lucas, in Noshpitz, J. D. (ed.): *Basic Handbook of Child Psychiatry*. Basic Books, New York, 1979.

Syndromes

MINOR CONGENITAL ANOMALIES

Head and face
  Head shape
    Brachycephaly
    Dolicoephaly
    Scaphocephaly
    Trigonocephaly
  Head circumference
    1.5 SD
    1.5 SD
  Long philthrum
  Depressed nasal bridge

Scalp hair configuration
  Multiple whorls, posterior and anterior
  Wry hair and cowlicks
  Low hairline
Telecanthus
Slanting palpebral fissures
Antiverted nares
Epicanthal folds

Ears
  Abnormalities of pinnae
    Low set
    Posterior rotation
    Pinna anatomy

Otic stenosis
Absent lobule
Asymmetry
Tags

Mouth
  Glossomandibular disproportion
  High arched palate

Nonspecific tooth abnormalities
Bifid uvula

Hands
  Short metacarpal
  Nails
    Hypoplastic
    Hyperconvex
  Camptodactly
  Hyperextensibility
  Transverse palmar crease (short hand)

Fifth digit: clinodactyly, missing flexion crease
Extra flexion crease (long digits)
First digit: triphalangeal low set
Supranumerary digits
Mild syndactyly

Feet
  Hypoplastic nails
  Lymphedema
  Low-set first or third and fourth digits

Mild syndactyly
Large gaps between first and second digits
Long third toe

Other
  Mild webbing of the neck
  Limitation of extension of knees and elbows

Nipples
  Widly spaced
  Supranumerary

SELECTED SYNDROMES ASSOCIATED WITH DEVELOPMENTAL DISABILITIES: CHARACTERISTIC CLINICAL FEATURES

Syndrome	Features

Alcohol embryopathy (fetal alcohol syndrome)	Facial features
	  Microcephaly
	  Microphthalmia, ptosis
	  Poorly developed philtrum
	  Short palpebral fissures
	  Flat nasal bridge
	  Thin upper lip
	  Micrognathia
	  Midface deficiency with prognathia
	Central nervous system involvement
	  Neurological abnormalities
	  Developmental delays
	  Mild to moderate mental retardation
	  Irritable infants
	  Hyperactivity (childhood)
	  Poor fine/gross motor coordination
	  Learning disabilities
	Organ system defects
	Prenatal and postnatal growth retardation
	Weight, height, and/or head circumference below 10th percentile

Alport syndrome	Familial nephropathy
	Nerve deafness (sensorineural); often noticed late in childhood
	  More common in males
	  Perceptive-type deafness
	Ocular changes
	  Bilateral anterior or posterior lenticonus
	  Cataracts
	  Rupture of lens capsule

Apert syndrome	Facial features
	  Brachycephaly
	  High forehead
	  Flattened occiput
	  Craniosynostosis of coronal, squamosal, and sphenoparietal sutures
	  Flat facies
	  Beaked nose
	  Antimongoloid slant to palpebral fissures
	  Ocular hypertelorism
	  Low-set ears
	  Dental malocclusion
	  Ocular changes
	Syndactyly (hands and feet)
	Congenital cardiac defects
	Mental retardation may occur
	Inherited as an autosomal dominant
	Majority of cases represent the appearance of a new mutation

Ataxia telangiectasia (Louis-Bar syndrome)	Intrauterine growth deficiency Linear growth deficiency Progressive neurological degeneration with ataxia Choreoathetosis Nystagmus

(continued)

SELECTED SYNDROMES ASSOCIATED WITH DEVELOPMENTAL DISABILITIES: CHARACTERISTIC CLINICAL FEATURES
(Continued)

Syndrome	Features
	Ocular apraxia Dysarthria Telangiectases of conjunctiva and skin (from 2 to 4 years of age) Recurrent infections Thin facies Café-au-lait spots Premature graying of hair Lymphopenia Inherited as an autosomal recessive

"Cat eye" syndrome	Facial features
	   Ocular coloboma
	   Upslanting eyes
	   Preauricular tags and fistulas
	Intelligence ranges from normal to mildly retarded
	Imperforate anus
	Congential heart disease
	Urinary tract abnormalities
	Extra chromosome 22

Cockayne syndrome	Facial features
	   Enophthalmos
	   Beaking of nose
	   Appearance of premature senility
	   Small mandible
	   High-arched palate
	   Gross dental caries
	Flexion deformities of knees, hips, elbows
	Kyphosis
	Limbs appear disproportionately long
	Hands and feet large
	Dimunition of muscle mass
	Delayed puberty
	Nystagmus, ataxia, tottering gait
	Hyporeflexia
	Microencephaly
	Intracranial calcifications
	Perceptive deafness
	Atrophic retinopathy and optic atrophy
	Mental retardation

Congential hypothyrodism (cretinism)	Little or no clinical evidence at birth
	Facial features
	   Protuberant, thick tongue
	   Course facial features
	   Flattened nasal bridge
	   Puffy edema of face
	Hoarse cry (myxedema of vocal cords)
	Marked muscular hypotonia
	Mental retardation
	Umbilical hernia
	Constipation
	Bradycardia, poor cardiac output
	Mottled, dry skin
	Coarse, dry, brittle hair
	Low hairline ($\pm$ hirsutism)
	Delayed dental development

SELECTED SYNDROMES ASSOCIATED WITH DEVELOPMENTAL
DISABILITIES: CHARACTERISTIC CLINICAL FEATURES
(Continued)

Syndrome	Features
	Growth retardation
	Excessive sleepiness
	Suggestions during newborn period
	Prolonged physiological jaundice
	Mottling of skin
	Excessive sleeping and inactivity
	Poor feeding
	Constipation
Congenital rubella syndrome	Neonatal manifestation (self-limiting)
	Low birth weight
	Neonatal thrombocytopenic purpura
	Radiolucencies, metaphysis long bones
	Hepatosplenomegaly
	Hemolytic anemia
	Bulging anterior fontanelle
	Developmental disorders
	Delayed psychomotor development
	Mental retardation (mild to profound)
	Deafness and communication disorders
	Eye defects
	Cataracts (unilateral or bilateral)
	Congenital glaucoma
	Microphthalmia
	Retinopathy (patchy black pigmentation)
	Cardiac defects
	Patent ductus arteriosus
	Ventricular septal defects
	Other defects
	Microcephaly ($\pm$)
	Risk of insulin-dependent diabetes mellitus
Cornelia deLange syndrome	Facial features
	Microbrachycephaly
	Hirsutism involving forehead, eyebrows
	Eyebrows extend across nasion without interruption
	Short nose
	Anteverted nares
	Thin lips; midline breaking of upper lip and notch in lower lip
	Downward curve of angles of mouth
	Severe mental retardation
	Autisticlike behaviors
	Increased muscle tone
	Limb defects (micromelia to oligodactyly)
	Cry is low, weak, and growling
Crouzon syndrome (craniofacial dystosis)	Facial features
	Froglike appearance
	Exophthalmos, bilateral
	Hypertelorism
	Divergent strabismus
	Maxillary hypoplasia
	Beaked nose
	Short upper lip
	High arched, narrow palate
	Brachycephaly
	Dental anomalies

(continued)

SELECTED SYNDROMES ASSOCIATED WITH DEVELOPMENTAL DISABILITIES: CHARACTERISTIC CLINICAL FEATURES
(Continued)

Syndrome	Features
	Ectrodactyly, syndactyly Mental retardation (±) Inherited as an autosomal dominant trait 25–40% mutations

Down syndrome	Facial features
	  Oblique palpebral fissure
	  Redundant nuchal skin
	  Abnormally shaped palate
	  Hypoplastic nose
	  Brushfield spots
	  Open mouth with protruding tongue
	  Epicanthal folds
	  Flattened occiput
	  Abnormal size and position of ears
	Moderate to severe mental retardation
	Wide space between 1st and 2nd toes
	Hyperflexibility and hypotonia
	Single (simian) palmar crease
	Short, spadelike hands
	Clinodactyly
	Abnormality of chromosome 21

Fragile X syndrome	Facial features
	  Normal or increased head circumference
	  High or prominent forehead
	  Elongated face with heavy features
	  High arched palate
	  Midfacial hypoplasia
	  Prominent chin
	  Large or prominent ears
	Mild to severe mental retardation
	Verbal disability
	Macroorchidism
	Behavioral dysfunction (hyperactivity, self-mutilation, psychosis, autism in some)
	Fragile site on long arm of X chromosome

Goldenhar syndrome	Facial features
	  External ear malformations
	  Ocular dermoids
	  Upper lid colobomas
	  Asymmetrical facial underdevelopment
	  Macrostomia
	Vertebral defects
	Congenital heart disease
	Sporadic, genetic transmission reported

Hallermann-Streiff syndrome	Facial features
	  Brachycephaly
	  Hypoplasia of mandible and maxilla
	  Thin nose, beaked
	  Hypoplasia of nasal cartilages
	  Frontal bossing
	  Small mouth

SELECTED SYNDROMES ASSOCIATED WITH DEVELOPMENTAL
DISABILITIES: CHARACTERISTIC CLINICAL FEATURES
(Continued)

Syndrome	Features
	High-arched palate Blue sclerae Nystagmus, strabismus Congential cataracts Coloboma of optic disc Low-set ears Atrophic scalp skin with alopecia or hypotrichosis Deficiency of eyebrows and eyelids Dwarfism Underdeveloped external genitalia Atrophied, wrinkled skin Intellectual retardation, slight ($\pm$)
Hunter syndrome (iduronate sulfatase deficiency)	Features similar (but less severe) than in Hurler syndrome Short stature Skeletal abnormalities Cardiovascular abnormalities Recurrent otitis media Pigmentary retinal degeneration Nodular dermal infiltrations Mental retardation ($\pm$) Laryngeal abnormalities (hoarsnness and airway obstructions) Chronic pseudopapilledema Mortality usually in early teens Transmitted as an X-linked recessive trait

Hurler syndrome (α-L-iduronidase deficiency)	Signs may not be detected at birth
	Facial features
	   "Gargoylelike"
	   Progressively coarsened features
	Marked diminution of growth after first year of life
	Severe psychomotor retardation
	Hepatosplenomegaly
	Progressive joint deformity
	Corneal opacification (blindness)
	Deafness
	Hydrocephalus
	Progressive heart disease
	Hirsutism
	Progressive disease due to intracellular mucopolysaccharide accumulation (death usually <10 years of age)

Klinefelter syndrome	Seldom diagnosed before puberty Small percentage are mentally retarded Failure of adolescent virilization Gynecomastia Azospermia One or more X-chromatin masses in phenotypic male (e.g., XXY)
Menke syndrome (kinky hair disease)	Confined to males, death in first 3 years Intrauterine growth retardation Linear growth is limited Cerebral deterioration in infancy Depigmentation of hair

(continued)

SELECTED SYNDROMES ASSOCIATED WITH DEVELOPMENTAL DISABILITIES: CHARACTERISTIC CLINICAL FEATURES
(Continued)

Syndrome	Features
	Hair stands on end and becomes tangled
	Hair twisted about longitudinal axis
	Hair fractures
	Seizures during infancy
	Focal cerebral and cerebellar degeneration
	Wormian bones in sagittal and lambdoid sutures
	Flared metaphyses of femora and ribs
	Transmitted as an X-linked recessive trait
Morquio syndrome	Symptoms usually between 1 and 2 years of age
	Severe skeletal deformities
	Pectus carinatum
	Severe kyphoscoliosis
	Shortened neck
	Genu valgum
	Short trunk
	Neurosensory deafness (progressive)
	Neurological complications secondary to hypoplasia of odontoid process
	Aortic insufficiency
	Respiratory compromise
	Slightly coarse facies
	Normal intelligence
	Autosomal recessive inheritance (keratin sulfate accumulation)
Noonan syndrome	Facial features
	Low-set or malformed ears
	Ptosis of eyelid ($\pm$)
	Hypertelorism
	Downward slant of palpebral fissures
	High or narrow palate
	Micrognathia
	Low posterior scalp hairline
	Short stature
	Mental retardation, mild to moderate
	Shield-shaped chest
	Congenital heart disease (pulmonary valvular or infundibular stenosis)
	Unilateral or bilateral cryptorchidism
	(?) Inherited as an autosomal dominant trait with variable expressivity
Oculocerebrorenal syndrome (Lowe syndrome)	Facial features
	Frontal bossing
	Enophthalmos
	Bilateral congenital cataracts
	Megalocornea
	Glaucoma
	Nystagmoid movements
	Diminished pupillary responses to light
	Mental retardation (severe)
	Hypotonia
	Cryptorchidism
	Renal tubular acidosis

SELECTED SYNDROMES ASSOCIATED WITH DEVELOPMENTAL
DISABILITIES: CHARACTERISTIC CLINICAL FEATURES
(Continued)

Syndrome	Features
	Aminoaciduria Growth failure Inherited as an X-linked autosomal recessive trait

Opitz syndrome	Facial features
	    Ocular hypertelorism
	    Brachycephaly
	    Facial asymmetry (±)
	    Cleft lip and palate (±)
	    Antimongoloid slant to palpebral fissures
	    Low-set posteriorly rotated ears
	    Epicanthus
	Hypospadius
	Cryptorchidism (±)
	Congenital cardiac defects
	Mental retardation (mild to moderate)
	Inherited as an autosomal dominant trait
	Cases reported were males

Pierre Robin syndrome	Facial features
	    Micrognathism
	    Cleft palate
	    Glossoptosis
	Associated congenital cardiac defects; ocular and skeletal abnormalities may occur
	Mental retardation in about 20%

Prader-Willi syndrome	Birth through 2 years
	    Growth failure
	    Feeding difficulty
	    Infantile central hypotonia
	Over 2 years of age
	    Hyperphagia and decreased feeling of satiety
	    Obesity
	    Short stature
	    Hypogonadism
	    Dysfunctional CNS performance
	Abnormality of chromosome 15

Rett syndrome	Appears to occur exclusively in girls
	Autistic behavior and dementia
	Apraxia of gait
	Loss of facial expression
	Stereotyped use of hands
	Progrssive course usually beginning during first 3 years of life
	    Deterioration of behavioral and mental status
	    Delayed onset of walking
	    Truncal ataxia
	    Deceleration of head growth (acquired microcephaly)
	Hyperammonemia (+/−)
	No clear-cut genetic explanation

Rubinstein-Taybi syndrome	Facial features
	    Hypoplasia of maxilla and mandible
	    Antimongoloid slant to palpebral fissures

(continued)

SELECTED SYNDROMES ASSOCIATED WITH DEVELOPMENTAL DISABILITIES: CHARACTERISTIC CLINICAL FEATURES
(*Continued*)

Syndrome	Features
	Beaked nose
	Nasal septum extends beyond alae nasi
	High-arched palate
	Limited growth
	Delayed bone development
	Hirsutism
	Cryptorchidism
	Scoliosis
	Congenital heart defects
	Abnormally broad thumbs and great toes
	Mental retardation (IQ below 50 in 75%)
Seckel syndrome (bird-headed dwarfism)	Facial features
	Microcephaly
	Craniosynostosis
	Facial hypoplasia (mandible, palate, and malar bones)
	Large bulging eyes
	Prominent nose
	Micrognathia
	Lobeless, low-set ears
	Small face with small or absent forehead
	Multiple malformations of bones and joints of axial skeleton and of extremities
	Mental retardation
	Low birth weight
	Small stature
	Inherited as an autosomal recessive trait
Silver syndrome (Russell-Silver dwarfism)	Facial features
	Pseudohydrocephalus (head appears large)
	Small triangular-shaped face
	Small, narrow jaw
	Thin lips
	"Carp-like" mouth
	Fine hair
	Prenatal dwarfism associated with low birth weight
	Café-au-lait spots
	Asymmetry of body (hemiatrophy)
	Scoliosis
	Slight hyperextensibility of some joints
	Delayed bone age
	Syndactyly of toes
	Clinodactyly of fifth finger with considerable shortening
	Hypospadias
	Mental retardation (moderate in a significant number of cases)
Smith-Lemli-Opitz syndrome	Facial features
	Scaphocephaly and microcephaly
	Bilateral ptosis
	Epicanthus
	Broad nasal tip and anteversion of nares
	Strabismus
	Low-set posteriorly rotated ears
	Broad maxillary alveolar ridge
	Hypertelorism
	Synophris

SELECTED SYNDROMES ASSOCIATED WITH DEVELOPMENTAL DISABILITIES: CHARACTERISTIC CLINICAL FEATURES
(Continued)

Syndrome	Features
	Hypotonia Partial syndactyly of second and third toes Clenched fist, index finger overlies the third finger Shield-shaped chest, wide-spaced nipples Cryptorchidism, hypospadias, very small penis Hypoplastic labia majora Spasticity with seizures Small brain Mental retardation
Soto syndrome (cerebral gigantism)	Large size present from birth Linear growth is excessvie Head circumference proportional to expected height Very large hands and feet Large nose and ears Advanced bone age Clumsiness Dysarthria, inane laughter Drooling of saliva Insensitivity to pain Hyperkinesis and short attention span Mild to moderate ventricular dilatation Intellectual retardation

Treacher Collins syndrome	Facial features
	    Antimongoloid slant to palpebral fissures
	    Supraorbital ridges underdeveloped
	    Marked hypoplasia of malar and mandibular bones
	    "Fishlike" mouth
	    Coloboma of lateral third of lower eyelid
	    May have absence of external auditory canals (agenesis of auditory ossides)
	Occasional skeletal defects
	Congenital cardiac defects
	Mental retardation (less than 5%)
	Inherited as an autosomal dominant with variable expressivity
	Fresh mutations in more than 55%

Tuberous sclerosis	Seizures (infantile spasms in young children and grand mal seizures in older children) Adenoma sebaceum; classically found in butterfly pattern over nasal bridge Café-au-lait spots Shagreen patches Subungual fibroma Intracranial tumors and foci of intracranial calcifications Normal intelligence to profound mental retardation Inherited as an autosomal dominant trait Diagnosis can be based on a triad of seizures, mental retardation and adenoma sebaceum

Turner syndrome	Facial features
	    Congential webbed neck
	    Low posterior hairline
	    Micrognathia
	    Low-set ears (occasionally malformed)

(continued)

SELECTED SYNDROMES ASSOCIATED WITH DEVELOPMENTAL
DISABILITIES: CHARACTERISTIC CLINICAL FEATURES
(Continued)

Syndrome	Features
	Shield-chest deformity
	Hypoplastic nipples
	Congenital heart disease
	Anomalies of urinary tract
	Cubitus valgus
	Dysplasia of fingernails and toenails
	Congenital lymphedema of limbs
	Absence of normally occurring growth spurts
	Absence of sexual development at puberty (primary amenorrhea and sterility)
	Normal intelligence (mental retardation in a few cases)
	Sex chromosome abnormality: 45,X
Waardenburg syndrome	Facial features
	Lateral displacement of medial canthi and inferior lacrimal puncta
	Broad nasal root
	Heterochromia iridum
	White forelock
	Congenital deafness
Williams syndrome	Facial features
	Medial eyebrows flare
	Flat nasal bridge
	Short nose with anteverted nares
	Long philtrum
	Prominent lips
	Mouth open
	Severe postnatal growth retardation
	Mild microcephaly
	Average IQ: 50–60
	Hoarse voice
	Supravalvular aortic stenosis

G

Office Management of
Developmental Disabilities

Parent Questionnaire*

This questionnaire concerns your child and family. It will help us understand some of the concerns which you have. Some of the information requested may not seem directly related to your child. However, the information requested is very important in appreciating your child and your concerns.

Although you may not recall all of the information requested, assistance can often be obtained from baby books, your physician, or relatives. Please try to answer as many of the questions as possible. This questionnaire was made for children of various ages and backgrounds. If a question does not apply to your child because of age, write N/A in the space provided. If there is not enough space to answer a question, please use the last page.

We appreciate your cooperation in completing this questionnaire to the best of your ability. The information you provide will be most helpful in evaluating your child.

Marvin I. Gottlieb, M.D., Ph.D.
Director, Institute for Child Development

*Modified from a sample questionnaire designed for parents of children with developmental disabilities. Prepared by Marvin I Gottlieb, MD, PhD, Director, and John E Williams, MD, Associate Director, Institute for Child Development, Hackensack Medical Center, Hackensack, New Jersey 07601

General Information

Date _____

Child's Name _____ Birthdate _____ Age _____ Sex: M F

Home Address _____ Phone_____

_____
County   City   State   Zip Code

Natural Father _____ Birthdate _____

    Occupation _____ Religion _____

    Ethnic Background _____ Years of Schooling_____

    Health _____

Natural Mother _____ Birthdate _____

    Occupation _____ Religion _____

    Ethnic Background _____ Years of Schooling_____

    Health _____

Who referred you to the ICD for evaluation? _____

What is it about your child that concerns you? _____

_____

_____

_____

When was it first noticed?_____

What have you been told with regard to this problem?_____

_____

_____

_____

What things do you presently **not** understand about your child's problem?_____

_____

_____

_____

How do you think that we might be able to help you? _____

_____

_____

_____

How do **you** feel your child can best be helped? _____

_____

_____

_____

Pregnancy

Questions in this and the following section refer to the pregnancy of the child whose problem has caused you to seek assistance.

Hospital where born _____

Address _____

How old were you when you became pregnant? _____

Did you have any problems getting pregnant? _____

Was this a planned pregnancy? _____ Feelings about being pregnant _____

_____

During which month did you start prenatal care? _____ Where? _____

Weight before pregnancy _____ Weight gain _____

Any weight loss in any part of pregnancy? _____ If so, when? _____

Medicines taken and when (include all medications, such as vitamins, birth control pills, etc., including aspirin if taken frequently) _____

Did you smoke during the pregnancy? _____ If so, when? _____

How many cigarettes per day? _____

Number of alcoholic drinks per week _____ If so, when? _____

Any narcotic drugs during or prior to this pregnancy? _____

Any illnesses? _____ If so, when? _____

Please list any antibiotics taken during pregnancy. _____

_____

Did you have any fever during pregnancy? 1st 3 mo. _____ 2nd 3 mo. _____ last 3 mo. _____

If so, how high was the fever? _____ For how long did it persist? _____

X-rays during or shortly before pregnancy? _____ Vaginal bleeding? _____

High blood pressure? _____ Much morning sickness? _____ Much swelling? _____

Hospitalizations? _____

When _____, Address _____

Operations? _____

Accidents? _____

Unusual worries? _____

Special diet? _____

When did you first feel the baby move? _____

How were the baby's movements during pregnancy?

_____ Stronger than expected

_____ Weaker than expected

_____ About the same as expected

Birth History

Was the baby born on time, early, or late? _____

Was any stimulation of labor used? _____ Type _____

Length of labor in hours _____ Length of hard labor _____

Length of time before delivery that "bag of waters" broke _____

Type of anesthesia or pain relief:

    Sedative _____ Shot for pain relief _____

    Spinal or caudal _____ Gas or Pentothal _____

Were you awake when the baby was born? _____

Type of delivery:

    Natural (vaginal) _____ Breech _____

    Cesarean section _____ Forceps _____

Mother's blood group (ABO) _____ Mother's Rh factor _____

Baby's blood group (ABO) _____ Baby's Rh factor _____

Baby's birth weight _____ Birth length _____ Head circumference _____

Infant's condition:

Breathed immediately _____ Cried immediately _____

Required oxygen _____ Length of stay in nursery _____

Seizures or fits _____ Apgar score _____

Other difficulties _____

Problems during the first week (i.e., incubator, hyaline membrane disease, oxygen therapy, prematurity, yellow skin, feeding difficulties, bleeding tendency, infection, antibiotics, etc.) _____

_____

Medicines given during hospital stay _____

Previous Pregnancies

Past pregnancies of child's mother: Number of times pregnant (include miscarriages) _____

Longest period of difficulty getting pregnant _____

Live births _____ Stillbirths _____ Miscarriages _____ Abortions _____

List dates of past pregnancies. Indicate if there was: a miscarriage; threatened miscarriage (bleeding); premature birth; twins; deformity or other difficulty with live-born children; or any other complications. Please list any birth defects, however unimportant you consider them.

Name	Birthdate	Birth Weight	Grade in School	Any School or Health Problems

Are the mother and father cousins, or in any other way related? _____

_____

Previous marriage of either parent? If so, to whom, date, and date of divorce _____

_____

Please list children of either parent born prior to this marriage:

Name	Birthdate	Birth Weight	Grade in School	Any School or Health Problems

Health

Breast or bottle fed _____   Did child eat well? _____

Sleep patterns _____

Childhood diseases (list age and anything unusual about any of them):

  Mumps _____   3-day (or German) measles _____

  Chicken pox _____   7-day (or red) measles _____

  Roseola _____   Scarlet fever _____

  Whooping cough _____   Serious illness _____

Immunizations (dates or ages received and any unusual reactions):

  DPT series _____   Smallpox_____

  DPT booster _____   Measles _____

  Polio (oral)_____   Mumps _____

If your child has had any of the following, please indicate and explain details:

Accidents_____

High fever, unknown cause _____

Pneumonia _____

Anemia _____

Urine infection or disease_____

Problem in bladder or bowel control (i.e., bedwetting, soiling) _____

Constipation _____

Does your child have trouble seeing? _____

Do your child's eyes turn in or out, or are they ever not straight? _____

Crossed eyes _____

Speech problems_____

Difficulty eating or feeding self _____

Difficulties in: Swallowing _____   Chewing _____   Drooling _____

Does your child watch TV with the volume on excessively loud? _____

Hearing problems _____

Does your child speak excessively loud? _____

Frequent ear infections _____   Most recent ear infection_____

  Treated with _____   Treated by _____

Foot problems (any special shoes, braces, etc.) _____

Skin disease or abnormality _____

Allergies _____

Seizures or convulsions _____

Poor coordination _____

Aggressive behavior _____

Unusual fears _____

Sleeping difficulties and night terrors _____

Head banging _____

Rocking _____

Breath holding _____

Temper tantrums_____

Discipline problem _____

Ingestion of drugs, cleaners, or non-food items _____

Other illnesses _____
_____

Please list present medication(s) and dosages _____
_____
_____

Later hospitalizations of child:

Name of Hospital	Address	Date	Age	Reason

Dental History

Has your child ever been examined by a dentist?_____

For what reason? _____

When was your child's last visit to the dentist? _____

Name and office address of your child's dentist _____
_____

Development

We would like to have information about some of the developmental milestones of your child. Indicate the age in months when your child first did each of the following. (Indicate that the child has not yet done it by writing "No." If you do not remember write "NR.") Please be as specific as possible in pinpointing the age.

Held head erect _____   Crawled _____

Rolled over front to back_____   Pulled to stand _____

Rolled over back to front_____   Fed self cookie _____

Stood alone _____   Drank from cup _____

Walked holding on furniture _____   Played pat-a-cake, peek-a-boo, or bye-bye

Walked without holding _____   _____

Ran with good control_____   Used spoon without spilling much _____

Walked up steps_____   Toilet training started _____

Rode tricycle _____   Toilet training finished _____

Said "ma-ma" or "da-da" _____   Took off clothing alone _____

Repeated sounds others made _____   Put on clothing alone _____

Sat Alone _____

Is your child left- or right-handed? _____

When did you first notice a hand preference? _____

Indicate age at which:

_____ Used single words with meaning

_____ Used words to make request

_____ Used words to comment or share information

_____ Used two or more different words together

Please answer yes or no (as applicable):

_____ Does your child use too many general terms (this, that, thing, stuff)

_____ Does your child interrupt himself before finishing what he's started, that is, revising a thought many times?

_____ Does your child change topics too quickly for listeners to follow?

_____ Can your child answer questions adequately without help from an adult?

Schools

Has child ever been in preschool? _____ When and where? _____

Please describe any problems _____

List schools that child has attended:

Name of School	Address	Grade(s)	Problems

Has your child ever been held back in school? _____

Has your child ever been in special education? If so, when, address, and what kind? _____

Has child ever been in remedial classes? Is so, when, address, and what kind? _____

Has child ever had special tutoring? If so, when, address, and by whom? _____

Has child ever received speech therapy? If so, when, address, and by whom? _____

Has child ever received any other type of therapy? If so, please describe: Name _____

Type _____ When _____ Address _____

Describe any school problems that you are presently aware of _____

_____

_____

_____

_____

Activities

What things does your child like to do? _____

_____

_____

What things does your child do well? _____

_____

What things present the greatest difficulty for your child?_____

_____

_____

Describe play indoors _____

_____

Does your child play alone? _____

Does your child play well with other children? _____

Describe play outdoors _____

_____

Does your child enjoy swings _____ slides _____ climbing equipment _____

Does your child recognize dangerous situations?_____

How does your child play and/or get along with other children? _____

_____

_____

Does your child act inappropriately or speak inappropriately? Often _____ Sometimes _____ Rarely _____

Give detailed description of an average day_____

_____

_____

_____

_____

_____

_____

_____

Does your child enjoy being touched or cuddled? _____

Does your child enjoy roughhouse play? _____

Does your child enjoy bath time? _____

Family History

Please indicate whether there are any relatives of the child (including parents, grandparents, aunts, uncles, and cousins), who have the same or a similar problem for which you are seeking evaluation. Also indicate for these persons whether there are serious, chronic, or recurrent illnesses or abnormalities such as birth defects, miscarriages, diabetes, convulsions or epilepsy (fits), mental or emotional disorders, slow development, mental retardation, school problems, cerebral palsy, muscular disorders, cancers, leukemia, thyroid disease (goiter), deafness or blindness, speech or language problems, reading or learning disorders. (Please be as specific as possible giving relationship to child, age of relative and problem.)

Mother_____

Mother's mother _____

Mother's father _____

Mother's brothers and sisters _____

Mother's maternal grandmother _____

Mother's maternal grandfather _____

Mother's paternal grandmother _____

Mother's paternal grandfather _____

Mother's aunts and uncles _____

Mother's cousins _____

Father _____

Father's mother _____

Father's father _____

Father's brothers and sisters _____

Father's maternal grandmother _____

Father's maternal grandfather _____

Father's paternal grandmother _____

Father's paternal grandfather _____

Father's aunts and uncles _____

Father's cousins _____

Describe any family tensions _____

_____

_____

Future goals of child's father _____

_____

Future goals of child's mother _____

_____

List, if available, sources of support outside your immediate family:

      Financial _____

      Transportation _____

      Babysitting _____

      Emotional _____

Environment

Who lives in home besides child, parents, brothers, and sisters?
List age, relation, and health:

_____

List members of the family not living at home, where living, and reason:

_____

Has your child ever been separated from the family? If so, list age, duration, and reason:

_____

Any recent major family problem such as death, illness, separation, or accident?_____

_____

Do you speak more than one language at home? _____

Date of marriage of child's parents _____

If appropriate, date of separation _____   Date of divorce _____

Step- or adopted father _____   Birthdate _____

    Occupation _____   Religion _____

Ethnic background _____   Years of schooling _____

Health _____

Step- or adopted mother _____   Birthdate _____

Occupation _____   Religion _____

Ethnic background _____   Years of schooling _____

Health _____

Would you describe your relationship with your husband/wife as:

Very good _____   Good _____   Average _____   Poor _____

Please list below any previous evaluations (e.g. psychological, IQ, educational or achievement tests, speech/language) that your child had.

Place and Type of Evaluation   Address   Date

_____

_____

_____

_____

Please list below the physicians who have seen your child.

Physician   Address   Date(s)   Reason for Consultation

_____

_____

_____

_____

Informant: (history giver): _____   Relationship to Child _____

Has your child been registered with Special Health Services?

No _____   Yes _____   When _____

Additional Information

Guidelines for Health Supervision*

GUIDELINES FOR HEALTH SUPERVISION

Each child and family is unique therefore these **Guidelines for Health Supervision of Children and Youth**[1] are designed for the care of children who are receiving competent parenting have no manifestations of any important health problems and are growing and developing in satisfactory fashion **Additional visits may become necessary** if circumstances suggest variations from normal These guidelines represent a consensus by the Committee on Practice and Ambulatory Medicine in consultation with the membership of the American Academy of Pediatrics

through the Chapter Chairmen

The Committee emphasizes the great importance of **continuity of care** in comprehensive health supervision[2] and the need to avoid **fragmentation of care**[3]

A **prenatal visit** by the parents for anticipatory guidance and pertinent medical history is strongly recommended

Health supervision should begin with medical care of the newborn in the hospital

	INFANCY						EARLY CHILDHOOD					LATE CHILDHOOD					ADOLESCENCE			
AGE[4]	By 1 mo	2 mos	4 mos	6 mos	9 mos	12 mos	15 mos	18 mos	24 mos	3 yrs	4 yrs	5 yrs	6 yrs	8 yrs	10 yrs	12 yrs	14 yrs	16 yrs	18 yrs	20+ yrs
HISTORY Initial/Interval	●	●	●	●	●	●	●	●	●	●	●	●	●	●	●	●	●	●	●	●
MEASUREMENTS Height and Weight	●	●	●	●	●	●	●	●	●	●	●	●	●	●	●	●	●	●	●	●
Head Circumference	●	●	●	●	●	●														
Blood Pressure									●	●	●	●	●	●	●	●	●	●	●	●
SENSORY SCREENING Vision	S	S	S	S	S	S	S	S	S	O	O	O	O	O	S	O	O	S	O	O
Hearing	S	S	S	S	S	S	S	S	S	S	O	O	S[5]	S[5]	S[5]	O	S	S	O	S
DEVEL./BEHAV. ASSESSMENT[6]	●	●	●	●	●	●	●	●	●	●	●	●	●	●	●	●	●	●	●	●
PHYSICAL EXAMINATION[7]	●	●	●	●	●	●	●	●	●	●	●	●	●	●	●	●	●	●	●	●
PROCEDURES[8] Hered./Metabolic Screening[9]	●																			
Immunization[10]		●	●	●		●	●					●					●			
Tuberculin Test						●	←— 11 —→					←— 11 —→					←— 11 —→			
Hematocrit or Hemoglobin[12]	←——————— ● ———————→						←——————— ● ———————→					←——————— ● ———————→					←——————— ● ———————→			
Urinalysis[13]	←——————— ● ———————→						←——————— ● ———————→					←——————— ● ———————→					←——————— ● ———————→			
ANTICIPATORY GUIDANCE[14]	●	●	●	●	●	●	●	●	●	●	●	●	●	●	●	●	●	●	●	●
INITIAL DENTAL REFERRAL[15]									●											

1 Committee on Practice and Ambulatory Medicine 1981
2 Statement on Continuity of Pediatric Care Committee on Standards of Child Health Care 1978
3 Statement on Fragmentation of Pediatric Care Committee on Standards of Child Health Care 1978
4 If a child comes under care for the first time at any point on the Schedule or if any items are not accomplished at the suggested age the Schedule should be brought up to date at the earliest possible time
5 At these points history may suffice if problem suggested a standard testing method should be employed
6 By history and appropriate physical examination if suspicious by specific objective developmental testing
7 At each visit a complete physical examination is essential with infant totally unclothed older child undressed and suitably draped
8 These may be modified depending upon entry point into schedule and individual need
9 PKU and thyroid testing should be done at about 2 wks Infants initially screened before 24 hours of age should be rescreened
10 Schedule(s) per Report of Committee on Infectious Disease ed 18 1982

11 The Committee on Infectious Diseases recommends tuberculin testing at 12 months of age and every 1-2 years thereafter In some areas tuberculosis is of exceedingly low occurrence and the physician may elect not to retest routinely or to use longer intervals
12 Present medical evidence suggests the need for reevaluation of the frequency and timing of hemoglobin or hematocrit tests One determination is therefore suggested during each time period Performance of additional tests is left to the individual practice experience
13 Present medical evidence suggests the need for reevaluation of the frequency and timing of urinalyses One determination is therefore suggested during each time period Performance of additional tests is left to the individual practice experience
14 Appropriate discussion and counselling should be an integral part of each visit for care
15 Subsequent examinations as prescribed by dentist

N B **Special chemical, immunologic, and endocrine testing** are usually carried out upon specific indications Testing other than newborn (e g inborn errors of metabolism sickle disease lead) are discretionary with the physician

Key ● = to be performed, S = subjective by history, O = objective, by a standard testing method

*Modified from Pediatric patient education Challenge for the '80s *Pediatrics* **74(5):**925, 1984

SELECTIONS FROM A "PHYSICIAN'S DEVELOPMENTAL SCREENING. TEST"

Visuospatial Orientation and Visual Discrimination*

Ask the child to circle the *one* most like the sample in left-hand column.

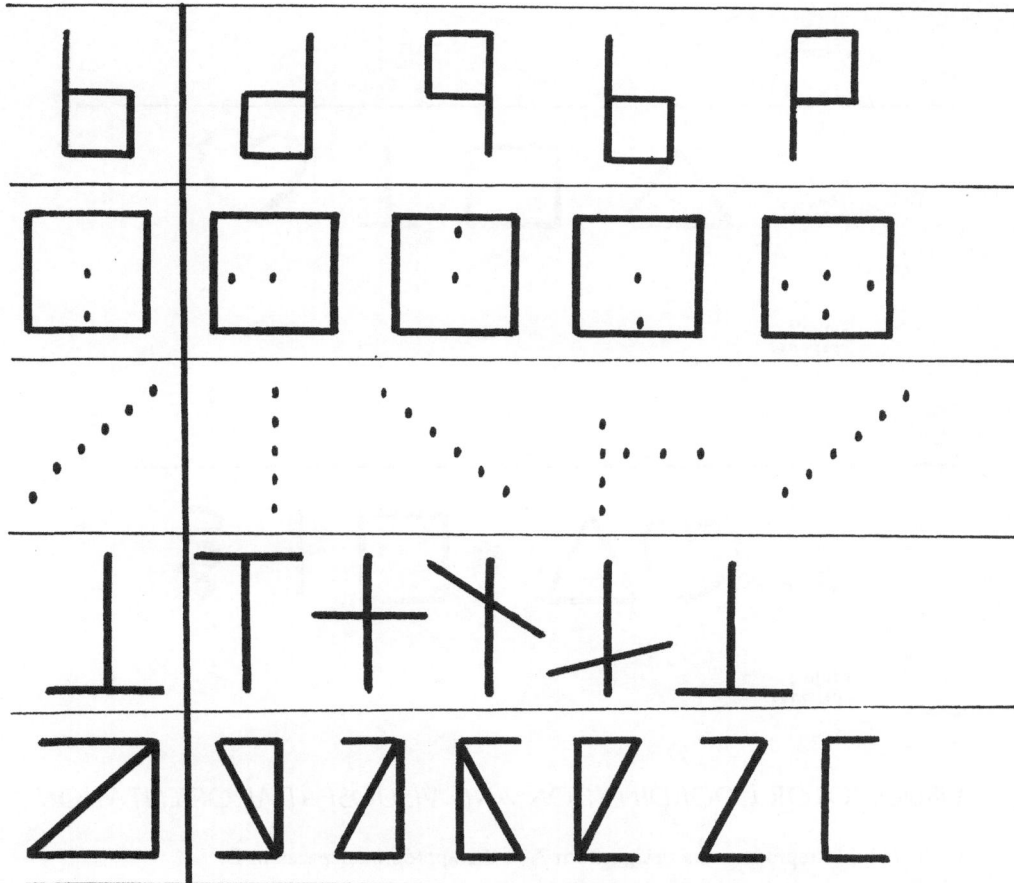

*Adapted from Physician's Developmental Screening Test. Copyright M. I. Gottlieb, MD, 1979.

Visual Sequential Memory

Ask the child to study a row of symbols for 15 seconds, cover *all* designs and ask the child to draw the designs in sequence from memory. Test one row at a time starting with the three-figure line.

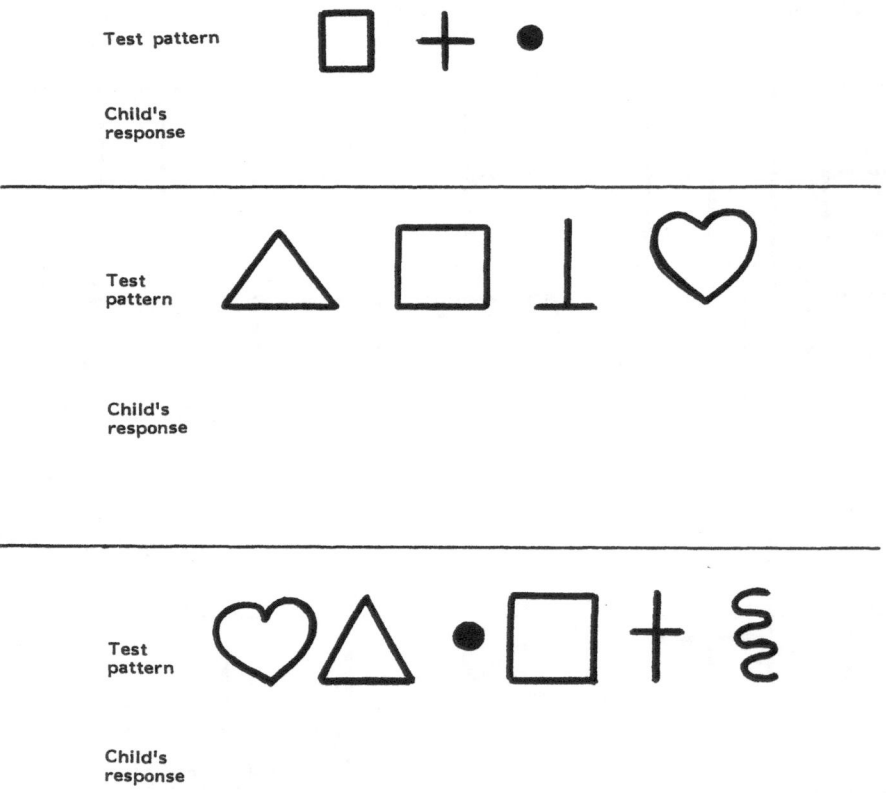

VISUOMOTOR COORDINATION AND VISUOSPATIAL ORIENTATION

Ask the child to reproduce the design from A to the appropriate spaces in B.

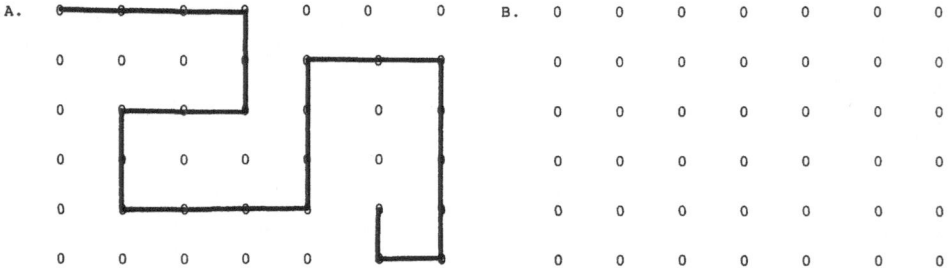

AUDITORY–VISUAL MEMORY

Ask the child to touch figures in sequence (e.g., "Touch the star, then the square"). Vary the length of sequence based on ability.

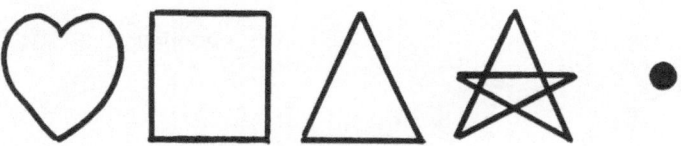

Visual Attention

Ask the child to complete the drawings of the puppets so that they are identical.

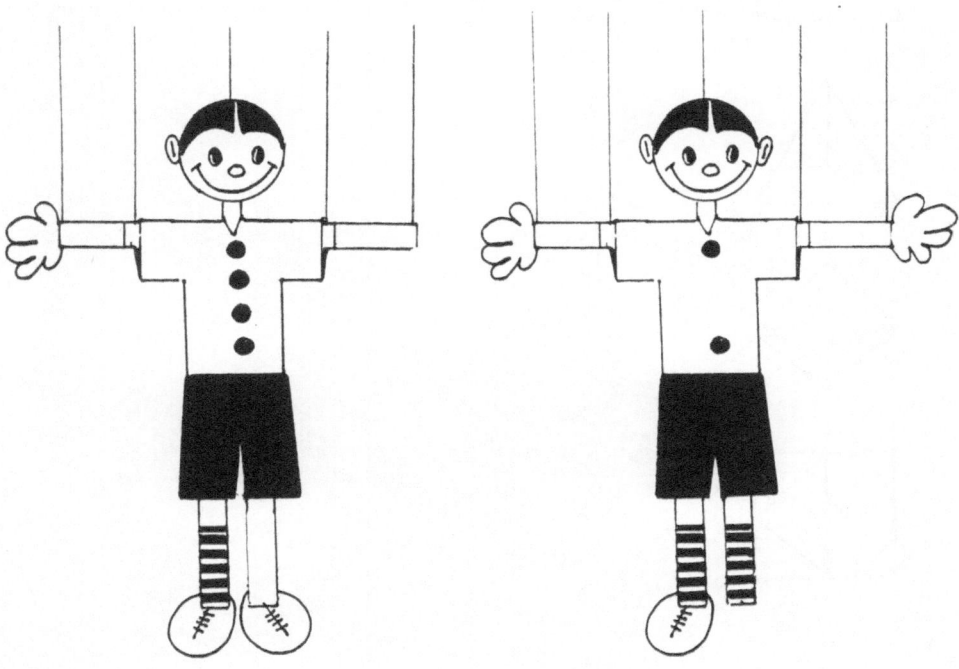

Visual Memory and Visuomotor Coordination

Ask the child to draw each figure from memory. Allow 15 seconds for each figure. Cover *all* figures; expose one at a time.

Figure   **Drawing**

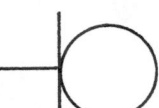

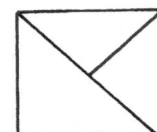

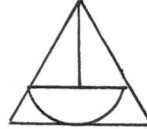

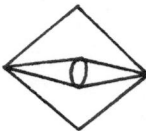

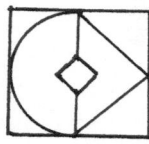

Controversies in Management

CONTROVERSIAL THERAPIES: CONTRIBUTING FACTORS[a]

"Vulnerability" of patients and parents (desire for quick cures)

Professional apathy, misunderstanding, and inadequate counseling

Reliance on individual case reports or advocacy group testimonials

Acceptance because of professional endorsement

Publicity in the media (despite lack of scientific proof in peer-review journals)

Statements that cannot be documented by the scientific method and ignoring placebo effects

Testimonials despite having utilized *multiple* therapies spontaneously; ignoring spontaneous remissions and cures

Explaining failures on "poor patient compliance"

"Prove me wrong" challenge

"It cannot hurt so try it" philosophy

Translating a low percentage of cures into a universal (100%) effectiveness

Failure to provide patient with facts and information about the traditional and acceptable therapy modalities

[a]Adapted in part from Gottlieb, M. I., Zinkus, P. W., and Bradford, L. J. (eds.): Brown, G. W.: Learning disabilities: Fads, fallacies and fictions, in *Learning Disabilities: An Audio Journal for.Continuing Education*, Grune & Stratton, New York, 1979.

CONTROVERSIAL THERAPIES: ASSESSING THE TRUTH ABOUT THERAPY[a]

Are the *definitions* of the conditions delineated clearly?

Are the *variables* considered?

Does the scientific protocol include *random* selection of controls and patients?

Does the scientific design for the *controls* include alternative therapies, placebos, untreated individuals, double-blind and crossover studies?

Has *experimenter bias* been eliminated?

Are *measurements* objective, replicable, statistically analyzed, and peer reviewed before publication?

[a]Adapted in part from Gottlieb, M. I., Zinkus, P. W., and Bradford, L. J. (eds.): Brown, G W.: Learning disabilities: FadS, fallacies and fictions, in *Learning Disabilities: An Audio Journal for Continuing Education*, Grune & Stratton, New York, 1979.

AMERICAN ACADEMY OF PEDIATRICS: DOMAN-DELACATO TREATMENT OF NEUROLOGICALLY HANDICAPPED CHILDREN*

During the past decade the Institutes for the Achievement of Human Potential and their affiliates have made increasing claims for the efficacy of their methods of treatment for brain damage and other disorders.[1,2] A few organizations have issued cautionary statements.[3-8] Information has recently become available that makes it important to review the current status of the controversy and to propose some recommendations.

The reasons for concern include the following:

1. Promotional methods[9,10] appear to put parents in a position where they cannot refuse such treatment without calling into question their adequacy and motivation as parents.
2. The regimens prescribed are so demanding and inflexible[9-11] that they may lead to neglect of other family members' needs.[12]
3. It is asserted that if therapy is not carried out as rigidly prescribed, the child's potential will be damaged, and that anything less than 100% effort is useless.[9,10]
4. Restrictions are often placed upon age-appropriate activities of which the child is capable, such as walking or listening to music,[12,13] although unwarranted by any supportive data and knowledge of long-term results published to date.
5. Claims are made for rapid and conclusive diagnosis[15] according to a Developmental Profile[16] of no known validity. No data on which construction of the Profile has been based have ever been published, nor do we know of any attempt or cross-validate it against any accepted methods.
6. Undocumented claims are made for cures in a substantial number of cases,[1,2] extending even beyond disease states to making normal children superior,[2,9,17,18] easing world tensions,[2] and possibly "hastening the evolutionary process."[2,19]
7. Without supporting data, Doman and Delacato have indicted many typical child-rearing practices as limiting a child's potential, thereby increasing the anxiety of already burdened and confused parents.[12,20]

The controversy over these claims and assertions has recently been reviewed in some detail.[12]

The Theory

The theory is alleged to be of universal applicability,[2,18] but is largely based on questionable and oversimplified concepts of hemispheric dominance and the relation of individual sequential development to phylogenesis.[21] Furthermore, it asserts that the great majority of cases of mental retardation, learning problems, and behavioral disorders are caused by brain damage or "poor neurological organization,"[15] and that all these problems lie somewhere on a single continuum of brain damage, for which the treatment advocated by the Institutes is the only effective answer.[2,9]

The available information does not support these contentions. In particular, the lack of uniform dominance or sidedness is probably not a significant factor in either the etiology or therapy of these conditions.[21-27]

Cultural and anthropological differences have also been "explained" by the theory. For example, the lack of a written language in some primitive tribes is attributed to restrictions on crawling and creeping,[28] an exceedingly narrow and questionable view.

A careful review of the theory has led to the conclusion that "the tenets are either unsupported or overwhelmingly contradicted when tested by theoretical, experimental, or logical evidence from

*Modified from *AAP Newsletter Supplement*, June 1, 1968. Copyright American Academy of Pediatrics, 1968. Approved by the American Academy of Cerebral Palsy; American Academy of Neurology; American Association on Mental Deficiency; Canadian Association for Children with Learning Disabilities; Canadian Association for Retarded Children; Canadian Rehabilitation Council for the Disabled; Congress of Rehabilitation Medicine; the National Association for Retarded Children (U.S.), and the American Academy of Pediatrics.

the relevant scientific literature. As a scientific hypothesis the theory of neurological organization seems to be without merit."[21]

Current Status of Claimed Therapeutic Results

Results published by the Institutes or their supporters are inconclusive.[15,29,30] Many reports of improvement in reading ability have been heralded as support for the theory,[19,31,32] but statistical analysis has shown no demonstrable benefit.[21,33]

It has been pointed out repeatedly that some young handicapped children have been misdiagnosed or given unduly pessimistic prognosis. The course of maturation in these children is quite varied and may result in an unwarranted claim that improvement was due to the specific form of treatment.[12,34,35] Some of the cases dramatically publicized by the Institutes have been children with traumatic brain damage, who often make substantial gains without any special treatment.

Some controlled studies of the Doman-Delacato claims with respect to reading have been carried out and have shown no benefit.[36–39]

Previous cautionary statements have emphasized the need for well-controlled studies. The theoretical and practical problems involved in carrying out a study of all aspects of the Institutes' claims present many difficulties.[40] A well-designed, comprehensive study (supported by both federal and private agencies) was in the final planning stage when the Institutes withdrew their original agreement to the design.[41] With the failure of this attempt, the burden of proof for claimed results lies with the Institutes.

No data are available that contradict the likelihood that any improvement observed with this method of treatment can be accounted for on the basis of growth and development, the intensive practice of certain isolated skills, or the nonspecific effects of intensive stimulation.

Summary

The Institutes for the Achievement of Human Potential appear to differ substantially from other groups treating developmental problems in (1) the excessive nature of their undocumented claims for cure, and (2) the extreme demands placed upon parents in carrying out an unproven technique without fail.

Advice to parents and professional workers cannot await conclusive results of controlled studies of all aspects of the method. Physicians and therapists should acquaint themselves with the issues in the controversy and the available evidence. We have done this and concur with the conclusion of Robbins and Glass[21]:

> There is no empirical evidence to substantiate the value of either the theory or practice of neurological organization. . . . If the theory is to be taken seriously. . . its advocates are under an obligation to provide reasonable support for the tenets of the theory and a series of experimental investigations, consistent with scientific standards, which test the efficacy of the rationale.

To date, we know of no attempt to fulfill this obligation.

References

1. Bird, J.: When children can't learn. *Saturday Evening Post* **240(15)**:27–31, 72–74, 1967.
2. Institutes for the Achievement of Human Potential: *Human Potential* **1(1)**, 1967.
3. American Academy of Pediatrics: Executive Board Statement. *AAP Newsletter* **16(11)**:1, 6, 1965.
4. American Academy for Cerebral Palsy: *Statement of Executive Committee*, Feb. 15, 1965.
5. United Cerebral Palsy Association of Texas: The Doman-Delacato Treatment of Neurologically Handicapped Children. Undated information bulletin.
6. Canadian Association for Retarded Children: Institutes for the achievement of human potential. *Mental Retardation* (Canada) **Fall:** 27–28, 1965.
7. American Academy of Neurology, Joint Executive Board Statement: The Doman-Delacato treatment of neurologically handicapped children. *Neurology* **17:**637, 1967.

8. American Academy of Physical Medicine and Rehabilitation: Statement on Doman-Delacato Treatment of Neurologically Handicapped Children, 1967.
9. Beck, J.: Unlocking the secrets of the brain. *Chicago Tribune Magazine* Sept. 13, 27, 1964.
10. Linton, T. S.: *A Parent's Guide to Patterning and Floor Activity*, The Neurosurgical Institute and the Neurosurgical Clinic for Children, Media, PA, Undated (processed).
11. Maisel, A. Q.: Hope for brain-injured children. *Reader's Digest* Oct.: 135–140, 1964.
12. Freeman, R. D.: Controversy over "patterning" as a treatment for brain damage in children. *J.A.M.A.* **202(5):**385–388, 1967.
13. Institutes for the Achievement of Human Potential: Instruction Sheets, *The Romper*, 1963; *The Harness*, 1964.
14. LeWinn, E. B., Doman, G., Doman, R. J., Delacato, C. H., Spitz, E. B., and Thomas, E. W.: Neurological organization: The basis for learning, in: J. Hellmuth (ed.): *Learning Disorders*, Vol. 2. Special Child Publication, Seattle, pp. 48–93, 1966.
15. Institutes for the Achievement of Human Potential: *A Summary of Concepts, Procedures and Organization*, 1964.
16. Institutes for the Achievement of Human Potential: *The Doman-Delacato Profile and the Doman-Moran Graphic Summary*, 1963 (revised 1965).
17. Institutes for the Achievement of Human Potential: *Bulletin* **12(1):**57–58, 1967.
18. Institutes for the Achievement of Human Potential: *Statement of Objectives*. Undated.
19. Delacato, C. H.: *The Treatment and Prevention of Reading Problems: The Neuro-Psychological Approach*. Charles C. Thomas, Springfield, Illinois, 1959.
20. Doman, G., and Delacato, C. H.: Train Your Baby to be a Genius. *McCall's* **65:**169–170, 172, 1965.
21. Robbins, M. P., and Glass, G. V.: The Doman-Delacato rationale: A critical analysis, in J. Hellmuth (ed.): *Educational Therapy*, Vol. 2. Special Child Publication, Seattle, 1968.
22. Money, J.: Dyslexia: A postconference review, in J. Money (ed.): *Reading Disability: Progress and Research Needs in Dyslexia*. Johns Hopkins Press, Baltimore, 1962, pp. 9–33.
23. Money, J.: Reading Disorders in Children, in *Brenneman-Kelley Practice of Pediatrics*. Vol. 4. Hoeber–Harper, Hagerstown, Maryland, pp. 1–14, 1967.
24. Belmont, L., and Birch, H. G.: Lateral dominance, lateral awareness, and reading disability. *Child Dev.* **36:**57–71, 1965.
25. Spitzer, R. L., Rabkin, R., and Kramer, Y.: The relationship between mixed dominance and reading disabilities. *J. Pediatr.* **54:**76–80, 1959.
26. Stephens, W. E., Cunningham, E. S., and Stigler, B. J.: Reading readiness and eye–hand preference patterns in first grade children. *Except. Child.* **33:**481–488, 1967.
27. Bettman, J. W., Jr., Stern, E. L., Whitsell, L. J., et al.: Cerebral dominance in developmental dyslexia. *Arch. Ophthalmol.* **78:**722–729, 1967.
28. Green, L. J.: Functional neurological performance in primitive cultures. *Hum. Potential* **1(1):**19–26, 1967.
29. Doman, R. J., Spitz, E. B., Zucman, E., et al.: Children with severe brain injuries: Neurological organization in terms of mobility. *J.A.M.A.* **174:**257–262, 1960.
30. Freeman, R. D.: Review of J. R. Kershner: An investigation of the Doman-Delacato theory of neuropsychology as it applies to trainable mentally retarded children in public schools. *J. Pediatr.* **71:**914–915, 1967.
31. Delacato, C. H.: *The Diagnosis and Treatment of Speech and Reading Problems*. Charles C. Thomas, Springfield, Illinois, 1963.
32. Delacato, C. H.: *Neurological Organization and Reading*. Charles C. Thomas, Springfield, Illinois, 1966.
33. Glass, G. V.: *A Critique of Experiments on the Role of Neurological Organization in Reading Performance*. University of Illinois College of Education, Urbana, Illinois, October 1966.
34. Koch, R., Graliker, B., Bronston, W., et al.: Mental retardation in early childhood. *Am. J. Diseases Child.* **109:**243–251, 1965.
35. Masland, R. L.: Unproven methods of treatment. *Pediatrics* **37:**713–714, 1966.
36. Robbins, M. P.: *The Delacato Interpretation of Neurological Organization: An Empirical Study*. Unpublished doctoral dissertation, University of Chicago, 1965.
37. Robbins, M. P.: A study of the validity of Delacato's theory of neurological organization. *Except. Child.* **32:**517–523, 1966.
38. Robbins, M. P.: Creeping, laterality and reading. *Acad. Ther. Q.* **1:**200–206, 1966.
39. Robbins, M. P.: Test of the Doman-Delacato rationale with retarded readers. *J.A.M.A.* **202:**389–393, 1967.
40. Rosner, B. S.: Outcomes of Treatment of Brain-damaged Children: Are Controlled Studies Possible? Unpublished manuscript, 1967.
41. Rosner, B. S.: Final Report on Planning Grant: Treatment of Brain-injured Children (to Vocational Rehabilitation Administration, National Association for Retarded Children, Given Foundation), 1967.

AMERICAN ACADEMY OF PEDIATRICS: THE EYE AND LEARNING DISABILITIES*,†

The problem of learning disability has become a matter of increasing public concern, which has led to exploitation by some practitioners of the normal concern of parents for the welfare of their children. A child's inability to read with understanding as a result of defects in processing visual symbols, a condition which has been called dyslexia, is a major obstacle to school learning and has far-reaching social and economic implications. The significance and magnitude of the problem have generated a proliferation of diagnostic and remedial procedures, many of which imply a relationship between visual function and learning.[1]

The eye and visual training in the treatment of dyslexia and associated learning disabilities have recently been reviewed‡ with the following conclusions by the American Academy of Pediatrics, the American Academy of Ophthalmology and Otolaryngology, and the American Association of Ophthalmology:

1. Learning disability and dyslexia, as well as other forms of school underachievement, require a multi-disciplinary approach from medicine, education, and psychology in diagnosis and treatment. *Eye care should never be instituted in isolation when a patient has a reading problem.* Children with learning disabilities have the same incidence of ocular abnormalities, e.g., refractive errors and muscle imbalance, as children who are normal achievers and reading at grade level.[2-4] These abnormalities should be corrected.

2. Since clues in word recognition are transmitted through the eyes to the brain, it has become common practice to attribute reading difficulties to subtle ocular abnormalities presumed to cause faulty visual perception. Studies have shown that *there is no peripheral eye defect that produces dyslexia and associated learning disabilities.*[5,6] Eye defects do not cause reversals of letters, words, or numbers.

3. No known scientific evidence supports claims for improving the academic abilities of learning-disabled or dyslexic children with treatment based solely on: (a) visual training (muscle exercises, ocular pursuit, glasses),[7-12] or (b) neurological organizational training (laterality training, balance board, perceptual training).[2-14] Furthermore, such training has frequently resulted in unwarranted expense and has delayed proper instruction for the child.

4. Excluding correctable ocular defects, glasses have no value in the specific treatment of dyslexia or other learning problems. In fact, unnecessarily prescribed glasses may create a false sense of security that may delay needed treatment.

5. The teaching of learning-disabled and dyslexic children is a problem of educational science. No one approach is applicable to all children. A change in any variable may result in increased motivation of the child and reduced frustration. Parents should be made aware that mental level and psychological implications are contributing factors to a child's success or failure. Ophthalmologists and other medical specialists should offer their knowledge. This may consist of the identification of specific defects, or simply early recognition. The precursors of learning disabilities can often be detected by 3 years of age. Since remediation may be more effective during the early years,[15] it is important for the physician to recognize the child with this problem and refer him to the appropriate service, if available, before he is of school age. Medical specialists may assist in bringing the child's potential to the best level, but the actual remedial educational procedures remain the responsibility of educators.

References

1. Optometric Extension Program. L. Manas, Duncan, Oklahoma.
2. Flax, N.: Visual functions in learning disabilities. *J. Learning Disab.* **1**:551, 1968.

*Modified from AAP. Joint Organizational Statement: The eye and learning disabilities, *Pediatrics* **49**:454, 1972.
†The Executive Committees and Councils of the American Academy of Pediatrics, the American Academy of Ophthalmology and Otolaryngology and the American Association of Ophthalmology have approved this statement.
‡This statement was prepared by an ad hoc committee of the American Academy of Pediatrics, the American Academy of Ophthalmology and Otolaryngology, and the American Association of Ophthalmology with the assistance of the President and the Past President of the Division for Children With Learning Disabilities.

3. Bettman, J. W., Jr., Stern, E. L., Whitsell, L. J., *et al.*: Cerebral dominance in developmental dyslexia: Role of ophthalmologist. *Arch. Ophthalmol.* **78:**722, 1967.
4. Norn, M. S., Rindziunsky, and Skydsgaard: Ophthalmologic and orthoptic examinations of dyslectics. *Acta Ophthal.,* **47:**147, 1969.
5. Goldberg, H. K. and Drash, P. W.: The disabled reader. *J. Pediatr. Ophthalmol.* **5:**11, 1968.
6. Goldberg, H. K.: The ophthalmologist looks at the reading problem. *Am. J. Ophthalmol.* **47:**67, 1959.
7. Robbins, M. P.: Test of the Doman-Delacato rationale with retarded readers. *J.A.M.A.* **202:**389, 1967.
8. Cohen, H. J., Birch, H. G., and Taft, L. T.: Some considerations for evaluating the Doman-Delacato "patterning" method. *Pediatrics* **45:**302, 1970.
9. Freeman, R. D.: Controversy over "patterning" as a treatment for brain damage in children. *J.A.M.A.* **202:**385, 1967.
10. Doman-Delacato Treatment of neurologically handicapped children. American Academy of Pediatrics. *Newsletter.* Committee on the Handicapped Child, June 1, 1968.
11. Goldberg, H. K.: Role of patching in learning. *J. Pediatr. Ophthalmol.* **6:**123, 1969.
12. Goldberg, H. K., and Arnott, W.: Ocular motility in learning disabilities. *J. Learning Disab.* **3:**160, 1970.
13. Rosen, C. L.: An experimental study of visual perceptual training and reading achievement in first grade. *Percept Mot. Skills* **22:**979, 1966.
14. Smith, H. M.: Motor activity and perceptual development. *J. Health-Physical-Recreation* 1968.
15. Children's Hospital Developmental and Evaluation Clinic. J. McMahon, Denver, Colorado.

I

Miscellaneous Information

OVERVIEW OF MAJOR SEQUENCES IN DEVELOPMENT

Age	Gross motor	Fine motor	Adaptive	Language	Personal-social
4 weeks	Asymmetrical tonic neck reflex positions predominate. Head sags forward in sitting.	Hands fisted. Hands clench on contact.	Regards object in line of vision only. Follows to midline. Drops toy immediately.	Vague indirect regard. Small throaty noises.	Stares indefinitely at surroundings. Regards observer's face and diminshes activity.
16 weeks	Symmetrical postures predominate. Head steady in sitting. Head lifted 90° when prone on forearms.	Hands engage. Scratches and clutches.	Eyes follow slowly moving object well. Arms activate on sight of dangling toy. Regards toy in hand and takes to mouth. Regard goes from hand to object when sitting.	Laughs aloud. Excites and breathes heavily.	Spontaneous social smile. Hand play with mutual fingering. Pulls dress over face. Anticipates food on sight.
28 weeks	Sits briefly leaning forward on hands. Supports large fraction of weight in standing. Bounces actively in supported standing.	Has radial palmar grasp of toy. Rakes at small pellet with whole hand.	One-hand approach and grasp of toy. Bangs and shakes rattle. Transfers toy from one hand to the other.	Vocalizes "m-m-m" when crying. Talks to toys.	Takes feet to mouth. Reaches for and pats mirror image.
40 weeks	Sits steady indefinitely. Creeps and pulls to feet at rail.	Crude release of toy. Plucks pellet easily with thumb and index finger.	Matches two objects in hand. Index finger approach. Spontaneously rings bell.	Says "mama" and "dada" with meaning. One other "word."	Waves "bye-bye" and pat-a-cake (or other nursery trick). Feeds self cracker and holds own bottle.
52 weeks	Walks with 1 hand held. Stands alone momentarily.	Neat pincer grasp of pellet.	Tries to build tower of two cubes. Releases cube in cup (after demonstration). Serial play with objects.	Two words besides "mama" and "dada." Gives toy on request or gesture.	Offers toy to image in mirror. Cooperates in dressing.
15 months	Toddles independently. Creeps upstairs.	Puts pellet into bottle.	Builds tower of two cubes in and out of cup. Incipient imitation of stroke.	Jargons. Four to six words, including names. Pats pictures in book.	Says "thank-you" or equivalent. Points or vocalizes wants. Indicates wet pants. Casts objects in play or refusal.

Age	Motor		Adaptive	Language	Personal-Social
18 months	Walks, seldom falling. Seats self in small chairs and climbs into adult chair. Hurls ball in standing position.	Turns pages of book two to three at a time.	Builds tower of three to four cubes. Imitates stroke with a crayon and scribbles spontaneously. Dumps pellet from bottle.	Has 10 words. Looks selectively at pictures and identifies 1. Names ball and carries out two directions ("on the table"; "to mother")	Pulls toy on string. Carries and hugs doll. Feeds self in part with spilling.
2 years	Runs well, no falling. Walks up and down stairs alone. Kicks large ball on request.	Turns pages of book singly.	Builds tower of six to seven cubes. Alignes cubes for train. Imitates vertical and circular strokes.	Uses pronouns. Three-word sentences; jargon discarded. Carries out four directions with ball ("on the chair," "to mother," "to me").	Verbalizes toilet needs consistently. Pulls on simple garment. Inhibits turning of spoon in feeding. Plays with domestic mimicry.
3 years	Alternates feet going upstairs. Jumps from bottom step. Rides tricycle, using pedals.	Holds crayon with fingers.	Builds tower of nine to ten cubes. Imitates three cubes bridge. Names own drawing. Copies circle and imitates cross.	Uses plurals. Gives action in picture book. Gives sex and full name. Obeys two prepositional commands ("on," "under").	Feeds self well. Puts on shoes and unbuttons buttons. Knows few rhymes or songs. Understands taking turns.
4 years	Walks downstairs alternating feet. Does broad jump. Throws ball overhand.		Draws man with two parts. Copies cross. Counts three objects with correct pointing. Imitates five-cube gate.	Names one or more colors correctly. Obeys five prepositional commands ("on," "under," "in back," "in front," "besides").	Washes and dries face and hands; brushes teeth. Distinguishes front from back of clothes. Laces shoes. Goes on errands outside of home.
5 years	Skips, alternating feet. Stands on 1 foot more than 8 sec.		Builds two steps with cubes. Draws unmistakable man with body, head, etc. Copies triangle. Counts 10 objects correctly.	Knows four colors. Names penny, nickel, dime. Descriptive comment on pictures. Carries out three commissions.	Dresses and undresses without assistance. Asks meaning of words. Prints a few letters.
6 years	Advanced throwing. Stands on each foot alternately, eyes closed.		Builds three steps with blocks. Draws man with neck, hands, and clothes. Copies diamond.	Uses Stanford-Binet items (vocabulary).	Ties shoelaces. Differentiates AM and PM. Knows right from left. Counts to 30.

MENTAL RETARDATION: FUNCTIONAL LEVELS

Level of mental retardation	Approx. IQ range	Preschool age: 0–5 years (maturation and development)	School age: 6–21 years (training and education)	Adults: 21 years and over (social and vocational adequacy)
Profound	<21	Gross mental retardation with minimal capacity for functioning in sensorimotor areas. Generally requires nursing care.	Obvious significant delays in all areas of development. Basic emotional responses. May respond to skillful training in use of legs, hands, and jaws. Generally requires supervision.	May walk but needs nursing care. Primitive speech. Usually benefits from regular physical activity. Incapable of self-maintenence.
Severe	20–35	Marked delay in motor development. Little or no comunication skills. May respond to training in elementary self-help (e.g., self-feeding)	Usually walks barring specific disability. Some understanding of speech. Profits from systemic habit training.	Conforms to daily routines and repetitive activities. Requires continuing direction and supervision in protected environment.
Moderate	35–55	Delays observed in motor development, especially in speech. Responds to training in various self-help activities.	Can learn simple communication, elementary health and safety habits and simple manual skills. Poor progress in functional reading or arithmetic.	Can perform simple tasks under sheltered conditions. Participates in simple interaction. Can travel alone in familiar places. Usually incapable of self-maintenance.
Mild	55–70	Often not recognized as "retarded" by a casual observer. Slower to walk, feed self and talk than most children.	Acquires practical skills and useful reading and arithmetic to third- to sixth-grade level with special education. Can be guided toward social conformity.	Can achieve social and vocational skills adequate for self-maintenance. May need occasional guidance and support when under unusual social or economic stress.
Borderline	70–85	As a rule not detected as "slow" until school age. Near average in physical development and acquisition of self-help skills.	Can acquire practical skills and useful academic skills to a seventh- or eighth-grade level with special education. "Slow learner" with good social skills.	Can achieve social vocational skills adequate to self-maintenance. Needs less guidance than mildly retarded group but may require support under unusual stress.

ORGANIZATIONS AND AGENCIES SERVING CHILDREN WITH DEVELOPMENTAL DISABILITIES

Alexander Graham Bell Association for the Deaf
3417 Volta Place, N.W.
Washington, D.C. 20007

American Association on Mental Deficiency
5101 Wisconsin Avenue
Washington, D.C. 20016

American Coalition of Citizens with Disabilities
1346 Connecticut Ave., N.W.
Suite 1124
Washington, D.C. 20036

American Council for the Blind
1211 Connecticut Avenue
Washington, D.C. 20006

American Foundation for the Blind, Inc.
15 West 16th Street
New York, New York 10011

American Occupational Therapy Association
1383 Piccard Drive
Rockville, Maryland 20580

American Physical Therapy Association
1156 15th Street, N.W.
Washington, D.C. 20005

American Printing House for the Blind
P.O. Box 6085
Louisville, Kentucky 40206

American Speech and Hearing Association
10801 Rockville Pike
Rockville, Maryland 20852

Association for Children with Learning Disabilities
4156 Library Road
Pittsburgh, Pennsylvania 15234

Association for Education of the Visually Handicapped
919 Walnut Street, Fourth Floor
Philadelphia, Pennsylvania 19107

Canadian Association for the Mentally Retarded
Kinsmen NIMR Building
York University Campus
4700 Keele Street, Downsview
Toronto, Ontario, Canada M3J1Pe

Canadian National Institute for the Blind
1929 Bayview Avenue
Toronto, Ontario, Canada M4G3F8

Canadian Rehabilitation Council for the Disabled
1 Young Street, Suite 2110
Toronto, Ontario, Canada M5E1A5

Council of Education of the Deaf
6 Gallaudet College
Seventh Street and Florida Avenue
Washington, D.C. 20002

Council for Exceptional Children
1920 Association Drive
Reston, Virginia 22091

Epilepsy Foundation of America
1828 L. Street, Suite 405
Washington, D.C. 20036

Federation of the Handicapped
211 West 14th Street
New York, N.Y. 10011

Foundation for Children with Learning Disabilities
99 Park Avenue, Second Floor
New York, N.Y. 10011

International Spinal Cord Research Foundation
4100 Spring Valley Road, Suite
104 LB3
Dallas, Texas 75234

John Tracy Clinic (deafness/hearing impairments, deaf-blind)
806 West Adams Boulevard
Los Angeles, California 90007

Juvenile Diabetes Association
23 East 26th Street
New York, N.Y. 10010

National Association of the Deaf
814 Thayer Avenue
Silver Spring, Maryland 20910

National Association for Down's Syndrome
Box 63
Oak Park, Illinois 60303

National Association for Mental Health, Inc.
1800 N. Kent Street, Second Floor
Arlington, Virginia 22209

National Association of the Deaf-Blind
2703 Forest Oak Circle
Norman, Oklahoma 73071

National Association of the Physically Handicapped
76 Elm Street
London, Ohio 43140

National Association of Private Residential Facilities for the Mentally Retarded
6269 Leesburg Pike
Falls Church, Virginia 22044

National Association of Private Schools for Exceptional Children
P.O. Box 34923
West Bethesda, Maryland 20817

National Association for Retarded Citizens
2501 Avenue J
Arlington, Texas 76011

National Association for the Visually Handicapped
305 East 24th Street, Room 17-C
New York, New York 10010

National Center for Law and the Handicapped
University of Notre Dame
P.O. Box 477
Notre Dame, Indiana 46556

National Congress of Organizations of the Physically
Handicapped, Inc.
1627 Deborah Avenue
Rockford, Illinois 61103

National Easter Seal Society for Crippled Children
and Adults
2023 West Ogden Avenue
Chicago, Illinois 60612

National Federation of the Blind
1346 Connecticut Avenue, N.W.
Suite 212, Dupont Circle Building
Washington, D.C. 20036

National Foundation of Dentistry for the
Handicapped
1726 Champa, Suite 422
Denver, Colorado 80202

National Foundation/March of Dimes
1275 Mamaroneck Avenue
White Plains, New York 10605

National Genetics Foundation
555 West 57th Street, Room 1240
New York, New York 10019

National Hearing Aid Society
20361 Middlebelt Road
Livona, Michigan 48152

National Society for Autistic Children
1234 Massachusetts Avenue, N.W.
Suite 1017
Washington, D.C. 20005

National Tay-Sachs and Allied Diseases Association
122 East 42nd Street
New York, New York 10068

National Tuberous Sclerosis Association
P.O. Box 159
Laguna Beach, California 92651

Orton Society (dyslexia)
8415 Bellona Lane
Towson, Maryland 21204

Quebec Association for Children with Learning
Disabilities
5003 Victoria Avenue
Montreal, Quebec, Canada H3W2NZ

Spina Bifida Association of America
343 South Dearborn Street
Room 327
Chicago, Illinois 60604

Tuberous Sclerosis Association of America
P.O. Box 44
Rockland, Massachusetts 02320

United Cerebral Palsy Association, Inc.
66 East 34th Street
New York, New York 10016

Government Agencies

Administration on Developmental Disabilities
Office of Human Development Services
Department of Health and Human Services
330 Independence Avenue, S.W., Room 3194
Washington, D.C. 20201

American Association of University Affiliated Programs for the Developmentally Disabled
(35 interdisciplinary facilities working with the Department of Health, Education and Welfare)
110 17th Street, N.W., Suite 908
Washington, D.C. 20026

National Information Center for Handicapped Children and Youth
1555 Wilson Blvd., Suite 600
Rosslyn, Virginia 22209

National Library for the Blind and Physically
Handicapped
Library of Congress
Washington, D.C. 20542

Office of Deafness and Communicative Disorders
Department of Education
Switzer Building, Room 3416
400 Maryland Avenue
Washington, D.C. 20202

President's Committee on Employment of the
Handicapped
Department of Labor
1111 20th Street, N.W.
Washington, D.C. 20036

Special Education and Rehabilitative Services Clear-
inghouse for the Handicapped
Department of Education
400 Maryland Avenue, S.W.
Switzer Building, Room 3106
Washington, D.C. 20202

COMPENDIUM OF SELECTED UNITED STATES GOVERNMENT AGENCIES INVOLVED WITH MENTAL RETARDATION AND DEVELOPMENTAL DISABILITY

Maternal and Child Health
Division of Maternal and Child Health
Offices of Health Services Administration
Parklawn Building
5600 Fishers Lane
Rockville, Maryland 20857

Administration on Developmental Disabilities
Office of Human Developmental Services
Switzer Building
330 C. Street, S.W.
Washington, D.C. 20201

Office of Special Education
Department of Education
400 Maryland Avenue, S.W.
Washington, D.C. 20202

National Institute of Child Health and Human
Development
Mental Retardation and Developmental Disabilities
Branch
Landow Building
National Institute of Health
Bethesda, Maryland 20205

National Institute for Handicapped Research
Hubert M. Humphrey Bldg., Room 305F
200 Independence Avenue, S.W.
Washington, D.C. 20201

President's Committee on Mental Retardation
U.S. Department of Health and Human Services
Office of Human Development Services
Washington, D.C. 20201

ROSTER OF UNIVERSITY-AFFILIATED FACILITIES

Chauncey M. Sparks Center for Developmental and
Learning Disorders
University of Alabama at Birmingham
1720 Seventh Avenue South
Birmingham, Alabama 35233

Division of Clinical Genetics and Developmental
Disabilities
Department of Pediatrics
College of Medicine
University of California at Irvine
Irvine, California 92717

University Affiliated Facility
Mental Retardation Program
University of California at Los Angeles
760 Westwood Plaza
Los Angeles, California 90024

University Affiliated Program
Children's Hospital of Los Angeles
University of Southern California
4650 Sunset Boulevard
Los Angeles, California 90027

John F. Kennedy Child Development Center
University of Colorado Health Sciences Center
4200 East 9th Avenue
Box C234
Denver, Colorado 80262

Georgetown University
Child Development Center
Bles Building, Room CG-52
3800 Reservoir Road, N.W.
Washington, D.C. 20007

Child Development Center and Multidisciplinary
Training Facility
Mailman Center for Child Development
University of Miami
P.O. Box 016820
Miami, Florida 33101

University Affiliated Facility
Georgia Retardation Center
Athens
850 College Station Road
Athens, Georgia 30610

Illinois Institute for Developmental Disabilities
1640 West Roosevelt Road
Chicago, Illinois 60608

Developmental Training Center
Indiana University
2853 East Tenth Street
Bloomington, Indiana 47405

Riley Child Development Center
Indiana University Medical Center
1100 West Michigan Street
Indianapolis, Indiana 46223

University Hospital School
The University of Iowa
Iowa City, Iowa 52242

Kansas University Affiliated Facility, Kansas City
Children's Rehabilitation Unit
Kansas University Medical Center
39th and Rainbow Boulevard
Kansas City, Kansas 66103

Kansas University Affiliated Facility
Central Office
Bureau of Child Research
223 Haworth Hall
University of Kansas
Lawrence, Kansas 66045

Kansas University Affiliated Facility at Parsons
2601 Gabriel
Parsons, Kansas 67357

University of Kentucky Human Development
Program
114 Porter Building
730 South Limestone
Lexington, Kentucky 40506

Developmental Disability Center for Children
Louisiana State University Medical Center
1100 Florida Avenue
Building #138
New Orleans, Louisiana 70119

The John F. Kennedy Institute for Handicapped
Children
707 North Broadway
Baltimore, Maryland 21205

Developmental Evaluation Clinic
Children's Hospital Medical Center
300 Longwood Avenue
Boston, Massachusetts 02115

Eunice Kennedy Shriver Center for Mental
Retardation
Walter E. Fernald State School
200 Trapelo Road
Waltham, Massachusetts 02254

Eastern Maine Medical Center
Bangor, Maine

Institute for the Study of Mental Retardation and
Related Disorders
University of Michigan
130 South First Street
Ann Arbor, Michigan 48104

Child Development Section
St. Paul–Ramsey Medical Center
640 North Jackson
St. Paul, Minnesota 55101

University Affiliated Program of Mississippi
1100 Robert E. Lee Building
Jackson, Mississippi 39201

University Affiliated Facility for Developmental
Disabilities
University of Missouri at Kansas City
Institute for Community Studies, School of Graduate
Studies
2220 Holmes Street
Kansas City, Missouri 64108

Meyer Children's Rehabilitation Institute
University of Nebraska Medical Center
444 South 44th Street
Omaha, Nebraska 68131

Institute for Human Services
Kean College of New Jersey
Morris Avenue
Union, New Jersey 07083

University Affiliated Facility
Rose F. Kennedy Center
Albert Einstein College of Medicine
Yeshiva University
1410 Pelham Parkway South
Bronx, New York 10461

Developmental Disabilities Center
St. Lukes–Roosevelt Hospital
Columbia University, College of Physicians and
Surgeons
428 West 59th Street
New York, New York 10019

University Affiliated Diagnostic
Clinic for Developmental Disorders
University of Rochester Medical Center
Box 671
601 Elmwood Avenue
Rochester, New York 14642

Mental Retardation Institute
New York Medical College at Valhalla
Valhalla, New York 10595

Division for Disorders of Development and Learning
The University of North Carolina at Chapel Hill
Biological Sciences Research Center 220H
Chapel Hill, North Carolina 27514

University Affiliated Program Center for Human
Development
Ohio University
Convocation Center
Athens, Ohio 45701

University Affiliated Cincinnati Center for Develop-
mental Disorders
Pavilion Building
Elland and Bethesda Avenues
Cincinnati, Ohio 45229

Nisonger Center for Mental Retardation and Developmental Disabilities
The Ohio State University McCampbell Hall
1580 Cannon Drive
Columbus, Ohio 43210

Center on Human Development
University of Oregon
901 East 18th Street
Eugene, Oregon 97403

Child Development and Rehabilitation Center
Crippled Children's Division
University of Oregon Health Sciences Center
P.O. Box 574
Portland, Oregon 97207

Developmental Disabilities Program
Temple University
Ritter Annex
13th Street and Columbia Avenue
Philadelphia, Pennsylvania 19122

Child Development Center
Rhode Island Hospital
593 Eddy Street
Providence, Rhode Island 02902

U.A.F. Program of South Carolina
Human Development Center
Winthrop College
Rock Hill, South Carolina 29733

U.A.F. Program of South Carolina, U.S.C.
Center for Developmental Disabilities
Benson Building, Pickens Street
University of South Carolina
Columbus, South Carolina 29208

Center for the Developmentally Disabled
University of South Dakota
Julian Hall
Vermillion, South Dakota 57069

Child Development Center
University of Tennessee
711 Jefferson Avenue
Memphis, Tennessee 38105

University Affiliated Center for Developmentally
Disabled Children
Department of Pediatrics
University of Texas Health Sciences Center at Dallas
5323 Harry Hines Blvd.
Dallas, Texas 75235

Exceptional Child Center
Utah State University
UMC 68
Logan, Utah 84322·

Child Development and Mental Retardation Center
University of Washington
Seattle, Washington 98195

University Affiliated Center for Developmental
Disabilities
807 Allen Hall
West Virginia University
Morgantown, West Virginia 26506

Harry A. Waisman Center on Mental Retardation
and Human Development
University of Wisconsin
1500 Highland Avenue
Madison, Wisconsin 53706

Dine Center for Human Development
Navajo Satellite Center
Navajo Community College
Tsaile, Arizona

Hawaii Affiliated Facility
Satellite Program
1319 Punahou Street
Bingham 106
Honolulu, Hawaii 98626

Montana University Affiliated Program Satellite
Social Science Building
University of Montana
Missoula, Montana 59812

Center for Developmental Disabilities
University Affiliated Facility Satellite
449C Waterman Building
University of Vermont
Burlington, Vermont 05405

AAP STUDIES PEDIATRIC ROLE IN EDUCATION FOR HANDICAPPED LAW*

With grant funding from the federal Bureau of Education for the Handicapped (BEH), the Academy has acquired a special resource consultant for one year to help chapters participate in the implementation of P.L. 94-142, the Education for All Handicapped Children Act of 1975.

P.L. 94-142 is intended to "assure that all handicapped children have available to them free, appropriate public education designed to meet their unique needs, to insure that the rights of handicapped children and their parents or guardians are protected, to assist states and localities to provide for the education of all handicapped children and to assess and assure the effectiveness of efforts to educate handicapped children."

The law provides a timetable to which states must adhere in their implementation of educational services for all handicapped children. Target dates in that schedule are as follows:

*Modified from AAP Studies Pediatric Role in Education for Handicapped Law, News and Comment. American Academy of Pediatrics, October 1978. Copyright American Academy of Pediatrics, 1978.

1. By Oct. 1, 1977, states were required to have completed individualized educational plans (IEPs) for each handicapped child being served by the state educational system at that time.
2. By September 1, 1978, states were required to have identified all unserved handicapped children between the ages of 3–18 and have developed IEPs for each of these additional children who were then added to the educational system.
3. The program will reach its full potential September 1, 1980. By that date, states are required to offer appropriate individualized education to all handicapped children and youth between the ages of 3–21.

These all-encompassing regulations were qualified in some instances. For example, programs for individuals in the 3–5 and 18–21 age groups need not be provided if they are not available to nonhandicapped children.

Because education is a state responsibility, individual states cannot be forced to comply with P.L. 94-142. However, to receive federal funding for education for the handicapped, states must adhere to the law's regulations. Even without this law, states are bound to provide appropriate education for the handicapped by the Rehabilitation Act of 1973, Section 504. Failure to comply with Section 504 regulations jeopardizes a state's federal assistance. Only one state, New Mexico, has elected to draft its own educational program for the handicapped rather than participate in P.L. 94-142.

The P.L. 94-142 related project in which the Academy is participating is directed by Melvin Levine, FAAP, who specializes in learning problems and developmental pediatrics. Dr. Levine is chief of the Division of Ambulatory Pediatrics at Children's Hospital Medical Center in Boston. The project has two objectives: to educate pediatricians and other practitioners about P.L. 94-142, and to increase knowledge of pediatricians and other practitioners about developmental disabilities in general.

For its part in the grant project, the Academy will work with William T. Twarog, the resource consultant, in providing to chapters state by state information on education for the handicapped.

Twarog began his job in August, reviewing individual state plans for implementation of P.L. 94-142, checking for ways in which pediatricians could become involved. This information will be sent to each chapter chairman or designated liaison representative for education of the handicapped. As more detailed information becomes available throughout the year, this also will be sent out.

The AAP resource consultant for P.L. 94-142 also will serve as a consultant to the individual chapters, traveling to chapter and district meetings on request to explain the intricacies of P.L. 94-142, offer suggestions for chapter involvement in state programs and relate information on progress being made in other states.

A second assignment for the resource consultant is to assist in the development of an AAP syllabus/core curriculum, including written materials and audiovisual programs, designed to train practitioners in evaluation and medical management of children with developmental disabilities. A grant request for this project will be submitted to BEH this month, for funding to begin in June 1979.

As of this writing, Twarog is working in the AAP Central Office, before being stationed in Boston and traveling to chapter and district meetings.

Reaching and providing suitable education for each handicapped child under the regulations of P.L. 94-142 is an ongoing three-stage process, as explained by Twarog: .

1. *Child identification:* The pediatrician, as often the first professional to see a child's handicap, plays a key role in identification and referral of children in need of special educational services. Pediatricians may make the initial referral by contacting the identification program in their state directly (program names vary—"Child Find" "Search and Serve"—but most have a hot line for referral). Referrals also may be made directly to the local school district or to a variety of cooperating agencies in each state which serve handicapped children, such as the Easter Seal Foundation, Association for Retarded Citizens, etc.

2. *Evaluation:* All children identified with suspected handicapping conditions must undergo a total assessment by an evaluation team. P.L. 94-142 regulations do not mandate the membership of this multidisciplinary team. The regulations, however, suggest several professions that should be represented on the team. Although the law itself does not require that a physician be a member of the

evaluation team, some states, Massachusetts for example, stipulate that a physician must be involved in the evaluation and must perform a physical exam. Other states require examination by a physician only for certain specific handicapping conditions.

3. *Individualized educational plan:* An individualized educational plan (IEP) must be developed for each handicapped child each year. Using information from the child's evaluation, a child study team drafts his IEP, which contains annual goals and several short-term objectives for the child's education, and identifies related services that should be made available to the child, such as speech therapy, occupational therapy, and counseling.

"Pediatricians can play an effective role at every stage in the process in insuring that each child receives education appropriate to his or her needs," according to AAP resource consultant Twarog.

He explained that, "First, the pediatrician has a primary responsibility to identify children with handicaps at an early age and guide these children and their families to the proper educational agencies. Next, having performed the initial examination on a handicapped child, the pediatrician can offer to supply information to the child's evaluation team, or to serve on that team. Finally, when an IEP is developed, the child's pediatrician may request a copy, with the parents' permission, so that he may be fully informed as to the child's educational program."

Twarog, who was a school administrator prior to taking his current post, sees P.L. 94-142 as the common cause which can foster cooperation between physicians and school officials. "Physicians and educators should be working hand in hand to provide appropriate care for handicapped children."

Following a provision of P.L. 94-142, each state appoints an advisory panel to regulate implementation of the state's plan. These panels are comprised of a mix of professionals and consumers. Twarog urged that pediatricians work with state panels and familiarize themselves with their individual states' plans. He stressed that, "It is at the state and local level that the role of the pediatrician in the special education process will be defined and implemented."

GUIDELINES FOR HOME CARE OF INFANTS, CHILDREN, AND ADOLESCENTS WITH CHRONIC DISEASE*

Many infants, children, and adolescents with long-term, serious health problems are confined to hospitals for prolonged treatment during recovery, and such patients are rehospitalized frequently. Hospitalized patients usually lack the normal, interpersonal family relationships that are important to growth and development. Combining the benefits of home care with optimal medical treatment and support is a challenge requiring development of innovative programs among hospitals, physicians, parents, and communities.

Although home care programs for patients with chronic diseases have been implemented, objective data about the efficiency, risks, benefits, and cost of these programs are limited. Careful planning and coordination of family, hospital, and community resources are essential for home care programs, and initial guidelines for program development and assessment are needed.

The goal of a home care program for infants, children, or adolescents with chronic conditions is the provision of comprehensive, cost-effective health care within a nurturing home environment that maximizes the capabilities of the individual and minimizes the effects of the disabilities.

Program Development

Comprehensive planning for all aspects of home health care is essential to minimize physical and emotional risk to the patient, adverse effects on the family members, or unforseen financial burdens. Because of the many factors to be considered, a multidisciplinary team interested in implementation

---

*Modified from AAP. Ad Hoc Task Forces on Home Care of Chronically Ill Infants and Children: Guidelines for home care of infants, children and adolescents with chronic disease. *Pediatrics* **74**:434, 1984. Copyright American Academy of Pediatrics, 1984.

of home health care should be organized. The team should include a pediatrician and may include other physicians (e.g., generalists, community physicians, neonatologists, intensivists); nurses; occupational, physical, and speech therapists; developmentalists; child life workers; nutritionists; social workers; teachers; home care providers (e.g., nursing providers outside the hospital and equipment providers); parents; and insurers. The team must develop and implement comprehensive care recommendations and arrangements based on the patient's demonstrated needs. Many of the resources used in home care programs may be an extension of existing hospital services. After the program is developed, it must be individualized for each patient and family, and the family should play a major role in the program. A primary case coordinator to oversee the program and coordinate it should be selected for each patient. The coordinator must be known to the family and work closely with them.

Implementation

Patient Selection

Criteria should be established to determine candidates for home health care based on comprehensive analysis of the existing program capabilities, potential benefit, risks, care needs, and resources. The following factors should be included:

1. *Patient factors:* Underlying any potential for home care in chronic disease is the patient's medical stability vis-à-vis the capacity of the program to provide back-up and emergency care. When the patient's condition is as stable as possible, plans should be made to maintain this optimal state. A successful trial of care by the home care providers within the hospital setting (using emergency back-up by the regular hospital staff) is essential prior to discharge.

2. *Family factors:* Whenever possible, the availability of at least two members of the extended family—trained and fully able to care for the child in the home—is desirable. This is essential in some situations. There should be evidence of parental involvement, safety in performing medical and nursing tasks, and an appropriate home situation (e.g., physical environment, safety, and geographical location) for the medical safety to be reasonably assured. There should not be excessive pressure on families to take children home if this move would be detrimental.

3. *Community factors:* An interested local physician should provide primary care and participate in the home care program. This physician should oversee the plan and its medical safety. Availability of appropriate home health care providers, equipment, and special needs (e.g., gas suppliers) must be assured. Reasonable contingency plans for emergencies (e.g., power backup for those with life-support equipment and appropriate transportation) also must be available.

Care Plan Development

Careful review of the patient's status and needs in the hospital should be made by each discipline participating in the patient's care. Each of these disciplines should formulate goals and objectives for the patient and develop a daily program to meet these goals in the home. Thereafter, an interdisciplinary meeting to formulate an integrated daily home care plan should be developed. This plan must include (1) case coordinator, (2) a defined back-up system for medical emergency, (3) family access to a telephone, (4) a plan for monitoring the care plan and a mechanism for making adjustments when needed, (5) a primary care physician, and (6) educational services for school-age children. No child should be disqualified from a home care program because of eligibility to attend an out-of-home school, if home care is otherwise deemed necessary. Many schools are willing and able to make special arrangements (e.g., ventilator or tracheostomy care). However, a safe medical plan must exist for the school as well as the home.

Equipment and Supplies

Equipment and supplies that are appropriate for use in the home must be selected and secured according to each patient's needs. Community suppliers must guarantee continuous availability, maintenance, and replacement of this equipment. Equipment and supplies to be used in the home should be used in the hospital first so the family can become familiar and proficient with their use. Financial reimbursement for necessary equipment and supplies should not be denied because of transfer of care from the hospital to the home.

Education and Training

Education and training for the family as well as professional and paraprofessional health care givers in the home care program (including pertinent school members if the child will be attending school) is important and should proceed according to the care plan. Participation of the family physician should be sought early in the development of the program. Prior to discharge from the hospital, the family rather than the hospital staff should provide as much of the child's care as possible. The family should be taught to recognize changes in the child's condition that would require consultation and/or modification of care. Although it may require restraint and patience, the hospital staff should assume a supportive, rather than primary, role in this stage of the child's care. Outreach education for local referring and back-up hospitals should be integrated into the home care plan.

Cost

Projected cost of the home care program and methods of payment should be evaluated. In addition, the projected cost for each patient's home care plan must be evaluated in light of available resources. Problems must be resolved prior to discharge of the patient. There should be continuing activity between the home care committee and insurers and public programs to assure the coverage of home care.

Program Maintenance

At intervals prior to discharge and during the home care program, there should be a coordinated review of the patient, the patient's needs, how the family is managing, and other available findings. A coordinator for the program and for individuals in the program is needed for program identification and resolution.

Program Evaluation and Outcome

A review of all patients in home care programs and an assessment of data from similar programs should be done by the multidisciplinary team on an ongoing basis. Data for review must be obtained from several sources (e.g., the parents, the community, local care providers, the schools, and so forth). By sharing experiences, a better program can be developed for each child. Follow-up and outcome assessments should be based on (1) survival, (2) need for subsequent hospitalizations, (3) development progress, (4) course of the underlying disease, (5) actual utilization of resources v expected utilization, (6) financial experience (cash flow and continued availability of benefits), and (7) effects on family members, including siblings.

Alternatives

The use of intermediate or chronic care facilities instead of acute care medical institutions is an alternative that may be considered. Separate program development and evaluation of alternate types of care also are needed.

Conclusion

Home care programs for infants, children, or adolescents with chronic disease may offer the advantages of family living and optimal, comprehensive health care in a cost-effective manner.

Careful analysis, shared experience, and controlled studies will help determine the appropriateness of home care programs in the care of patients with chronic disease.

Ad Hoc Task Force on Home Care of Chronically Ill Infants
Gerald B. Merenstein, MD, Chairman
Philip G. Rhodes, MD
John V. Hartline, MD
Heather Bryan, MD
Donald R. Moffitt, MD

Ad Hoc Task Force on Home Care of Chronically Ill Children
Paul S. Bergeson, MD, Chairman
Antoinette P. Eaton, MD
Arthur F. Kohrman, MD
Ivan B. Pless, MD
Ruth E. K. Stein, MD

In consultation with

Committee on Fetus and Newborn
George A. Little, MD, Chairman
    Committee on Hospital Care
Paul S. Bergeson, MD, Chairman

Selected Readings

Burr, B. H., Guyer, B., Todress, I. D., *et al*.: Home care for children on respirators. *N. Engl. J. Med.* **309:**1319, 1983.

Koop, C. E.: *Report on the Surgeon General's Workshop on Children with Handicaps and Their Families.* US DHHS (DHHS Publication PHS-83-50194), 1983.

Koop, C. E.: The Surgeon General's Workshop on Children with Handicaps and Their Families: Keynote address. *Clin. Pediatr.* **22:**567, 1983.

Koops, B. L., Abman, S. H., and Accurso, F. S.: Outpatient management and follow-up of bronchopulmonary dysplasia. *Sem. Perinatol.* 1984.

Hammond, J.: Home health care cost effectiveness: An overview of the literature. *Publ. Health Rep.* **94:**305, 1979.

Stein, R. E. K., and Jessop, D. J.: A noncategorical approach to chronic childhood illness. *Publ. Health Rep.* **97:**354, 1982.

Index